The Encyclopaedic Companion to Medical Statistics

The Encyclopaedic Companion to Medical Statistics

Edited by

Brian S. Everitt and Christopher R. Palmer

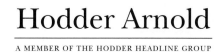

Hodder Arnold

A MEMBER OF THE HODDER HEADLINE GROUP

First published in Great Britain in 2005 by
Hodder Education, a member of the Hodder Headline Group,
338 Euston Road, London NW1 3BH

www.hoddereducation.com

Distributed in the United States of America by
Oxford University Press Inc.
198 Madison Avenue, New York, NY10016

Hodder Headline's policy is to use papers that are natural, renewable and
recyclable products and made fromwood grown in sustainable forests.
The logging and manufacturing processes are expected to conform to the
environmental regulations of the country of origin.

The advice and information in this book are believed to be true and
accurate at the date of going to press, but neither the authors nor the publisher
can accept any legal responsibility or liability for any errors or omissions.

British Library Cataloguing in Publication Data
A catalogue record for this book is available from the British Library

Library of Congress Cataloging-in-Publication Data
A catalog record for this book is available from the Library of Congress

ISBN-10: 0 340 80998 1
ISBN-13: 978 0 340 80998 3

1 2 3 4 5 6 7 8 9 10

Typeset in 9 on 10 Plantin by Phoenix Photosetting, Chatham, Kent
Printed and bound in Great Britain by Martins the Printers Ltd., Berwick upon Tweed

What do you think about this book? Or any other Hodder
Education title? Please send your comments to the feedback
section on www.hoddereducation.com

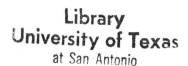

Contents

Foreword

This encyclopaedia contains no entry for 'Peer review'. In my small corner of the medical statistical universe, this seems like a gross sin of omission. Instead, the process of evaluating research papers is discussed under 'Critical appraisal'. Are these two procedures synonymous? And, irrespective of whether they are or are not, should anybody care?

I believe that peer review and critical appraisal do differ, that these differences matter a great deal when considering the ways in which readers should interpret the medical literature, and that an understanding of these differences helps to place medical statistics in its proper context when surveying the wide horizon of clinical and public health research.

The editors of this quite wonderfully rewarding treatise on statistical terms have defined critical appraisal as 'the process of evaluating research reports and assessing their contribution to scientific knowledge'. This statement follows naturally from the meaning of the words 'criticism' (the art of judging) and 'appraisal' (the estimation of quality). That is to say, critical appraisal is an estimation of worth followed by some kind of judgment – a judgment that leans more towards an art than a science. As a non-statistician, I rather warm to the precise imprecision of this definition.

Now consider the more commonly embedded term 'peer review'. And look how inferior it is! Who is this anonymous idealised peer? Generally, one would consider a peer to be an equal, somebody who comes from a group comparable to that from which the person under scrutiny has emerged. And this intellectual egalitarian is subsequently set the task of viewing again (to take 'review' at its most literal meaning) the work under consideration. But to view with what purpose? None is specified.

Despite these practical shortcomings, editors of biomedical journals remain wedded to 'peer review'. We feel uncomfortable with the notion of critical appraisal. The embodiment of peer review as a distinct scientific discipline is the series of international congresses devoted to peer review in biomedical publication, organised jointly by *JAMA* and the *BMJ*. These congresses have spawned hundreds of abstracts, dozens of research papers, and four theme issues of *JAMA*. They are entirely commendable in every way. For the editors of *JAMA* and the *BMJ*, peer review encompasses a broad range of activities: mechanisms of editorial decision making, together with their quality, validity, and practicality, online peer review and publication, pre-publication posting of information, quality assurance of reviewers and editors, authorship and contributorship, conflicts of interest, scientific misconduct, peer review of grant proposals, economic aspects of peer review, and the future of scientific publication.

In other words, peer review is a tremendously elastic concept, allowing editors to stretch it to mean whatever interests them at a given (whimsical) moment in time and place. Indeed, its elasticity is seen by many of us as its great strength. The concept grows in richness and understanding as our own appreciation of its complexity and nuance soars. The impenetrable nature of peer review and the obscure and hard-to-learn expertise it demands, feeds our brittle egos. The notion of critical appraisal, by contrast, is far thinner in meaning, with much less room for editorial manipulation and aggrandisement.

Even if peer review and critical appraisal do differ, should anyone actually care? Yes, they should, and for a very simple reason: the idea of peer review is now bankrupt. Its retention as an operation within the biomedical sciences reflects the interests of those who wish to preserve their own power and position. Peer review is fundamentally anti-democratic. It elevates the mediocre. It asphyxiates originality. And it kills careers. How so?

Peer review is not about intelligent engagement with a piece of research. It is about defining the margins of what is acceptable and unacceptable to the reviewer. The mythical 'peer' is being asked to view again, after the editor, the work in question and to offer a comment about the geographical location of that work on the map of existing knowledge. If there is space on this map, and provided the work does not disrupt (too much) the terrain established by others, its location can be secured and marked by sanctioning publication. If the disruption is too great, the work's wish to seek a place of rest must be vetoed. Peer review is about the agency of power to preserve established orthodoxy. It has nothing to do with science. It has everything to do with ideology. And the maintenance of a quiet life of privilege and mystique.

Instead, critical appraisal is about incrementally working one's way towards truth[1]. It can never be about truth itself. The essence of biomedical research is estimation. Our world resists certainty. Critical appraisal is about transparent, measurable analysis that cuts a path towards greater precision. Critical appraisal refuses to veil itself in the gaudy adornments that editors pin to peer review in order to embellish their own importance in the cartography of scientific inquiry. And a far more robust instrument critical appraisal is for that refusal.

What do these differences tell us about the proper place of medical statistics in biomedicine today? In my view, as a lapsed doctor and a now wrinkled editor, medical statistics is the most important aspect of our critical appraisal of any piece of new research. The evaluations by so-called peers in the clinical specialties that concern a particular research paper provide valuable insight into how that work will be received by a community of practitioners or scholars. But as an editor I am less interested in reception than I am in meaning[2].

I want a tough interrogation of new work before its publication, according to commonly agreed standards of

---

1. Horton, R. 2002: Postpublication criticism and the shaping of clinical knowledge. *JAMA* 287, 2843-7.
2. Horton, R. 2000: Common sense and figures: the rhetoric of validity in medicine. *Statist Med* 19, 3149-64.

questioning, standards that I can see and evaluate for myself. To return to my personal definition of critical appraisal, I want an estimation of quality combined with a judgment. I do not want a view from the club culture of one particular academic discipline. The rejection of peer review by the editors of this encyclopaedia is therefore a triumph of liberty against the forces of conformity.

Yet still today, too much of medicine takes medical statistics for granted. Time and again, we see research that has clearly not been within a hundred miles of a statistical brain. Physicians usually make poor scientists, and physicians and scientists together too often play the part of amateur statistician – with appalling consequences. The future of a successful biomedical research enterprise depends on the flourishing of the discipline we call medical statistics. It is not at all clear to me that those who so depend on medical statistics appreciate either that dependence or the fragility of its foundation.

If this magnificent encyclopaedia can be deployed in the ongoing argument about the future of twenty-first century academic medicine, then not only the research enterprise but also the public's health and well-being will be far stronger tomorrow than it is today.

Richard Horton
Editor, *Lancet*

Preface

Statistical science plays an important role in medical research. Indeed a major part of the key to the progress in medicine from the 17th century to the present day has been the collection and valid interpretation of evidence, particularly quantitative evidence, provided by the application of statistical methods to medical investigations. Current medical journals are full of statistical material, both relatively simple (for example, t-tests, p-values, linear regression) and, increasingly, more complex (for example, generalised estimating equations, cluster analysis, Bayesian methods). The latter material reflects the vibrant state of statistical research with many new methods having practical implications for medicine being developed in the last two decades or so. But why is statistics important in medicine? Some possible answers are:

(1) Medical practice and medical research generate large amounts of data. Such data are generally full of uncertainty and variation, and extracting the 'signal' from the 'noise' is usually not trivial.
(2) Medicine involves asking questions that have strong statistical overtones. How common is the disease? Who is especially likely to contract a particular condition? What are the chances that a patient diagnosed with breast cancer will survive more than five years?
(3) The evaluation of competing treatments or preventative measures relies heavily on statistical concepts in both the design and analysis phase.

Recognition of the importance of statistics in medicine has increased considerably in recent years. The last decade, in particular, has seen the emergence of evidence-based medicine, and with it the need for clinicians to keep one step ahead of their patients, many of whom nowadays have access to virtually unlimited information (much of it being virtual, yet some of it being limited in its reliability). Compared with previous generations of medical students, today's pre-clinical undergraduates are being taught more about statistical principles than their predecessors. Furthermore, today's clinical researchers are faced (happily, in our view) with growing numbers of biomedical journals utilising statistical referees as part of their peer review processes (see CRITICAL APPRAISAL and STATISTICAL REFEREEING). This enhances the quality of the papers journal editors select, although from the clinical researcher's perspective it has made publication in leading journals more challenging than ever before.

So statistics is (and are) prevalent in the medical world now and is set to remain so for the future. Clearly, clinicians and medical researchers need to know something about the subject, even if only to make their discussion with a friendly statistician more fruitful. The article on consulting a statistician quotes one of the forefathers of modern statistics, R.A. Fisher who, back in 1938, observed wryly: '*To consult the statistician after an experiment is finished is often merely to ask him to conduct a post-mortem examination. He can perhaps say what the experiment died of.*' Thus, one of our hopes for the usefulness and helpfulness of the *Encyclopaedic Companion to Medical Statistics* is that it may serve to encourage both productive and timely interactions between medical researchers and statisticians. Another sincere hope is that it fills a gap between, on the one hand, textbooks that delve into possibly too much theory and, on the other hand, shorter dictionaries that may not necessarily focus on the needs of medical researchers, or else have entries that are tantalisingly succinct. To meet these ends, the present reference work contains concise, informative, relatively non-technical, and hence, we trust, readable accounts of over 350 topics central to modern medical statistics.

Topics are covered either briefly or more extensively, in general, in accordance with the subject matter's perceived importance, although we acknowledge there will be disagreement, inevitably, about our choice of article lengths. Many entries benefit from containing real-life, clinical examples. Each has been written by an individual chosen not only for subject-matter expertise in the field but, just as importantly, also by ability to communicate statistical concepts to others.

The extensive cross-referencing supplied using SMALL CAPITALS to indicate terms that appear as separate entries should help the reader to find his or her way around and also serves to point out associated topics that might be of interest elsewhere within the *Encylopaedic Companion*. All but the shortest entries contain references to further resources where the interested reader can learn in greater depth about the particular topic.

Thus, while hoping this work is found to be mostly comprehensible we do not claim it to be fully comprehensive. As co-editors we take joint responsibility for any errors ('sins of commission') and would positively welcome suggestions for possible new topics to consider for future inclusion to rectify perceived missing entries ('sins of omission').

Our thanks are due to numerous people – first, to all of the many contributors for providing such excellent material, mostly on time (mostly!) with particular gratitude extended to those who contributed multiple articles or who handled requests for additional articles so gracefully. Next, we appreciated the tremendous and indispensable efforts of staff at Arnold, especially Liz Gooster and Liz Wilson, and not least for their remaining calm during an editor's moments of anxiety and neurosis about the entire project. In addition we would like to thank Harriet Meteyard for her constant support and encouragement throughout the preparation of this book. Finally, our family members deserve especial thanks for having been extra tolerant of our time spent on developing and executing this extensive project from beginning to end. It is our hope that the *Encyclopaedic Companion* proves all these efforts and sacrifices to be well worthwhile, becoming a useful, regularly-thumbed reference added to the bookshelf of many of those involved in contemplating, conducting or contributing to medical research.

Brian Everitt and Christopher R. Palmer
January 2005

Biographical Information on the Editors

B. S. Everitt – Professor Emeritus, King's College London. After 35 years at the Institute of Psychiatry, University of London, Brian Everitt retired in May 2004. Author of approximately 100 journal articles and over 50 books on statistics, and also co-editor of *Statistical Methods in Medical Research*. Writing continues apace in retirement but now punctuated by tennis, walks in the country, guitar playing and visits to the gym, rather than by committees, committees and more committees.

Chris Palmer, founding Director of Cambridge University's Centre for Applied Medical Statistics, regularly teaches and collaborates with current and future doctors. His first degree was from Oxford, while graduate and post-doctoral studies were in the USA (at UNC-Chapel Hill and Harvard). He has shifted from mathematical towards applied statistics, with particular interest in the ethics of clinical trials and the use of flexible designs whenever appropriate. Fundamentally, he likes to promote sound statistical thinking in all areas of medical research and hopes this volume might help towards that end. Chris served as Deputy or Acting Editor for *Statistics in Medicine*, 1996–2000, and is a long-standing statistical reviewer for *The Lancet*. He and his wife have three children they consider to be more than statistically significant.

List of Contributors

K.R. Abrams (KRA), Centre for Biostatistics and Genetic Epidemiology, Department of Health Sciences, 22—28 Princess Road West, Leicester LE1 6TP, UK

Colin Baigent (CB), Clinical Trial Service and Epidemiological Studies Unit, Radcliffe Infirmary, Woodstock Road, Oxford OX2 6HE, UK

Alun Bedding (AB), Statistics and Information Sciences, Eli Lilly and Company, Lilly Research Centre, Erl Wood Manor, Sunninghill Road, Windlesham, Surrey GU20 6PH, UK

Tijl De Bie (TDB), ISIS Research Group, Building 1, University of Southampton, SO17 1BJ, UK

J. Martin Bland (JMB), Professor of Health Sciences, Department of Health Sciences, University of York, Heslington, York YO10 5DD, UK

Michelle Bradley (MMB), Centre for Applied Medical Statistics, Department of Public Health and Primary Care, Institute of Public Health, University Forvie Site, Robinson Way, Cambridge CB2 2SR, UK

Sara Brookes (SB), Department of Social Medicine, University of Bristol, Canynge Hall, Whiteladies Road, Clifton, Bristol BS8 2PR, UK

Marc Buyse (MB), International Drug Development Institute, 430 avenue Louise B14, 1050 Brussels, Belgium

M.J. Campbell (MJC), School of Health and Related Research, University of Sheffield, Regent Court, 30 Regent Street, Sheffield S1 4DA, UK

James R. Carpenter (JRC), Medical Statistics Unit, London School of Hygiene and Tropical Medicine, Keppel Street, London WC1E 7HT, UK

Lucy Carpenter (LC), Nuffield College, Oxford OX1 1NF, UK

Susan Chinn (SC), Department of Public Health Services, King's College London, 5th Floor Capital House, 42 Weston Street, London SE1 3QD, UK

Tim Cole (TJC), Centre for Paediatric Epidemiology and Biostatistics, Institute of Child Health, 30 Guilford Street, London WC1N 1EH, UK

Chris Corcoran (CCo), Department of Mathematics and Statistics, Utah State University, Logan, UT 84322-3900, USA

Nello Cristianini (NC), UC Davis Department of Statistics, 360 Kerr Hall, One Shields Ave., Davis, CA 95616, USA

Sarah Crozier (SRC), MRC Epidemiology Resource Centre, University of Southampton, Southampton SO16 6YD, UK

Carole Cummins (CLC), The University of Birmingham, Division of Reproductive and Child Health, Institute of Child Health, Whittall Street, Birmingham B4 6NH, UK

George Davey-Smith (GDS), Department of Social Medicine, University of Bristol, Canynge Hall, Whiteladies Road, Bristol BS8 2PR, UK

Simon Day (SD), Licensing Division, Medicines and Healthcare Products Regulatory Agency, Market Towers, 1 Nine Elms Lane, London SW8 5NQ, UK

Daniela De Angelis (DDA), Statistics, Modelling and Economics Department, Health Protection Agency, Centre for Infections, London and MRC Biostatistics Unit, Institute of Public Health, University Forvie Site, Robinson Way, Cambridge CB2 2SR, UK

Jonathan Deeks (JD), Centre for Statistics in Medicine, Old Road Campus, Headington, Oxford OX3 7LF, UK

Graham Dunn (GD), Biostatistics Group, Division of Epidemiology and Health Sciences, Stopford Building, Oxford Road, Manchester M13 9PT, UK

Doug Easton (DE), Strangeways Research Laboratory, Worts Causeway, Cambridge CB1 8RN, UK

Jonathan Emberson (JE), Clinical Trials Service Unit, Harkness Building, Radcliffe Infirmary, Oxford OX2 6HE, UK

Brian S. Everitt (BSE), PO 20, Biostatistics and Computing, Institute of Psychiatry, Denmark Hill, London SE5 8AF, UK

David Faraggi (DF), Department of Statistics, University of Haifa, Haifa 31905, Israel

W. Harper Gilmour (WHG), Section for Public Health and Health Policy, Division of Community Based Sciences, University of Glasgow, Glasgow G12 8RZ, UK

Els Goetghebeur (EG), Department of Applied Mathematics and Statistics, Ghent University, Krijgslaan 281-S9, 9000 Ghent, Belgium

Andrew Grieve (AG), Biometrics Division, Pfizer Central Research, Ramsgate Road, Sandwich, Kent CT13 9NJ, UK

Julian P.T. Higgins (JPTH), MRC Biostatistics Unit, Institute of Public Health, University Forvie Site, Robinson Way, Cambridge CB2 2SR, UK

Theodore R. Holford (TRH), Public Health and Statistics, Yale, New Haven, CT 06520, USA

Sally Hollis (SH), AstraZeneca, Parklands, Alderley Park, Macclesfield, Cheshire SK10 4TF, UK

Hazel Inskip (HI), MRC Epidemiology Resource Centre, University of Southampton, Southampton General Hospital, Tremona Road, Southampton SO16 6YD, UK

Tony Johnson (TJ), MRC Biostatistics Unit, Institute of Public Health, University Forvie Site, Robinson Way, Cambridge CB2 2SR, UK

Karen Kafadar (KKa), Department of Mathematics, University of Colorado at Denver, PO Box 173364, Campus Box 170, Denver, CO 80217-3364, USA

Kyungmann Kim (KK), Department of Biostatistics and Medical Informatics, University of Wisconsin Medical School, 600 Highland Ave., Madison, WI 53792-4675, USA

Ruth King (RK), School of Mathematics and Statistics, Mathematical Institute, University of St Andrews, Fife KY16 9SS, UK

Wojtek Krazanowski (WK), School of Mathematical Sciences, Laver Building, North Park Road, Exeter EX4 4QE, UK

Ranjit Lall (RL), Warwick Emergency Care and Rehabilitation, Division of Health in the Community, Warwick Medical School, University of Warwick, The Farmhouse, Gibbet Hill Campus, Coventry CV4 7AL, UK

Sabine Landau (SL), Biostatistics and Computing Department, Institute of Psychiatry, King's College, Denmark Hill, London SE5 8AF, UK

Andrew B. Lawson (AL), Department of Epidemiology and Biostatistics, Arnold School of Public Health, University of South Carolina, Columbia, SC 29208, USA

Morven Leese (ML), Health Services Research, Institute of Psychiatry, King's College, Denmark Hill, London SE5 8AF, UK

Andy Lynch (AGL), Centre for Applied Medical Statistics, Institute of Public Health, University Forvie Site, Robinson Way, Cambridge CB2 2SR, UK

Cyrus Mehta (CM), President, Cytel Software Corporation, 675 Massachusetts Avenue, Cambridge, MA 02139, USA

Richard Morris (RM), Department of Primary Care and Population Sciences, Royal Free and University College Medical School, Hampstead Campus, London NW3 2PF, UK

Paul Murrell (PM), Department of Statistics, The University of Auckland, Private Bag 92019, Auckland, New Zealand

Christopher R. Palmer (CRP), Department of Public Health and Primary Care, Institute of Public Health, University Forvie Site, Robinson Way, Cambridge CB2 2SR, UK

Max Parmar (MP), MRC Clinical Trials Unit, 222 Euston Road, London NW1 2DA, UK

Nitin Patel (NP), Cytel Software Corporation, 675 Massachusetts Avenue, Cambridge, MA 02139-3309, USA

John Powles (JP), Department of Public Health and Primary Care, Institute of Public Health, University Forvie Site, Robinson Way, Cambridge CB2 2SR, UK

P. Prescott (PP), Faculty of Mathematical Studies, University of Southampton, Southampton SO17 1BJ, UK

Sophia Rabe-Hesketh (SRH), Graduate School of Education and Graduate Group in Biostatistics, University of California, Berkeley, 3659 Tolman Hall, California 94720, USA

Ben Reiser (BR), Department of Statistics, University of Haifa, Haifa 31905, Israel

Shaun Seaman (SRS), Max-Planck Institute of Psychiatry, Kraeplinstr. 2—10, 80804 Munich, Germany

Mark Segal (MRS), Division of Biostatistics, University of California, 500 Parnassus Avenue, San Francisco, CA 94143-0560, USA

Pralay Senchaudhuri (PSe), Cytel Software Corporation, 675 Massachusetts Avenue, Cambridge, MA 02139-3309, USA

Stephen Senn (SS), Department of Statistics, The University of Glasgow, Glasgow G12 8QQ, UK

Pak Sham (PS), Genetic Epidemiology, Institute of Psychiatry, Decrespigny Park, London SE5 8AF, UK

Charlie Sharp (CS), Biostatistics and Computing Department, Institute of Psychiatry, Denmark Hill, London SE5 8AF, UK

Anders Skrondal (AS), Department of Statistics, London School of Economics, Houghton Street, London WC2A 2AE, UK and Division of Epidemiology, Norwegian Institute of Public Health, PO Box 4404 Nydalen, N-0403 Oslo, Norway

Nigel Smeeton (NCS), Department of Public Health Sciences, Division of Population Sciences and Health Research, King's College, London, 5th Floor Capital House, 42 Weston Street, London SE1 3QD, UK

Nigel Stallard (NS), Medical and Pharmaceutical, Statistics Research Unit, The University of Reading, PO 240, Earley Gate, Reading RG6 6FN, UK

Jonathan Sterne (JS), Department of Social Medicine, University of Bristol, Canynge Hall, Whiteladies Road, Bristol BS8 2PR, UK

Elisabeth Svensson (ES), Department of Statistics, Örebro University, SE-701 82 Örebro, Sweden

Matthew Sydes (MS), MRC Clinical Trials Unit, 222 Euston Road, London NW1 2DA, UK

Jeremy Taylor (JMGT), Department of Biostatistics, University of Michigan, 1420 Washington Heights, M4041 Ann Arbor, MI 48109-2029, USA

Kate Tilling (KT), Department of Social Medicine, University of Bristol, Canynge Hall, Whiteladies Road, Bristol BS8 2PR, UK

Brian Tom (BT), MRC Biostatistics Unit, Institute of Public Health, University Forvie Site, Robinson Way, Cambridge CB2 2SR, UK

Rebecca Turner (RT), MRC Biostatistics Unit, Institute of Public Health, University Forvie Site, Robinson Way, Cambridge CB2 2SR, UK

Andy Vail (AV), Biostatistics Group, University of Manchester, Oxford Road, Manchester M13 9PL, UK

Stijn Vansteelandt (SV), Ghent University, Dept. of Applied Mathematics and Computer Science, Krijgslaan 281, S9, B-9000 Ghent, Belgium

Sarah L. Vowler (SLV), Centre for Applied Medical Statistics, Department of Public Health and Primary Care, Institute of Public Health, University Forvie Site, Robinson Way, Cambridge CB2 2SR, UK

Stephen J. Walters (SJW), Medical Statistics Group, School of Health and Related Research, University of Sheffield, Regent Court, 30 Regent Street, Sheffield S1 4DA, UK

J.G. Wheeler (JGW), Department of Public Health and Primary Care, Institute of Public Health, University Forvie Site, Robinson Way, Cambridge CB2 2SR, UK

Brandon Whitcher (BW), Translational Medicine and Genetics, GlaxoSmithKline, Greenford Road, Greenford UB6 0HE, UK

Ian White (IW), MRC Biostatistics Unit, Institute of Public Health, University Forvie Site, Robinson Way, Cambridge CB2 2SR, UK

Janet Wittes (JW), 1710 Rhode Island Ave. NW, Suite 200, Washington DC 20036, USA

Mark Woodward (MW), The George Institute for International Health, PO Box M201, Missenden Road, Sydney NSW 2050, Australia

Ru-Fang Yeh (RFY), University of California San Francisco, Campus Box Number 0560, 500 Parnassus, 420 MU-W, San Francisco, CA 94143-0560, USA

Abbreviations and Acronyms

ACES	Active control equivalence study
ACET	Active control equivalence test
AD	Adaptive design
AI	Artificial intelligence
AIC	Akaike's information criterion
ANCOVA	Analysis of covariance
ANOVA	Analysis of variance
AR	Autoregressive
ARMA	Autoregressive moving average
AUC	Area under curve
BIC	Bayesian information criterion
BUGS	Bayesian inference Using Gibbs Sampling (software)
CACE	Complier average causal effect
CART	Classification and regression tree
CAT	Computer-adaptive testing
CBA	Cost-benefit analysis
CEA	Cost-effectiveness analysis
CI	Confidence interval
CONSORT	Consolidation of standards of reporting trials
COREC	Central Office for Research Ethics Committees
CPMP	Committee for Proprietary Medicinal Products
CPO	Conditional predictive ordinate
CrI	Credible interval
CRM	Continual reassessment method
CSM	Committee on Safety of Medicines
CUE	Cost-utility analysis
CV	Coefficient of variation
CWT	Continuous wavelet transform
DAG	Directed acyclic graph
DALY	Disability adjusted life-year
DAR	Dropout at random
DCAR	Dropout completely at random
DDD	Data-dependent design
df	Degrees of freedom
DIC	Deviance information criterion
DM	Data mining
DMC	Data monitoring committee
DSMC	Data and safety monitoring committee
DWT	Discrete wavelet transform
DZ	Dizygotic
EBM	Evidence-based medicine
EDA	Exploratory data analysis
EM	Expectation-maximisation
EMEA	European Medicines Evaluation Agency
FDA	Food and Drug Administration
GAM	Generalised additive model
GEE	Generalised estimating equations
GFR	General fertility rate
GIS	Geographical information system
GLIM	Generalised linear interactive modelling (software)
GLIMM	Generalised linear mixed model
GLM	Generalised linear model
GLMM	Generalised linear mixed model
GRR	Gross reproduction rate
HALE	Health-adjusted life expectancy
HMM	Hidden Markov model
HPDI	Highest posterior density interval
HREC	Human research ethics committee
HRQoL	Health-related quality of life
IBD	Identity-by-descent
ICC	Intraclass (or intracluster) correlation coefficient
ICER	Incremental cost-effectiveness ratio
ICH	International Conference on Harmonization
IRB	Institutional review board
ITT	Intention-to-treat
IV	Instrumental variable
KDD	Knowledge discovery in databases
KM	Kaplan-Meier
kNN	k-nearest neighbour
LDF	Linear discriminant function
LR	Likelihood ratio
LREC	Local research ethics committee
LS	Least squares
LST	Large simple trial
MA	Moving average
MANOVA	Multivariate analysis of variance
MAR	Missing at random
MCA	Medicines Control Agency
MCAR	Missing completely at random
MCMC	Markov chain Monte Carlo
MHRA	Medicines and Healthcare Products Regulatory Agency
MLE	Maximum likelihood estimate (or estimation)
MREC	Multi-centre research ethics committee
MSE	Mean square error
MTD	Maximum tolerated dose
MZ	Monozygotic
NI	Non-ignorable (or non-informative)
NMB	Net monetary benefit
NNH	Number needed to harm
NNT	Number needed to treat
NPV	Negative predictive value
NRR	Net reproduction rate
OLS	Ordinary least squares
OR	Odds ratio
PCA	Principal component analysis
pdf	Probability density function
PEST	Planning and Evaluation of Sequential Trials (software)
PGM	Patient generated measure
PH	Proportional hazards
PK/PD	Pharmacokinetics/pharmacodynamics
POP	Persuade-the-optimist probability
PP	Per protocol
P-P	Percentile-percentile
PPP	Persuade-the-pessimist probability

PPV	Positive predictive value	SEM	Standard error of the mean; structural equation model
QALY	Quality adjusted life-year		
QoL	Quality of life	SMR	Standardised mortality ratio
Q-Q	Quantile-quantile	SPM	Statistical parametric map
QTL	Quantitative trait loci	SPRT	Sequential probability ratio test
RCT	Randomised controlled trial	SS	Sum of squares
REB	Research ethics board	SSE	Sum of squares due to error
REC	Research ethics committee	SVM	Support vector machine
REML	Restricted maximum likelihood	TDT	Transmission distortion test
ROC	Receiver operating characteristic	TFR	Total fertility rate
ROI	Region of interest	TSM	Tree-structured method
RPW	Randomised play-the-winner	TT	Triangular test
RR	Relative risk	VAS	Visual analogue scale
SD	Standard deviation	WLSE	Weighted least squares estimate (or estimation)
SE	Standard error		

Dedications

Brian S. Everitt
To: Mary-Elizabeth

Christopher R. Palmer
To: Cathy-Joan, Laura, Carolyn and David

A

***

accelerated factor See SURVIVAL ANALYSIS

accelerated failure time models See SURVIVAL ANALYSIS, TRANSFORMATION

active control equivalence studies The classic randomised CLINICAL TRIAL seeks to prove superiority of a new treatment to an existing one and a successful conclusion is one in which such proof is demonstrated. The famous MRC trial of streptomycin is a case in point (Medical Research Council Streptomycin in Tuberculosis Trials Committee, 1948). The trial concluded with a significant difference in outcome in favour of the group given streptomycin compared to the group that was not. In recent years, however, there has been an increasing interest in trials whose objective is to show that some new therapy is no worse as regards some outcome than an existing treatment. Such trials have particular features and difficulties that were described in an important paper by Makuch and Johnson (1989) in which they used the term 'active control equivalence studies' (ACES).

Actually, the term is not ideally chosen since, unlike bioequivalence studies, where the object is to show that the bioavailability of a new formulation is not only at least 20% *less* than that of an existing formulation, but also at most 25% *more*, and hence where *equivalence* to some degree is genuinely the aim, in ACES it is almost always the case that only non-inferiority is the goal. It may be questioned as to why the rather modest goal of non-inferiority should be of any interest in drug regulation. There are several reasons. The first is that the new drug may have advantages in terms of tolerability. Second, the new drug, while showing no net advantage to the existing one, may increase patient choice and this can be useful. For example, many people have an aspirin allergy. Hence, it is desirable to have alternative analgesics, even if no better on average than aspirin. Third, it may become necessary to withdraw treatments from the market and one can never predict when this may happen. There are now several statins on the market. The fact that this is so means that withdrawal of cerivastatin does not make it impossible for physicians to continue to treat their patients with this class of drug. Fourth, introduction of further equivalent therapies before patent expiry of an innovator in the class may permit price competition to the advantage of reimbursers. (Although such competition is probably not particularly effective, Senn and Rosati, 2003.) However, the fifth reason is probably the most important. Drug regulation is designed to satisfy some minimum requirements for pharmaceuticals: that they are of sufficient quality, are safe and efficacious. Efficacy is demonstrated if the treatment is better than PLACEBO, even if it is not as good as some other treatments. The comparison of a new drug to an active treatment may be dictated by ethics but the object of the trial may simply be an indirect proof that the treatment is better than placebo through comparison to an agent whose efficacy is accepted.

Recently the issue of the indirect comparison to placebo has been taken more seriously. Consider the case where we have a single effective treatment on the market, say A, whose efficacy has been demonstrated in a series of trials comparing it to placebo. We now run some new trials comparing a further treatment, B, to A. Taking all these trials together, they then have the structure of an incomplete blocks design. The effect of B compared to placebo can then be estimated using the double contrast of B compared to A and A compared to placebo. This approach has been examined in detail by Hasselblad and Kong (2001). A consequence of taking this particular view of matters is that the precision with which the effect of A was established compared to placebo cannot be exceeded by the indirect comparison of B to placebo, since the variance of this indirect contrast is the sum of the variances of the two direct contrasts.

This is, however, not the only difficulty with such studies. The following are some of those that apply.

Establishing a clinically irrelevant difference. If the route of a formal analysis compared to placebo via an indirect contrast is taken, this particular difficulty may be finessed. The new treatment is shown to be 'significantly' better than placebo, albeit using an indirect argument, and the extent of its inferiority to the comparator is only of relevance to the extent that it impinges on the proof of efficacy compared to placebo. If this proof is provided, then the comparison to the active comparator is 'water under the bridge'. If this particular approach is *not* taken, however, then any proof of efficacy of the new treatment rests on a demonstration that it is not 'substantially inferior' to the comparator, which comparator is accepted as being efficacious. This raises the issue as to what it means for a drug to be not substantially inferior to another one. This appears to require that some margin Δ, $\Delta > 0$ be adopted such that if τ is the extent by which the new treatment is inferior to the standard (where $\tau < 0$ indicates inferiority) then it is judged *substantially* inferior if $\tau \leq -\Delta$ and not substantially inferior or 'equivalent' if $\tau > -\Delta$.

Technical statistical aspects. In a Neyman-Pearson framework (see Salsbury, 1998) the test of non-inferiority requires one to use a shifted null hypothesis. One might, therefore, adopt $H_0 : \tau \leq -\Delta$. The situation is not as controversial as that for true bioequivalence, where the fact that two hypotheses have to be rejected, that of inferiority and that of superiority, means that an intuitive approach of seeing that the confidence limits for the difference lie within the limits of equivalence is not 'optimal' (Berger and Hsu, 1996), although the 'optimal' test may in practice be worse (Perlman and Wu, 1999; Senn, 2001). In practice, in the case of ACES if the lower conventional $1-\alpha$ *two-sided* CONFIDENCE INTERVAL for τ exceeds $-\Delta$, the hypothesis of substantial inferiority may be rejected at the level α and non-inferiority asserted. It might be thought that a one-sided confidence interval would be sufficient for this purpose. However, the general regulatory convention is that all tests designed to show superiority are two-sided (despite apparent purpose) and, since such tests are a special case of a non-inferiority test with $\Delta = 0$, use of one-sided tests for non-inferiority would lead to inconsistencies (Committee for Proprietary Medicinal Products, 2000; Senn, 1997). In a Bayesian framework (see BAYESIAN METHODS) one might require that the posterior probability of non-inferiority were less than some specified amount. Alternatively, use of a loss function would permit a decision analytic method, such as has been proposed for bioequivalence (Lindley, 1998), to be used.

Power of trials. Note that the reason one does not employ a value of $\Delta = 0$ in practice is that unless it is expected that the new treatment really is better than the standard, the POWER of the resulting test could never exceed 50%. However, the clinically irrelevant difference is likely to be less than the clinically relevant difference used in conventional trials. Hence, if the new treatment is actually no better than the standard treatment, then, for a given sample size, the non-centrality parameter, $\delta = \Delta/SE(\hat{\Delta})$ is likely to be smaller for ACES than for trials designed to show superiority. Consequently, ACES either have lower power or higher sample sizes than conventional trials.

Assay sensitivity. A problem with ACES is that if the trial appears to show non-inferiority of the new treatment, then there are three plausible explanations. The first, that of chance, is one that statistical analysis is designed to address. The second, that the new treatment is indeed non-inferior, is what was desired to prove. However, a third possibility, that the experiment was not sensitive to find a difference, is difficult to exclude. This issue has been referred to as one of 'competence' (Senn, 1993) and affects whatever inferential framework one decides to use. An analogy may be useful here. In a game of hunt the thimble, a found thimble renders the quality of the strategy used for finding it irrelevant. It is no more 'found' if a good strategy were used than if a bad one were. However, a failure to find a thimble does not automatically justify the conclusion that the room does not contain one and the quality of the search employed is a crucial consideration in any judgement that it does not.

The effect of DROPOUTS, NON-COMPLIANCE *and the role of* INTENTION-TO-TREAT *analysis.* It is plausible that in many circumstances in conventional superiority trials if non-compliance or dropouts are a problem an intention-to-treat analysis will give a more modest estimate of the treatment effect than will a PER PROTOCOL analysis. In ACES, it is at least plausible that this may not be the case.

Conflict of requirements of additivity and clinical relevance. It may be that the clinically irrelevant difference is most meaningfully established on a scale that is not additive. For example, in a trial of an anti-infective, it could be most appropriate to establish that the difference in cure rate on the probability scale was not greater than some specified amount. Contrariwise, the log-odds scale might lend itself more readily to statistical modelling. This can lead to considerable difficulties (Holmgren, 1999), in particular because a trial does not recruit a random sample from the target population. It may be that further modelling using additional data may be necessary (Senn, 2000).

A common circumstance likely to make regulatory authorities ask questions is that a trial that was designed

with optimism to show superiority to an active comparator fails to do so, but then is used to attempt to demonstrate non-inferiority. This particular set of circumstances has become the subject of one of the European Medicine Evaluation Agency's 'points to consider' (Senn, 1997; Committee for Proprietary Medicinal Products, 2000). This stresses the desirability of establishing the trial's purpose pre-performance and also warns against establishing the clinically irrelevant difference, Δ, after the trial is complete. It regards putting a trial that was designed to show superiority to the purpose of non-inferiority as an unacceptable use but accepts the converse. The guideline recognises that there are no issues of multiple testing involved with such switches (Bauer and Kieser, 1996) but that establishing values of Δ retrospectively may be biasing. Thus, it is preferable for investigators to specify in advance (e.g. by means of formal change to the CLINICAL TRIALS PROTOCOL) their intended switch of purpose and to fix the value of Δ prior to data unblinding. This however, raises, the issue as to whether the value of Δ is not something the regulator should declare for given indications rather than relying on the sponsor to do so. Otherwise, a regulator could be faced with the following position. Drug B is registered on the basis of comparison to a standard treatment A because the lower confidence interval for the treatment effect, τ_{B-A}, exceeds some pre-specified value Δ. However, a further drug, C, which has also been compared to A, is not granted a licence because a superiority trial was planned. Although superiority to A was not proven, the lower confidence interval for the treatment effect τ_{C-A} excludes a smaller possible difference between C and A than is excluded for the difference between B and A by the trial that has led to registration of B.   *SS*

Bauer, P. and Kieser, M. 1996: A unifying approach for confidence intervals and testing of equivalence and difference. *Biometrika* 83, 4, 934–7. **Berger, R.L. and Hsu, J.C.** 1996: Bioequivalence trials, intersection-union tests and equivalence confidence sets. *Statistical Science* 11, 4, 283–302. **Committee for Proprietary Medicinal Products** 2000: Points to consider on switching between superiority and non-inferiority. **Hasselblad, V. and Kong, D.F.** 2001: Statistical methods for comparison to placebo in active-control studies. *Drug Information Journal* 35, 435–49. **Holmgren, E.B.** 1999: Establishing equivalence by showing that a specified percentage of the effect of the active control over placebo is maintained. *Journal of Biopharmaceutical Statistics* 9, 4, 651–9. **Lindley, D.V.** 1998: Decision analysis and bioequivalence trials. *Statistical Science* 13, 2, 136–41. **Makuch, R. and Johnson, M.** 1989: Issues in planning and interpreting active control equivalence studies. *Journal of Clinical Epidemiology* 42, 6, 503–11. **Medical Research Council Streptomycin in Tuberculosis Trials Committee** 1948: Streptomycin treatment for pulmonary tuberculosis. *British Medical Journal* ii, 769–82. **Perlman, M.D. and Wu, L.** 1999: The emperor's new tests. *Statistical Science* 14, 4, 355–69. **Salsbury, D.** 1998: Hypothesis testing. In Armitage, P. and Colton, T. (eds), *Encyclopedia of Biostatistics*. Chichester: John Wiley & Sons. **Senn, S.J.** 1993: Inherent difficulties with active control equivalence studies. *Statistics in Medicine* 12, 24, 2367–75. **Senn, S.J.** 1997: *Statistical issues in drug development.* Chichester: John Wiley & Sons. **Senn, S.J.** 2000: Consensus and controversy in pharmaceutical statistics (with discussion). *The Statistician* 49, 135–76. **Senn, S.J.** 2001: Statistical issues in bioequivalence. *Statistics in Medicine* 20, 17–18, 2785–99. **Senn, S.J. and Rosati, N.** 2003: Editorial: Pharmaceuticals, patents and competition – some statistical issues. *Journal of the Royal Statistical Society Series A – Statistics in Society* 166, 271–7.

adaptive designs CLINICAL TRIALS that are adaptive are modified in some way by the data that have already been collected within that trial. The most common way the designs adapt is in the allocation of treatment, as a function of the response. For example, if we were interested in a dose that gives a 20% chance of toxicity, where excesses to this level of toxicity would be harmful. Therefore, we may want to design the trial in such a way that, as more information is gathered, doses are allocated to optimise the estimate of that dose. If we were to use a traditional fully randomised approach to running the trial, which is not adaptive, we would probably not look at the data until the end of the trial, thereby risking exposing subjects to toxic doses and also possibly failing to produce an optimal estimate of the required dose. Another such example of an adaptive design is given in Rosenberger and Lachin (1993), whereby there are two treatments in the study, A and B, and as information emerges from the trial the treatment assignment probabilities are adapted in an attempt to assign more patients to the treatment performing better thus far. Therefore, when a patient enters the study, if treatment A appears to be better than treatment B, a patient has a greater than 50% chance of being allocated treatment A – and vice versa.

Because adaptive designs modify the allocation of treatment on an ongoing basis, and thus protect patients from ineffective or toxic doses, they can be said to be more ethical than traditional designs. Rosenberger and Palmer (1999) consider the ethical dilemma between collective and individual ethics (see ETHICS AND CLINICAL TRIALS) and argue that in a clinical trial setting individual ethics should be uppermost. That is, consideration should be towards doing what is best for patients in the current trial as opposed to doing what is best for future patients who stand to benefit from the results of current trial. The Declaration of Helsinki of October 2000 outlines the tension between these two types of ethics by stating: 'Considerations related to the well-being of the human subject should take precedence over the interests of science and society.' It is adaptive designs that address the individual ethics, as opposed to fully randomised designs, which address those collective ethics.

We will be dealing primarily with response-adaptive designs here, such as those just outlined and will not be describing those designs that attempt dynamically to balance the randomisation for covariate information, such as outlined by Pocock and Simon (1975). (See DATA-DEPENDENT DESIGNS, MINIMISATION.)

The randomised play the winner (RPW) design attempts to allocate treatments to patients sequentially based on a simple probability model. Rosenberger (1999) emphasises that the RPW design specifically applies to the situation where the outcome from a trial is binary, i.e. either 'success' or 'failure' and where there are only two treatments, e.g. Drug A and Drug B. At the start of the trial there is an assumed urn of α balls of type A (which relate to Drug A) and β balls of type B (which relate to Drug B). When a subject is recruited, a ball is drawn from the urn and then replaced. If the ball is type A then the subject is allocated to Drug A, if type B then the subject is allocated to Drug B. When the subject's outcome is available (and we assume that the outcome is available before the next subject is randomised), the urn is updated. If the response is a success on Drug A, then a ball of type A is put into the urn, similarly for a success on Drug B. If the outcome is a failure on Drug A, then a ball of type B is put into the urn, again similarly for a failure on Drug B. In this way, the balls build up such that a new subject has a better chance of being allocated to a better treatment.

Rosenberger (1999) concludes with a table of conditions under which the RPW rule is reasonable and provides a realistic alternative to the standard clinical trial design. These are given in the table.

Traditional dose-response studies, where patients are allocated to a limited number of doses along an assumed dose-response curve, are limited and, some would say, wrong. For example, if the assumed dose-response model is incorrect then patients may be allocated to ineffective or unsafe doses. One answer could be to increase the number of doses. However, this would result in many patients allocated to wasted doses. It would be much better to increase the number of doses and allocate doses to a subject based on current knowledge of the dose-response curve, which best optimises some pre-specified criteria. This is precisely what Bayesian response adaptive designs attempt to do, by employing Bayesian DECISION THEORY to a utility function. Thus, the dose that most optimally addresses the utility is allocated to the next available subject or cohort of subjects.

One of the first BAYESIAN METHODS described was the continual reassessment method (CRM), introduced by O'Quigley, Pepe and Fisher (1990), and originally devised for dose-escalation studies in oncology. Whitehead *et al.* (2001a) suggest that the method could also be used for applications in other serious diseases. The CRM envisages a study whereby human volunteers are treated sequentially, in order to detect a dose with a probability of toxicity of 20%, i.e. TD20. The response is a binary response, 'toxicity' or 'no toxicity'. Before the study starts, investigators are asked to provide what their best guess is of a probability of toxicity at each of the series of doses. The first patient is then treated with the dose that is considered to be the closest to the TD20. Once the outcome is observed the PROBABILITY of toxicity at each of the doses is recalculated using the Bayesian method of statistics. The procedure continues in this way until it settles on a single dose. Whitehead *et al.* (2001a) point out that the CRM does home in on the TD20 quickly and efficiently, however, there has been concern that early on in the trial subjects could be allocated to too high a dose, leading to potential toxicity problems. This has led to a number of modifications, such as starting at the lowest dose and never skipping a dose during the escalation.

---

adaptive designs *Conditions under which the RPW is reasonable (Rosenberger and Palmer, 1999)*

- The therapies have been evaluated previously for toxicity
- The response is binary
- Delay in response is moderate, allowing adapting to take place
- Sample sizes are moderate (at least 50 subjects)
- Duration of the trial is limited and recruitment can take place during the entire trial
- The trial is carefully planned with extensive computations done under different models and initial urn compositions
- The experimental therapy is expected to have significant benefits to public health if it proves effective

Whitehead *et al.* (2001b) suggest practical extensions to the CRM for pharmacokinetic data, employing the use of Bayesian decision theory to allocate treatments optimally to subjects. They argue that conventional dose-escalation studies carried out in healthy volunteers do not normally employ statistical methodology or formal guidelines for dose escalation. As such the studies can take a long time to complete with little opportunity to skip doses. The methods proposed allocate doses in order to maximise the information about the dose-response curve, given a pre-specified safety constraint. They use two simple utility or gain functions, one that allocates the highest allowable dose under the safety constraint and the other that allocates doses in order to optimise the shape of the dose-response curve.

Krams *et al.* (2003) also use a Bayesian decision theory approach with sequential dose allocation to a Phase II study in acute stroke therapy by inhibition of neutrophils (ASTIN), which employs up to 15 dose levels. They use a response-adaptive procedure in order to find a dose that gives an improvement over that of placebo in the primary ENDPOINT, allocating the next subject either to the optimal dose or PLACEBO. Stopping rules were employed by which if the posterior probability of an effective drug or ineffective drug were greater than 0.9 then the decision would be made either to go onto a confirmatory trial (effective drug) or to stop development (ineffective drug). In this way, they were able to stop development of a compound more quickly than would have been possible under the traditional paradigm. *AB*

Krams, M., Lees, K., Hacke, W., Grieve, A.P., Orgogozo, J.-M. and Ford, G.A. 2003: Acute stroke therapy by inhibition of neutrophils (ASTIN). An adaptive dose-response study of UK-279,276 in acute ischemic stroke. *Stroke* 34, 2543–8. **Pocock, S. and Simon, R.** 1975: Sequential treatment assignment with balancing of prognostic factors in controlled clinical trials. *Biometrics* 31, 103–15. **Rosenberger, W.F.** 1999: Randomized play-the-winner clinical trials: review and recommendations. *Controlled Clinical Trials* 20, 328–42. **Rosenberger, W.F. and Lachin, J.M.** 1993: The use of response-adaptive designs in clinical trials. *Controlled Clinical Trials* 14, 471–84. **Rosenberger, W.F. and Palmer, C.R.** 1999: Ethics and practice: alternative designs for Phase III randomised clinical trials. *Controlled Clinical Trials* 20, 172–86. **Whitehead, J., Yinghui, Z., Patterson, S., Webber, D. and Francis, S.** 2001a: Easy-to-implement Bayesian methods for dose-escalation studies in healthy volunteers. *Biostatistics* 2, 47–61. **O'Quigley, J., Pepe, M. and Fisher, L.** 1990: Continual reassessment method: a practical design for Phase I clinical trials in cancer. *Biometrics* 46, 33–48. **Whitehead, J., Zhou, Y., Stallard, N., Todd, S. and Whitehead A.** 2001b: Learning from previous responses in Phase I dose-escalation studies. *British Journal of Clinical Pharmacology* 52, 1–7.

adaptive randomisation See ADAPTIVE DESIGNS, RANDOMISATION

adjustment for non-compliance in randomised controlled trials In clinical medicine, 'non-compliance' occurs when a patient does not fully follow a prescribed course of treatment. The alternative terms 'adherence' and 'concordance' attempt to avoid the authoritarian overtones of 'compliance'. In randomised CLINICAL TRIALS, we are concerned with any departure from a randomised treatment, whether due to non-compliance or a treatment change agreed with medical staff. In a trial to compare two types of medication (Drug A and Drug B) for the treatment of heart disease, for example, patients may refuse or forget to take any of their medication or forget to take it some of the time (partial compliance). Patients allocated to receive Drug A might switch to Drug B and vice versa. Some of the patients may even finish up taking another medication altogether (Drug C, say) or, particularly if the therapy appears to be failing, receive a much more radical intervention such as surgery. A further complication for the estimation of treatment effects arises when patients who fail to comply with their prescribed treatment are also those who are more likely to be lost to follow-up.

Conventionally, trials with departures from randomised treatment are analysed by INTENTION-TO-TREAT. This directly compares the *effectiveness* of the different treatment policies as actually implemented in the trial – for example, 'Drug A plus changes' versus 'Drug B plus changes'. Unlike effectiveness, *efficacy* relates to the effects of the treatments themselves and is not estimated by an intention-to-treat analysis. Researchers may also be interested in the effectiveness of an intervention in other circumstances, for example, if public suspicion of the intervention had been reduced by the positive results of a clinical trial. In these circumstances, the rates of compliance may be improved and adjustment for this change may be attempted.

It is important to define the aim of adjustment for non-compliance. For example, in a trial of immediate versus deferred zidovudine in asymptomatic HIV infection, the initial plan was to defer zidovudine until the onset of symptomatic disease. However, following a protocol amendment, some individuals started zidovudine before the onset of symptomatic disease (White *et al.*, 1997). There was interest in estimating the effect that would have been observed under the original protocol. Zidovudine before the onset of symptomatic disease was therefore regarded as 'non-compliance'. Other individuals stopped zidovudine treatment because of adverse events. Additional adjustment for stopping treatment would not answer a clinically relevant question, so the analysis did not aim to estimate efficacy.

Adjustment for non-compliance is useful in a variety of situations. If a treatment effect is observed to vary with time or between subgroups in a trial, or between trials in a META-ANALYSIS, this may be explained by differences in compliance. Reconciling trial data with observational data may require adjustment for non-compliance in the trial. Policy analysis may require projections for situations with improved compliance.

Most attempts to allow for non-compliance use on-treatment analysis or PER PROTOCOL analysis. This only provides a valid comparison of the treatments themselves (efficacy) if compliers and non-compliers do not systematically differ in their disease state or prognosis. In practice, this is unlikely to be the case, so SELECTION BIAS occurs. Heart disease patients who comply with their prescribed medication, for example, are also those who are likely to improve their diet or take more exercise and these changes, in turn, are likely to lead to a better outcome. Selection bias may often be reduced by adjustment for baseline covariates, but there is still no guarantee of an unbiased analysis. For example, in the placebo arm of the Coronary Drug Project, 5-year mortality of poor compliers was

28.2% compared with 15.1% in good compliers. Adjustment for 40 baseline factors only reduced the difference to 25.8% vs. 16.4% (Coronary Drug Project Research Group, 1980).

Newer methods can estimate efficacy while avoiding selection bias, by directly comparing the randomised groups as in an intention-to-treat analysis. This is made possible by considering the subgroup of 'compliers' who would have received their randomised treatment, whichever group they were randomised to. For example, a trial in Indonesian children compared vitamin A supplementation with no intervention, the outcome being 12-month mortality. Vitamin A supplementation was actually received by only 80% of the intervention arm and by none of the control arm. Sommer and Zeger (1991) considered the subgroup that did not receive vitamin A in the intervention arm and a corresponding subgroup of the control arm that *would not have received vitamin A if they had been allocated to receive it*. These 'non-complier' subgroups were assumed to be unaffected by allocation to vitamin A. It is then straightforward to estimate the number of non-compliers in the control arm and their MEAN outcome, and hence the risk difference, risk ratio or ODDS RATIO in compliers. This is often called the complier average causal effect (CACE) estimate (Little and Rubin, 2000).

A more general approach requires a model relating *potential outcomes* for each individual under different counterfactual treatments. A simple model might assume that each individual would have blood pressure b mm Hg lower if they took the drug with perfect compliance than if they did not take the drug, with proportional blood pressure reductions for partial compliance. Such a model may be fitted by assuming that untreated blood pressure has the same distribution in each randomised group (Fischer-Lapp and Goetghebeur, 1999). An important advantage of these methods is that no assumption is required about the relationship between compliance and potential outcomes.

The approaches just described are generally only able to estimate one treatment effect in a two-arm trial. They tend to be hopelessly imprecise in situations such as equivalence trials where patients may stop all treatment, so that the analysis requires estimation of the effect of both treatments. In this case it is possible to adjust the randomised comparison using an observational estimation of one or more treatment effects – that is, assuming there are no unmeasured confounders for treatment. Methods such as *marginal structural modelling* can work even when actual treatment is both a consequence of symptomatic deterioration and a cause of slower disease progression (see Little and Rubin, 2000, for references to this literature).

A trial with non-compliance has less POWER than one with perfect compliance (as a result of the reduced effect size as estimated in an intention-to-treat analysis) and it is natural to want to recover the lost power. However, many of the new procedures preserve the intention-to-treat SIGNIFICANCE LEVEL and therefore do not affect power. In some cases, it is impossible to regain power without making some assumption about comparability of non-compliers and compliers. In other situations, some gain in power is theoretically possible, but this is unlikely to be appreciable in practice. Significance testing should therefore rely

on intention-to-treat analysis even when other methods are used to estimate efficacy. *IW/GD*

Coronary Drug Project Research Group 1980: Influence of adherence to treatment and response to cholesterol on mortality in the Coronary Drug Project. *New England Journal of Medicine* 303, 1038–41. **Fischer-Lapp, K. and Goetghebeur, E.** 1999: Practical properties of some structural mean analyses of the effect of compliance in randomized trials. *Controlled Clinical Trials* 20, 531–46. **Little, R. and Rubin, D.B.** 2000: Causal effects in clinical and epidemiological studies via potential outcomes: concepts and analytical approaches. *Annual Review of Public Health* 21, 121–45. **Sommer, A. and Zeger, S.L.** 1991: On estimating efficacy from clinical trials. *Statistics in Medicine* 10, 45–52. **White, I.R., Walker, S., Babiker, A.G. and Darbyshire, J.H.** 1997: Impact of treatment changes on the interpretation of the Concorde trial. *AIDS* 11, 999–1006.

age-period cohort analysis To understand the effect of time on a particular outcome for an individual it is essential to realise the relevant temporal prospective. Age affects many aspects of life, including the risk of disease, so this is an essential component of any analysis of time trends. Period denotes the date of the outcome and if the outcome varies with period it is likely due to some underlying factor that affects the outcome and varies in the same way for the entire population under study. Cohort, contrariwise, refers to generational effects caused by factors that only affect particular age groups when their level changes with time.

An example of a period effect would be a potential effect of an air contaminant that affected all age groups in the same way. If the level of exposure to that factor increased/decreased with time exerting a change in the outcome in all age groups then we would expect a related pattern across all age groups in the study. In studies that take place over long periods of time, the technology for measuring the outcome may change, giving rise to an artifactual effect that was not due to change in exposure to a causative agent. For example, intensive screening for disease can identify disease cases that would not previously have been identified, thus artificially increasing the disease rate in a population that has had no change in exposure over time.

Cohort (also called birth cohort) effects may be due to factors related to exposures associated with the date of birth, such as the introduction of a particular drug or practice during pregnancy that was brought in at a particular point in time. For example, a pregnancy practice associated with increased risk and adopted by the population of mothers during a particular time period could affect the risk during the lifespan of the entire generation born during that period. While it is common to refer to these effects as being associated with year of birth, they could also be the result of changes in exposure that occurred after birth. In many individuals, lifestyle factors that may affect disease risk over a lifetime are fixed as they approach adulthood. A quantification of these effects on such a generation would give rise to a comparison of these cohort or generational effects.

An inherent redundancy among these three temporal factors arises from the fact that knowing any two factors implies the value of the third. For example, if we know an individuals age (a) at a given date or period (p), then the cohort is the difference, ($c = p - a$). This linear dependence gives rise to an identifiability problem in a formal regression model that attempts to obtain quantitative estimates of regression parameters associated with each temporal element:

$$E[Y] = \beta_0 + a\beta_a + p\beta_p + c\beta_c$$

Using the linear relationship between the temporal factors gives rise to:

$$E[Y] = \beta_0 + a\beta_a + p\beta_p + (p - a)\beta_c$$
$$= \beta_0 + a(\beta_a - \beta_c) + p(\beta_p + \beta_c)$$

which has only two identifiable parameters besides the intercept instead of the expected three. Another way of visualising this phenomenon is that all combinations of age, period and cohort may be displayed in the LEXIS DIAGRAM (see Figure), which is obviously a representation of a two-dimensional plane instead of the three dimensions expected for three separate factors.

In general, these analyses are not limited to linear effects applied to continuous measure of time, but instead they are applied to temporal intervals, such as disease rates observed for 5- or 10-year intervals of age and period. When the widths of these intervals are equal, the model may be expressed as:

$$E[Y_{ijk}] = \mu + \alpha_i + \pi_j + \gamma_k$$

where μ is the intercept, α_i the effect of age for the ith ($i = 1,...,I$) interval, π_j the effect of period for the jth ($j = 1,...,\mathcal{J}$) interval, γ_k and the effect of the kth cohort ($k = i - j + I = 1,...,K = I + \mathcal{J} - 1$). The usual constraints in

this model imply that $\sum \alpha_i = \sum \pi_j = \sum \gamma_k = 0$. The identifiability problem manifests itself through a single unidentifiable parameter (Fienberg and Mason, 1979), which can be more easily seen if we partition each temporal effect into components of overall linear trend and curvature or departure from linear trend. For example, age can be given by $\alpha_i = \ddot{i}\beta_a + \breve{\alpha}_i$, where $\ddot{i} = i - .5(I + 1)$, β_a is the overall slope and the $\breve{\alpha}_i$ curvature. The overall model can be expressed as:

$$E[Y_{ijk}] = \mu + (\ddot{i}\beta_a + \breve{\alpha}_i) + (\ddot{j}\beta_\pi + \breve{\pi}_i) + (\ddot{k}\beta_\gamma + \breve{\gamma}_k)$$
$$= \mu + \ddot{i}(\beta_a + \beta_\gamma) + \ddot{j}(\beta_\pi + \beta_\gamma) + \breve{\alpha}_i + \breve{\pi}_j + \breve{\gamma}_k$$

because $\ddot{k} = \ddot{j} - \ddot{i}$. Thus, each of the curvatures can be uniquely determined, but the overall slopes are hopelessly entangled so that only certain combinations can be uniquely estimated (Holford, 1983).

The implication of the identifiability problem is that the overall direction of the effect for any of the three temporal components cannot be determined from a regression analysis. Thus, we cannot even determine whether the trends are increasing or decreasing with cohort, for instance. The second Figure (see page 7) displays several combinations of age, period and cohort parameters, each set of which provides an identical set of fitted rates. Notice that as the period parameters are rotated clockwise, the age and cohort parameters are comparably rotated in the counterclockwise direction. Each of these parameters can be rotated a full 180°, but it is important also to realise that they cannot be rotated one at a time, only all together. Thus, even though the specific trends cannot be uniquely estimated, certain combinations of the overall trend can be uniquely determined, such as $\beta_\pi + \beta_\gamma$, which is called the *net drift* (Clayton and Schifflers, 1987a and b). Alternative drift estimates covering shorter timespans can also be determined and these have practical significance in that they describe the experience of following a particular age group in time, because both period and cohort will advance together. Curvatures, by way of contrast, are completely determined, including polynomial parameters for the square and higher powers, changes in slopes and second differences. The significance test for any one of the temporal effects in the presence of the other two will generally be a test of the corresponding curvature and not the slope. Holford provides further detail on how software can be set up for fitting these models (Holford, 2004).

TRH

Clayton, D. and Schifflers, E. 1987a: Models for temporal variation in cancer rates I: Age-period and age-cohort models. *Statistics in Medicine* 6, 449–67. **Clayton, D. and Schifflers, E.** 1987b: Models for temporal variation in cancer rates II: Age-period cohort models. *Statistics in Medicine* 6, 469–81. **Fienberg, S.E. and Mason, W.M.** 1979: Identification and estimation of age-period-cohort models in the analysis of discrete archival data. *Sociological Methodology* 1978, 1-67. **Holford, T.R.** 1983: The estimation of age, period and cohort effects for vital rates. *Biometrics* 39, 311–24. **Holford, T.R.** 2004: Temporal factors in public health surveillance: sorting out age, period and cohort effects. In Brookmeyer, R. and Stroup, D.F. (eds), *Monitoring the health of populations*. Oxford: Oxford University Press, 99–126.

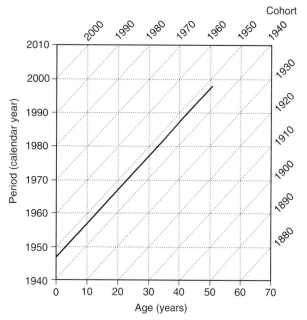

age-period cohort analysis *Lexis diagram showing the relationship between age, period and cohort. The diagonal line traces age-period lifetime for an individual born in 1947*

age-related reference ranges Ranges of values of a measurement that identify the upper and lower limit of normality in the population, where the range varies

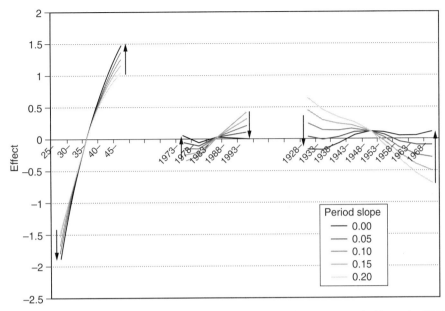

age-period cohort analysis *Age, period and cohort effects for pre-menopausal breast cancer incidence for SEER, 1973–1997*

according to the subject's age. Reference ranges are an important part of medical diagnosis, where a continuous measurement (for example blood pressure) needs converting to a binary variable for decision-making purposes. If the patient's value lies outside the measurement's reference range it is treated as abnormal and the patient is investigated further. The construction of reference ranges involves estimating the range of values that covers a specified percentage of the reference population, often 95%. Usually this is the central part of the distribution with equal tail area probabilities, although in some cases the reference range is bounded at zero or infinity. For normally distributed data the range can be derived from the population MEAN and STANDARD DEVIATION (SD), the 95% range, for example, being the mean plus or minus 2 SDs. For non-normal data the simplest approach is to use quantiles, i.e. rank and count the data, then the 2.5% and 97.5% points are the lower and upper limits of the 95% reference range. But this is inefficient and requires a large sample. If the data are skew they can be transformed e.g. to logarithms, then the reference range can be calculated from the mean and SD on the transformed scale and transformed back to the original scale. A more flexible variant is to use a Box-Cox power transformation (of which the logarithm is a special case), which adjusts for SKEWNESS more precisely (see TRANSFORMATION).

Age-related reference ranges are reference ranges that depend on age. They arise most commonly in paediatrics, notably for age-related measures of body size like height and weight, which can be displayed as GROWTH CHARTS. The principles of reference range estimation are essentially the same when they are age related, except that the ranges for adjacent age groups need to be consistent. To avoid discontinuities at the age group boundaries this requires the summary statistics defining the reference range (e.g. the mean and SD) to change smoothly with age and imposing this constraint complicates the fitting process. For normally distributed homoscedastic data,

where the SD is constant across age, the age-related mean can be estimated by LINEAR REGRESSION and the reference range constructed around the regression curve using the residual SD. The regression curve is estimated using a smoothing regression function, e.g. a polynomial, fractional polynomial or some form of SCATTERPLOT SMOOTHER. If the SD changes with age, as is often the case, a curve of the age-related SD also needs to be estimated by the regression methods of Aitkin (1987) or Altman (1993) and the age-related mean obtained using weighted linear regression with weights corresponding to the inverse square of the age-related SD. The age-related reference range is again constructed around the regression curve using the SD curve. When the data are skew it may be possible to adjust for the skewness using a single, e.g. logarithmic, transformation at all ages. But often the degree of skewness is itself age-related, although this needs a large sample to show it. In this case an age-related summary statistic for the skewness has to be estimated, along with the age-related mean and SD. Two main methods have been proposed, the LMS method and the EN method, both of which provide smooth curves plotted against age for the mean, SD and skewness parameter. The LMS method uses a Box-Cox power transformation to adjust for skewness and the skewness curve is the age-related power needed to transform the distribution to near-normality. It also estimates the SD in the form of the COEFFICIENT OF VARIATION or CV, which is relatively constant as the SD is often proportional to the mean. The EN method uses an exponential-normal transformation and the skewness parameter is again the corresponding power. For more extreme non-normal data, a non-parametric approach based on quantile regression is needed, where smooth curves are constructed for the age-related upper and lower limits of the reference range. The Figure on page 8 gives age-related reference ranges for systolic and diastolic blood pressure in boys aged 4–24, estimated by the LMS method.

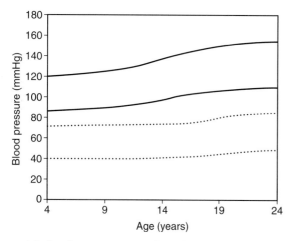

age-related reference ranges *Age-related 95% reference ranges for blood pressure in boys: systolic (solid lines); diastolic (dotted lines)*

age-specific rates *Population, number of deaths and death rates from all causes for Costa Rica and the United Kingdom for the year 1999*

	Costa Rica			
Age group	Population (100,000s)	% in age group	Deaths	Death rate/1000
0–15	10.7	32%	1296	1.2
15–49	17.4	52%	2766	1.6
50–69	3.9	12%	3447	8.8
70+	1.3	4%	7523	56.6
Total	33.4		15,032	4.5

	United Kingdom			
Age group	Population (100,000s)	% in age group	Deaths	Death rate/1000
0–15	113.9	19%	5850	0.5
15–49	288.0	48%	31228	1.1
50–69	126.1	21%	120,759	9.6
70+	67.0	11%	474,225	70.8
Total	595.0		632,062	10.6

There are two advantages of reference ranges based on an underlying frequency distribution, as opposed to those derived using quantile regression. The first is efficiency – the standard errors of the reference range limits are smaller. The second is analytical convenience – data for individuals can be converted to SD scores, indicating how many SDs they are above or below the median of the distribution, which is a convenient way of adjusting for age prior to further analysis. *TJC*

Aitkin, M. 1987: Modelling variance heterogeneity in normal regression using GLIM. *Applied Statistics* 36, 332–39. **Altman, D.G.** 1993: Construction of age-related reference centiles using absolute residuals. *Statistics in Medicine* 12, 917–24. **Cole, T.J. and Green, P.J.** 1992: Smoothing reference centile curves: the LMS method and penalized likelihood. *Statistics in Medicine* 11, 1305–19. **Koenker, R.W. and D'Orey, V.** 1987: Computing regression quantiles. *Applied Statistics* 36, 383–93. **Royston, P. and Wright, E.M.** 1998: A method for estimating age-specific reference intervals ('normal ranges') based on fractional polynomials and exponential transformation. *Journal of the Royal Statistical Society Series A* 161, 79–101.

age-specific rates Rates calculated within a number of relatively narrow age bands. A crude rate is the number of events occurring in a population during a specified time period divided by an estimate of the size of the population. However when comparing rates between populations with different age distributions, it is necessary to consider rates at specific ages separately.

In the Table, death rates are presented for Costa Rica and the United Kingdom for 1999, derived from data from the United Nations (2002). The final column gives the age-specific rates for broad age bands and the crude (total) rate. The age-specific rate is calculated as the number of deaths in the particular age group divided by the population in that age group. In Costa Rica, the death rate at ages 0–5 is calculated as 1296/1,070,000. The rate is expressed per 1000 persons so the result is multiplied by 1000 to give the rate of 1.2 per 1000 in the final column of the table.

The crude (total) rate for Costa Rica is less than half that for the UK. However, at no age is the rate in the UK double that for Costa Rica and for some age groups the rate is higher in Costa Rica than in the UK. Note that the percentages of the populations in each age group (third column) differ markedly. The UK population is much older (11% of the population are over 70 compared with 4% in Costa Rica). The different age structure explains the misleading comparison between the crude rates.

Age-specific rates are cumbersome to compare across a number of populations. Standardisation methods are often used to provide an age-adjusted summary rate for each population.

Many countries publish age-specific rates for all cause and specific causes of death, for example the annual publications of the Office of National Statistics (ONS) in England and Wales (ONS, 2002). Age-specific disease incidence rates are also published in various countries, most notably cancer incidence for which international data are compiled by the International Agency for Research on Cancer (Parkin *et al.*, 2003). Age-specific prevalence rates for exposures such as smoking can also be derived, but are more usually obtained from specific surveys such as the General Household Survey (Walker *et al.*, 2001). *HI*

[See also CAUSE-SPECIFIC DEATH RATE, STANDARDISED MORTALITY RATIO)

Office for National Statistics 2002: *Mortality statistics: cause. Review of the Registrar General on deaths by cause, sex and age, in England and Wales, 2001.* London: Office for National Statistics. **Parkin, M., Whelan, S., Ferlay, J., Teppo, L. and Thomas, D.B.** 2003: *Cancer incidence in five continents.* Vol. VIII. Lyon: IARC Scientific Publications. **United Nations** 2002: *2000 Demographic Yearbook.* New York: United Nations 2002. **Walker, A., Maher, J., Coulthard, M., Goddard, E. and Thomas, M.** 2001: *Living in Britain: results from the 2000 General Household Survey.* London: The Stationery Office.

Akaike's information criterion Akaike's information criterion (AIC) is an index used in a number of areas as an aid to choosing between competing models. It is widely used when there is the issue of model choice where we wish to find the most parsimonious model (see Akaike, 1974). Often there may be a number of possible models that can be fitted to the data, from which parameters can be estimated using, for example, MAXIMUM LIKELIHOOD ESTIMATION. Generally, complex models are more flexible, but contain a relatively large number of parameters, whereas simpler models with fewer parameters may compromise the fit of the model to the data. Essentially, the AIC statistic compares competing models by considering the trade-off between the complexity of the model and the corresponding fit of the model to the data.

Let x denote the data and $\hat{\theta}$ the corresponding maximum likelihood estimates (MLEs) of the parameters. Then, the AIC for a given model is denoted by:

$$AIC = -2 \log L(\hat{\theta}; x) + 2p$$

where p denotes the number of parameters in the given model being fitted to the data and $\log L(\hat{\theta}; x)$ the corresponding likelihood evaluated at the MLEs of the parameters. The AIC statistic is calculated for each possible model being considered. The model deemed optimal is the one with smallest AIC value; i.e. a model with a relatively small number of parameters, which adequately fits the data. The AIC is generally easy to calculate given the maximum of the likelihood function and very versatile, allowing us to compare, for example, non-nested models. We note that corrections have been suggested to the AIC statistic to allow for data with overdispersion (denoted by QAIC) and small sample sizes (AIC_c). See for example Burnham and Anderson (2002), Sections 2.4–5.

The AIC statistic has also been used to compare the performance of different models, relative to each other (Buckland, Burnham and Augustin, 1997; Burnham and Anderson, 2002, Section 2.6). Then, it is not the absolute values of the AIC statistics that are important, but their relative values, in particular their difference. For each model the term $\Delta AIC = AIC - \min AIC$ is calculated, where min AIC is the value of the AIC statistic for the model deemed optimal. Clearly, $\Delta AIC = 0$ for the model deemed optimal; the larger the value of ΔAIC the poorer the model. The relative penalised likelihood weights w_i can also be calculated for each model $i = 1, ..., m$, where:

$$w_i = \frac{\exp(-\Delta AIC_i/2)}{\sum_{j=1}^{m} \exp(-\Delta AIC_j/2)}$$

where AIC_i is the corresponding AIC value associated with model i. The weights provide a scale to interpret the difference in values for the models.   *RK*

[See also DEVIANCE, LIKELIHOOD RATIO]

Akaike, H. 1974: A new look at the statistical model identification. *IEEE Transactions on Automatic Control AC* 19, 716–72. **Buckland, S.T., Burnham, K.P. and Augustin, N.H.** 1997: Model selection: an integral part of inference. *Biometrics* 53, 603–18. **Burnham, K.P. and Anderson, D.R.** 2002: *Model selection and multimodel inference*, 2nd edition. Heidelberg: Springer Verlag.

all subsets regression A form of regression in which all possible models are considered and compared

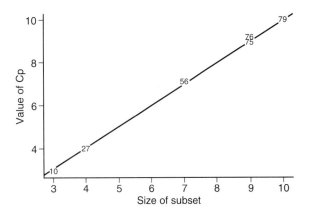

all subsets regression *Some of the models fitted to the cystic fibrosis data in all subsets regression*

using some appropriate criterion useful in indicating the best models for consideration. One such possibility is MALLOWS C_p STATISTIC. If there are P explanatory variables, there are a total of 2^P-1 possible regression models since each explanatory variable can be in or out of the model and the model containing no explanatory variables is excluded. To illustrate this approach we will use data that arise from a study of 25 patients with cystic fibrosis reported in O'Neill *et al.* (1983), also given in Altman (1991). The data are given in the first Table. The dependent variable in this case is a measure of malnutrition (*PEmax*). Some of the models considered in the all subsets regression of these data are shown in the second Table, together with their associated C_p values. Often useful is a plot of C_p against p, labelling the points by subset number, particularly if plotting is restricted to subsets lying close to

all subsets regression *Some of the models fitted in all subsets regression (size is one more than the number of variables, to include the intercept)*

Model	Size	Variables	C_p
7	2	Sex	17.24
10*	3	Weight, BMP	2.88
14	3	Sex, weight	4.63
21	4	Age, FEV, RV	2.62
27*	4	Age, FEV, FRC	3.94
35	5	Sex, weight, BMP, FEV	2.95
42	6	Age, weight, BMP, FEV, RV	2.8
49	6	Age, sex, height, FEV, TLC	6.99
56*	7	Age, sex, height, FEV, RV, TLC	7.06
63	8	Sex, weight, BMP, FEV, RV, FRC, TLC	6.49
70	9	Age, height, weight, BMP, FEV, RV, FRC, TLC	8.06
75*	9	Age, sex, height, weight, BMP, RV, FRC, TLC	8.95
76*	9	Age, sex, height, weight, BMP, FEV, FRC, TLC	9.12
77	9	Age, sex, height, BMP, FEV, RV, FRC, TLC	10.29
79*	10	Age, sex, height, weight, BMP, FEV, RV, FRC, TLC	10.00

* Models close to the line shown in the figure

the line $C_p = p$. Such a plot is shown in the Figure on page 9.   *BSE*

[See also MULTIPLE LINEAR REGRESSION]

Altman, D.G. 1991: *Practical statistics for medical research.* London: CRC/Chapman & Hall. **O'Neill, S., Leahy, F., Pasterkamp, H. and Tal, A.** 1983: The effects of chronic hyperfunction, nutritional status and posture on respiratory muscle strength in cystic fibrosis. *American Review of Respiratory Disorders* 128, 1051–4.

allelic association

An association between two alleles (at two different loci), or between an allele and a phenotypic trait, in the population. Since humans are diploid a more technical definition of the former is necessary: two alleles are associated if their frequency of co-occurrence in the same haplotype (i.e. the genetic material transmitted from one parent) is greater than the product of the marginal frequencies of the two alleles.

Association between two alleles is also known as *linkage disequilibrium*. The reason is that, in a large population under random mating, the extent of association between two alleles (as measured by the difference between the frequency of the haplotype containing the two alleles and the product of the frequencies of the two alleles), decreases by a factor equal to one minus the recombination fraction (see GENETIC LINKAGE) between the two loci, per generation. Thus allelic association represents a state of disequilibrium that tends to dissipate at a rate determined by the strength of linkage between the two alleles.

Associations between two alleles can arise in a population for a number of reasons. The mutation that gave rise to the more recent allele may have occurred on a chromosome containing the older allele. Random genetic drift during a population bottleneck may have led to the over-representation of some haplotypes. The mixing of two populations with different allele frequencies may have resulted in associations between alleles in the overall population. When, for any of these reasons, such allelic associations arose many generations ago, only those occurring between tightly linked loci are likely to have persisted to the current generation. We would therefore expect an imperfect inverse relationship between the extent of association between two alleles and the distance between them.

An association between an allele and a disease may be the result of a direct causal relationship. In other words, the allele is a causal variant that is functional and increases the risk of the disease. However, it could also be indirect, with the allele being in linkage disequilibrium with a causal variant. The presence of linkage disequilibrium between tightly linked loci means that it is possible to screen a chromosomal region for a causal variant without examining all the alleles, only a sufficient number to ensure that any causal variant in the region is likely to be in linkage disequilibrium with one or more of the alleles examined.

Classical epidemiological designs (CASE-CONTROL, COHORT, CROSS-SECTIONAL STUDIES) are readily applicable to the study of disease-allele associations, as are the statistical methods developed for these designs (e.g. LOGISTIC REGRESSION, SURVIVAL ANALYSIS). These designs are potentially susceptible to the problem of hidden population stratification, which can lead to spurious associations or mask true associations. Family-based association designs are robust to population stratification and usually consist of the use of either parental or sibling controls. Methods for the analysis of matched samples, such as the MCNEMAR'S TEST (also called the transmission disequilibrium test in the context of parental controls) and CONDITIONAL LOGISTIC REGRESSION are applicable to these designs.

The study of disease-allele associations is a complementary to linkage analysis as the localisation and identification of genes that increase the risk of disease. In general, allelic association is unlikely to be detected when the marker locus is quite far (> 1 megabase) from the disease locus, but can be much more powerful than linkage when the marker locus is close enough to the disease locus to be in substantial linkage disequilibrium with it, particularly when the effect size of the disease locus is small. For this reason, allelic association is particularly appealing for searching regions that demonstrate linkage to the disease or to the investigation of specific candidate genes.   *PS*

Sham, P. 1997: *Statistics in human genetics.* London: Arnold.

analysis of covariance (ANCOVA, ANOCOVA)

An extension of the ANALYSIS OF VARIANCE (ANOVA) that incorporates a continuous explanatory variable. Where ANOVA aims to detect if there is a change in the mean value of a variable across two or more groups, ANCOVA (or rarely ANOCOVA) does the same but adjusts for a continuous covariate.

Most commonly this covariate will be a baseline measurement, allowing the analysis to adjust for initial variation between participants and isolate the effects due to the treatment factor. However, sometimes a different covariate is used. For example, Karhune *et al.* (1994) consider the association between alcohol intake (divided into four categories) and numbers of Purkinje cells. In doing so they introduce age as a continuous covariate in order to 'control' or 'adjust' for the effects of age on cell numbers.

Under other circumstances the authors could have been interested in the effects of age, and wanting to adjust for alcohol intake. Despite being the same analysis computationally, this is not typically what is thought of as analysis of covariance and might more commonly be presented as a 'regression'. Indeed the various analysis of variance methods can all be viewed from within a regression framework, which demonstrates that ANCOVA can be extended to cope with much more than one continuous covariate.

Mathematically, ANCOVA follows a similar path to that for ANOVA and the output is usually summarised in a similar table, although the details may vary.

The promised benefits of the analysis of covariance are clear. If one has an unbalanced observational study, then ANCOVA can adjust for differences in baseline values and remove a potential bias from the results. By the same token, if one has a randomised trial that is naturally balanced, then ANCOVA reduces the amount of unexplained variation in the data and thus increases the power of the test.

However, ANCOVA can only be employed if the appropriate assumptions are met. These include those of ANOVA (i.e. normality of residuals, homoscedasticity) as well as the appropriateness of the ANCOVA model. Is the relationship with the covariate truly linear? Does the effect of the covariate vary between groups? Failing to meet these assumptions can lead to the introduction of important but subtle biases. It is a frequent concern that medical research papers report a covariate as having been 'controlled' or 'adjusted' for, with no evidence that the control or adjustment was appropriate. *AGL*

[See also GENERALISED LINEAR MODEL]

Altman, D.G. 1991: *Practical statistics for medical research.* London: Chapman & Hall. Karhune, P.J., Erkinjutti, T. and Laippala, P. 1994: Moderate alcohol consumption and loss of cerebellar Prikinje cells. *British Medical Journal* 308, 1663–7. Miller, G.A. and Chapman, J.P. 2001: Misunderstanding analysis of covariance. *Journal of Abnormal Psychology* 110, 40–8. Owen, S.V. and Froman, R.D. 1998: Uses and abuses of the analysis of covariance. *Research in Nursing and Health* 21, 557–62. Vickers, A.J. and Altman, D.G. 2001: Analysing controlled trials with baseline and follow-up measurements. *British Medical Journal* 323, 123–4.

analysis of variance (ANOVA)

Often referring to one-way analysis of variance; a test for a common MEAN in multiple groups. Despite the confusion sometimes caused by the name, ANOVA is a method for testing to see whether multiple samples come from populations that share the same mean. In this respect it can be viewed as an extension to the t-test, which assesses whether samples from two populations share a common mean. An analysis of variance performed on two samples is equivalent to performing a t-test.

ANOVA assumes that all the samples come from populations with a NORMAL DISTRIBUTION that share the same VARIANCE. It can be viewed in a number of ways, but essentially compares the estimate of the variance obtained within samples (that makes no assumption that the populations have a common mean) with an estimate of the variance from the sample means (which will require the assumption that the populations have the same mean). If the two estimates of the variance are different, then this is evidence that our assumption of equality failed and, therefore, that the populations do not all have the same mean.

Note that the variance of a single sample is estimated as the sum of squared differences from the mean divided by the sample size minus one. The sum of squared differences term is interpretable as a measure of the total variation in the sample. In the analysis of variance, by combining all groups together, one can calculate this measure for all the data. This is termed the 'Total Sum of Squares' or 'Total SS'.

Variation in the data is either 'Between' or 'Within' the samples. The 'Within groups Sum of Squares' or 'Within SS' can be calculated as the sum of squared differences from the individual sample means (rather than the differences from the overall mean that produced the Total SS). 'Between groups Sum of Squares' or 'Between SS' can be calculated directly, but is most easily calculated by subtraction of the Within SS from the Total SS minus.

The two estimates of the variance (or 'mean square' as it is often termed in this context) can then be calculated. The Between groups mean square is equal to the Between SS divided by the number of groups minus one. The Within groups mean square is equal to the Within SS divided by the number of observations minus the number of groups.

An F-statistic is then calculated as the Between groups variance divided by the Within groups variance. Under the assumptions of normality and homoscedasticity (common variance) this statistic will be an observation from an F-DISTRIBUTION if the groups come from populations with a common mean. The DEGREES OF FREEDOM of the F-distribution are the number of groups minus one and the number of observations minus the number of groups.

From the F-distribution, we can calculate the probability of observing such an extreme value of the F-statistic if the populations have a common mean. This is a *one-tailed test*. If the value is unusually small, this suggests the Between groups variance is unusually small and so is not evidence of variation between the groups. Therefore, the test is to find the probability, if the populations do have a common mean, of observing a value greater than that observed.

A natural way of presenting ANOVA is the ANOVA table. Given N observations that fall into k groups, it is necessary to calculate the Total SS and the Within SS as described earlier and then the analysis can be completed as presented in the first Table on page 12.

Murphy *et al.* (1994) conducted an analysis of variance to see if milk consumption before the age of 25 affects bone density of the hip in later life. A total of 248 women participated in this part of their study ($N = 248$) and were divided into groups that represent low, medium and high milk consumptions ($k = 3$). The samples had similar variances and so at least one of the assumptions for ANOVA was satisfied. As is common for reasons of space, the ANOVA table was not presented in the published paper, just the P-VALUE, but enough data were presented for an approximate reconstruction.

We can infer that the Within SS is approximately 4.4 and the Between SS is approximately 0.15. This leads to an F-statistic of approximately 4. From the reported P-value (0.023), it can be calculated from the F-distribution (with 2 and 245 degrees of freedom) that the F-statistic was 3.8. The conclusion then is that there is evidence that these samples do not come from populations that share a common mean. The reconstructed table is presented in the second Table on page 12 (entries in bold in this table were inferred from the paper, the rest simply follow from the calculations).

It is preferable to conduct an analysis of variance rather than to conduct t-tests between all pairs of groups. ANOVA avoids problems of multiple testing and thus keeps control of the SIGNIFICANCE LEVEL. Having conducted an ANOVA and rejected the hypothesis of common means, it may then be desired to test to see which groups are responsible (although a plot of the data might be as informative). In this case, care must be taken to correct for the problems of multiple testing, for example by utilising the BONFERONNI CORRECTION.

It is important to take note of the assumptions being made, rather than simply ignoring them. ANOVA can be quite robust to variations from normality, but heteroscedasticity can be a serious problem. Residual plots can be used to help assess the normality and BOX PLOTS can be used to help assess the heteroscedasticity. Possible formal tests for the assumptions are the KOLMOGOROV-SMIRNOV TEST and LEVENE'S TEST respectively.

If the assumptions do not hold, then TRANSFORMATION of the data might correct this. Otherwise a number of non-parametric alternatives to ANOVA exist, the most commonly used being the KRUSKAL-WALLIS TEST and the FRIEDMAN TEST.

analysis of variance *The analysis of variance table: general form*

Source of variance	Degrees of freedom	Sums of squares	Mean squares	F	P-value
Between groups	$k-1$	Between SS = Total SS – Within SS	Between MS = Between SS/$(k-1)$	$\dfrac{\text{Between MS}}{\text{Within SS}}$	p
Within groups	$N-k$	Within SS	Within MS = Within SS/$(N-k)$		
Total	$N-1$	Total SS			

analysis of variance *Approximate reconstruction of the analysis of variance table (from Murphy et al., 1994)*

Source of variance	Degrees of freedom	Sums of squares	Mean squares	F	P-value
Between groups	2	**0.15**	0.075	3.8	0.023
Within groups	245	**4.4**	0.018		
Total	247	4.6			

The one-way analysis of variance is appropriate when our data are simply divided into a number of groups. There are many other forms of analysis of variance. The TWO-WAY ANALYSIS OF VARIANCE should be used when the groups are defined by two factors. Suppose, for example, we had six groups: the three groups of women in Murphy *et al.* (1994) and three groups of men at the same levels of milk consumption. Rather than a one-way analysis of variance, a two-way analysis of variance with gender and milk consumption as the two factors would be appropriate in this instance.

If the data are multiple observations from the same subjects, perhaps measurements of cholesterol levels 0, 7, 14, 21 and 28 days after starting a new diet on several individuals, then a REPEATED MEASURES ANALYSIS OF VARIANCE would be appropriate. This is a special case of the two-way ANOVA and is an extension of the paired sample t-test.

If there are observations of more than one characteristic from the individuals in several groups, i.e. measures of both the diastolic and systolic blood pressure, then a multivariate analysis of variance (MANOVA) can be used. Or if it is desired to correct for a measured baseline covariate, such as body mass index, in the analysis, then an ANALYSIS OF COVARIANCE (ANCOVA) may be used.

All these techniques could be implemented through a regression framework, in most cases MULTIPLE LINEAR REGRESSION. The advantages of doing so would be the transition from use of a HYPOTHESIS TEST to an actual estimate of effect sizes. This approach would also allow more flexibility, for instance in the case of Murphy *et al.* (1994) we could account for the natural ordering of the levels of milk consumption that ANOVA ignores. As a general principle, estimation and modelling are usually preferred to testing of hypotheses. *AGL*

Altman, D.G. 1991: *Practical statistics for medical research.* London: Chapman & Hall. Altman, D.G. and Bland, J.M. 1996: Statistics notes: comparing several groups using analysis of variance. *British Medical Journal* 312, 1472–3. Murphy, S., Khaw, K.-T., May, H. and Compston, J.E. 1994: Milk consumption and bone mineral density in middle aged and elderly women. *British Medical Journal* 308, 939–41.

area under the curve (AUC) A simple and useful method of obtaining a summary measure from plotted data. Medical research is frequently concerned with serial data, as in repeated measurements (see REPEATED MEASURES ANALYSIS OF VARIANCE) on a subject over time; for example, blood aspirin concentration measured at various times over a 2-hour interval (Matthews *et al.*, 1990). Say we have n measurements y_i taken at times t_i ($i = 1 ,..., n$). Such data are frequently exhibited by plotting y_i versus t_i and joining the resulting points by straight-line segments resulting in a 'curve'. The resulting area under the curve (AUC) is often used as a single-number summary measure for the individual subject. Further analysis of the subjects or comparison of groups of subjects is carried out

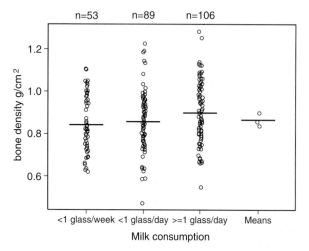

analysis of variance *Milk consumption and bone density*

based on the summary measures. The AUC for the set of points (y_i, t_i) $i = 1, \ldots, n$ is typically calculated by the trapezium rule:

$$\text{AUC} = \frac{1}{2} \sum_{i=1}^{n-1} (t_{i+1} - t_i)(y_i + y_{i+1})$$

The AUC is used as a summary measure in many areas of medical research including bioequivalence and pharmacokinetics. It plays an especially important role in the analysis of RECEIVER OPERATING CHARACTERISTIC (ROC) CURVES. The area under the ROC curve of a diagnostic marker (test) measures the ability of the marker to discriminate between healthy and diseased subjects. It is the most commonly used measure of performance of a marker. We use the convention that larger marker values are more indicative of disease. Then if we randomly pick one subject from the healthy population and one from the diseased population we would 'expect' that the value of the marker for the healthy subject would be smaller than the corresponding value for the diseased. AUC is the probability that this, in fact, occurs. The larger the AUC, the better the overall discriminatory accuracy of the marker. An area of 1 represents a perfect test while an area of 1/2 represents a worthless test having a discriminatory ability, which is the equivalent of differentiating between healthy and diseased subjects by a fair coin toss. Consider the example discussed in the entry for the ROC curve. The points on the curve are given in the Table.

area under the curve *Summary data used in an ROC curve*

Specificity	(y_i)	0	0.56	0.84	0.94	0.98	1.00
1-Sensitivity	(t_i)	0	0.04	0.12	0.32	0.60	1.00

The data presented result in an AUC as follows:

$$\begin{aligned}\text{AUC} = {} & 0.5[(0.04 - 0) \times (0 + 0.56) + (0.12 - 0.04) \times \\ & (0.56 + 0.84) + (0.32 - 0.12) \times (0.84 + 0.94)) + \\ & (0.60 - 0.32) \times (0.94 + 0.98) + (1.00 - 0.60) \times \\ & (0.98 + 1.00)] \\ = {} & 0.91\end{aligned}$$

An area of 0.91 indicates the high discriminatory ability of the marker.

For the ROC curve estimating the area by the trapezium rule is equivalent to computing the WILCOXON or MANN-WHITNEY statistic divided by the products of the sample sizes on the healthy and diseased populations. For smoothed ROC curves alternative estimates of the AUC are available (Faraggi and Reiser, 2002). The effectiveness of alternative diagnostic markers is usually studied by comparing their AUCs (Wieand *et al.*, 1989). Adjustments of these areas for covariate information, selection bias and pooling effects are discussed in the references given in the entry for the ROC curve. Schisterman *et al.* (2001) consider corrections of the AUC for MEASUREMENT ERROR. *DF/BR*

Faraggi, D. and Reiser, B. 2002: Estimation of the area under the ROC curve. *Statistics in Medicine* 21, 3093–106. **Hanley, J.A. and McNeil, B.J.** 1982: The meaning and use of the area under the receiver operating characteristic (ROC) curve. *Radiology* 143, 29–36. **Matthews, J.N.S., Altman D.G., Campbell, M.J. and Royston, P.** 1990: Analysis of serial measurements in medical research. *British Medical Journal* 300, 230–5. **Schisterman, E., Faraggi, D. Reiser, B. and Trevisan, M.** 2001: Statistical inference for the area under the ROC curve in the presence of random measurement error. *American Journal of Epidemiology* 154, 174–9. **Wieand, S., Gail, M.H., James, B.R. and James, K.L.** 1989: A family of nonparametric statistics for comparing diagnostic markers with paired or unpaired data. *Biometrika* 76, 585–92.

artificial intelligence (AI) Branch of computer science devoted to the simulation of intelligent behaviour in machines. Traditional focus areas of AI are machine vision, MACHINE LEARNING, natural-language processing and speech recognition. Historically an interdisciplinary field, hence characterised by the presence of several competing paradigms and approaches, recently AI has started developing a more unified conceptual framework, based largely on the convergence of statistical and algorithmic ideas.

A constant theme of AI throughout its history has been 'pattern recognition', the crucial task of detecting 'patterns' (regularities, relations, laws) within data. This task has emerged as a roadblock in all the traditional areas mentioned earlier and hence has attracted significant attention. Since most current approaches to pattern recognition involve significant use of statistics, this has become an important tool in AI in general.

Recently, AI has been applied to a new series of important problems and this, in turn, has heavily affected general AI research. Important applications of modern AI include: intelligent data analysis (see also DATA MINING IN MEDICINE); information retrieval and filtering from the web; bioinformatics; and computational biology.

Traditional application areas, by way of contrast, included the design of EXPERT SYSTEMS for medical or industrial diagnosis, methods for scheduling in logistics and creation of other decision-making assistant software.

The imprecise definition of what AI actually is has made it harder in time to gauge the impact of this research field on everyday applications. A number of widely used computer programs would have met early definitions of artificial intelligence, for example popular web-based recommendation systems or air travel planning advisors.

Popular techniques for pattern recognition such as NEURAL NETWORKS, decision trees and cluster analysis (see CLUSTER ANALYSIS IN MEDICINE) have made their way into the standard toolbox of data analysis and are commonly found in the toolbox of any biology lab. Machine vision methods are routinely used in analysing medical images, as well as parts of systems such as microarray machines for collecting gene expression data. Web retrieval and email filtering software also incorporate several ideas from natural-language processing and pattern recognition and the modern sequence analysis of genomic data heavily relies on techniques originally developed for speech recognition. Intelligent web agents exist to find, assess and retrieve relevant information for the user and speech-recognition systems are routinely used in automatic phone information systems. The field of artificial intelligence has clearly produced a number of practical applications, but – the critics say – these have been achieved without solving the general problem of building intelligent machines. Maybe for this reason, generally the main success story of AI is reported to be the defeat of the chess world champion Gary Kasparov by an IBM algorithm in 1997.

The origin of the field of AI is often identified with a paper by A.M. Turing, which appeared in 1950 in the journal *Mind*, and with a workshop held at Dartmouth College in the summer of 1956, although many key ideas had already been debated before, during the early years of cybernetics.

Modern techniques of artificial intelligence include Bayesian belief networks, part of the more general field of probabilistic graphical models; pattern-recognition algorithms such as SUPPORT VECTOR MACHINES, which represent the convergence of ideas from classical statistics and from neural networks analysis; statistical analysis of natural language text and machine vision algorithms; reinforcement learning algorithms which represent a connection with control theory; and many other methods.

NC/TDB

Bishop, C. 1996: *Neural networks for pattern recognition*. Oxford: Oxford University Press. **Mitchell, T.** 1995: *Machine learning*. Maidenhead: McGraw Hill. **Russell, S. and Norvig, P.** 2002: *Artificial intelligence: a modern approach*, 2nd edn. Harlow: Prentice Hall. **Shawe-Taylor, J. and Cristianini, N.** 2004: *Kernel methods for pattern analysis*. Cambridge: Cambridge University Press.

as treated   See INTENTION-TO-TREAT

association   The statistical dependence between two variables. Measures of association, unlike descriptive statistics of a single variable, summarise the extent to which one variable increases or decreases in relation to a change in a second variable. The basic graphical analysis of two variables is the SCATTERPLOT, which provides evidence of association in the shape and direction of the scatter of points. In the example given here, there appears to be an association between body mass index and systolic blood pressure values in a sample of a few thousand middle-aged men and women: higher values of body mass index tend to be associated with higher values of systolic blood pressure, suggesting a 'positive' association. A 'negative' association, in contrast, would describe a situation where an increase in one variable tends to be related to a decrease in the second variable.

Various statistical measures can be used to interpret the degree of association.

Correlation coefficient. Specifically measures the degree of *linear* association between two quantitative variables on a scale from negative one to positive one. A value of zero indicates a total absence of linear association, while a value of positive or negative one indicates a perfect linear relationship. The correlation coefficient between body mass index and systolic blood pressure in our example was 0.25, indicating a positive association that is less than perfectly linear. However, adherence to a linear relationship is only one form of association and it is easy to imagine other plausible patterns of association, such as a parabolic scatter, in which the change in one variable may be perfectly reflected in the change in the second variable, but the correlation coefficient might be close to zero.

Regression coefficient. In the case of simple linear regression, there is a complete correspondence between the correlation coefficient and the regression coefficient for the slope (β). The regression coefficient, therefore, also measures association, but its value is interpreted as the magnitude of change in the dependent variable that arises, on average, from a unit change in the independent variable. In our example, an estimate of $\hat{\beta} = 1.37$ indicated a 1kg/m^2 increase in body mass index was associated with an average increase of 1.37mmHg systolic blood pressure. However, in more complex regression models, the regression coefficient can measure other forms of association beyond linear dependence. For example, either the dependent or independent variable may be mathematically transformed, such as raising to a higher power, taking logarithms, etc., and the association measured by the regression coefficient would express a non-linear change in one variable in response to a change in the second variable.

Relative risk. In the special case of two binary variables, various ratio measures are often used to quantify the degree of association. For example, one variable might be a measure of disease occurrence, the other a biological or environmental quantity. Most commonly the ratio would compare probability of disease expressed as an odds, a risk or some other relevant approximation to the risk. A relative risk value of 1, indicating equal risks in both groups, suggests that no association exists between the biological or environmental quantity and disease.

If a statistical measure suggests positive or negative association, this should not immediately be taken to imply that the association is valid and generalisable. Several considerations might lead us to question the importance of an observed statistical association.

First, consideration of the STANDARD ERROR of the measure of association, generally reflecting the size of the sample, places the magnitude of association in perspective with the magnitude of random error. Apparently strong associations may in fact be poorly estimated and fall short of statistical significance.

Second, an apparent association may be entirely spurious (i.e. 'confounded') due to the influence of other measured, or unmeasured, variables that have not be accounted for in the analysis. For example, in a preliminary statistical enquiry, risk of coronary heart disease may appear to be associated with watching television, although consideration of the underlying relationship with obesity and physical exercise would probably suggest that the preliminary finding was spurious. An association may alter after adjustment for the interdependence of other variables and the general validity of a measure of association would often depend on the extent to which such potential interdependencies have been taken into account. Studies measuring several variables often utilise multiple regression models to estimate adjusted regression coefficients and partial correlation coefficients by including all relevant variables in the model. However, even after allowing for such interdependencies, the much stronger claim of CAUSALITY between two variables would generally require examination of more stringent criteria.

Third, an observed association may be specific to the chosen range of the variables or to the particular group of subjects studied and any inference beyond the range of the data to hand would require careful consideration of the method of sample selection. Various forms of selection bias may limit the generalisability of the association.   *JGW*

attenuation due to measurement error A bias reducing the size of a correlation or a regression coefficient due to imprecision of data measurement. Consider an analytical epidemiological study in which the aim is to estimate the correlation between true average consumption of alcohol (mg per day) and true average systolic blood pressure (mm Hg). Blood pressure measurements are well known to be variable within individuals and a single measurement is likely to be rather imprecise (see MEASUREMENT PRECISION AND RELIABILITY). Such imprecision is even stronger for a single day's intake of alcohol used as a measure of the true average daily intake of alcohol (even if that day's intake were found to be measured without error). Now, suppose we chose to measure each participant's systolic blood pressure once and asked him/her to recall alcohol intake of the previous day. If we calculate the Pearson product-moment correlation between the two measures we are likely to get a positive value that may be statistically significant (assuming we have a large enough sample) but will not be particularly high (i.e. not far above zero). Let us suppose we have found a value of this correlation to be 0.20. It should be fairly obvious that as the measures of systolic blood pressure and alcohol become less precise (equivalent for a fixed population to lowering their reliabilities) the correlation will tend to zero. This is attenuation due to measurement error.

Let the observed measurement of blood pressure for the ith participant be Y_i and the corresponding true average blood pressure be τ_i. Similarly let the measured alcohol intake be X_i with a true average of η_i. We have estimated the correlation between Y and X, ρ_{YX}, when we are really interested the correlation between the true values, $\rho_{\eta\tau}$. If the errors of measurement for blood pressure are uncorrelated with those for alcohol consumption then it can be shown that the following relationship holds:

$$\rho_{YX} = \rho_{\eta\tau}\sqrt{(\kappa_Y\kappa_X)}$$

Here, κ_Y and κ_X are the reliabilities of the blood pressure and alcohol consumption measurements, respectively. It follows that:

$$\rho_{\eta\tau} = \rho_{YX}/\sqrt{(\kappa_Y\kappa_X)}$$

Provided we know the reliabilities for the two measurements, this equation can be used to adjust the observed correlation between Y and X to obtain the required correlation between their true average values. If we know that $\kappa_X = 0.3$ and $\kappa_Y = 0.7$, for example, the required correlation is $0.2/\sqrt{(0.3 \times 0.7)} = 0.44$.

If, instead of a correlation, the linear regression coefficient for the effect of blood pressure on alcohol consumption were of key interest then:

$$\beta_{YX} = \beta_{\eta\tau}\kappa_X$$

Again, the required adjustment is straightforward. This last equation also holds approximately if were to use a logistic regression to predict presence/absence of hypertension.

These calculations are fine as long as we have valid estimates of the reliabilities. But they are only valid in very simple situations such as those described here. Epide-miologists almost always wish to adjust their estimates to allow for confounding and some of these confounders are inevitably prone to measurement errors. Under these circumstances the situation is considerably more complicated!

We cannot even be certain that the estimate of the required parameter will be attenuated, never mind being attenuated in a way described by our third equation. Readers are referred elsewhere to these much more challenging but more realistic situations (see Carroll, Ruppert and Stefanski, 1995; Cheng and Van Ness, 1999; Gustafson, 2003). *GD*

Carroll, R.J., Ruppert, D. and Stefanski, L.A. 1995: *Measurement error in nonlinear models*. London: Chapman & Hall. **Cheng, C.-L. and Van Ness, J.W.** 1999: *Statistical regression with measurement error*. London: Arnold. **Gustafson, P.** 2003: *Measurement error and misclassification in statistics and epidemiology*. London: Chapman & Hall/CRC.

attributable risk As a measure of the public health significance of exposure to a risk factor for disease, the attributable risk provides an estimate of the proportion of diseased subjects that may be attributed to the exposure. It is defined by:

$$\lambda = \frac{\Pr\{D\} - \Pr\{D|\bar{E}\}}{\Pr\{D\}}$$

where $\Pr\{D\}$ is the probability that an individual develops disease and E and $\bar{E}$ represent whether an individual is exposed or not exposed to the factor of interest (Levin, 1953). Ideally, one would like to know both $\Pr\{D\}$ and $\Pr\{D|\bar{E}\}$ for the population under study, but for some study designs this is not possible, so if one wishes to use the measure, care is needed to design a study that will provide as good an estimate as possible, especially when one employs an observational study. Using BAYES THEOREM, and rearranging the equation, we can obtain an expression expressed in terms of the RELATIVE RISK (*RR*):

$$\lambda = \frac{\Pr\{E\}(RR - 1)}{1 + \Pr\{E\}(RR - 1)}$$

where $\Pr\{E\}$ is the prevalence of exposure in the population at large. This is a convenient way of expressing the measure of association, because *RR* is often estimated using alternative study designs, including CASE-CONTROL, COHORT and CROSS-SECTIONAL STUDIES.

Attributable risk is most easily interpreted when the factor of interest increases risk, i.e. *RR* > 1, and in these cases the possible range of the measure is from 0 to 1. An attributable risk of zero can occur when no individuals in the population are exposed to the factor of interest, or if the factor is not related to risk of disease, *RR* = 1. The measure is not easily interpreted when the exposure is protective, *RR* < 1, so it is generally not used in this case. By redefining the reference group, one can always express the results of a study in a form in which *RR* is greater than 1, so this is not a serious limitation. In addition, the measure is often expressed as a percent. As *RR* become large, λ goes to 1, but λ goes to zero either as the proportion exposed, $\Pr\{E\}$, becomes small or as the relative risk, *RR*, approached the null value of 1. If an entire population is exposed to a particular factor, $\Pr\{E\} = 1$, then the second equation (above) reduces to $\lambda = (RR - 1)/RR$.

The Table shows a typical 2×2 table that can be used to display the results from an epidemiological study. In a case-control study, the column totals are generally regarded as being fixed by design and the odds ratio or cross-product ratio is used as a good approximation to the estimate of RR when the disease is rare. In addition, the exposure distribution in the controls, $\Pr\{E\} = \Pr\{E \mid \bar{D}\}$, is considered to be representative of the exposure distribution in the overall population. Substituting in the sample estimates of these quantities gives rise to what is the maximum likelihood estimate of λ:

$$\hat{\lambda} = \frac{ad - bc}{d(a + c)}$$

When setting a confidence interval about the estimate, Walter (1975) suggests using the normal approximation on the log transformation of the complement of the estimate:

$$\mathrm{Var}\left[\log(1 - \hat{\lambda})\right] = \frac{a}{c(a + c)} + \frac{b}{d(b + d)}$$

Alternatively, Leung and Kupper (1981) have suggested using a LOGIT transformation in which:

$$\mathrm{Var}\left[\log\frac{\hat{\lambda}}{1 - \hat{\lambda}}\right] = \left[\frac{a}{c(a + b)} + \frac{b}{d(b + d)}\right]\left[\frac{d(b + d)}{a(b + d) - b(a + c)}\right]^2$$

In a cohort study, the row totals in the table are regarded as fixed, therefore such a study does not provide a good internal estimate of the exposure distribution neither does it provide a good estimate of the unconditional estimate of the probability of disease. In this case, the proportion exposed is usually derived from another study, perhaps an earlier case-control study or a survey of the entire population. A cross-sectional study provides both an estimate of the relative risk and the overall population distribution, so in that sense it is ideal for estimating attributable risk. However, a cross-sectional study suffers in other ways (see CROSS-SECTIONAL STUDIES). Walter (1976) discusses the properties of estimates of attributable risk using these alternative study designs.

Methods for estimating attributable risk for a particular exposure while adjusting for potential confounding factors depends on whether the effect is constant over the levels of the covariates under consideration. When the effect is constant, it can be represented as having a common relative risk over the strata when using a stratified approach,

such as the MANTEL-HAENSZEL METHOD, or it can be represented by a main effect only in a model, such as the linear logistic model. In these situations, one can directly use the adjusted estimator or the relative risk, along with an estimate of the exposure distribution in the diseased group in the second equation (above) to obtain an estimate of adjusted attributable risk (Greenland, 1987; Walter 1976). However, the assumption that the association can be described without the inclusion of an interaction term is a strong one and it is critical in that a seriously biased estimate can result if it is not true.

An estimate of attributable risk that can be used either in a stratified analysis in which the effect is not homogeneous across strata or in a GENERALISED LINEAR MODEL that includes interaction terms can be expressed as:

$$\lambda = 1 - \sum_{i,j}\frac{p_{ij}}{RR_{i|j}}$$

where j represents the levels of the factor(s) being adjusted, i represents the levels of exposure, p_{ij} is the proportion of diseased individuals in (i,j), and $RR_{i|j}$ the relative risk for exposure level i for individuals with level j of the covariates being adjusted (Benichou, 1993; Walter, 1976).   *TRH*

Benichou, J. 1993: Methods of adjustment for estimating the attributable risk in case-control studies: a review. *Statistics in Medicine* 10, 1753–73. **Greenland, S.** 1987: Variance estimators for attributable fraction estimates, consistent in both large strata and sparse data. *Statistics in Medicine* 6, 701–8. **Leung, H.K. and Kupper, L.L.** 1981: Comparison of confidence intervals for attributable risk. *Biometrics* 37, 293–302. **Levin, M.L.** 1953: The occurrence of lung cancer in man. *Acta Unio Internationalis contra Cancrum* 9, 531–41. **Walter, S.D.** 1975: The distribution of Levin's measure of attributable risk. *Biometrika* 62, 371–4. **Walter, S.D.** 1976: The estimation and interpretation of attributable risk in health research. *Biometrics* 32, 829–49.

AUC   See AREA UNDER THE CURVE

autocorrelation   See CORRELATION

automatic selection procedures   Procedures for identifying a parsimonious model in regression in general and MULTIPLE LINEAR REGRESSION in particular. A number of methods are available.

Forward selection. This method starts with a model containing *none* of the explanatory variables and then considers variables one by one for possible inclusion. At each step the variable added is the one that results in the largest increase in the regression sum of squares (for multiple linear regression; for other regression techniques, for example, LOGISTIC REGRESSION, some other more suitable criterion would be used to judge whether or not a variable should be entered into the model. An F-TEST is used to judge when further additions would not represent a significant improvement in the model.

Backward elimination. This method starts with a model containing all the explanatory variables and eliminates variables one by one, at each stage selecting the variable for exclusion as the one leading to the smallest decrease in the regression sum of squares. Once again an F-test is used to judge when further exclusions would represent a significant deterioration in the model.

attributable risk *Results from an epidemiological study with two levels of exposure and disease status*

Exposed	Disease status		Total
	D	$\bar{D}$	
E	a	b	$a + b$
$\bar{E}$	c	d	$c + d$
Total	$a + c$	$b + d$	N

Stepwise regression. This method is, essentially, a combination of the preceding two. Starting with no variables in the model, variables are added as with the forward selection approach, but now with the addition of a variable a backward elimination process is considered to assess whether variables entered earlier might now be removed, since they no longer contribute significantly to the model.

None of the automatic procedures for selecting subsets of variables is foolproof and it is possible for them to be seriously misleading in some circumstances (see Agresti, 1996). That said, at least one can be more confident in a chosen model if all three procedures converge onto the same set of variables, as occurs quite frequently, but not always, in practice. When different subsets of variables are indicated, judgement is necessary to decide on a preferred model, such judgement being based on the desire to create a parsimonious model that is likely to be generalisable, not overly complex as if modelling mere quirks of the particular dataset on which it is based, and yet including important or standard parameters deemed to be of clinical relevance. *BSE*

[See also ALL SUBSETS REGRESSION]

Agresti, A. 1996: *Introduction to categorical data analysis.* New York: John Wiley & Sons.

(See COVARIANCE MATRIX).

available case analysis

An approach to multivariate data containing missing values on a number of variables, in which MEANS, VARIANCES and covariances (see COVARIANCE MATRIX) are calculated from all available subjects with non-missing values on the variable (means and variances) or pair of variables (covariances) involved. Although this approach makes use of as much of the observed data as possible, it does have disadvantages. For example, the summary statistics for each variable may be based on different numbers of observations and the calculated variance–covariance matrix may now not be suitable for methods of multivariate analysis such as PRINCIPAL COMPONENTS ANALYSIS and FACTOR ANALYSIS for reasons described in Schafer (1997). *BSE*

[See also MISSING DATA, MULTIPLE IMPUTATION]

Schafer, J.L. 1997: *Analysis of incomplete multivariate data.* Bacon Raton, Florida: Chapman & Hall/CRC.

average age at death

A flawed statistic sometimes used for summarising life expectancy and other aspects of mortality. For example, Andersen (1990), comments on a study that compared average age at death for male symphony orchestra conductors and for the entire US male population and showed that, on average, the conductors lived about 4 years longer. The difference is, however, largely illusory because as age at entry was birth, those in the US male population who died in infancy and childhood were included in the calculation of the average lifespan, whereas only men who survived long enough to become conductors could enter the conductor cohort. The apparent difference in longevity disappeared after accounting for infant and perinatal mortality.

And, in the other direction, a study in the USA that used average age at death of rock stars (which, on the basis of 321 such deaths, they found to be 36.9 years) to warn of the perils of rock music also got it wrong. It took no account of the rock stars still alive.

Proper analysis of mortality involves the determination of AGE-SPECIFIC mortality RATES, which requires denominator data on the age distribution of the population (see Colton, 1974). *BSE*

Andersen, B. 1990: *Methodological errors in medical research.* Oxford: Blackwell Scientific. **Colton, T.** 1974: *Statistics in medicine.* Boston: Little, Brown and Co.

B

back-calculation Also known as back-projection, this is a means of estimating, for example, past HIV infection rates and predicting the number of new AIDS cases in the future and was first proposed in the mid-1980s (Brookmeyer and Gail, 1986). The essence of the method is contained in the equation:

$$d(t) = \int_0^t h(s) \, p(t - s) \, ds$$

where $d(t)$ and $h(s)$ denote the disease diagnosis rate at time t and the infection rate at time s; and $p(.)$ indicates the probability distribution (density) of the incubation time (or INCUBATION PERIOD). This expression states that the rate of disease diagnosis at time t depends on the rate of new infections at time s and on the distribution of the incubation time $t - s$. Therefore, if any two of these three components are known, the third can be *inferred*. Typically, the disease diagnosis rate for t up to the current time T and the distribution of the incubation time are assumed known and the infection rate is estimated.

The Figure explains the idea in a discrete time framework using the HIV epidemic as an example. Here the interest is in estimating HIV incidence and in predicting future AIDS cases. Suppose data on new AIDS cases over time up to the current time T are available together with the information on the distribution of the incubation time. It is then possible to reconstruct the number of past infections that have resulted in the observed AIDS cases. The estimated incidence of HIV can be used in conjunction with the distribution of the incubation time to produce short-term projections of new AIDS diagnoses. Note that in this particular case, the MEDIAN length of the incubation time is of the order of 10 years, with very few individuals

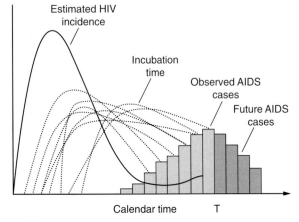

back-calculation *Back-calculation using HIV incidence and prediction of future AIDS cases*

developing AIDS within a short time period from infection. The observed AIDS cases therefore provide information on infections that occurred in the distant past, rather than in recent years. Estimates of incidence of infection for the years just preceding T will necessarily be quite inaccurate, as they are based on little information. Care should then be taken in the interpretation of recent trends in the number of infections. However, this problem will not affect projections of AIDS cases as long as they are short term.

A number of formulations of the back-calculation equation have been proposed. To give a flavour of the estimation problem, it is convenient to use a discrete version of our first equation. Let t_0 be the beginning of the epidemic and y_k the number of individuals that develop the disease end point of interest (e.g. AIDS in an HIV context) in the kth time interval $[t_{k-1}, t_k]$ for $k = 1,...,K$. Suppose that f_{ij}, the probability of developing the disease end point in the jth time interval given infection in the ith interval, is also known. Then the expected number of new disease cases in $[t_{k-1}, t_k]$ can be expressed as:

$$E(y_k) = \sum_{i=1}^{k} E(h_i) f_{ik}$$

where h_i is the unobserved number of new infections in the ith time interval. Assuming that the h_i are independently distributed according to a POISSON DISTRIBUTION with parameter $E(h_i)$, then the y_k are also Poisson distributed with parameter $E(y_k)$. From this the likelihood for the observed data can be constructed and maximised to obtained estimates of the number of new infections over time (see MAXIMUM LIKELIHOOD DISTRIBUTION). In practice, estimation of $\mathbf{h}=(h_1,..h_k)$ is not so straightforward. The high dimensionality of $\mathbf{h}$ can lead to unstable estimates. In order to avoid lack of identifiability, some structure needs to be imposed on the shape of $\mathbf{h}$. This has typically been achieved by choosing fully parametric models for $\mathbf{h}=\mathbf{h}(\boldsymbol{\theta})$. The problem is then reduced to estimation of $\boldsymbol{\theta}$, conveniently chosen to be of a lower dimension than $\mathbf{h}$. Alternatively, to retain some flexibility, weakly parametric models (i.e. step functions constant over a long period of time) have been specified or smoothness constraints on $\mathbf{h}$ have been introduced. This has created a rich literature, especially in the HIV field (see Brookmeyer and Gail, 1994).

Attractive in principle, given the simplicity of the idea, the method does require precise knowledge of at least two of the three components introduced already. However, perfect information is rarely available. For example, as in HIV, the incidence of the disease end point, typically acquired from surveillance schemes, might be affected by reporting delay or underreporting. Further, the distribution of the incubation time may also be imprecisely known. Results can be highly sensitive to misspecification of the inputs. It is therefore important that data are appropriately adjusted for delay in reporting before they are used in the back-calculation. Equally, it is essential that sensitivity analyses to the model chosen for the distribution of the incubation time are carried out. One more limitation of the method is the inability to provide precise estimates of incidence of infection in recent times. This is a particularly serious problem for diseases with long incubation times, as seen in the HIV example.

These limitations notwithstanding, the back-calculation method has been widely used and developed in various ways, especially in the HIV area. Notably, the original methodology assumed a fixed distribution for the incubation time, independent of calendar time or age at infection. However, therapeutic changes over time and the discovery of a clear dependence of HIV progression on age at infection have made the time–age independence assumption untenable. This has led to the development of age-time specific versions of back-calculation. Equally, the need to estimate the number of individuals at different stages of the development of HIV has resulted in the development of 'staged' back-calculations, where the incubation time is divided into stages according to the value of markers of HIV disease. A final example is given by the need to refine estimation of HIV incidence, especially in the recent years, and AIDS projections. This has resulted in a further development of the method, now able to incorporate external information on the disease spread as well as other surveillance data, in addition to AIDS diagnoses (see Becker, Lewis and Li, 2003; De Angelis, Gilks and Day, 1998).

The method and its developments have found important application in other contexts besides HIV. Examples include the assessment of the bovine spongiform encephalopathy epidemic in cattle and the consequent Creutzfeldt-Jakob disease epidemic in humans in Great Britain; the estimation of the Hepatitis C virus epidemic in France; and the estimation of the number of new injecting drug users in Australia.   *DDA*

Bacchetti, P. 1998: Back-calculation. In Armitage, P. and Colton, T. (eds), *Encyclopedia of biostatistics*, Chichester: John Wiley & Sons. Vol. 1, 235–42. **Becker, N.G., Lewis, J.J.C. and Li, Z.F.** 2003: Age-specific back-projection of HIV diagnosis data. *Statistics in Medicine* 22, 2177–90. **Brookmeyer, R. and Gail, M.H.** 1986: Minimum size of the acquired immunodeficiency syndrome (AIDS) epidemic in the United States. *Lancet* 2(8519), 1320–2. **Brookmeyer, R. and Gail, M.H.** 1994: *AIDS epidemiology: a quantitative approach.* New York: Oxford University Press. **De Angelis, D., Gilks, W.R. and Day, N.E.** 1998: Bayesian projection of the acquired immune deficiency syndrome epidemic. *Journal of the Royal Statistical Society C – App* 47, 449–81.

back-projection   See BACK-CALCULATION

backwards regression   See LOGISTIC REGRESSION, MULTIPLE LINEAR REGRESSION

balance   See RANDOMISATION

bar chart   A graphical display of data classified into a number of (usually unordered) categories. Equal width rectangular bars are used to represent each category, with the heights of the bars being proportional to the observed frequency in the corresponding category. An example is shown in the first Figure.

An extension of the simple bar chart is the component

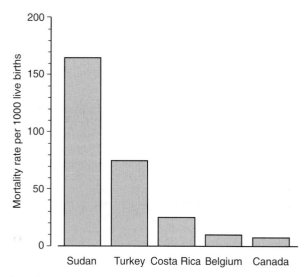

bar chart *Mortality rates per 1000 live births for children under 5 in five different countries*

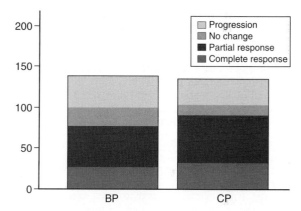

bar chart *Response to treatment*

bar chart (also known as stacked bar chart) in which particular lengths of each bar are differentiated to represent a number of frequencies associated with each category forming the chart. Shading or colour can be used to enhance the display. An example is given in the second Figure; here the numbers of patients in the four categories of a response variable for two treatments (BP and CP) are displayed.   *BSE*

[See also HISTOGRAM, PIE CHART]

baseline measurements   These are measurements taken at the beginning of a study. (This section, however, concentrates on their role within the context of a CLINICAL TRIAL.) Baseline measurements come in different varieties and may also have a variety of purposes (Senn, 1998). First are *demographic characteristics* of the patient, which either do not change such as, for example, sex, change slowly, if at all, such as height, or change at the same rate for all patients, such as age. The second and simplest sort is a measurement of the same type as the outcome variable, but taken one or more occasions prior to RANDOMISATION: these might be referred to as *true baselines*. Third, one has *baseline correlates*, measurements taken before randomisation on variables other than the true outcome variable but predictive of it and which may vary during the trial.

Some such measurements are invariably collected as part of the process of deciding which patients may enter the trial. For example, it may be required in a trial of asthma that patients be aged 18–65, have a baseline forced expiratory volume in 1 second (FEV_1) no more than 75% of that predicted by age, sex and height, can demonstrate 20% reversibility when given a bronchodilator and are normotensive. Simply fulfilling these requirements will necessitate taking at least two FEV_1 measurement prior to randomisation, as well as diastolic and systolic blood pressures and recording height, sex and age of patients, the last two being variables that are always recorded anyway. In practice, many other things, such as, for example, concomitant medication and the centre in which the patient is treated, will also be recorded and such things are also potential candidates for any model.

All three sorts of baseline may be used for four further common purposes. First, to help characterise the patients in the trial; second, to compare the groups in various arms of the trials; third, to provide conditional estimates, which will generally have greater precision and will be conditionally unbiased given the observed baseline measurements; and fourth, to investigate the constancy or otherwise of the treatment effect as patients vary. There is a fifth purpose to which true baselines can be put: as part of a general repeated-measures framework, such as for example the random slopes approach of Laird and her co-writers (Laird and Wang, 1990; Laird and Ware, 1982).

The following are some issues that arise.

Generalising results. Using the actual baseline measurements observed is clearly superior to using the inclusion criteria to characterise the trial, as the latter simply define values the patients might have had, rather than values they did have. It is unclear, however, to what extent the baseline characteristics measured can be used as a basis for generalising the results, since many things that might be important have not been measured. In any case, the logic of clinical trials is comparative rather than representative. In many areas it is accepted that the patients in a clinical trial will be unrepresentative. It is hoped rather that an additive scale of measurement may permit useful application of the results. This may require use of additional covariate information from the target population (Lane and Nelder, 1982).

Comparing groups. This suggests perhaps that the second use of comparing the groups is more valuable. However, from another point of view, the comparison of groups is simply an unimportant resting point on the road to adjustment. If the baseline measurement is prognostic a superior inference will be made by conditioning on it, whether or not it is imbalanced. Particularly questionable is the common practice of comparing groups at baseline in terms of significance tests (Altman, 1985; Senn, 1989; Senn, 1994). This has no useful role as part of a general strategy for analysis but could possibly have some limited use as a test of the randomisation process itself (to detect fraud, for example) as part of some general quality control of the trial. That being so, however, the commonly employed significance levels of 5% seem inappropriate.

Covariate adjustment. This in turn suggests that the third use of baseline measurements, to provide conditional estimates by stratification or adjustment using analysis of covariance, is the most important of these purposes. However, many trialists appear to have a strong (one might say unreasonably strong) preference for simple analyses over more complicated ones, preferring simple t-TESTS to ANALYSIS OF COVARIANCE and the log-rank test to PROPORTIONAL HAZARDS regression.

Effects in subgroups. The fourth use of baselines is also controversial. An issue of bias VARIANCE trade-off arises. Some, the 'splitters', are more worried about bias and consider that it is important to report treatment effects by subgroups defined by baseline measurements, others, the 'poolers', regard variance as being the bigger concern and point to the unreliability of inferences based on small groups.

Use of true baselines in repeated measures analysis. A controversial matter here is that the baselines are sometimes explicitly measured as part of the outcome despite the fact that, obviously, the treatments cannot affect the baselines. If the baselines, or some function of them, are also included as covariates this may lead to causally acceptable inferences. The simplest example is where change scores are used and baselines are fitted as covariates. Inferences as to the effect of treatment are then identical to those that would be made using raw outcomes and baselines as covariates (Laird, 1983).

Non-linear models. For the general linear model, the expected value of the estimator conditioning on the covariate is the same as the unconditional estimator. This is not generally true for non-linear cases. Gail, Waind *et al.* (1984) have considered where this does and does not hold for a variety of models. Robinson and Jewel have concentrated on the case of LOGISTIC REGRESSION (Robinson and Jewell, 1991) and Ford *et al.* on the proportional hazards model (Ford *et al.*, 1995). It is usually the case where non-linear models are involved that fitting covariates leads to an increase in variance. However, there is a biasing of the treatment effect towards the null if prognostic covariates are not fitted so it does not follow that fitting such covariates necessarily leads to a loss of power. There are many arguments, in fact, as to why the conditional estimators should be preferred (Lindsey and Lambert, 1998), however so-called marginal approaches using working correlations matrices have also become extremely popular, in particular via the GENERALISED ESTIMATING EQUATION approach of Liang and Zeger (1986).

Measurement error. It is well known that where a covariate is measured with error, the estimate of its effect on outcome is attenuated (see ATTENUATION TO MEASUREMENT ERROR). The false conclusion is sometimes drawn that under such circumstances, analysis of covariance does not yield conditionally unbiased estimators (Chambless and Roeback, 1993). What has been overlooked is a second attenuation: that of the true baseline difference on the observed baseline difference (Senn, 1994; Senn, 1995). The variance of the observed covariate will exceed that of the 'true' covariate. The covariance of the two can be shown to be the variance of the true covariate. Hence, since the regression of observed on true is the covariance divided by the variance of true this regression is one.

However, the regression of true on observed is the covariance divided by the variance of observed and hence is less than 1. On average the true baseline difference is closer to zero than the observed baseline difference. The two attenuations exactly cancel out and so it turns out that correcting for an imbalance in observed covariates using the observed covariates is the right thing to do.

Correcting for true baselines. It has also been claimed that, in the case where the covariate is of the same sort as the outcome measure, in other words is a true baseline, analysis of covariance is only appropriate if the baselines are balanced and that unadjusted change scores provide an unbiased estimate in the more general case (Liang and Zeger, 2000). This is incorrect as the following counterexample shows. Imagine a trial in hypertension in which, quite irrationally, but as is theoretically possible, we include only patients who have diastolic blood pressures (DBP) of either 95mm Hg or 105mm Hg (to the nearest mm Hg). Forty patients of each sort are recruited and are allocated, otherwise at random, but in proportions 3:1 in the first stratum and 1:3 in the second stratum. In the absence of any further knowledge, a perfectly reasonable estimate under these unreasonable circumstances would be obtained by subtracting mean DBP under the active treatment from mean DBP under PLACEBO separately in each of the two strata and averaging the results. What would be misleading would be to take DBP at baseline from DBP at outcome and compare the average over both strata under active treatment with that under placebo. Yet, since we can recode 95 and 105 to a dummy variable with values 0 and 1 by dividing by 10 and subtracting 9.5, the first approach is formally equivalent to analysis of covariance and the second approach is simply that of change-scores.

Choice of covariates. Regulatory authorities are naturally nervous that sponsors may unfairly manipulate results by choosing the model most favourable to them and journal editors ought to have similar fears about their authors. One way of protecting the Type I error rate is to prespecify the model and this is common practice with the pharmaceutical industry and recommended by various guidelines (International Conference on Harmonisation, 1999). A model-checking approach based on randomisation tests not using the treatment information is an alternative (Edwards, 1999). From the Bayesian point of view, however, this is simply a formal and pointless game. Having a variable in a model is equivalent to saying that one knows nothing about its effects. An excluded variable is one for which the effect is known to be zero. Other positions are possible. If users cannot agree which model is appropriate, then even given a fiction of prior ignorance about the treatment effect, different posterior opinions will obtain. This may give a sort of justification for frequentist sensitivity analysis. However, it should not be forgotten that whereas little may be known about the effect of treatment in advance of a trial, the same cannot be said for covariates and such prior knowledge is an important guide in choice of model (Senn, 2000).

Choice of true baseline to fit. It sometimes happens that in a run-in period a number of measurements are made of the eventual outcome variable. Often the last only is used as a covariate, although this is in fact wasteful as it implicitly assumes, which is unlikely, an autoregressive process. Better is either to fit the mean baseline or, more generally, each of the baseline measurements (Senn, 1997).

Subgroup analysis and treatment by covariate interactions. Such analyses are sometimes undertaken to examine the constancy of the treatment effects. The former is the natural extension of the stratification approach and the latter of analysis of covariance. Once such analyses have been undertaken a problem of combining results from individual strata arises. This issue arises frequently in the analysis of multi-centre trials where centre specific effects may be examined. If such effects are weighted by precision, this is equivalent to using SAS Type II sums of squares. If unweighted averages are used, the equivalence is to Type III sums of squares (Gallo, 2001). From one point of view, once an interaction has been fitted an overall effect is no longer of interest, however, it can also be maintained that this attitude naively maintains the claims of reducing bias against reducing variance. Compromise positions involving random effects are sometimes used but not nearly as commonly in combining effects from various centres as in the analogous problem in meta-analysis of combining effects from various trials and hardly ever when other sorts of covariate are involved. Great care must be taken in interpreting effects when interactions are involved (Chuang-Stein and Tong, 1996) and it may be wise to fit a model without interactions as a check (Senn, 2000). This is recommended by international guidelines (International Conference on Harmonisation, 1999). Note that it is the interaction of covariates with the treatment effect that causes problems in this way. The interaction of covariates with each other is not an issue of the same importance, since it is merely the joint effect of these for which one seeks adjustment.

Of course, there are also very many technical issues to be confronted when considering adjustment for baseline measurements. A particular instructive case to consider is that where a number, say k, of binary covariates have been measured. One approach is that of stratification. One creates 2^k strata based on these covariates, forms a treatment contrast within each and then a combination, usually weighted, of them all. In the case of a linear model, if within-stratum variances are assumed constant and combined efficiently, this is equivalent to carrying out analysis of covariance using ordinary least squares having formed a factor for each binary covariate and fitting all interactions between covariates up to and including the highest. Note that if we characterise an interaction by the number of covariates r involved, with $r = 1$ corresponding to main effects and $r = 0$ to the general intercept, then there are in general $\binom{k}{r}$ such terms and that since $\sum_{r=0}^{k} \binom{k}{r} = 2^k$ one is fitting the same number of degrees of freedom in both cases, as is indeed necessary, since the two are equivalent. If there are q treatments in the trial, fitting the treatment effect as a main effect only, removes a further $q - 1$ degrees of freedom. Most trials have two treatments and so $q = 2$, $q - 1 = 1$ and one further degree of freedom is removed. Going further and considering interactions between covariates and the treatment is moving a step along the road to splitting the treatment effect by subgroup.

Interactions between treatment and covariates will not be considered here and instead the issue of interactions of covariates among themselves is considered.

The approach via analysis of covariance has greater flexibility than that using strata, since it is possible to fit main effect of covariates only or a limited degree of interactions between them. Furthermore, if we move to covariates with more than two levels, models with reduced degrees of freedom are possible. Suppose, for example, that we have measured baseline severity on a three-point scale as 1, 2, 3. We can code this using two dummy variables. This is equivalent to fitting a linear and a quadratic covariate. Possible schemes for both approaches are illustrated in the Table. Note that these are equivalent since $Z_1 = X_2 + 2X_3 - 1$ and $Z_2 = 1 - 3X_2$. The circumstances under which one would wish to fit X_3 alone and especially X_2 alone are fewer than those where one might choose to fit Z_1 alone. Thus, there is an attractive flexibility and economy of the analysis of covariance approach. Of course, where truly continuous measures are involved the advantages for the covariate modelling approach increase as arbitrary cut-points have to be used if stratification is employed.   *SS*

Altman, D.G. 1985: Comparability of randomized groups. *Statistician* 34, 1, 125–36. **Chambless, L.E. and Roeback, J.R.** 1993: Methods for assessing difference between groups in change when initial measurements is subject to intra-individual variation. *Statistics in Medicine* 12, 13, 1213–37. **Chuang-Stein, C. and Tong, D.M.** 1996: The impact of parametrization on the interpretation of the main-effect terms in the presence of an interaction. *Drug Information Journal* 30, 421–4. **Edwards, D.** 1999: On model prespecification in confirmatory randomized studies. *Statistics in Medicine* 18, 7, 771–85. **Ford, I. *et al.*** 1995: Model inconsistency, illustrated by the Cox proportional hazards model. *Statistics in Medicine* 14, 735–46. **Gail, M. H. *et al.*** 1984: Biased estimates of treatment effects in randomized experiments with nonlinear regressions and omitted covariates. *Biometrika* 71, 431–44. **Gallo, P.** 2001: Center-weighting issues in multicenter clinical trials. *Journal of Biopharmaceutical Statistics* 10, 2, 145–63. **International Conference on Harmonisation** 1999: Statistical principles for clinical trials (ICH E9). *Statistics in Medicine* 18, 1905–42. **Laird, N.** 1983: Further comparative analyses of pre-test post-test research designs. *The American Statistician* 37, 329–30. **Laird, N.M. and Wang, F.** 1990: Estimating rates of change in randomized clinical trials. *Controlled Clinical Trials* 11, 6, 405–19. **Laird, N.M. and Ware, J.H.** 1982: Random-effects models for longitudinal data. *Biometrics* 38, 4, 963–74. **Lane, P.W. and Nelder, J.A.** 1982: Analysis of covariance and standardization as instances of prediction. *Biometrics* 38, 3, 613–21. **Liang, K.Y. and Zeger, S.L.** 1986: Longitudinal data-analysis using generalized linear models. *Biometrika* 73, 1, 13–22. **Liang, K.Y. and Zeger, S.L.** 2000: Longitudinal data analysis of continuous and discrete responses for pre-post designs. *Sankhya – the Indian Journal of Statistics*

baseline measurements *Coding schemes for a three-point severity scale*

	Intercept	Dummy variables		Covariates	
		Severity level 2	Severity level 3	Linear	Quadratic
Severity		X_2	X_3	Z_1	Z_2
1	1	0	0	−1	1
2	1	1	0	0	−2
3	1	0	1	1	1

Series B 62, 134–48. **Lindsey, J.K. and Lambert, P.** 1998: On the appropriateness of marginal models for repeated measurements in clinical trials. *Statistics in Medicine* 17, 4, 447–69. **Robinson, L.D. and Jewell, N.P.** 1991: Some surprising results about covariate adjustment in logistic regression models. *International Statistical Review* 58, 227–40. **Senn, S.J.** 1994: Testing for baseline balance in clinical trials. *Statistics in Medicine* 13, 17, 1715–26. **Senn, S.** 1995: In defence of analysis of covariance: a reply to Chambless and Roeback. *Statistics in Medicine* 14, 20, 2283–5. **Senn, S.J.** 1997: *Statistical issues in drug development*. Chichester: John Wiley & Sons. **Senn, S.J.** 1998: Baseline adjustment in longitudinal studies. In Armitage, P. and Colton, T. (eds), *Encyclopedia in Biostatistics*. New York: John Wiley & Sons. Vol.1, 253–7. **Senn, S.J.** 2000: The many modes of meta. *Drug Information Journal* 34, 535–49.

basic reproduction number A term used in the theory of infectious diseases for the average number of secondary cases that an infectious individual produces in a completely susceptible population. The basic reproduction number (R) of an infectious agent is a key factor determining the rate of spread and the proportion of the host population affected. The number depends on the duration of the infectious period, the probability of infecting a susceptible individual during one contact and the number of new susceptible individuals contacted per unit time; consequently, it may vary considerably for different infectious diseases and also for the same disease in different populations. The value of R has implications for whether there is a positive probability that an epidemic may occur and the proportion of the population infected were an epidemic to take place. The larger the value of R, the larger the fraction of the population that must be immunised to prevent an epidemic.   *BSE*

Bayes' theorem Bayes' theorem is a method by which conditional probabilities (see CONDITIONAL PROBABILITY) may be manipulated. In particular, it provides a means of reversing the conditioning in order to obtain probability statements regarding specific events of interest. Bayes' theorem itself was described originally in 'An essay …' and published two years after the death of the Reverend Thomas Bayes in 1761 (Bayes, 1763). The use of Bayes' theorem in manipulating conditional probabilities is used widely, even if users may not be aware of it, but its use for more general quantities, for example relative risks, gives rise to considerable controversy (see BAYESIAN METHODS).

Following Spiegelhalter, Abrams and Myles (2004) consider two events a and b, using the *multiplication rule* of probability (*see* PROBABILITY), the probability of both a and b occurring, denoted '$a \wedge b$' is given by:

$$P(a \wedge b) = P(a|b) \times P(b) = P(b|a) \times P(a) \qquad (1)$$

rearranging (1) yields an expression for $P(b|a)$:

$$P(b|a) = \frac{P(a|b) \times P(b)}{P(a)} \qquad (2)$$

Considering the events '$a \wedge b$' and '$a \wedge \bar{b}$', where $\bar{b}$ represents the event 'not b', then these are mutually exclusive and using the *addition rule* of probability (see probability), we can 'extend the argument' for a to include b:

$$P(a) = P(a \wedge b) + P(a \wedge \bar{b}) = P(a|b) \times P(b) + P(a|\bar{b}) \times P(\bar{b}) \quad (3)$$

Combining (2) and (3) yields Bayes' theorem which expresses $P(b|a)$ in terms of conditional probabilities for a and the probability of b:

$$P(b|a) = \frac{P(a|b) \times P(b)}{P(a|b) \times P(b) + P(a|\bar{b}) \times P(\bar{b})} \quad (4)$$

Conversely, (4) could be considered in terms of $\bar{b}$, i.e.:

$$P(\bar{b}|a) = \frac{P(a|\bar{b}) \times P(\bar{b})}{P(a|b) \times P(b) + P(a|\bar{b}) \times P(\bar{b})} \quad (5)$$

Dividing (4) by (5) yields:

$$\frac{P(b|a)}{P(\bar{b}|a)} = \frac{P(a|b) \times P(b)}{P(a|\bar{b}) \times P(\bar{b})} = \frac{P(a|b)}{P(a|\bar{b})} \times \frac{P(b)}{P(\bar{b})} \quad (6)$$

Hence, (6) is Bayes' theorem in terms of the odds of event b, in which the prior odds of b, i.e. $P(b)/P(\bar{b})$, are modified in the light of the data, i.e. the LIKELIHOOD RATIO, to yield the posterior odds of b, conditional on knowing a. In the case when b is not a simple event, i.e. b or $\bar{b}$ and $b_1, ..., b_n$ are in fact n mutually exclusive events, (5) can be generalised so that the probability of $b_1|a$ is given by:

$$P(b_1|a) = \frac{P(a|b_1) \times P(b_1)}{\sum_j P(a|b_j) \times P(b_j)}$$

Consider the case of wishing to determine whether a patient has a particular disease, D, that the background prevalence of the disease in the population is 30%, but a test is available. The characteristics of the test are such that a patient who has disease D will test positive with probability 0.8, i.e. the sensitivity (see SENSITIVITY), while the probability of a positive test result for non-diseased patients is 0.2, i.e. one minus the specificity (see SPECIFICITY). Using Bayes' theorem we can calculate the probability that a patient who has tested positive does have disease D as:

$$P(D|T+) = \frac{P(T+|D) \times P(D)}{P(T+|D) \times P(D) + P(T+|\bar{D}) \times P(\bar{D})}$$
$$= \frac{0.8 \times 0.3}{0.8 \times 0.3 + 0.2 \times 0.7} = 0.63$$

In terms of odds, the prior odds of having the disease are $0.3/0.7 = 0.43$, i.e. just under 1 in 2, while the likelihood ratio is 4 for a positive test result, i.e. $0.8/0.2$, and the posterior odds therefore of having the disease, having tested positive, is 1.72. *KRA*

Bayes, T. 1763: An essay towards solving a problem in the doctrine of chances. *Philosophical Transactions of the Royal Society*, 53, 418. **Spiegelhalter, D.J., Abrams, K.R. and Myles, J.P.** 2004: *Bayesian approaches to clinical trials and health-care evaluation.* Chichester: John Wiley & Sons.

Bayesian methods The use of Bayes' theorem for manipulating conditional probabilities of specific events of interest is used widely without controversy (see BAYES'

THEOREM). However, Bayes' theorem may also be applied to more general quantities, for example relative risks, and in such settings the inclusion of *external* information in the form of the unconditional probability distribution (see CONDITIONAL PROBABILITY) for the quantity of interest, the PRIOR DISTRIBUTION, rather than the prevalence as in diagnostic testing, *is* controversial and has attracted considerable debate (Spiegelhalter, Abrams and Myles, 2004).

In short, a Bayesian approach (generally) has been described as 'the explicit quantitative use of external evidence in the design, monitoring, analysis, interpretation and reporting of a health-care evaluation' (Spiegelhalter, Abrams and Myles, 2004). As such, it has been argued that a Bayesian approach is often more *flexible* than traditional methods as it can adapt to each unique situation; is more *efficient* in that it uses all available evidence thought to be relevant; is more *useful* in providing predictions and inputs for making decisions about individual patients and summarising evidence regarding a problem, e.g. making direct probability statements that are clinically relevant; and more *ethical* in both clarifying the basis for randomisation and fully exploiting the experience provided by past patients.

There are three elements of a Bayesian approach to medical statistics: subjective probability, assessment of evidence and decision theory. While the second is the one that is most often thought of as a Bayesian approach per se, i.e. the use of external evidence, the first underpins many of the purported advantages of a Bayesian approach, while the third illustrates the wider perspective that a Bayesian approach can give. A frequentist view of probability relies on a long-run view of the world, with probability being defined as the long-run frequency of events occurring (see PROBABILITY). While such a view is entirely consistent with replicable events, when considering unique events, such as the probability that a patient has a particular disease, such a reliance on repeatability makes little sense. A Bayesian approach views probability as a degree of belief in an event occurring, which not only does not rely on repeatability but also encompasses a subjective nature of probability, we all bring own experiences and background information in making probability assessments (Lindley, 1985). The use of a decision theoretic approach to statistical inference places the decision regarding a parameter within the context of the potential loss/gain in utility associated with making decisions (Lindley, 1985).

Fundamental in both frequentist and Bayesian approaches to statistical inference is the likelihood function (see LIKELIHOOD). From a frequentist perspective the likelihood function summarises how plausible different values of a parameter are by using an inverse argument, i.e. for a given value of the unknown parameter how plausible are the data that have been observed. A Bayesian approach uses the likelihood function, $P(y|\theta)$, in the same manner, i.e. as a summary of the relationship between data observed (y) and unknown parameter (θ), but using Bayes' theorem reverses the conditioning to obtain the probability distribution for the unknown parameter conditional on both the data and any background information summarised in the prior distribution, $P(\theta)$. Thus:

$$P(\theta|y) = \frac{P(\theta)P(y|\theta)}{P(y)} = \frac{P(\theta)P(y|\theta)}{\int P(\theta)P(y|\theta)d\theta} \quad (1)$$

Although (1) is applicable whether the model contains a single unknown parameter or multiple unknown parameters, the specification of $P(\theta)$ (see PRIOR DISTRIBUTIONS) and the computation of $P(y)$ (see COMPUTATIONAL METHODS) can be more difficult, but an added complexity is that we are often only interested in certain key parameters, e.g. a treatment effect, and wish to consider the other parameters as nuisance parameters. Thus, in addition to obtaining the joint posterior distribution, we often obtain the *marginal posterior distribution* for one or more parameters, say $\theta = (\delta, \phi)$ then the marginal posterior distribution for δ is given by:

$$P(\delta|y) = \int P(\theta|y)d\phi \qquad (2)$$

As with the computation of $P(y)$ in (1) the integration out of the remaining model parameters in (2) is very rarely analytically tractable.

The prior distribution does not necessarily have to be temporally prior to the study in question, but rather is a summary of the pertinent external information, i.e. either based on other studies, subjective beliefs or a combination of the two. When there are multiple sources of external evidence in the form of other study results then the prior distribution may be based on a synthesis of such evidence using meta-analysis or generalised evidence synthesis techniques, which may downweight some sources of external evidence, e.g. observational studies, or may adjust the results for potential confounders or in order to make the synthesis of more relevance to the study in question (Spiegelhalter, Abrams and Myles, 2004). In terms of using subjective prior beliefs, there have been a number of methods advocated for the elicitation of such beliefs using a variety of methods, ranging from informal discussion, through the use of structure questionnaires possibly using a 'trial roulette' format to the use of interactive computer elicitation techniques (Chaloner *et al.*, 1993; Spiegelhalter, Freedman and Parmar, 1994). When the beliefs of multiple individuals are elicited then consideration has to be given as to whether these should be pooled in a formal manner or used independently (Genest and Zidek, 1986).

A particular type of prior distribution that is often used is what is termed a 'non-informative' or 'vague/prior' distribution. Such a distribution is deemed to be 'vague' relative to the likelihood so that the data from the study in question dominate the analysis. While such an analysis appeals to analysts wishing to maintain a sense of objectivity but nevertheless take advantage of other aspects of adopting a Bayesian approach, e.g. the ability to make direct probability statements, when considering prior distributions for parameters in complex models other than main effects, e.g. variance components, careful consideration has to be given to what 'vague' really means and this should be assessed as part of a sensitivity analysis (Spiegelhalter, Abrams and Myles, 2004). A related issue is that of whether a 'vague' prior distribution is invariant to transformations, i.e. what is vague on one scale may in fact be informative on another, and in such circumstances Jeffreys' priors may be considered, which, although not necessarily 'vague', are invariant to transformations (Bernardo and Smith, 1994). In complex multi-parameter models the specification of a joint prior distribution can be a difficult task in itself, since assuming independence

between all parameters, and thus being able to specify a series of univariate prior distributions, is usually unreasonable. A consequence is that we often have to specify conditional prior distributions.

In summary, there is no such thing as a 'correct' or single prior distribution, and consideration of a range (or 'community') of prior distributions is advocated (Spiegelhalter, Abrams and Myles, 2004; Spiegelhalter, Freedman and Parmar, 1994). Such a 'community' could contain; a 'vague' prior distribution, a 'sceptical' prior distribution, i.e. one which places only a small probability on an intervention being beneficial, an 'enthusiastic' prior distribution and a prior essentially based at the null (Spiegelhalter, Abrams and Myles, 2004; Spiegelhalter, Freedman and Parmar, 1994).

Having obtained the posterior distribution using Bayes' theorem (1) all subsequent inference is based on it. Standard measures of location and uncertainty may be obtained, e.g. posterior mean and variance, and the posterior density itself may be plotted, which is especially important when it exhibits unusual behaviour, e.g. multi-modal. CREDIBLE INTERVALS (CrIs) can also be calculated which are analogous to CONFIDENCE INTERVALS, but which have the interpretation often incorrectly ascribed to CIs, namely that they are intervals in which the unknown parameter lies with a specific posterior probability. CrIs can be obtained in a number of ways, either as equal-tail area intervals or as highest posterior density intervals (HPDIs), which have the property that no point outside the interval has higher point probability than a point inside the interval and are particularly informative when the posterior distribution is either skew or multimodal (Spiegelhalter, Abrams and Myles, 2004). In addition to obtaining CrIs, a particularly appealing advantage of a Bayesian approach is that direct probability statements can be made that are of direct clinical relevance, for example the posterior probability that a relative risk is above a certain value or is within a certain specified range (Spiegelhalter, Abrams and Myles, 2004).

Another advantage of adopting a Bayesian approach is the ability to make predictive statements regarding future data by obtaining the posterior predictive distribution. The posterior predictive distribution for future data is obtained by integrating the likelihood function for the future data over the posterior distribution, i.e. current state of knowledge regarding the parameter, so that the predictive distribution for future data, x, having observed data y is given by:

$$P(x|y) = \int P(x|\theta)P(\theta|y)d\theta \qquad (3)$$

This equation can be used specifically in the monitoring of studies, since having obtained the posterior predictive distribution, direct probability statements can therefore be made regarding the eventual 'observed' study result and thus decisions made as to whether to continue or not (see CLINICAL TRIALS).

An alternative form of the predictive distribution is to use the prior distribution rather than the posterior distribution and so the resulting predictive distribution is in fact that for the data observed. Comparison of this with the observed data has been advocated a means by which prior-data conflict can be assessed, although this raises fundamental questions when subjective beliefs are used (Spiegelhalter, Abrams and Myles, 2004).

In many biomedical settings data accumulates sequentially over time and an important advantage in the use of a Bayesian approach is the ability of Bayes' theorem to naturally accommodate such scenarios (Bernardo and Smith, 1994). Essentially, the posterior distribution at one time point becomes the prior distribution for the subsequent time point, assuming that the data can be considered to be conditionally independent. Thus, if data y_1 are observed first, followed by data y_2 then:

$$P(\theta|y_1, y_2) \propto P(y_1|\theta)P(y_2|\theta)P(\theta) \propto P(y_2|\theta)\, P(\theta|y_1) \quad (4)$$

Of fundamental importance to the practical application of Bayesian methods in a medical setting are the assumptions made regarding model parameters. In many situations specific model parameters may represent subgroups of individuals within a single study (see SUBGROUP ANALYSIS), studies within a meta-analysis or units within an institutional comparison setting, such multiplicity of parameters requires assumptions to be made regardless of whether a frequentist or Bayesian approach is adopted. From a Bayesian perspective three possibilities exist: the parameters can be thought to be identical and therefore all the data pooled and the common parameter estimated; the parameters can be thought to be independent and therefore each subgroup/study/unit analysed separately (specifying an independent prior distribution for each); or the parameters can be thought to 'similar' in the sense that we thought them not to be systematically different, in which case are termed 'exchangeable'. If the assumption of exchangeability *a priori* is thought to be a reasonable one then the parameters are assumed to be drawn from a common distribution (with unknown hyper-parameters) – this specifies a hierarchical or multilevel model (see MULTI-LEVEL MODELS). Consequently, in estimating a specific parameter, i.e. the underlying effect in a subgroup/study/unit, we 'borrow strength' from the other parameters via the common distribution. In practical terms, this means that a Bayesian approach to problems of multiplicity ensures that individual parameters are shrunk towards some overall common effect and that the 'borrowing of strength' ensures that there is less uncertainty surrounding the underlying effect within an individual subgroup/study/unit than had been originally observed in the data (Spiegelhalter, Abrams and Myles, 2004). Specification of prior distributions for the unknown hyper-parameters in the model then encompass the *degree* to which we believe individual subgroups/studies/units may be different to one another.

As with statistical modelling generally, model criticism can take the form of answering these questions: if a different statistical model were used would different conclusion be reached? How well does the model perform, i.e. how well does it model the data? In terms of different statistical models, obviously different models could be used and results compared or some form of model selection process may be used (see later). Regarding 'model fit' one approach is to consider prediction of the observed data based on the model and to compare this with the actual observed data using a cross-validation approach to produce the conditional predictive ordinate (CPO) (Gilks, Richardson and Spiegelhalter, 1996). Alternatively, an overall assessment of model performance can be calculated deviance information criterion (DIC) (Spiegelhalter

et al., 2002). In addition, the use of specific prior distributions raises the question of whether different conclusions would be drawn, legitimately, by individuals holding different prior beliefs? However, sometimes equally important is the specific specification of prior distributions even though they may be intended to be 'vague' (see PRIOR DISTRIBUTIONS). Consequently, the use of a Bayesian approach dictates the need for careful and conscientious sensitivity analyses and this may appear daunting to the uninitiated analyst.

Model selection, whether relating to the specific parametric form or covariates included in a model, can be achieved either by qualitatively comparing aspects of model fit, e.g. CPOs and DIC discussed earlier or quantitatively via the use of Bayes' factors (Bernardo and Smith, 1994). Bayes' factors provide a means of assessing the relative plausibility of the two competing models, in an analogous manner to LIKELIHOOD RATIO, but having integrated over the prior distributions for model hyper-parameters. Consequently, the specification of improper prior distributions, which often arise when attempting to represent 'vague' beliefs, causes computational difficulties (Bernardo and Smith, 1994). While Bayes' factors themselves can be used to compare competing models directly, and which do not have to be nested, they can also be used in conjunction with prior model probabilities to obtain the posterior model probabilities, i.e. the plausibility of the competing models based on both data and subjective prior beliefs, and which can, in turn, be used to average across models, so that the estimation of a treatment effect for example takes into account both the within and between model uncertainty present (Kass and Raftery, 1995).

As has already been mentioned the application of Bayesian methods to realistic biomedical problems can be computationally intensive, with only highly stylised examples being analytically tractable. In order to evaluate integrals such as those in equations (1) and (2) three broad techniques have been considered; asymptotic approximations, quadrature (numerical integration) techniques and simulation methods (Bernardo and Smith, 1994). The development of MARKOV CHAIN MONTE CARLO (MCMC) simulation methods together with user-friendly software such as WinBUGS (see BUGS AND WINBUGS) has enabled the use of a Bayesian approach to be a realistic choice for many analysts regardless of philosophical credence.

The Table on page 26 summarises the differences between a frequentist and a Bayesian approach to many of the issues that arise in the design, monitoring, analysis and interpretation of RCTs and which are now discussed briefly.

Although in practice Bayesian methods have been applied more frequently in the analysis of RCTs, use of Bayesian methods in specifically the design of early phase trails in which decisions as to appropriate dose level or whether to initiate a confirmatory trial have to be taken as data accumulates has received attention (Gatsonis and Greenhouse, 1992; Stallard, 1998). The role that elicitation of prior beliefs and demands from various stakeholders (clinicians, patients and policymakers) has to play in confirming (or refuting) the need for a randomised trial on the basis of equipoise has also been advocated, whether or not these are used in a formal assessment of whether a

Bayesian methods *Comparison of frequentist and Bayesian approaches to design, monitoring and analysis/interpretation of RCTs (adapted from Spiegelhalter, Abrams and Myles, 2004)*

Issue	Frequentist	Bayesian
External information	Informally used in design	Used formally to specify prior
Sample size	Required to detect minimum clinically significant difference at pre-specified level of Type I and II error	Assumed fixed, but assessment of probability of final CrI excluding clinically significant difference, allowing for uncertainty in inputs
Parameter of interest	Fixed state of nature	Unknown quantity
Randomisation	Justifies hypothesis testing	Not necessary due to subjective nature of probability
Basic question	How likely are data given value of parameter?	How likely is value of parameter given data?
Presentation of results	Likelihood functions, P-values and CIs	Plots of posterior, posterior probabilities of quantities of interest, CrIs, posterior used in decision model
Interim analyses	P-values and estimates adjusted for #analyses	Inference not affected by #analyses
Interim predictions	Conditional power	Use posterior predictive distribution
Subsets	Adjusted P-values, e.g. Bonferroni	Subset effects 'shrunk' using 'sceptical' prior

proposed RCT is likely to lead to a definitive answer given the resources available and uncertainty in for example the event rate in the control group (Spiegelhalter, Abrams and Myles, 2004).

A crucial aspect of conducting large scale PHASE III TRIALS is the issue of monitoring the trial as data accumulate in order to minimise exposure of patients to less effective (or even harmful) interventions. From a frequentist perspective such monitoring raises issues of multiplicity and for which methods to adjust for this exist. The use of a Bayesian approach to accumulating evidence is entirely natural, in that at various stages during a trial the posterior distribution for the outcome is an assessment of the current state of knowledge and on which decisions regarding continuation/termination should be based without the need for adjustment (Fayers, Ashby and Parmar, 1997). An additional advantage is the ability to predict, using the posterior predictive distribution at interim inspections, what the consequences of continuation would be in terms of the eventual posterior distribution, conditional on the data so far (Abrams, 1998). An alternative approach that has been suggested extends the consideration of the posterior distribution to incorporate the potential losses of making (Spiegelhalter, Abrams and Myles, 2004).

One key question, however, is what prior to use in such monitoring situations? As regards the situation in which a difference in favour of one intervention has been detected, then a 'sceptical' prior (see PRIOR DISTRIBUTION) has been advocated, on the grounds that if the data so far are sufficient to convince a sceptic of the merits of a particular intervention then continuation would appear inappropriate (Fayers *et al*, 1997). Similarly, when no difference has been detected at an interim analysis, an enthusiastic prior distribution could be used to assess whether there is sufficient evidence for a proponent of an intervention to rule out a benefit.

Having conducted an RCT, how should the results be analysed and interpreted from a Bayesian perspective and what advantages do they confer? Ultimately, a Bayesian approach allows an exploration of how and why individuals interpreting the same RCT evidence may reach differing conclusions – namely, that they held different *a priori*

beliefs, although in the light of substantial evidence even 'sceptics' and 'enthusiasts' should converge to a consensus. The use of Bayesian methods also focuses attention on estimation and/or decision making and enables direct probability statements to be made that are of clinical relevance. It also enables the inclusion of pertinent external information, which in the case of RCTs that are relatively small, but which have produced large effects and appear to be 'too good to be true', provide a means by which such results can be ameliorated (Spiegelhalter *et al*, 2004). An alternative approach in such circumstances is to ask the question: what prior beliefs would I have to hold in order not to accept the findings of a RCT? If the prior beliefs required to overturn such findings are so 'extreme' that it is unlikely for them to be held by a rational individual then the RCT results are accepted at 'face value'.

Frequently in RCTs, interest focuses on subgroups of patients (see SUBGROUP ANALYSIS) and interpretation of the effects of an intervention within such subgroups raises issue of multiplicity. A Bayesian approach to subgroup analyses considers the simultaneous analysis of the subgroups within a hierarchical model, in which a 'sceptical' prior distribution is placed on the degree to which the estimates of effectiveness within individual subgroups differ from one another – a consequence of such an approach is that aberrant effects in relatively small subgroups of patients are 'shrunk' towards a common overall effect, the degree of shrinkage depending on both size of the subgroup and degree of scepticism expressed. Such an approach thus reduces the possibility that spurious findings are accepted unwittingly.

Bayesian approaches to the analysis of RCTs other than two-group parallel designs have also been advocated, including CROSS-OVER TRIALS, FACTORIAL DESIGNS and CLUSTER RANDOMISED TRIALS (Spiegelhalter, 2001).

The growth of EVIDENCE-BASED MEDICINE and healthcare is based on the systematic searching for and synthesis of research evidence. Meta-analysis, the quantitative pooling of evidence from 'similar' studies, raises a number of methodological issues and for which a Bayesian approach has been advocated.

The most fundamental issue in meta-analysis is *heterogeneity* – statistical, clinical and methodological. Statistical heterogeneity refers to the study-to-study variability in terms of the estimates associated with each study. When excessive statistical heterogeneity exists attempts should be made to explain it in terms of study- and patient-level covariates, however, this is not always possible and so random effects models, which allow for such heterogeneity, are often used (Spiegelhalter *et al*, 2004). Estimation of the variance components within such models can be problematic, especially when the number of studies is small and Bayesian methods have the advantage of not only allowing for the uncertainty in variance component estimates, but also allow for the possibility of informative prior distributions on variance components based on other external evidence.

Clinical heterogeneity refers to the fact that different studies may have used different doses, may have had different patient populations, e.g. in terms of age and may have considered different comparators. In particular, studies that compare different interventions only provide indirect evidence for other comparisons and the use of multi-parameter evidence synthesis methods within a Bayesian framework have been advocated in order that the appropriate correlation and uncertainty is taken into account. A specific issue for which Bayesian methods are advantageous is when *baseline risk* is considered as a possible treatment modifier, i.e. the event rate in the control group. Clearly regression techniques have to allow for the correlation induced between control group event rate and treatment effect and this is most easily accomplished by using effectively a multivariate meta-analysis model. Such multivariate models can also be used when multiple or surrogate outcomes are considered.

Methodological heterogeneity often refers to study design and Bayesian methods for the synthesis of evidence from a variety of disparate sources have been developed, for example; randomised and observational studies, epidemiological and toxicological and qualitative and quantitative studies. These methods can allow for both heterogeneity between different sources of evidence and can be extended to allow for differing levels of bias associated with different study designs and quality.

Specific methodological issues in EPIDEMIOLOGY for which Bayesian methods have been advocated are: MEASUREMENT ERROR, MISSING DATA and pharmaco-epidemiology, when assessing evidence on potentially rare but serious adverse events. One specific area of epidemiology for which Bayesian and empirical Bayes methods have been used for some considerable time is SPATIAL EPIDEMIOLOGY and in which interrelationships between geographical areas are considered.

The comparison of institutions in terms of health outcomes, often referred to as profiling, raises a number of methodological issues, most notably multiplicity and issues concerned with interpreting the outcome in individual 'units' that appear aberrant and for which Bayesian methods have been applied.

In evaluating healthcare interventions interest often focuses not only on clinical effectiveness but also on cost-effectiveness (see COST-EFFECTIVE ANALYSIS), with both clinical outcomes and resource use/cost data collected as part of study. Methodological issues arise when analysing both outcomes simultaneously, most notable of which is the correlation between the two and for which Bayesian methods have been advocated.

Although collection of both clinical and cost data within an RCT is highly desirable, such studies are often of relatively short duration and extrapolation to the longer term and to include other outcomes is often required. Such extrapolation is most frequently achieved within a decision-modelling framework, which decomposes the intervention/disease pathway into a finite number of transitions or states between which patients can move (see DECISION THEORY and MARKOV CHAIN MONTE CARLO). Decision models can assess either clinical or cost-effectiveness of competing interventions or policies, with different parts of the model being populated by either different sources of evidence or the same source, e.g. study, by using a common metric for different health states, usually a utility or quality of life outcome (see QUALITY OF LIFE MEASUREMENT). The key advantages that a Bayesian approach confers on such models are the ability to infer indirectly key model inputs and on which there may be no direct evidence and allow for appropriate sources of uncertainty and correlation in the model inputs. The development of economic decision models can also play an important role in identifying aspects of the model (and therefore intervention/disease process) about which there is considerable uncertainty and on which further research may need to be commissioned.

While the areas of application above have concentrated on epidemiological and evaluation studies, Bayesian methods are beginning to be developed in other areas of biomedical research, most notably image analysis, time series and genetics, especially the analysis of gene expression data.

While the use of Bayesian methods in many areas of biomedical research conveys numerous advantages, their use requires careful and conscientious application, which places considerable emphasis on the role of sensitivity analyses with respect to statistical model, prior distributions and computational methods (see Markov chain Monte Carlo and BUGS and WinBUGS). In order to improve and harmonise the reporting of analyses using Bayesian methods a checklist *BayesWatch* (Spiegelhalter, Abrams and Myles, 2004) has been developed.   *KRA*

Abrams, K.R. 1998: Monitoring randomised controlled trials – Parkinson's disease trial illustrates the dangers of stopping early. *British Medical Journal* 316, 7139, 1183–4. **Bernardo, J.M. and Smith, A.F.M.** 1994: *Bayesian theory.* Chichester: John Wiley & Sons. **Chaloner, K., Church, T., Louis, T.A. and Matts, J.P.** 1993: Graphical elicitation of a prior distribution for a clinical trial. *Statistician* 42, 341–53. **Fayers, P.M., Ashby, D. and Parmar, M.K.B.** 1997: Tutorial in biostatistics: Bayesian data monitoring in clinical trials. *Statistics in Medicine* 16, 1413–30. **Gatsonis, C. and Greenhouse, J.B.** 1992: Bayesian methods for Phase I clinical trials. *Statistics in Medicine* 11, 1377–89. **Genest, C. and Zidek, J.** 1986: Combining probability distributions: a critique and an annotated bibliography (with discussion). *Statistical Science* 1, 114–48. **Gilks, W.R., Richardson, S. and Spiegelhalter, D.J.** 1996: *Markov chain Monte Carlo methods in practice.* New York: Chapman & Hall. **Kass, R. and Raftery, A.** 1995: Bayes' factors and model uncertainty. *Journal of the American Statistical Association* 90, 773–95. **Lindley, D.V.** 1985: *Making decisions,* 2nd edn. Chichester: John Wiley & Sons. **Parmar, M.K.B., Spiegelhalter, D.J. and Freedman, L.S.** 1994: The CHART trials: Bayesian design and monitoring in practice. *Statistics in Medicine* 13, 1297–312. **Spiegelhalter, D.** 2001: Bayesian methods for cluster randomized trials with continuous responses. *Statistics in Medicine* 20, 435–52. **Spiegelhalter, D.J., Best, N.G., Carlin, B.P. and van der Linde, A.** 2002: Bayesian measures of model complexity and fit (with discussion). *Journal of the Royal Statistical Society B* 64, 583–640. **Spiegelhalter, D.J., Abrams, K.R. and Myles, J.P.** 2004: *Bayesian approaches to clinical trials and health-care evaluation.* Chichester: John Wiley & Sons. **Spiegelhalter, D.J., Freedman, L.S. and Parmar, M.K.B.** 1994: Bayesian approaches to randomised trials (with discussion). *Journal of the Royal Statistical Society Series A* 157, 357–87. **Stallard, N.** 1998: Sample size determination for Phase II clinical trials based on Bayesian decision theory. *Biometrics* 54, 279–94.

Bayesian networks   See GRAPHICAL MODELS

Bayesian persuasion probabilities

Posterior probabilities that a new treatment being tested in a Phase II clinical trial is better than or no better than a standard treatment. In a Phase II trial INTERIM ANALYSES are carried out to determine whether or not to stop the trial early because, on the basis of the data already accrued, the new treatment appears either unlikely to be better than the standard treatment or unlikely not to be better than it.

One method of determining whether or not to stop the trial is that of persuasion probabilities. The persuade-the-pessimist probability (PPP) is defined as the posterior probability that the new treatment is better than the standard treatment.

The persuade-the-optimist probability (POP) is the posterior probability that the new treatment is no better than the standard.

Prior to commencement of the trial, two pairs of prior distributions for the effectiveness of the standard and new treatments are chosen. One pair is that of an investigator who is optimistic that the new treatment is better than the standard. The other pair is that of someone who is pessimistic (or sceptical) about the effectiveness of the new treatment. Also pre-specified are thresholds PPP_{CRIT} and POP_{CRIT}.

At each interim analysis PPP and POP are calculated using the data collected so far.

If $POP > POP_{CRIT}$, the trial is stopped, because even an optimist should be persuaded that the new treatment is no better than the standard. Similarly, if $PPP > PPP_{CRIT}$, the trial is stopped because even a pessimist should be persuaded that the new treatment is better.   *SRS*

[See also BAYESIAN METHODS]

Heitjan, D.F. 1997: Bayesian interim analysis of Phase II cancer clinical trials. *Statistics in Medicine* 16, 1791–802.

benchmarking

A procedure for adjusting a less reliable series of observations to make it consistent with more reliable measurements known as *benchmarks*. For example, data on hospital bed occupation collected monthly will not necessarily agree with figures collected annually and the monthly figures (which are likely to be less reliable because the annual figures will probably originate from a census, exhaustive administrative records or a larger sample) may be adjusted at some point to agree with the more reliable annual figures. Benchmarking is often used to adjust time-series data to annual benchmarks while preserving as far as possible the month-to-month movement of the original series – see, for example, Cholette and Dagum (1994).   *BSE*

Cholette, P.A. and Dagum, E.B. 1994: Benchmarking time series with autocorrelated survey errors. *International Statistics Review* 62, 365–77.

Berkson's fallacy

Sometimes a spurious relationship can be concluded because the data from which the conclusion was derived came from a special source, which is not representative of the general population. Such bias is known as Berkson's fallacy and it can only be avoided by careful study design.

A classic example of this bias is the study of autopsies by Pearl (1929). Fewer autopsies than expected found both tuberculosis and cancer to occur together; the frequency of cancer was thus lower among tuberculosis victims than others. This led Pearl to the erroneous conclusion that tuberculosis might be offering people some kind of protection against cancer, even leading to the suggestion that cancer patients might be treated with the protein of the tuberculosis bacterium. The problem with this line of thinking is that not every death is autopsied; in this case it turned out that people who died with both diseases were less likely to be autopsied, leading to an artificial lack of numbers with both diseases in Pearl's autopsy series.

Berkson's fallacy is a particular problem with CASE-CONTROL STUDIES. For example, suppose that both the case and control series are derived from hospitals. If it happened that anyone with both the 'case' disease and some other disease were more likely to be hospitalised than someone with only one of the pair, we may well see a relationship between the prevalence of the two diseases in the case-control study, even when there is really no such relationship in the general population. Exactly the same situation may also give rise to spurious relationships between any risk factor for the 'second' disease and the disease that defines cases. For instance, consider a hospital-based case-control study of coffee drinking and angina among the elderly. Suppose that coffee drinking is a risk factor for Parkinson's disease. If someone has Parkinson's disease she or he is unlikely to be hospitalised unless she or he develops a potentially life-threatening condition, such as angina. Most individuals with angina will be treated in the community, the exception, perhaps, being when there is a disabling co-morbidity. The result of these hypothetical conditions might be a disproportionate number with Parkinson's disease (who tend to drink coffee) among the angina cases in hospital than among the controls (people with other illnesses). The case-control study would thus find coffee drinking to be a risk factor for angina, even if this were not actually true.   *MW*

[See also BIAS IN OBSERVATIONAL STUDIES]

Feinstein, A.R., Walter, S.D. and Horwitz, R.I. 1986: An analysis of Berkson's bias in case-control studies. *Journal of Chronic Diseases* 39, 495–504. **Pearl, R.** 1929: Cancer and tuberculosis. *American Journal of Hygiene* 9, 97–159. **Walter, S.D.** 1980: Berkson's bias and its control in epidemiological studies. *Journal of Chronic Diseases* 33, 721–5. **Woodward, M.** 2005: *Epidemiology: study, design and data analysis*, 2nd edn. Boca Raton: Chapman & Hall/CRC Press.

beta distribution

A member of a flexible family of PROBABILITY DISTRIBUTIONS commonly used to describe a proportion. Whereas most of the distributions we encounter are non-zero over an infinite range of values, this versatile distribution is non-zero only in the range 0 to 1. By rescaling it can be useful any time that a distribution is required over a finite range. The distribution is defined by two parameters, r and s and has the density function:

$$f(x) = x^{r-1} (1 - x)^{s-1}/\beta(r,s)$$

where the $\beta(r,s)$ term can be viewed as a constant to ensure that the total probability is equal to one.

The MEAN of the beta distribution is $r/(r + s)$, and the VARIANCE is $rs/((r + s)^2(r + s + 1))$. The parameters r and s define the shape of the distribution. This shape can be wide ranging, with u-shaped curves, n-shaped curves, strictly increasing/decreasing curves and triangular distributions all possible. Some of the possible distributions are illustrated in the Figure. If r and s are equal then the distribution will be symmetric.

Note the similarities to the BINOMIAL DISTRIBUTION. Where the binomial models the distribution of the number of successes, when given the probability of a success, the beta can model the probability of a success given the number of successes. Indeed, in a Bayesian analysis (see BAYESIAN METHODS), the beta distribution is the conjugate prior for the binomial distribution.

The beta distribution is related to a number of other distributions. It contains the uniform distribution over [0,1] as a special case (when $r = 1$ and $s = 1$), it is increasingly well approximated by a NORMAL DISTRIBUTION as r and s increase and it can result from constructions of the form $A/(A+B)$ where A and B are both random variables with GAMMA DISTRIBUTIONS.

The beta distribution is most commonly used to model proportions. Suppose that we wish to estimate the speci-

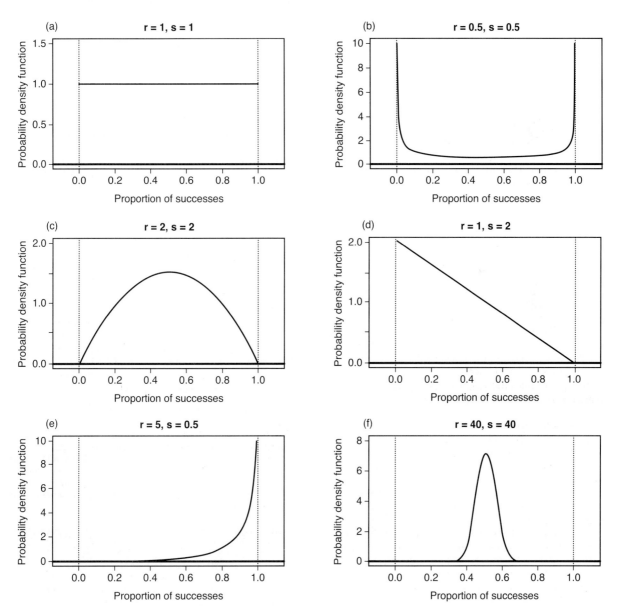

beta distribution *Illustrating the variety of forms that the beta distribution can take: (a) the uniform distribution over (0,1), (b) a bimodal concave distribution (in this case the Jeffrey's prior), (c) a curve with a single mode, (d) a linear function of the proportion, (e) a non-linear but still strictly increasing distribution, (f) an example that is well approximated by the normal distribution*

ficity of a test that in trials correctly identifies 50 of the 52 participants that do not have the condition. The usual technique of using a normal approximation suggests a CONFIDENCE INTERVAL from 0.91 to 1.01. Since a value greater than 1 makes no sense and a value of 1 is not possible with these data, this is unsatisfactory.

There are a number of ways to use the beta distribution to estimate the interval (see Brown, Cai and DasGupta, 2001). For this example, we give the Jeffrey's interval, which is a Bayesian CREDIBLE INTERVAL from 0.90 to 0.99.

AGL

Brown, L.D., Cai, T.T. and DasGupta, A. 2001: Interval estimation for a binomial proportion. *Statistical Science* 16, 101–33. **Leemis, L.M.** 1986: Relationships among common univariate distributions. *The American Statistician* 40, 2, 143–6.

bias Any experiment, study or measuring process is said to be biased if it produces an outcome which differs from the 'truth' in a systematic way. Bias can occur at any stage of the research process from the literature review through to the publication of the results (Armitage and Colton, 1998).

It is important to distinguish between bias or systematic error, on the one hand, and random error, on the other hand. For example, suppose that we had a population of subjects with a MEAN weight of 80kg and a STANDARD DEVIATION of 10kg. If we select a simple random sample of 25 subjects from this population and measure their weights using a well-calibrated set of scales, then it is possible that the mean weight for this sample will be substantially different from 80kg. In fact, there is about a 1 in 20 chance that the sample mean will be more than 4kg below or 4kg above the true mean of 80kg.

However, simple random sampling produces an unbiased estimate of the true mean weight because, if the process of selecting a simple random sample of 25 subjects and computing the sample mean weight were repeated a large number of times, the distribution of the sample means would be centred around the true mean of 80kg. The larger the sample size, the closer the sample means will be clustered around the true population mean. In other words, the expected value of the sample mean equals the population mean. In this scenario, there is no bias and any deviation of the observed sample mean from the true value can be accounted for by pure chance, known as random variation or random error.

If, however, the weights of a random sample of subjects were measured using a *poorly* calibrated set of scales that weighed each subject as being 2kg heavier than his actual weight, this would lead to a biased estimate of the true population mean weight. The size of this bias, or systematic error, would not be reduced by increasing the sample size and the distribution of the sample mean will be centred around 82kg rather than 80kg. The systematic error in this example is a measurement bias due to a faulty measuring instrument.

More generally, measurement bias could be due to such diverse causes as poor questionnaire design, faulty equipment, observer error or respondent error (McNeil, 1996). Examples of observer error include misreading the scale on an instrument, bias in reporting results by an unblinded evaluator in a clinical trial or bias in eliciting information about the exposure history of cases and controls in a CASE-CONTROL STUDY. Examples of respondent error include biased reporting of symptoms by unblinded

patients in a clinical trial, bias in recall of exposure history by cases and controls in a case-control study.

All types of study are susceptible to design bias. This can arise from many sources, such as SELECTION BIAS (when the subjects selected for study are not representative of the target population), non-response bias (when there is a systematic difference between the characteristics of those who choose to participate and those who do not), non-comparability bias (when groups of subjects chosen for comparison in, for example, a case-control study are not in fact comparable). Randomised trials (see CLINICAL TRIALS) are generally regarded as being least susceptible to design biases. The scope for BIAS IN OBSERVATIONAL STUDIES, especially case-control studies, is much greater. Armitage and Colton (1998), Ellenberg (1994), Last (2001) and Sackett (1979) all provide a comprehensive description of sources of design bias.

Analysis bias arises from errors in the analysis of data. This covers such issues as confounding bias (in which confounding factors have not been appropriately adjusted for in the analysis), analysis method bias (including inappropriate assumptions about the distribution of variables, faulty strategies for handling MISSING DATA or OUTLIERS, unplanned SUBGROUP ANALYSIS and *data dredging*) (Armitage and Colton, 1998; Davey Smith and Ebrahim, 2002).

Ensuring that the interpretation of data is unbiased is just as important as ensuring that the processes of design, measurement and analysis are unbiased. Bias in the interpretation of data can be conscious or unconscious and is particularly difficult to address because it involves subjective judgements on the part of the researchers. Kaptchuk (2003) provides an overview of the issues involved.

Publication bias (see SYSTEMATIC REVIEWS AND META-ANALYSIS) arises from two main sources. First, researchers are more likely to submit papers for publication if the research produces a statistically and clinically significant result rather than an inconclusive result. Second, journal editors are more likely to publish papers reporting statistically and clinically significant results (Begg and Berlin, 1988).

Finally, there is recent evidence to suggest that the source of funding for drug studies is related to the outcome. A systematic review by Lexchin *et al.* (2003) demonstrated a systematic bias in favour of the products made by the company funding the research. The main sources of this bias were thought to be inappropriate selection of treatments to compare against the product being investigated and publication bias.

WHG

[See also NON-RESPONSE BIAS, SELECTION BIAS]

Armitage, P. and Colton, T. (eds) 1998: *Encyclopaedia of biostatistics*. New York: John Wiley & Sons. **Begg, C.B. and Berlin, J.A.** 1988: Publication bias: a problem in interpreting medical data. *Journal of the Royal Statistical Society Series A* 151, 419–63. **Davey Smith, G. and Ebrahim, S.** 2002: Data dredging, bias or confounding. *British Medical Journal* 325, 1437–8. **Ellenberg, J.H.** 1994: Selection bias in observational and experimental studies. *Statistics in Medicine* 13, 557–67. **Kaptchuk, T.J.** 2003: Effect of interpretive bias on research evidence. *British Medical Journal* 326, 1453–5. **Last, J.M.** 2001: *A dictionary of epidemiology*, 4th edn. Oxford: Oxford University Press. **Lexchin, J., Bero, L.A., Djulbegovic, B. and Clark, O.** 2003: Pharmaceutical industry sponsorship and research outcome and quality: systematic review. *British Medical Journal* 326, 1167–76. **McNeil, D.** 1996: *Epidemiological research methods*. New York: John Wiley & Sons. **Sackett, D.L.** 1979: Bias in analytic research. *Journal of Chronic Diseases* 32, 51–63.

bias in observational studies In an ideal study, an investigator seeks to estimate the effect of an exposure to a factor on an outcome of interest. We might like to be able to look at what happens to a population when the factor is at one level and then turn back time and rerun things at the second level; but that is impossible, of course.

Very often it is not even possible or practical to conduct an experiment in which the levels of exposure are controlled, so that one is left with analysing observational data that occur naturally. Bias is any systematic departure from this idealised construct, which is distinct from purely random error that is zero on average. The latter can be dealt with by reducing variability in the measure of association, which can be accomplished in a variety of ways including the increase of the overall sample size. However, bias cannot be reduced by increasing the sample size and it can only be controlled through carefully conducted research by an investigator. There have been attempts to catalogue the types of bias that can occur and these broadly fall into three sources: the selection of study subjects; errors in the information collected; and confounding or entangling the effects with other causes of the outcome (Hill and Kleinbaum, 1998).

In order to discuss the sources of bias in an observational study in more concrete terms, consider a hypothetical epidemiological study in which the results are summarised in a 2×2 table (shown in the Table). We are interested in studying the association between exposure and disease in a manner that avoids bias. Among the choices of study design from which data for this 2×2 table may have arisen are a CROSS-SECTIONAL STUDY, a COHORT STUDY or a CASE-CONTROL STUDY. In a cross-sectional study, N subjects are sampled and the four cell frequencies determined, but in a cohort study, a groups of exposed and unexposed subjects are chosen, essentially fixing the row totals and then the column frequencies are determined by what transpires during the course of follow-up. For a case-control study, the column totals are regarded as fixed and subjects distributed to each row within a column depending on their exposure history that would usually be gleaned by interview. Fundamental to each of these study designs is the realisation of a random sample, either overall, or within the rows or columns.

Selection bias occurs when the proportion recruited from the target population that is counted in a cell of the 2×2 table depends on both the row and the column. One way in which this can occur in a cohort study is if there are differential diagnoses depending on the exposure status. For example, suppose that an exposure of interest occurs in a manufacturing plant that provides health insurance for its employees, but among the unexposed are substan-

tial numbers who are uninsured. If the insured receive regular checkups from their physicians, this may increase the likelihood of a correct diagnosis among those exposed, while similar cases may have been missed for the unexposed that are uninsured. Clearly, this would bias an estimate of the odds ratio that would be calculated from such a study. Another potential source of such bias in a cohort study may arise from loss to follow-up. For example, if instead of exposure, the investigator is interested in whether a person is using a particular type of treatment. However, suppose that the treatment is not only ineffective but it also causes unpleasant symptoms in patients who are related to the occurrence of the disease outcome. If the individuals so affected drop out of the study, this would artificially lower the count in this cell of the 2×2 table and bias the estimate. Notice that the magnitude of the effect of this selection bias may be substantial, even if the number lost represents a small proportion of the total. This is especially true when the proportion that develops the disease is small, so that the portion lost in a cell of the table is relatively high, even though the proportion lost represents a small proportion of the overall sample.

In a case-control study, a common source of bias when selecting cases can occur when subjects with prevalent disease are enrolled into the study, some of which may have had the disease for some time. Those who have been ill for a long period of time will be more likely to be enrolled if such a study design is used, a phenomenon known as LENGTH-BIASED SAMPLING. If the primary aims of the study are to study the association between exposure and the occurrence of disease, this will clearly lead to a biased estimate of association, but this could have been avoided by only enrolling newly diagnosed cases instead.

The choice of appropriate controls in a case-control study can be an especially common source of bias. If the cases are selected from among those who are diagnosed at a collaborating set of hospitals, then the controls should ideally be a representative sample of those who are healthy in the catchment areas of those hospitals. If all hospitals in an area are cooperating with a study, then this could be accomplished by recruiting a random sample of the overall population in the geographic area. Random digit dialling is one approach that has been useful in populations well covered by telephones, but it is becoming more difficult to employ the method with the increasing use of current technologies such as cell phones, caller ID and no-call lists. In some studies, controls are selected using subjects who have been admitted into the same hospital for a disease that is unrelated to the exposure of interest. This would result in a group of subjects from the same catchment area as the cases, thus avoiding one source of potential selection bias. The estimate of association in such a study would be the difference between the effect of exposure on the disease of interest and its effect on the 'control disease' (Breslow, 1978, 1982). If one has chosen a control disease that is not related to exposure, i.e., the effect is zero, then the estimate of association will be an unbiased estimate of the effect on disease risk. However, it is often difficult to be certain that this is the case because the assumption may just be the result of a lack of knowledge about the aetiology of disease affecting the controls.

A cross-sectional study can be a useful way of obtaining a snapshot of the association between two or more variables at a single point in time, especially if the population

bias in observational studies *Tabulated results from an epidemiological study with two levels of exposure and disease status*

Exposed	Diseased		Total
	Yes	No	
Yes	a	b	$a + b$
No	c	d	$c + d$
Total	$a + c$	$b + d$	N

chosen for study is of broad interest and a carefully planned method for drawing a random sample has been put in place. Some national health surveys are good examples of such studies, such as those conducted by the National Center for Health Statistics. However, if the aim is to study disease aetiology or other outcomes that evolve over time, then the single snapshot in time can be a serious limitation. For example, in an epidemiological study, subjects with a disease who have been identified by a survey conducted at a single point in time would necessarily be a prevalent case, which is a potential source of bias here as it is in a case-control study.

Information bias in an observational study arises from error in the variables that have been collected as part of the data for each subject in a study. Such errors can either be differential or non-differential, i.e. random. Differential error in reporting values summarised in a 2×2 table would arise if the error rate for reporting the variable in the column depended on the row or vice versa. This would obviously be a potentially important source of bias when estimating an association. However, bias can also arise when the error is non-differential or purely random.

Case-control studies can be prone to information bias because someone with a serious illness may remember their history of exposure to the factor of interest quite differently from a healthy control. This RECALL BIAS can be especially significant when other studies of the exposure of interest have entered the public's consciousness or been reported in the news. One technique for minimising its effect is to use a well-structured interview in which the questions have been clearly and unambiguously phrased and posed in an identical manner to all subjects in the study. This requires considerable effort on the part of an investigator, in that the questionnaire would need to be pre-tested and the interviewers well trained.

Information bias can potentially also affect a study by subconsciously influencing evaluations by interviewers, professional diagnosticians or even laboratory technicians. This could happen if the individual has a preconceived idea of what the results of a study will be or of the way the results are going. Thus, it is generally preferred that the study hypotheses not be known to those responsible for collecting the data or that the status of a subject be masked, a procedure in which the person recording the data is said to be blind with respect to the outcome. These measures should reduce the possibility for differential errors, but not non-differential errors.

While it is intuitively easy to appreciate that differential error of measurement can bias the results of an observational study, non-differential error can also have an effect, as well. If only a single variable is affected by non-differential error, then the effect is generally to attenuate the effect, i.e. to bias the estimated association toward the null value of no association. This would tend to make the results of a study with non-differential error in one of the variables conservative in the sense that it would make it more difficult to establish that an estimated association was not due to chance alone. Contrariwise, it would also result in an underestimate of an effect, which can be important when trying to determine the public health significance of exposure to a particular factor.

It is most desirable to minimise information bias during the design and data collection phase of a study by min-

imising measurement error, but it is generally not possible to be entirely successful in these efforts. One approach to correcting for bias at the data analysis phase is to introduce a correction factor that takes into account the measurement error. In the case of a 2×2 table, formulae have been provided for this (Barron, 1977; Copeland et al., 1977) and similar approaches are also available for use in LOGISTIC REGRESSION (Rosner, Spiegelman and Willett, 1990). There is now a rich variety of statistical techniques for dealing with errors in variables, many of which are described in the text by Carroll, Ruppert and Stefanski (1995).

Confounding arises when the estimated effect for an association of interest is entangled with another factor, perhaps one that is well known to be associated with the outcome. It is conceptually related to aliasing in design of experiments, in which two effects are completely entangled, and *collinearity* in other contexts. The potential for confounding in an observational study of two variables exists when each is associated with a third variable, the confounder, in the presence of the factor of interest. Precise definitions of confounding go to the heart of the objectives of observational studies and various models have been proposed as a theoretical basis for its effect (Rubin, 1974; Wickramaratne and Holford, 1987). Alternatively, *collapsability* is sometimes used as a simple and practical alternative to more formal definitions of confounding (Bishop, Fienburg and Holland, 1973). An association is collapsible with respect to a putative confounder if the estimated association is unchanged when adjusting for the confounder in the analysis.

Approaches for dealing with a potential confounder are in essence to estimate the association holding the value of the confounder constant. In a designed experiment, this would be accomplished by selecting strata or blocks of subjects with identical values of the confounder and only vary the exposure of interest within the strata. One way of accomplishing a similar effect in an observational study is to stratify the data by the potential confounder and then combine information across the strata, if the effect is constant, using the MANTEL-HAENSZEL METHOD or something similar (Mantel and Haentszel, 1959). Alternatively, one can adjust for one or more putative confounders by including them in a model, such as the linear logistic model (Hosmer and Lemeshow, 1989) or an alternative GENERALISED LINEAR MODEL (McCullagh and Nelder, 1989) for a binary response.

It is entirely possible that an observational study will not be able to separate out the effect of an exposure of interest from the effect of another exposure that it thought to be a confounder. This is not unlike the more general problem of collinearity that arises in the context of regression analysis. In these situations, it may only be possible to conduct a new study in which the design has been carefully constructed so that one can tease apart the separate contributions of a factor of interest from its confounder.

TRH

Barron, B.A. 1977: The effects of misclassification on the estimate of relative risk. *Biometrics* 33, 414–18. **Bishop, Y.M.M., Fienburg, S.E. and Holland, P.W.** 1973: *Discrete multivariate analysis: theory and practice.* Cambridge, MA: MIT Press. **Breslow, N.** 1978: The proportional hazards model: applications in epidemiology. *Communications in Statistics-Theory and Mathematics* A7, 4, 315–32. **Breslow, N.** 1982: Design and analysis of case-control studies. *Annual Review of Public Health* 3, 29–54. **Carroll, R.J., Ruppert, D. and Stefanski, L.A.** 1995: *Measurement error in nonlinear models*. London: Chapman & Hall. **Copeland, K.T., Checkoway, H., McMichael, A.J. and Holbrook, R.H.** 1977: Bias due to misclassification in the estimation of relative risk. *American Journal of Epidemiology* 105, 488–95. **Hill, H.A. and Kleinbaum, D.G.** 1998: Bias in observational studies. In Armitage, P. and Colton, T. (eds), *Encyclopedia of Biostatistics*. Chichester: John Wiley & Sons. **Hosmer, D.W. and Lemeshow, S.** 1989: *Applied logistic regression*. New York: John Wiley & Sons. **Mantel, N. and Haenszel, W.** 1959: Statistical aspects of the analysis of data from retrospective studies of disease. *Journal of the National Cancer Institute* 22, 719–48. **McCullagh, P. and Nelder, J.A.** 1989: *Generalised linear models*. London: Chapman & Hall. **Rosner, B., Spiegelman, D. and Willett, W.C.** 1990: Correction of logistic regression relative risk estimates and confidence intervals for measurement error: the case of multiple covariates measured with error. *American Journal of Epidemiology* 132, 734–45. **Rubin, D.B.** 1974: Estimating causal effects of treatments in randomized and nonrandomized studies. *Journal of Educational Psychology* 66, 688–701. **Wickramaratne, P.J. and Holford, T.R.** 1987: Confounding in epidemiologic studies: the adequacy of the control group as a measure of confounding. *Biometrics* 43, 751–65.

bimodal distribution

A PROBABILITY DISTRIBUTION, or a FREQUENCY DISTRIBUTION, with two modes. Often the two modes in the distribution correspond to the data arising from two distinct populations. The first figure shows a bimodal density function arising from a weighted sum of two NORMAL DISTRIBUTIONS (a FINITE MIXTURE DISTRIBUTION). An example of a HISTOGRAM with two distinct modes is shown in the second figure. The data here correspond to the sizes of myelinated lumbosacral ventral root fibres taken from a kitten of a particular age. The first mode is associated with axons of gamma neurons and the second with alpha neurons. *BSE*

binomial distribution

The PROBABILITY DISTRIBUTION of the number of 'successes', X, in a series of n independent trials, where the probability of a success is p for each trial. Specifically the distribution is given by:

$$\Pr(X = x) = \frac{n!}{x!(n-x)!}\,p^x(1-p)^{n-x}\ x = 0,1,2,...,n$$

where $n!$ (factorial n) is the product of all the integers up to and including n, and 0! is defined to be one. The mean of the distribution is np and its variance $np(1-p)$. Some binomial distributions with $n = 10$ and different values of p are shown in the Figure on page 34. The distribution often occurs in medicine as the basis for testing the hypothesis that the probability of some event of interest takes a particular value. For example, a researcher may postulate that 10% of a population is infected with a virus and, on sampling 20 people at random from the population, finds that 6 people have the virus. Is there any evidence that the infection rate is higher than the hypothesised value of 10%? To answer this question a *P*-value can be computed from the binomial distribution as the probability that 6 or more people in the 20 sampled have the virus when the probability that a person is infected is 0.1, i.e. the sum:

$$\sum_{x=6}^{20} \frac{20!}{x!(20-x)!}(0.1)^x(0.9)^{20-x}$$

The resulting value is 0.01, giving strong evidence that the infection rate is larger than 10%. As well as testing for a specific proportion, the binomial distribution can be used in calculating CONFIDENCE INTERVALS for a proportion. Villanueva *et al.* (2003) use the binomial distribution to estimate confidence intervals for the proportion of adverts in medical journals with inaccurate claims. *BSE/AGL*

Altman, D.G. 1991: *Practical statistics for medical research.* London: Chapman & Hall. **Villanueva, P., Peiró, S., Librero, J. and Pereiró, I.** 2003: Accuracy of pharmaceutical advertisements in medical journals. *Lancet* 361, 27–32.

birth cohort studies

Studies established to examine growth, development and health of children from birth. However, given sufficient follow-up they also provide longer term insights into influences on adult disease that operate throughout the life course.

In principle, a birth cohort study is one in which all study participants are recruited at birth and then followed over time. The cohort is defined by the location and the time period in which the participants were born; this may be those born in one week or over a period of a year or more. The members of the cohort are then followed up at various time points to ascertain risk factors and health

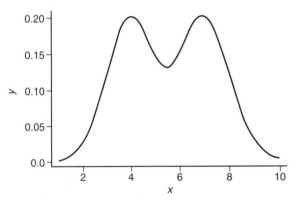

bimodal distribution *Finite mixture distribution*

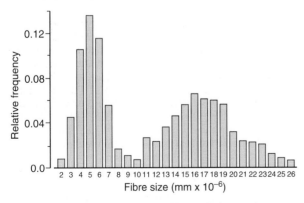

bimodal distribution *Histogram with two distinct modes*

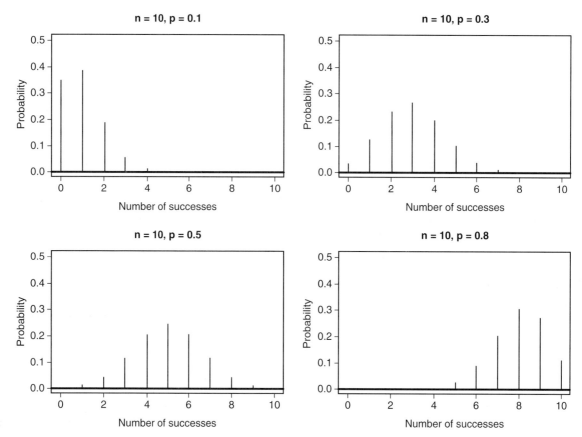

binomial distribution *Binomial distributions for various values of* n *and* p

outcomes. As the cohort ages the focus of the research tends to shift. In the early years, the emphasis tends to be on childhood growth and development and risk of childhood illness but as the cohort matures adult risk factors such as smoking and obesity and health measures such as blood pressure start to be of greater interest. Outcome variables in childhood such as height can later be considered as risk factors when assessing chronic disease in adult life.

The first birth cohort study to be established was the National Survey of Health and Development, which studied all babies born in Britain in the first week of March 1946 (Wadsworth *et al.*, 2003). The cohort has since been followed up on more than 20 occasions since birth. Many of the contacts with the participants have been by postal questionnaire or home visit, although, in the earlier years, contact was also made through schools. Use was also made of the statutory services in that health visitors, school nurses and doctors and teachers were asked to collect the required data.

Britain has two other birth cohort studies conducted on similar lines: all births born between 3 and 9 March 1958 (Power, 1992) and those born between 5 and 11 April 1970 (Bynner, Ferri and Shepherd, 1997). Both studies have included a number of follow-ups that have given insights into the growth and development of these cohorts through childhood adolescence and into adulthood. Cross-cohort comparisons have also been possible and have allowed examination of secular trends, for example

into Crohn's disease, ulcerative colitis and irritable bowel syndrome (Ehlin *et al.*, 2003).

Birth cohort studies are not, of course, confined to Britain, although such comprehensive national coverage has rarely been attempted elsewhere. Frequently, birth cohorts are located in one town or city. For example, the Pelotas Birth Cohort Study in Brazil recruited all births born in the city of Pelotas during 1982. It represents a rare example of a birth cohort study with long-term follow-up in a developing country (Victora *et al.*, 2003).

Many birth cohorts have been defined retrospectively. Thus births in a defined geographical area during a specified time period are identified from established records. The data can then be linked to other standard records such as death indices, or the study population can be traced and those still alive can be assessed by post or by interview. An example of this is the birth records of the 1920s and 1930s from the English county of Hertfordshire that were extracted in the 1980s. The population was traced through the National Health Service Central Register and details of deaths and current general practitioner addresses obtained. This allowed not only an analysis of mortality in relation to birth and infant weight but also enabled follow-up of the survivors to examine them for risk factors for chronic conditions such as cardiovascular disease (Osmond *et al.*, 1993).

Some retrospectively defined birth cohorts have focused on particular events that gave rise to extreme living conditions. For example, those born in Amsterdam in 1944–5 around the time of the famine imposed by the German occupation have been followed up to assess the impact of famine at key stages of pregnancy and early life (Roseboom *et al.*, 2001). Similarly, a cohort of men born between 1916 and 1935 were identified from one district in Leningrad, one-third of whom had experienced starvation during the siege of Leningrad in 1941–4, when they were around the age of puberty (Sparén *et al.*, 2003). The whole cohort was followed up and invited to take part in health examinations to assess the long-term effects of the famine.

Increasingly there has been a trend towards defining birth cohorts at an earlier time point than birth. A child's growth and development begins before birth and so characterisation of aspects of pregnancy is considered important in determining the long-term influences on the offspring's health. A good example of this is the Avon Longitudinal Study of Parents and Children (ALSPAC), which recruited 14,000 pregnant women resident in the English county of Avon whose expected dates of delivery were between 1 April 1991 and 31 December 1992. The women and their offspring have been followed up by means of postal questionnaires on many occasions and a sub-sample known as Children in Focus has been seen at clinics at least 10 times. From the age of 7 years clinics began for the entire cohort (Golding *et al.*, 2001). The United States of America is undertaking a similar study, recruiting women before birth, but on a larger scale, planning 100,000 births (see www.nichd.nih.gov/despr/cohort).

Taking this one step further, with an increasing focus on the very early origins of life, two cohort studies have recruited women before pregnancy. The first of these recruited some 2500 women in six villages near Pune in India. Of these, over 1000 became pregnant and full data were obtained on nearly 800 births. This cohort has now been followed up to age 8 (Rao *et al.*, 2001). In the UK, the Southampton Women's Survey recruited 12,500 women aged 20 to 34 years when they were not pregnant and the women are studied throughout their subsequent pregnancies and the children followed through infancy and beyond (Inskip, 1999).

Birth cohort studies have many strengths. Usually they capture a cross-section of the population and they have all the advantages of longitudinal studies. However, the weakness is that over the life course a large percentage of prospectively defined birth cohorts tends to drop out. Many DROPOUTS are due to death as the cohort ages or to migration out of the region or country of study. Persistent questioning and requests to attend clinics or be visited at home adds to the attrition as participants feel that they have contributed enough and their motivation wanes. The remaining cohort may no longer represent the general population. Retrospectively defined cohorts can suffer less from this problem but then they often lack data on the early years.   *HI*

[See also COHORT STUDIES]

Bynner, J.M., Ferri, E. and Shepherd, P. (eds) 1997: *Twenty-something in the 1990s: getting on, getting by, getting nowhere.* Aldershot: Ashgate. **Ehlin, A.G.C., Montgomery, S.M., Ekbom, A., Pounder, R.E. and Wakefield, A.J.** 2003: Prevalence of gastrointestinal diseases in two British national birth cohorts. *Gut* 52, 1117–21. **Golding, J., Pembrey, M., Jones, R. and the ALSPAC Study Team** 2001: ALSPAC – the Avon Longitudinal Study of Parents and Children 1: study methodology. *Paediatric and Perinatal Epidemiology* 15, 74–87. **Inskip, H.** 1999: The Southampton Women's Survey. *MIDIRS Midwifery Digest* 9, 445–7. **Osmond, C., Barker, D.J.P., Winter, P.D., Fall, C.H. and Simmonds, S.J.** 1993: Early growth and death from cardiovascular disease in women. *British Medical Journal* 307, 1519–24. **Power, C.** 1992: A review of child health in the 1958 birth cohort: National Child Development Study. *Paediatric and Perinatal Epidemiology* 6, 81–110. **Rao, S., Yajnik, C.S., Kanade, A., Fall, C.H.D., Margetts, B.M., Jackson, A.A., Shier, R., Joshi, S., Rege, S., Lubree, H. and Desai, B.** 2001: Intake of micronutrient-rich foods in rural Indian mothers is associated with the size of their babies at birth: Pune Maternal Nutrition Study. *Journal of Nutrition* 131, 1217–24. **Roseboom, T.J., van der Meulen, J.H.P., Osmond, C., Barker, D.J.P., Ravelli, A.C.J. and Bleker, O.P.** 2001: Adult survival after prenatal exposure to the Dutch famine 1944–45. *Paediatric and Perinatal Epidemiology* 15, 220–25. **Sparén, P., Vågerö, D., Shestov, D.B., Plavinskaja, S., Parfenova, N., Hoptiar, V., Paturot, D. and Galanti, M.R.** 2003: Long-term mortality after severe starvation during the siege of Leningrad: prospective cohort study. *British Medical Journal* 10, 1136. **Victora, C.G., Barros, F.C., Lima, R.C., Behague, D.P., Gonçalves, H., Horta, B.L., Gigante, D.P. and Vaughan, J.P.** 2003: The Pelotas Birth Cohort Study, Rio Grande do Sul, Brazil, 1982–2001. *Cad Saude Publica* 19, 1241–56. **Wadsworth, M.E.J., Butterworth, S.L., Hardy, R.J., Kuh, D.J., Richards, K., Langenberg, C., Hilder, W.S. and Connor, M.** 2003: The life-course prospective design: an example of benefits and problems associated with study longevity. *Social Science and Medicine* 57, 2193–205.

bivariate distribution   For each and every pair of feasible values, the probability that a pair of variables will take those values. This then is a natural extension of the idea of a univariate probability distribution, applicable when we are measuring two paired variables, e.g. a person's height and weight.

If the two variables are independent then the bivariate distribution will not be of particular interest. When they are correlated, as with height and weight, however, it becomes important to consider the bivariate distribution. If we were to look at a sample we might see that 20% of the sample are over 6 feet tall and 20% of the sample are under 50kg in weight, but only by looking at the bivariate distribution would we know that there were no (or few) people who were both over 6 feet tall and under 50kg in weight.

Whereas univariate distributions can usually be depicted in a BAR CHART or HISTOGRAM, bivariate distributions due to their additional dimension cannot. If the two variables are categorical then a simple cross-tabulation will probably be most informative, while if the two variables are continuous a SCATTERPLOT will probably be appropriate.

For example, whereas in previous univariate work (McLaren *et al.*, 2000) have separately looked at the distributions of red-blood cell volume and haemoglobin levels when identifying anaemia, in a more sophisticated approach, McLaren *et al.* (2001) employ a bivariate distribution of red cell volume and haemoglobin.

The most commonly encountered bivariate distribution is the BIVARIATE NORMAL DISTRIBUTION, a special case of the MULTIVARIATE NORMAL DISTRIBUTION.   *AGL*

McLaren, C.E., Kambour, E.L., McLachlan, G.J., Lukaski, H.C., Li, X., Brittenham, G.M. and McLaren, G.D. 2000: Patient-specific analysis of sequential haematological data by multiple linear regression and mixture distribution modelling. *Statistics in Medicine* 19, 1, 83–98. **McLaren, C.E., Cadez, I.V.,**

Smyth, P. and McLachlan, G.J. 2001: Classification of disorders of anemia on the basis of mixture model parameters. Technical Report No. 01–56. Irvine: Information and Computer Science Department, University of California.

bivariate normal distribution

A special case of the multivariate normal distribution with two variables and the most common example of a bivariate distribution. The bivariate normal distribution is worthy of mention because of multivariate normal distributions, it is the most commonly used, the easiest to illustrate and the easiest to write out in mathematical notation.

Given two variables, X and Y, the probability density function of the bivariate normal distribution is defined by the means of X and Y (here denoted μ_X and μ_Y respectively), the STANDARD DEVIATIONS of X and Y (here denoted σ_X and σ_Y respectively) and the CORRELATION of X and Y (denoted ρ). Given these values, the probability that X and Y take values x and y respectively, $f(x,y)$, is:

$$f(x,y) = \frac{1}{2\pi\sigma_X\sigma_Y\sqrt{1-\rho^2}} \exp\left\{-\frac{1}{2(1-\rho^2)}\left[\left(\frac{x-\mu_X}{\sigma_X}\right)^2 \right.\right.$$
$$\left.\left. -2\rho\left(\frac{x-\mu_X}{\sigma_X}\right)\left(\frac{y-\mu_Y}{\sigma_Y}\right)+\left(\frac{y-\mu_Y}{\sigma_Y}\right)^2\right]\right\}$$

This formula may not appear particularly pleasant, but is easier to handle than for higher-variate normal distributions because of the single correlation involved.

When graphed as a SCATTERPLOT, data from this distribution will appear as a cluster of points in an approximately elliptical shape with the density of the points being greatest at the centre of the ellipse. The location of the ellipse will be dependent on the two means, while the standard deviations and correlation determine the angle and spread of the ellipse. The ellipse gets 'narrower' as the magnitude of the correlation increases and approaches a straight line at $\rho = 1$ or -1.

Suryapranata *et al.* (2001) use the bivariate normal distribution so as to compare simultaneously the clinical effectiveness and cost-effectiveness of two treatments for patients with acute myocardial infarction. By drawing a graph of difference in effect against difference in cost they were able to illustrate a CONFIDENCE INTERVAL for the differences between the two treatments as an ellipse.

A convenient property of the bivariate normal distribution is the fact that the marginal distributions of the two variables are univariate normal. That is, if Y is ignored, then X by itself has a NORMAL DISTRIBUTION (and vice versa). Also, the conditional distributions of X and Y are normal. Or to put it another way, if Y is observed to take a particular value, then the unknown value of X still has a normal distribution given this knowledge. *AGL*

Chatfield, C. and Collins, A.J. 1980: *Introduction to multivariate analysis*. London: Chapman & Hall. **Grimmet, G.R. and Stirzaker, D.R.** 1992: *Probability and random processes*, 2nd edition. Oxford: Clarendon Press. **Suryapranata, H., Ottervanger, J.P., Nibbering, E., van't Hof, A.W.J., Hoorntje, J.C.A., de Boer, M.J., Al, M.J. and Zijlstra, F.** 2001: Long-term outcome and cost-effectiveness of stenting versus balloon angioplasty for acute myocardial infarction. *Heart* 85, 667–71.

Bland–Altman plot   See LIMITS OF AGREEMENT

blinding   See CLINICAL TRIALS

blocked randomisation   See RANDOMISATION

Bonferroni correction

A correction used when performing multiple significance tests in order to avoid an excess of false positives (Schaffer, 1995). Suppose, for example, STUDENT'S T-TEST is to be applied to sample data on six variables to assess mean differences in two populations of interest. If the null hypothesis of no difference in means holds for each of the six variables, and each of the six tests is performed at the 5% SIGNIFICANCE LEVEL, the probability of falsely rejecting the equality of at least one pair of means is 0.26 (this assumes the variables are independent), a fivefold increase over the nominal significance level. The Bonferroni correction approach to this problem involves using a significance level of α/n rather than α for each of the n tests to be performed. For a small number of multiple tests (up to about 5) this method provides a simple and acceptable answer to the problem of inflating the Type I error. The correction is, however, highly conservative and not recommended if large numbers of tests are to be applied, particularly since its use can lead to the rather unsatisfactory situation where many tests are significant at the α level but none at level α/n (Perneger, 1998). In addition, the Bonferroni correction ignores the degree to which the variables may be correlated, which again leads to conservatism when such correlations are substantial. *BSE*

[See also MULTIPLE COMPARISON PROCEDURES]

Perneger, T.V. 1998: What's wrong with Bonferroni adjustments? *British Medical Journal* 316, 1236–8. **Schaffer, J.P.** 1995: Multiple hypothesis testing. *Annual Review of Psychology* 46, 561–84.

bootstrap

The bootstrap is a computationally intensive technique for statistical inference, which can be used when the assumptions that underpin much of classical statistical inference are questionable. This may be because the data are not normally distributed, or the dataset is small so that theoretical results based on large sample theory are inapplicable. For example, the bootstrap can be used to estimate the BIAS and STANDARD ERROR of parameter estimates together with CONFIDENCE INTERVALS.

In effect, as we illustrate in the Figures, the bootstrap is a data re-sampling technique. It was formally introduced by Efron (see discussion in Efron and Tibshirani, 1993) and although it has a sound theoretical basis, the idea there is something magical about is reflected in its name. The term bootstrap derives from the phrase to pull oneself up by one's bootstrap, widely thought to be based on one of the 18th-century adventures of Baron Munchausen. The Baron found himself at the bottom of a deep lake and saved himself by hauling himself up by his bootstraps.

We describe the idea using the Figure on page 37. Suppose we have a population, in which the true value of a quantity of interest, say adult height, is denoted by θ. We wish to estimate θ and take a sample of 12 individuals from this population. In the Figure, the population is denoted by the large rectangle in the first row (note the numbers identify population members and are not their

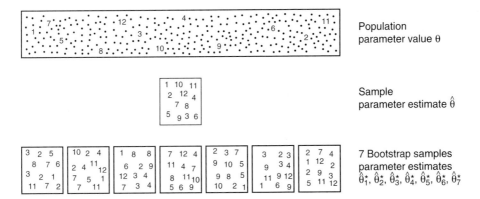

Population
parameter value θ

Sample
parameter estimate $\hat{\theta}$

7 Bootstrap samples
parameter estimates
$\hat{\theta}_1^\star, \hat{\theta}_2^\star, \hat{\theta}_3^\star, \hat{\theta}_4^\star, \hat{\theta}_5^\star, \hat{\theta}_6^\star, \hat{\theta}_7^\star$

bootstrap *Schematic illustration of bootstrapping*

adult heights). In this population, the 12 individuals to be included in the sample are numbered. They comprise the actual sample, which is shown in the second row. Our estimate of adult height, calculated from this sample, is denoted by $\hat{\theta}$.

In order to quantify how close $\hat{\theta}$, the estimate of adult height in our sample, is likely to be to θ, the actual adult height in the population, we need at the very least to estimate the variance of $\hat{\theta}$.

Imagine doing this in the following way. Take a large number, say B, samples of size 12 from the population. In each of these samples, calculate an estimate of adult height. Call these estimates $\hat{\theta}_1, \ldots, \hat{\theta}_B$. Then estimate the variance of $\hat{\theta}$ by the sample variance of $(\hat{\theta}_1, \ldots, \hat{\theta}_B)$.

Of course, this approach is impossible in practice; if we could afford to draw B extra samples of size 12, we would have drawn a much larger sample initially! However, an approximation to it can be achieved as follows.

Suppose we sample with replacement from the 12 observations in the data (second row in the Figure) to form a 'sub-sample', also of size 12. Seven possible such 'sub-samples' are shown in the third row of the figure. For example, the first sub-sample, shown in the first rectangle in the third row, consists of the following observations (note some observations will occur more than once, and some not at all): {1, 2, 2, 2, 3, 3, 5, 6, 7, 7, 8, 11}. These 'sub-samples' are known as *bootstrap samples*.

Using each of these bootstrap samples we calculate an estimate of adult height. By convention, these are denoted with a '$\star$', to indicate they have been calculated from a bootstrap sample. From the 7 bootstrap samples in the third row of the Figure, we therefore get $\hat{\theta}_1^\star, \ldots, \hat{\theta}_7^\star$.

Now we simply estimate the variability of the estimate of adult height calculated from the actual data, $\hat{\theta}$, by the sample variance of the bootstrap estimates $\hat{\theta}_1^\star, \ldots, \hat{\theta}_7^\star$. Of course, in practice we would need many more than 7 bootstrap estimates.

Another way of looking at this is as follows. We wish to learn about the relationship between the true population parameter value, θ, and estimates of θ obtained from samples from the population, denoted $\hat{\theta}$. To do this, we pretend the observed data are the population and repeatedly sample from the data to learn about the relationship between $\hat{\theta}$ and estimates obtained from the re-sampled data, denoted $\hat{\theta}^\star$. In other words, we say:

$$\text{Distribution of estimates } \hat{\theta} \text{ given } \theta$$

$$\text{is approximated by}$$

$$\text{Distribution of estimates } \hat{\theta}^\star \text{ given } \hat{\theta} \qquad (1)$$

This is known as the *bootstrap principle*. It is important to separate this principle from simulation, which is used to estimate the distribution of estimates $\hat{\theta}^\star$ given $\hat{\theta}$. In fact, there are two potential sources of error in bootstrap procedures. The first arises because the bootstrap principle does not hold true, i.e. the two distributions in equation (1) are not equal. The second arises because we only use a finite number of bootstrap samples, B, to estimate the distribution of the $\hat{\theta}$'s. However, this error can be made as small as we like by simply increasing B, whereas the bootstrap error is fixed. One of the arts of bootstrapping is to consider simple functions of θ, such as $(\hat{\theta} - \theta)/\hat{\sigma}$, (where $\hat{\sigma}$ is the sample standard error of $\hat{\theta}$) for which the bootstrap principle is more nearly true.

To make things more concrete, we illustrate how to use the bootstrap to estimate VARIANCE.

Consider the data in the Table. We are interested in estimating the average change in the carbon monoxide transfer factor. The obvious estimate is the MEAN: $(33+2+24+27+4+1-6)/7 = 12.14$. Suppose we were able to draw a large number, B, samples of the same size as that in the table from the 'population' of smokers with chickenpox and estimate the average change on each. Denote the resulting estimates by $\hat{\theta}_1, \ldots, \hat{\theta}_B$, and recall the true

bootstrap *Data on the carbon monoxide transfer factor for 7 smokers with chickenpox, measured on admission to hospital and after a stay of one week (Davison and Hinkley, 1997:67)*

Patient	Entry	Week	Change=(Week − Entry)
1	40	73	33
2	50	52	2
3	56	80	24
4	58	85	27
5	60	64	4
6	62	63	1
7	66	60	−6

value in the population is called θ. Then an estimate of the variance would be:

$$\frac{1}{B} \sum_{i=1}^{B} (\hat{\theta}_i - \theta)^2 \qquad (2)$$

Using the bootstrap principle (1), we estimate this by (i) replacing θ by its estimate from the data, $\hat{\theta}$, and (ii) replacing the $\hat{\theta}_i$ by $\hat{\theta}_i^{\star}$, where each $\hat{\theta}_i^{\star}$ is the mean carbon monoxide transfer in the ith bootstrap sample.

The second Table shows the bootstrap in action. The first row shows the observed differences, corresponding to the fourth column of the first table. The second row shows the frequency of these observations in the data in the first table; they all occur once. Rows 3–11 show the frequency of the observations in bootstrap samples 1–9. Thus, in the first bootstrap data set, observation one does not appear, observation two appears 3 times, observation 3 appears twice, observation 4 once, observation 5 does not appear, observation 6 appears once and observation 7 does not appear: the mean is then 11.71. The table shows $B = 9$ bootstrap samples. We thus have $\hat{\theta}_1^{\star}, \ldots, \hat{\theta}_9^{\star}$, each of which stands in approximately the same relationship to $\hat{\theta}$ as $\hat{\theta}$ does to the true parameter θ. We can use these to learn about the relationship between $\hat{\theta}$ and θ.

Specifically, the bootstrap estimate of variance is:

$$\frac{1}{B} \sum_{i=1}^{B} (\hat{\theta}_i^{\star} - \hat{\theta})^2 \qquad (3)$$

Comparing with (2), we see the bootstrap version (3) is derived by (i) putting '*'s next to everything with a 'hat' and (ii) putting a 'hat' on what is left. This rule of thumb is very useful in practice.

Substituting the bootstrap estimates from the second table gives:

$$\frac{1}{9} \begin{aligned}[t] &[(11.71 - 12.14)^2 \\ &+ (7.00 - 12.14)^2 \\ &+ (18.57 - 12.14)^2 \\ &+ (15.43 - 12.14)^2 \\ &+ (15.71 - 12.14)^2 \\ &+ (26.43 - 12.14)^2 \\ &+ (13.29 - 12.14)^2 \\ &+ (24.29 - 12.14)^2 \\ &+ (16.43 - 12.14)^2] = 7.17^2 \end{aligned}$$

However, $B = 9$ is not nearly enough. Typically we may need around $B = 800$ bootstrap samples to estimate the variance accurately (Booth and Sarkar, 1998). Taking $B = 1000$, we obtain the bootstrap variance of the mean is 5.39^2, which compares with the maximum likelihood estimate of 5.38^2. The bootstrap estimate of the standard error of the mean, 12.14, is thus 5.39. Of course, this example is only illustrative; we know the answer anyway. However, in many circumstances we may not, for example if the data are not normally distributed and we want the standard error of the median or some other non-standard measure of the data's 'centre'.

The bootstrap principle can clearly be applied much more widely. It is probably most often used to calculate confidence intervals (Carpenter and Bithell, 2000) where it avoids the need to rely on large sample theory or assumptions concerning the distribution of the data. For example, the distribution of individual patients' hospital costs is usually very skew and the bootstrap has been applied to calculate confidence intervals for average cost of hospitalisation.

Other applications include hypothesis tests, power calculations and estimating the predictive performance a statistical model will have when applied to a new dataset that was not used in formulating or estimating the model.

In order for the bootstrap principle (1) to hold, it is necessary for the bootstrap sampling to mimic the actual data sampling. So, if we are bootstrapping a clinical trial with two treatments, we should sample with replacement within each treatment group, to preserve the randomisation. Other situations require different approaches.

The bootstrap re-sampling illustrated here does not depend on any statistical model and is an example of the *non-parametric bootstrap*. An alternative, the parametric bootstrap, is less widely used. This samples data from a parametric statistical model, such as a regression model, rather than with replacement from the observed data.

Lastly, note the bootstrap, although it uses simulation, is characterised by the bootstrap principle (1). It is thus quite distinct from two other common uses of simulation, randomisation tests and MARKOV CHAIN MONTE CARLO (for fitting BAYESIAN MODELS).　　　*JRC*

[**Acknowledgement**: James R. Carpenter was supported by ESRC Research Methods Programme grant H333250047, titled 'Missing data in multi-level models'.]

bootstrap *Frequencies with which each difference from the original data in the first table appear in each of 9 non-parametric bootstrap samples*

	33	2	24	27	4	1	−6	Statistic (mean)
Observed differences								
Frequency in observed data	1	1	1	1	1	1	1	$\hat{\theta} = 12.14$
1st bootstrap sample		3	2	1		1		$\hat{\theta}_1^{\star} = 11.71$
2nd bootstrap sample	1	1	1			2	2	$\hat{\theta}_2^{\star} = 7.00$
3rd bootstrap sample	3	1		1		2		$\hat{\theta}_3^{\star} = 18.57$
4th bootstrap sample	1	1	1	2		1	1	$\hat{\theta}_4^{\star} = 15.43$
5th bootstrap sample		2	2	2	1			$\hat{\theta}_5^{\star} = 15.71$
6th bootstrap sample	4	1	1	1				$\hat{\theta}_6^{\star} = 26.43$
7th bootstrap sample	1	2	1	1	1	1		$\hat{\theta}_7^{\star} = 13.29$
8th bootstrap sample	2	1	2	2				$\hat{\theta}_8^{\star} = 24.29$
9th bootstrap sample	1	1	1	2		2		$\hat{\theta}_9^{\star} = 16.43$

Booth, J.G. and Sarkar, S. 1998: Monte-Carlo approximation of bootstrap variances. *The American Statistician* 52, 354–7. **Carpenter, J. and Bithell, J.** 2000: Bootstrap confidence intervals: when, which, what? A practical guide for medical statisticians. *Statistics in Medicine* 19, 1141–64. **Davison, A.C. and Hinkley, D.V.** 1997: *Bootstrap methods and their application.* Cambridge: Cambridge University Press. **Efron, B. and Tibshirani, R.** 1993: *An introduction to the bootstrap.* New York: Chapman & Hall.

box plot A graphical display useful for highlighting important distributional features of a variable. The diagram is based on the five-number summary of a dataset, the numbers being the minimum, the lower quartile, the MEDIAN, the upper quartile and the maximum. The box plot is constructed by first drawing a 'box' with ends at the lower and upper quartiles of the data, next a horizontal line (or some other feature) is used to indicate the position of the median within the box, then lines are drawn from each end of the box to the most remote observations. One convention modifies this last step by truncating the lines to within (unmarked) points given by the upper quartile plus 1.5 times the interquartile range (the difference between the upper and lower quartiles) and the lower quartile plus 1.5 times the interquartile range. In this case, any observations outside these limits are represented individually by some means in the finished graphic. Different computer packages may employ slightly different conventions for displaying extreme or outlying values.

The resulting diagram schematically represents the body of the data minus the extreme observations. Particularly useful for comparing the distributional features of a variable in different groups as illustrated in the Figure, which shows the birthweights of infants with severe idiopathic respiratory disorder, classified by whether or not the infant survived. For other examples see Altman (1991). *BSE*

[See also HISTOGRAM, STEM-AND-LEAF PLOT]

Altman, D.G. 1991: *Practical statistics for medical research.* London: Chapman & Hall.

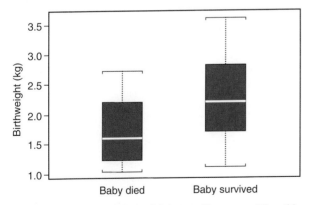

box plot *Birthweights (kg) of infants with severe idiopathic respiratory disease syndrome*

Box-Cox transformation See TRANSFORMATIONS

Bradford Hill criteria Guidelines for drawing conclusions about causal relationships, proposed by Sir Austin Bradford Hill, Professor Emeritus of Medical Statistics at the London School of Hygiene and Tropical Medicine, in his address to the Section of Occupational Medicine of the Royal Society of Medicine in 1965 (Bradford Hill, 1965). Bradford Hill's guidelines drew on his many contributions to chronic disease research in the post-war era, including the groundbreaking work with Richard Doll on the link between smoking and lung cancer. The following nine aspects were proposed for deciding whether a statistical association might be causal: strength – magnitude of the association, as observed by measures such as the ratio of incidence rates; consistency – repeated observation of the association in different populations and circumstances and by different researchers; specificity – whether a cause leads to a single effect in a given population; temporality – whether the cause precedes the effect in time; biological gradient – existence of a trend or dose-response curve between the cause and effect; plausibility – whether the association is consistent with current biological knowledge; coherence – ensuring that the interpretation of cause and effect does not conflict with what is known of the natural history of the disease; experiment – existence of experimental, rather than observational evidence, such as through conducting a randomised trial or by introduction of a preventive measure; analogy – comparison with previous research that identified similar effect mechanisms.

Bradford Hill did not intend these guidelines to be philosophically rigorous 'criteria' for causal inference, rather a basis for decision making that could lead to timely action for the good of public health. With further consideration, some of the guidelines (for example, 'specificity') are less than universal in their utility and some commentators have proposed alternative criteria more firmly rooted in deductive logic (Weed, 1986). However, in proposing these guidelines, Bradford Hill advocated an approach of making the best use of the totality of available evidence: 'All scientific work is incomplete – that does not confer upon us the freedom to ignore the knowledge we already have, or to postpone the action it demands.' *JGW*

Bradford Hill, A. 1965: The environment and disease: association or causation? *Proceedings of the Royal Society of Medicine* 58, 295. **Weed, D.L.** 1986: On the logic of causal inference. *American Journal of Epidemiology* 123, 965–79.

BUGS and WinBUGS The use of BAYESIAN METHODS in practical problems in medical statistics and other substantive areas of application has been hindered until relatively recently by computational aspects. In particular, the evaluation of integrals in order to obtain posterior marginal, conditional and predictive distributions in many multi-parameter problems are not usually analytically tractable and asymptotic, numerical integration techniques or simulation-based methods are required (Bernardo and Smith, 1994). In many practical problems in medical statistics the structure and nature of the models used have made parameter estimation particularly amenable to the use of MARKOV CHAIN MONTE CARLO (MCMC) simulation methods and it is these that the software packages Bayesian inference Using Gibbs Sampling (BUGS) and WinBUGS (Windows version of BUGS) implement. (Latest versions at the time of writing are BUGS 0.5 and WinBUGS 1.4 are freely available from www.mrc-bsu.cam.ac.uk.)

BUGS and WinBUGS use the BUGS syntax, which is

similar to that of S-PLUS & R, to specify the likelihood and prior distributions for the statistical model in question, together with initial starting values for the sampler (Gilks, Thomas and Spiegelhalter, 1994). Within WinBUGS specification of models may also be in terms of directed acyclic graphs (DAGs) using the Doodle feature [see GRAPHICAL MODELS], with the appropriate code being produced automatically.

Additions to the most recent version of WinBUGS (1.4) are the ability to use scripts so that WinBUGS may be used in 'batch mode' and improved graphics capabilities, together with calculation of the deviance information criterion (DIC) to assess model complexity and fit (see BAYESIAN METHODS). In addition, the suite of S-PLUS functions CODA (Best, Cowles and Vines, 1995) can be used to explore convergence issues with output from BUGS and WinBUGS.

Specific developments of WinBUGS are PKBUGS, which allows MCMC methods to be used for complex population *pharmacokinetic/pharmacodynamic* (PK/PD)

models and GeoBUGS, which is an add-on to WinBUGS that fits spatial models and produces a range of maps as output.

Since BUGS and WinBUGS require the user to specify statistical models in terms of the LIKELIHOOD and PRIOR DISTRIBUTIONS (see BAYESIAN METHODS), then to use MCMC methods in order to evaluate the model, it is only recommended for users skilled at undertaking Bayesian analyses and must therefore be used with considerable care – the manual even comes with a 'health warning'!

KRA

Bernardo, J.M. and Smith, A.F.M. 1994: *Bayesian theory.* Chichester: John Wiley & Sons. **Best, N.G., Cowles, M.K. and Vines, S.K.** 1995: CODA convergence diagnosis and output analysis software for Gibbs Sampler output: Version 0.3. MRC Biostatistics Unit, Cambridge. **Gilks, W.R., Thomas, A. and Spiegelhalter, D.J.** 1994: A language and program for complex Bayesian modelling. *The Statistician* 43, 169–78. **Spiegelhalter, D.J., Thomas, A. and Best, N.G.** 2001: *WinBUGS version 1.4 user manual.* Cambridge: MRC Biostatistics Unit.

C

---

calibration Consider a situation in which we wish to measure serum concentrations of hormones, enzymes and other proteins, for example, using such methods as radioimmunoassays (RIA) and enzyme-linked immunosorbent assays (ELIZA). Three key questions in the development of such assays are: how does the expected value (average) of the assay response change as a function of the true amount of the target material in the serum samples; how does the VARIANCE (or STANDARD DEVIATION) of the assay results change with the average assay result; and, subsequently, how might we use a particular assay result to determine the amount of the target material in a new sample of serum?

We leave the last question for the time being and concentrate on the first two. Let the assay response be Y and let the true level of the target material be X. We wish to determine the form of the functions F and G in the following two equations:

$$E(Y|X) = F(X) \qquad (1)$$

and

$$\mathrm{Var}(Y|X) = G(E(Y|X)) \qquad (2)$$

Here we assume that the values of X are known without MEASUREMENT ERROR. We are concerned with what is often referred to as *absolute calibration*. If we do not have access to the truth, but only have measurements using alternative assays, $Y1$ and $Y2$, say, then we are concerned with the problem of comparative calibration (for the latter, see METHOD COMPARISON STUDIES). Typically, such a univariate calibration study involves performing the assay procedure (ideally with full, independent, replications) on each of N training samples or specimens with known values of X and then, using various data analytic and modelling procedures, to evaluate the form of F and G. The statistical methods might be fully parametric (fitting linear or non-linear models, for example, with an assumed parametric model for the variance) or non-parametric (essentially fitting an arbitrarily shaped smooth dose-response curve).

Suppose an analytical chemist wishes to use some form of absorption spectroscopy to study the composition of say, certain body fluids. He or she is likely to use measurements of many peak heights from such spectra to measure several substances simultaneously. This activity is the multivariate analogue of the univariate case; that is, multivariate calibration. Technically, multivariate calibration is much more difficult than the simpler univariate problem, but the ultimate aims and logic are similar. We start with the latter and then briefly discuss the former.

Instead of dealing with the technical complexities of fitting non-linear models with heterogeneous error distributions, we will consider an example, which by comparison, appears to be quite simple. Suppose we have a simple colorimetric assay for urinary glucose. We obtain a series of specimens with known glucose concentrations (X) and

then measure the absorbance (Y) using the relevant assay procedure. We assume that the calibration function F is a straight line and that the variance of the Y measurements is independent of X (that is, the 'error' variance is constant). Fitting a simple linear regression model for Y using ordinary least squares gives us estimates of the intercept (α) and slope (β) of the straight line relating X to Y. Having answered our first two questions using the simple regression analysis, we now move on to our last question. Suppose we are presented with a new urine specimen and are asked to determine its glucose content.

The classical method of estimating the unknown X from our measurement, Y, involves using information from the regression of Y on X. The required estimate is given by:

$$X = (Y - \alpha)/\beta \qquad (3)$$

An alternative is the so-called inverse estimator suggested by Krutchkoff (1967). This involves using the original X, Y data to regress X on Y to obtain estimates of the intercept (γ) and slope (λ) and then simply using these parameter estimates to predict X given a new $Y1$. That is:

$$X = \hat{\gamma} + \hat{\lambda}Y \qquad (4)$$

For details of the properties of these two estimators, see the review by Osborne (1991).

To illustrate the ideas of multivariate calibration, consider a relatively simple example. Suppose we wish to measure the concentration of a particular metabolite in the blood (X) but we are now able to use, say, three different colorimetric assay procedures to obtain values $Y1$, $Y2$ and $Y3$. Assuming that the three corresponding calibration curves ($F1$, $F2$ and $F3$), as before, are all straight lines (but with different intercepts, slopes and 'error' VARIANCES) we can use multivariate linear regression (or three separate regressions) in order to estimate the parameters of the three calibration curves. The classical approach to the use of a new set of three measurements ($Y1$, $Y2$ and $Y3$) on a new specimen to predict an unknown X is the multivariate generalisation of the univariate problem. Details of multivariate calibration are well beyond the scope of the present article, however, and readers are referred to Thomas (1994) and Naes *et al.* (2002), for further information. Considering our present example, one simple approach (particularly if we are prepared to assume conditional independence of the Ys) might involve estimating the unknown X using each of the $Y1$, $Y2$ and $Y3$ separately (in each case using equation (3)) and then producing a weighted average of these three estimates, with weights proportional to their estimated precision. An example of the inverse approach would be to produce a multiple regression to predict the unknown X from the three Y measurements. This has obvious technical drawbacks, however, because of MULTICOLLINEARITY (high correlations between the three Ys). One possible solution involves the use of *principal components regression*. A PRINCIPAL COMPONENT ANALYSIS is carried out using the *Y*s and then one or more of the resulting components are used to predict the unknown *X*. Further details of principal components regression and alternative analytical strategies can be found in Thomas (1994) and Naes *et al.* (2002). Whatever method of prediction is used, however, it is important in both univariate and multivariate calibration problems that the performance of the predictions is adequately evaluated. This might involve validation using a test set of new *X*, *Y* values or internal cross-validation (use of the leave-one-out approach, for example) using the original training set. *GD*

Dunn, G. 2004: *Statistical evaluation of measurement errors.* London: Arnold. **Krutchkoff, R.G.** 1967: Classical and inverse regression methods of calibration. *Technometrics* 9, 425–39. **Naes, T., Isaksson, T., Fearn, T. and Davies, T.** 2002: *A user-friendly guide to multivariate calibration and classification.* Chichester: NIR Publications. **Osborne, C.** 1991: Statistical calibration: a review. *International Statistical Review* 59, 309–36. **Thomas, E.V.** 1994: A primer on multivariate calibration. *Analytical Chemistry* 66, 795A–804A.

caliper matching   See MATCHING

canonical correlation analysis

A technique for establishing whether relationships exist between *a priori* groups of variables in a study. For example, in a study of heart disease, we might ask if there is a connection between personal physical characteristics such as age, weight and height, on the one hand, and the systolic and diastolic blood pressures of the individuals, on the other. Or, in chronic depression, a study might be aimed at uncovering relationships between personal social and financial variables such as gender, age, educational level, income and a range of health variables including various indicators of depression. Another example, in a public health survey might be conducted to explore connections between housing quality variables and indicators of different illnesses.

A first attempt at analysing the strength of association between two *groups* of variables (e.g. between housing quality and illness) might involve examination of all correlations between pairs of variables, one from each group. However, if each group contains more than just a few variables, such an approach is bound to lead to confusion. Ideally, one would like to replace each set of original variables by a new set, in such a way that the new variables were mutually uncorrelated within sets and just a few of them exhibited correlation between sets. Canonical correlation analysis takes just such an approach, and finds optimal sets of *linear transformations* of the original variables, one for each original group of variables. Suppose that $u_1, u_2, ..., u_s$ are the transformed variables for one set (say, the housing quality variables), while $v_1, v_2, ..., v_s$ are the transformed variables for the other set (say, the illness variables).

'Optimality' is defined by requiring the correlation between u_1 and v_1 to be as large as possible among all linear combinations of the original variables, that between u_2 and v_2 to be the next largest, that between u_3 and v_3 the third largest and so on, subject to the following constraints: $u_1, u_2, ..., u_s$ are mutually uncorrelated; $v_1, v_2, ..., v_s$ are mutually uncorrelated; and any u_i, v_j pair is uncorrelated when $i \neq j$.

It is clearly not possible to have more (uncorrelated) transformed variables than there were original variables in a set, so the number *s* of pairs that can be derived is equal to the *smaller* of the numbers of original variables in the two groups.

The effect of canonical correlation analysis is thus to channel all the association between the two groups of variables through the resulting pairs of linear combinations $(u_1, v_1), (u_2, v_2), ...$ These derived variables are known as *canonical variates*. The only non-zero correlations remaining in the correlation matrix of the new variables are those between corresponding pairs of canonical variates, i.e. between u_i and v_i for $i = 1, ..., s$; they are known as the *canonical correlations* of the system. Most computer software packages that contain multivariate statistical procedures will conduct such an analysis. They will also quote a significance level against each canonical correlation, appropriate for testing the null hypothesis that all succeeding population canonical correlations are zero. Such significance levels should be treated with some caution, as they rely on the assumption that the data follow a MULTIVARIATE NORMAL DISTRIBUTION. Nonetheless, the number of significant canonical correlations is usually taken to indicate the number of (independent) connections that exist between the two groups of variables.

Inspection of the coefficients of each original variable in each canonical variate may also provide an interpretation of the canonical variate in the same manner as interpretation of principal components, which may help to identify the nature of the connection between the groups (see PRINCIPAL COMPONENT ANALYSIS). However, again a cautionary note is in order, because such interpretation is not quite as straightforward as for principal components. The reason for the complication is that there may be very diverse VARIANCES and covariances among the original variables in the two groups, which affects the sizes of the coefficients in the canonical variates, and there is no convenient normalisation to place all coefficients on an equal footing. This drawback can be alleviated to some extent by restricting interpretation to the *standardised* coefficients, i.e. the coefficients that are appropriate when the original variables have been standardised, but nevertheless the problem still remains.

To illustrate the technique, consider a canonical correlation analysis between the 'health' variables and the 'personal' variables in the Los Angeles depression study of 294 respondents presented by Afifi and Clark (1984, Chapter 15). The four 'personal' variables were: gender, age, income, education level (numerically coded from the lowest, 'less than high school', to the highest, 'finished doctorate'), while the two 'health' variables were: CESD (the sum of 20 separate numerical scales measuring different aspects of depression) and health (a numerical score measuring 'general health'). The correlation matrix between these variables for the sample is shown in the Table on page 43.

Here the maximum number of canonical variate pairs is $s = min(2, 4) = 2$. The first canonical correlation turns out to be 0.405 and this gives a significance level $P < 0.00001$. It might be argued that gender and education are unlikely to have normal distributions, so this significance level should not be taken too literally. Nevertheless, there does seem to be strong evidence that the first canonical

canonical correlation analysis *Correlation matrix for two health and four personal variables in LA depression study*

	CESD	Health	Gender	Age	Education	Income
CESD	1.0	0.212	0.124	−0.164	−0.101	−0.158
Health		1.0	0.098	0.308	−0.270	−0.183
Gender			1.0	0.044	−0.106	−0.180
Age				1.0	−0.208	−0.192
Education					1.0	0.492
Income						1.0

correlation is significant. The corresponding canonical variates, in terms of standardised original variables, are:

$$u_1 = -0.490CESD + 0.982Health$$

$$v_1 = 0.025Gender + 0.871Age - 0.383Education + 0.082Income$$

High coefficients correspond to CESD (negatively) and health (positively) for the perceived health variables and to age (positively) and education (negatively) for the personal variables. Thus relatively older and uneducated people tend to score low in terms of depression, but perceive their health as relatively poor, while relatively younger but educated people have the opposite health perception.

The second canonical correlation is 0.266, which has a significance level $P<0.001$ so also carries interpretative worth. The corresponding canonical variates are:

$$u_2 = 0.899CESD + 0.288Health$$

$$v_2 = 0.396Gender - 0.443Age - 0.448Education - 0.555Income$$

Since the higher value of the gender variable is for females, the interpretation here is that relatively young, poor and uneducated females are associated with higher depression scores and, to a lesser extent, with poor perceived health. Thus there are two interpretable 'dimensions' of connection between the two sets of variables. A SCATTERPLOT of the scores of respondents against each pair of canonical variates would help to identify any anomalous individuals in the sample.

A further interesting application of canonical correlation analysis occurs when there is just a single set of variables, but they are measured on individuals in a number of *a priori* distinct groups or populations. For example, a set of signs or symptoms $x_1, x_2, ..., x_p$ is observed on a sample of patients suffering from jaundice and each patient is classified into one of g illnesses that have the external manifestation of jaundice. We can thus define a set of indicator variables $y_1, y_2, ..., y_g$ that specify a patient's illness, by setting the values $y_i = 1$, $y_j = 0$ ($j \neq i$) for a patient suffering from illness i. A canonical correlation analysis with the xs as one set of variables and the ys as the other set of variables will then produce the linear combinations of the xs that are most highly correlated with linear combinations of the group indicator variables. Since the latter define the best way to view group differences, the former are just the canonical variables that best discriminate between the g groups of individuals (see DISCRIMINANT FUNCTION ANALYSIS).

Finally, the variables in a study may fall into more than two *a priori* sets and some general between-set measure of

association is required. Various possible definitions of such association may be made and, consequently, the ideas of canonical correlation analysis may be generalised in various ways. However, such generalisation is quite complicated and interpretation of the results becomes much more problematic. Gnanadesikan (1997) provides a brief overview and further references.   *WK*

[See also DISCRIMINANT FUNCTION ANALYSIS, PRINCIPAL COMPONENT ANALYSIS]

Afifi, A.A. and Clark, V. 1984: *Computer-aided multivariate analysis*. California: Wadsworth. **Gnanadesikan, R.** 1997: *Methods for statistical analysis of multivariate observations*, 2nd edn. New York: John Wiley & Sons.

canonical variates See CANONICAL CORRELATIONS ANALYSIS

capture-recapture methods An alternative approach to a census for estimating population size that operates by sampling the population several times, identifying individuals who appear more than once. Capture-recapture methods have a long history dating back to 1786, when Laplace used such a technique to estimate the size of the total population of France. The original capture-recapture methodology was primarily focused on wildlife populations, but has increasingly been applied to human populations, particularly within epidemiological situations. Within the ecological field, capture-recapture experiments involve observers going into the field and recording all animals that are observed (either visual sightings or trappings) at a sequence of capture events. On the initial capture event, all animals that are observed are recorded, uniquely marked and released back into the population. At each subsequent capture event, all unmarked animals are recorded and uniquely marked; all marked animals are recorded; and all animals released. Then the data from such an experiment are simply the record of the capture histories for each individual animal observed within the study.

There are generally two forms of models: closed and open. Closed models assume that the population is constant throughout the study period, with no births, deaths or migrations, whereas open models allow for these transitions in the population. Generally speaking, the parameters of interest differ between the two models. For example, within closed populations, the total population size is generally of particular interest; conversely, for open populations, parameters of interest may include birth rates, death rates, migration rates and/or productivity rates. There have been a series of models proposed for analysing both closed and open populations. For closed populations, Otis *et al.* (1978) described a series of different capture-recapture models, relating to possible heterogeneity in the capture rates as a result of time, trap response or individual effects. Similarly, there have been a series of models proposed for open populations, dependent on the parameters of interest, with perhaps the most widely used being the Cormack-Jolly-Seber model, where the survival rates are of primary interest, and the Arnason-Schwarz model, which incorporates multi-strata data. Within the epidemiological literature, closed populations are usually modelled, with the total population size of particular interest – and this is what we shall focus on here.

Within the epidemiological field the capture-recapture approach is sometimes called 'multiple record systems' and the corresponding estimate of the total population referred to as 'Bernoulli census estimates' or 'ascertainment corrected rates'.

Many areas of scientific research focus on the estimation of population size: from the number of susceptibles to a given disease, to the number of drug addicts in a particular area or the number of injuries sustained in the workplace. However, it is usually impossible to enumerate each member of a population, possibly due to their number (for example, the number of web pages on the internet) or when the population is 'hidden' (such as the number of drug addicts). Thus, data are often collected in the form of a series of incomplete population counts using a variety of sources or lists. Each source corresponds to a capture event and an individual being recorded by a given source corresponds to being observed at that capture event. It is assumed that each individual is uniquely identifiable by each source. Then, the data are simply the capture histories of all individuals observed. This is represented by a series of 0s and 1s, where the 0 and the 1 denote the absence or presence of the individual on the given list. The data are usually summarised in the form of a 2^k contingency table, where k is the number of sources, and the cell entries correspond to the number of individuals that are observed by each combination of sources. Clearly, the contingency table is incomplete since the number of individuals belonging to the population but not observed within the study is unknown (see the table below, for example). Unlike the ecological application the sources do not usually have a temporal sequencing as for the capture events and so different models have been developed within the epidemiological application.

The most common approach to analysing epidemiological data of this sort is via the use of LOG-LINEAR MODELS, introduced by Fienberg (1972). In these models, the logarithm of the expected cell count is expressed as a linear function of parameters. These parameters represent main effect terms for individual sources; and associations between two or more sources. Thus, these models allow for interactions between different sources, and for which the model assuming independence between each source is a special case. There are usually a number of possible log-linear models that can be fitted to the data, each specifying different sets of interactions between the sources.

Traditionally, classical analyses consist of initially finding the model which provides the best fit to the data, using for example LIKELIHOOD RATIO TESTS and/or information criteria, such as AKAIKE'S INFORMATION CRITERION (AIC) or *Bayesian information criterion* (BIC). Once the given model has been selected, the total population is estimated

capture-recapture methods *Example of an incomplete contingency table, with three sources – A, B and C. The entries n_{ijk} denote the number of individuals observed in the given cell, where 0/1 represents absence/presence on the given list. The cell n_{000} is unobserved and hence unknown*

		C=1	C=0
A=1	B=1	n_{111}	n_{110}
A=1	B=0	n_{101}	n_{100}
A=0	B=1	n_{011}	n_{010}
A=0	B=0	n_{001}	n_{000}

using the MAXIMUM LIKELIHOOD ESTIMATOR for the missing cell, combined with the observed number of individuals (see, for example, Hook and Regal, 1995). Recently, Bayesian approaches have also been developed for fitting log-linear models to the data, and in particular the issue of model choice (King and Brooks, 2001). This approach also allows the calculation of a model-averaged estimate of the total population, removing the model-dependence problem that may arise when only a single model is chosen on which to base inference. Alternative approaches to using log-linear models include the use of Rasch model (see Carriquiry and Fienberg, 1998) in order to model possible heterogeneity in the population and also latent class models where the individuals can be categorised into different sub-populations. *RK*

Carriquiry, A.L. and Fienberg, S.E. 1998: Rasch models. In Armitage, P. and Colton, T. (eds), *Encyclopedia of biostatistics*. Chichester: John Wiley & Sons. **Fienberg, S.E.** 1972: The multiple recapture census for closed populations and incomplete 2^k contingency tables. *Biometrika* 59, 591–603. **Hook, E.B. and Regal, R.R.** 1995: Capture-recapture methods in epidemiology: Methods and limitations. *Epidemiological Reviews* 17, 243–64. **King, R. and Brooks, S.P.** 2001: On the Bayesian analysis of population size. *Biometrika* 88, 317–36. **Otis, D.L., Burnham, K.P., White, G.C. and Anderson, D.R.** 1978: Statistical inference from capture data on closed animal populations. *Wildlife Monographs* 62, 1–135.

carry-over See CROSS-OVER TRIALS

CART Acronym for classification and regression tree. See TREE-STRUCTURED METHODS

cartogram A diagram in which descriptive statistical information is displayed on a geographical map by means of shading, by using a variety of different symbols or by some more involved procedure. Two examples are given on page 45. *BSE*

[See also DISEASE CLUSTERING]

case-cohort studies See CASE-CONTROL STUDIES

case-control studies Studies in which a group of people with the disease of interest (the cases) is compared with a group without the disease (the controls). Exposure to the risk factor of interest is then ascertained in all those recruited to the study and the exposure levels of the cases are compared with those of the controls. Differing levels of exposure between the cases and controls indicate that the exposure is associated with the disease. Such studies are particularly appropriate for rare diseases for which follow-up studies are inappropriate, as insufficient cases of the disease would arise to provide sufficient statistical POWER.

It is important at the outset to have a clear definition of the type of person who is eligible to be a case. Issues that need to be considered include:

(1) *The definition of the disease.* Can this be broadly defined or is a specific subtype of the disease the focus of interest? For example, in a study of leukaemia a decision needs to be made as to whether all cases of leukaemia will be included or only a specific subtype such as chronic myeloid.

(2) *The age range of the cases*: some diseases are likely to have different causes at different ages.

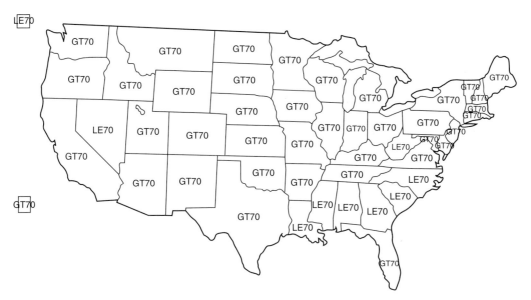

cartogram *Cartogram of life expectancy in the USA by state. <70 = 70 years or less, >70 = more than 70 years*

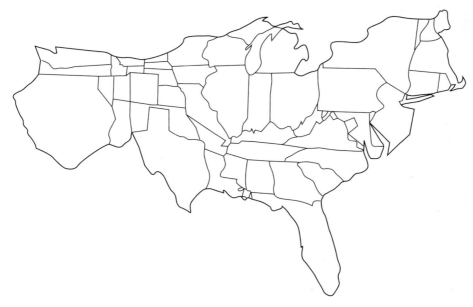

cartogram *1996 US population cartogram (all state are resized relative to their population)*

(3) *The sex of the cases*: for some disorders, it would be appropriate to restrict the sex of the cases. For example, while cases of breast cancer do arise in men, the aetiology of these is likely to be very different from that of the disease in women.

(4) *Incident, prevalent or dead cases*: it is usually preferable to recruit cases when they are diagnosed (incident cases). However, for diseases that are very rare it can take too long to recruit sufficient cases. They can therefore be supplemented by existing (prevalent) cases. However, for diseases that can lead to death, the prevalent cases will only represent the survivors. To avoid survivor bias, deceased cases can be included if the next of kin can provide the appropriate information on the exposure of interest.

(5) *Hospital or community cases*: a decision needs to be taken as to where the cases are to be found. If the disease is of such a nature that all cases are likely to come to hospital (e.g. breast cancer), then the hospital may be an appropriate recruitment location. For diseases that are often treated in the community such as back pain, recruitment from hospital would only include cases at the most severe end of the disease spectrum.

Equally, besides the choice of cases, there are important considerations for the selection of controls, who should be drawn from the population at risk of becoming cases. In theory, the cases and controls can be considered as being part of a large hypothetical cohort study. Those who

45

develop the disease are the cases and those who have not acquired it form the pool from which the controls are drawn. Thus, controls should be drawn carefully from the group of people who would be classified as cases if they happened to develop the disease.

Controls should be within the same age range as that chosen for the cases, and if only one sex is being considered for the cases, the same restriction should apply to the controls. If the cases are recruited in hospital then the controls may also be recruited from the hospital or from the community defined by the catchment area of the hospital. Any exclusion criteria applied to the cases must also be applied to the controls and the controls must be at risk of developing the disease. For example, in a case-control study of endometrial cancer, it was important that women who had had a hysterectomy and thus no longer had an endometrium, were not included as controls (Barbone, Austin and Partridge, 1993).

Increasingly, matched case-control studies are being conducted. One or more controls are chosen for each case, matched as closely as possible to the case for various factors that are not of intrinsic interest to the study. Common matching factors are age and sex. Thus for each case, a control of the same age (to perhaps within one year) and the same sex would be chosen. One-to-one matching gives rise to a matched pair study. To increase the statistical power of the study, more than one control can be chosen for each case. This is particularly useful if the disease is rare and it is hard to find sufficient cases. However, it is rarely worth studying more than 4 controls per case, as the effort spent in collecting the data on the extra controls tends to outweigh the minimal increase in power.

Frequently, the exposures will be assessed by QUESTION-NAIRES. This can present logistical difficulties if the cases are very sick and sometimes (as with deceased cases) the next of kin need to be questioned instead. For example, in a case-control study to examine the risk of sudden infant death syndrome in relation to used infant mattresses, all the exposure data were collected by questionnaire (Tappin et al., 2002). Exposure to a used infant mattress was assessed by asking parents about routine night and day sleeping place and ascertaining the state of the mattress and whether it was new for this baby. Other studies have been able to link records with data held on the individuals. For example, a study of Alzheimer's disease in relation to levels of aluminium in drinking water was able to utilise records from the water companies to ascertain the aluminium levels in water piped to each address at which the cases and controls had lived during their lives (Martyn et al., 1997).

A particular concern in case-control studies is the possibility of RECALL BIAS, particularly when obtaining information by questionnaire from the cases and controls. The cases are likely to have thought about the possible causes of their disease, whereas the controls will not. Thus the level of recall of past exposures may differ between cases and controls, which may lead to spurious differences in exposure between the two groups.

One of the most difficult aspects of a case-control study is ensuring that the choice of controls is appropriate. Controls that are not representative of the population at risk of the disease will lead to biased findings (see BIAS IN OBSERVATIONAL STUDIES). An example is when cases are asked to choose a friend to act as the control. Such an approach tends to maximise the response rate in the controls (as the controls are usually willing to help their sick friends). But, if the exposure of interest is related to work or leisure activities or lifestyle, then the friends will be more similar to the cases than the average person in the population at risk. Thus 'overmatching' of controls to cases takes place and little difference may be found between the exposures of the cases and the controls. Any association between the disease and the exposure can therefore be missed.

Issues of bias need to be addressed at the design stage of a case-control study as no adjustment can be made in the analysis to take account of it.

In common with all epidemiological studies, *confounding* is an issue that has to be considered in case-control studies. A confounding factor is one that is related both to the disease under study and the exposure of interest. Account can be taken of confounding factors at the analysis stage, but it is important at the design stage to identify and collect as much information as possible on all putative confounding factors. Common confounding factors are age and sex as these two factors are invariably related to any disease and to most exposures. Matching at the design stage on one or more confounders provides a way of removing the effect of these confounders and so adjustment for them is not needed in the analysis.

The appropriate method of analysis depends on the type of case-control study employed. The analytical methods for matched case-control studies differ from those for unmatched studies and it is important that the appropriate methods are employed to avoid bias in the results. Basic methods of analysis in unmatched studies are described next.

Estimates of risk of disease in the unexposed and exposed groups cannot be obtained from case-control studies, because the case-control ratio has been fixed in the design. However, it is possible to obtain an estimate of the relative risk of disease from the odds ratio. The simplest form of a case-control study arises when exposure is classified into two groups, namely exposed and unexposed. The data can then be presented in a 2×2 table.

case-control studies *2×2 table for comparing $a + c$ cases with $b + d$ controls*

	Cases	Controls
Exposed	a	b
Unexposed	c	d

Recall that the ODDS RATIO is the ratio of the odds of exposure in the cases (a/c) to the odds of exposure among the controls (b/d) and thus is calculated as ad/bc. Odds ratios above 1 imply that the exposure is associated with an increased risk of the disease whereas a value below 1 indicates that the exposure may be protective.

As an example, consider a study of cod liver oil in infancy in relation to child-onset Type I diabetes (Stene et al., 2003). The results are given in the second Table (see page 47).

The odds ratio is $197 \times 834/(777 \times 318) = 0.66$ indicating that cod liver oil appears to protect against child-onset diabetes.

Standard analysis of a 2×2 table using a CHI-SQUARE TEST can be performed to test whether the odds ratio dif-

case-control studies *Results of a case-control study in Type I diabetes*

Cod liver oil in 1st year of life	Cases	Controls
Yes	197	777
No	318	834

fers significantly from 1. 95% CONFIDENCE INTERVALS can be derived using a variety of approximate methods. The most sophisticated methods require iterative solutions but simple methods such as that proposed by Woolf in 1955 (see Breslow and Day, 1980; Schlesselman, 1982) provide reasonable approximations. Woolf's method involves calculating the approximate VARIANCE of the natural logarithm of the odds ratio as:

$$\frac{1}{a} + \frac{1}{b} + \frac{1}{c} + \frac{1}{d}$$

and then obtaining the 95% confidence interval of the natural logarithm of the odds ratio from:

$$\ln(OR) \pm 1.96 \times \sqrt{\mathrm{var}(\log(OR))}$$

Taking exponentials of the two resulting values gives the 95% confidence interval for the odds ratio.

In the example we have just seen the chi-square test gives a value of 15.3 indicating p<0.0001 and a 95% confidence interval for the odds ratio of 0.54 to 0.81. Thus the association between cod liver oil and diabetes appears to be strong.

However, odds ratios and their confidence intervals are usually derived using computer packages. One that is freely available and provides ready access to these forms of analysis is EPIINFO (www.cdc.gov/epiinfo/). This can be downloaded via the internet and is in the public domain.

More often we are interested in examining different levels of exposure. A trend in odds ratios across different levels of an ordered, categorical exposure provides more convincing evidence of a relationship between the exposure and the disease than results from the simple dichotomy of exposed versus unexposed.

Odds ratios can be calculated at each level of exposure compared with the baseline exposure level (usually the unexposed). A chi-square test for trend can be performed to test for linear trend in the odds ratios.

In our third Table, there is an apparent trend with more frequent consumption of cod liver oil leading to lower odds ratios. The chi-square test for trend leads to a significance level of *p*<0.001.

More sophisticated analyses are possible using LOGISTIC REGRESSION. This allows assessment of exposure on a continuous scale (rather than requiring grouping into levels) as well as allowing for the effects of confounding factors.

case-control studies *Case-control study data according to an ordinal exposure*

Cod liver oil in 1st year of life	Cases	Controls	Odds ratio
No	318	834	1 (reference)
Yes, 1–4 times per week	60	224	0.70
Yes, ≥5 times per week	137	553	0.65

The coefficients obtained in the logistic regression model are the logarithm of the odds ratios, thus allowing odds ratios and their confidence intervals to be readily obtained from such models.

In a matched study, the controls have deliberately been chosen to be more similar to the cases than those generally at risk of the disease. This has to be recognised in the analysis.

The analysis of matched studies is more complex than for unmatched studies and in the discussion of the basic analysis, only matched pairs analyses will be considered. The analysis focuses on the pairs rather than the individuals contributing to the pairs and the standard presentation of the data is as follows:

		Control	
		Exposed	Unexposed
Case	Exposed	r	s
	Unexposed	t	u

Thus each pair contributes to one of the cells and the total ($r+s+t+u$) is the total number of pairs rather than the total number of individual cases and controls in the study. Interest focuses on the ($s+t$) pairs that are discordant for exposure. A comparison is made, therefore, between those pairs where the case is exposed but the control is not and the pairs where the control is exposed and the case is not. The odds ratio is calculated as the ratio of the discordant pairs s/t. The odds ratio will therefore be high if the pairs with case exposed and control unexposed greatly outnumber the pairs where the control is exposed but the case is not.

As an example, consider a study on hip osteoarthritis by Cooper *et al.* (1998) that examined the risk associated with previous hip injury to the affected hip (or to the hip on the same side – right or left – for the matched control). The data from the study are given in the fourth Table.

case-control studies *Data from a matched case-control study in hip osteoarthritis*

		Control	
		Previous hip injury	No previous injury
Case	Previous hip injury	1	46
	No previous injury	11	553

The odds ratio is 46/11 = 4.2

Basic analysis of matched studies becomes difficult in anything other than the matched paired analysis of a simple dichotomous exposure. Nowadays, matched case-control studies are usually analysed using CONDITIONAL LOGISTIC REGRESSION. This is not the same as unconditional logistic regression mentioned earlier, as it takes account of the matching structure in the design of the study.

Conditional logistic regression enables us to test the odds ratio calculated already, giving *p*<0.0001 and a 95% confidence interval around the odds ratio of 2.2 to 8.1. This indicates that hip injury is associated with an increased risk of hip osteoarthritis later in life.

Unmatched case-control studies can be analysed in most standard statistical computing packages. Logistic regression is used in many forms of analysis not confined to case-control studies. Conditional logistic regression is somewhat more specialised and is not available in all packages. It is most readily available in STATA, but can be performed in SAS and SPLUS (see STATISTICAL PACKAGES). It cannot be done in SPSS. EPIINFO, mentioned earlier, does enable much of the basic analyses and this can be useful if one is examining data that are already tabulated (such as in a published paper) rather than in the raw form of data on individuals. *HI*

[See also NESTED CASE-CONTROL STUDIES, SAMPLE SIZE DETERMINATION IN OBSERVATIONAL STUDIES]

Barbone, F., Austin, H. and Partridge, E.E. 1993: Diet and endometrial cancer: a case-control study. *American Journal of Epidemiology* 137, 393–403. **Breslow, N.E. and Day, N.E.** 1980: *Statistical methods in cancer research.* Vol. 1: *The analysis of case-control studies.* Lyon: International Agency for Research on Cancer. **Cooper, C., Inskip, H., Croft, P., Campbell, L., Smith, G., McLaren, M. and Coggon, D.** 1998: Individual risk factors for hip osteoarthritis: obesity, hip injury, and physical activity. *American Journal of Epidemiology* 147, 516–22. **Martyn, C., Coggon, D., Inskip, H., Lacey, R. and Young, W.** 1997: Aluminium concentrations in drinking water and risk of Alzheimer's disease. *Epidemiology* 8, 281–6. **Schlesselman, J.J.** 1982: *Case-control studies. Design, conduct and analysis.* Oxford: Oxford University Press. **Tappin, D., Brooke, H., Ecob, R. and Gibson, A.** 2002: Used infant mattresses and sudden infant death syndrome in Scotland: case-control study. *British Medical Journal* 325, 1007–12.

categorising continuous variables

The process of converting a continuous variable such as age, into a categorical variable with a number of categories, for example, 'young' (<40 years), 'middle aged' (40–60 years) and 'old' (>60). The practice is very common in medical research where clinicians appear to have a general preference for categorising individuals (see Altman, 1991). And when used to simplify or improve the presentation and description of the data, grouping individuals into categories may often be useful, although the choice of category boundaries and number of categories may not be easy. When, however, the categorical variables created by the process are used in data analysis, rather than the original continuous variables, problems arise (see, for example, Hunter and Schmidt, 1990; Streiner, 2002).

Categorisation introduces an extreme form of MEASUREMENT ERROR; splitting a continuous variable into categories results in lost information and an inevitable loss of POWER in analysis. The apparent simplicity of the categorical variables and the ability to use proportions and odds ratios, which are more familiar to many clinicians, are unlikely to compensate for the lost power. Retaining the continuous variable and analysing the data using the appropriate statistical methodology will always be a far better strategy. *BSE*

Altman, D.G. 1991: Categorising continuous variables. *British Journal of Cancer* 64, 975. **Hunter, J.E. and Schmidt, F.L.** 1990: Dichotomisation of continuous variables: the implications for meta-analysis. *Journal of Applied Psychology* 75, 334–49. **Streiner, D.L.** 2002: Breaking up is hard to do: heartbreak of dichotomizing continuous data. *Canadian Journal of Psychiatry* 47, 262–6.

causal diagram See CAUSAL MODELS

causal models

Models attempting to discover whether an observed association between an exposure (e.g. cigarette smoking) and an outcome (e.g. high blood pressure) arises because the exposure causes the disease or whether it is a *spurious association*. A spurious association can arise if both the exposure and the disease have one (or more) common cause – for example, if socioeconomic status is a cause of both high blood pressure and cigarette smoking. There are four major types of causal model (see Greenland and Brumback, 2002) and many definitions of 'causal' in an epidemiological context (see Parascandola and Weed, 2001).

One type of causal model is the *causal diagram* (Greenland and Brumback, 2002; Hernan *et al.*, 2002). Such diagrams link exposure, outcome and other variables by arrows representing direct causal effects. A hypothetical example for smoking and high blood pressure is shown in the first Figure.

Such diagrams can be drawn from prior knowledge of causal mechanisms. Uses include deciding whether adjusting for confounding variables would increase or decrease bias. For example, from the figure, one would adjust for socioeconomic status in analysing the relationship between smoking and high blood pressure (as it is a common cause). (For more details, see Hernan, *et al.*, 2002.)

A second type of causal model, the *counterfactual model*, arises from a definition of CAUSALITY: 'Exposure makes a difference in outcome (or the probability of an outcome) when it is present, compared with when it is absent' (Parascandola and Weed, 2001). Thus the 'counterfactual' arises because the definition hypothesises about what 'might have been' if conditions had been other than those actually observed (Maldonado and Greenland, 2002). The definition also specifies that all other conditions should have remained constant, that is, it is only the exposure that was (hypothetically) changed. For example, we could say that smoking causes high blood pressure if blood pressure is higher when a person smokes compared to what it would be if that same person were a non-smoker. The causal effect of smoking on blood pressure for an individual could then be estimated by the difference between their blood pressure when they smoked and their blood pressure if they did not smoke. However, only one of these outcomes for each person is actually observed. The unobserved quantities are estimated using substitutes (Maldonado and Greenland, 2002). This could be by using unexposed individuals to estimate the outcomes if exposed individuals had in fact been unexposed (Greenland and Brumback, 2002) or by imputing the outcome from observed covariates. In a randomised trial, we assume that treatment and control groups are balanced in all respects except the exposure and therefore the outcome

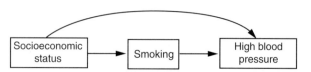

causal models *Causal diagram showing a possible relationship between smoking, high blood pressure and socioeconomic status*

in the exposed group can be used as a substitute for the outcome in the control group were it to have been exposed (Mandolado and Greenland, 2002).

The third type of causal model discussed in the 2002 review, the *sufficient-component cause* model, assumes that the outcome is caused by several causes, none of which is necessary and sufficient alone to cause the disease (Greenland and Brumback, 2002). Such models are often shown as pie charts, with each slice representing one of the components of the overall cause. For example, high blood pressure could be caused by presence of any two of smoking, low socioeconomic status and being overweight (see second Figure).

One disadvantage of such models is that in order to explain relationships such as that of smoking with lung cancer, it is necessary to assume that 'smoking is one element in a sufficient cause and that the other elements simply have not been identified yet' (Parascandola and Weed, 2001). This is clearly a strong assumption to make in many areas of medical statistics.

The fourth type of causal model, the STRUCTURAL EQUATION MODEL, may be thought of as a parameterisation of the causal graph (Greenland and Brumback, 2002). Here, each relationship on the graph is expressed as an equation, with each variable occurring as an outcome in only one of the equations. All parameters are estimated simultaneously and can include error terms and underlying LATENT VARIABLES (as unobserved variables) and correlation between any of the variables.

Singh-Manoux, Richards and Marmot (2003) used causal diagrams and structural equation models to analyse the causal relationship between leisure activities and cognitive function. The causal diagram showed 8 measured variables (including the outcome) and 7 unobserved variables and included correlation between leisure activities entailing low and high cognitive effort. Participation in leisure activities, particularly social or high cognitive effort activities, was positively associated with cognitive function. *KT*

Greenland, S. and Brumback, B. 2002: An overview of relations among causal modelling methods. *International Journal of*

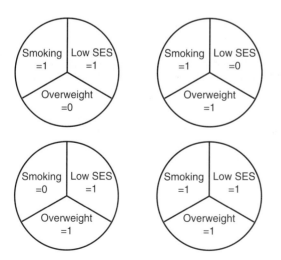

causal models *Sufficient-component cause model showing hypothetical causes of high blood pressure*

Epidemiology 31, 1030–7. **Hernan, M.A., Hernandez-Diaz, S., Werler, M.M. and Mitchell, A.A.** 2002: Causal knowledge as a prerequisite for confounding evaluation: an application to birth defects epidemiology. *American Journal of Epidemiology* 155, 176–84. **Maldonado, G. and Greenland, S.** 2002: Estimating causal effects. *International Journal of Epidemiology* 31, 422–9. **Parascandola, M. and Weed, D.L.** 2001: Causation in epidemiology. *Journal of Epidemiology and Community Health* 55, 905–12. **Singh-Manoux, A., Richards, M. and Marmot, M.** 2003: Leisure activities and cognitive function in middle age: evidence from the Whitehall II study. *Journal of Epidemiology and Community Health* 57, 907–13.

causality The two fundamental principles for establishing evidence for a cause and effect relationship are deduction and induction. The first, with its roots in early Greek philosophy, encompasses mathematical reasoning: starting with a premise formulated without reference to the outside world, a general theory is developed through logical reasoning and subsequently confirmed by statistical observation. Induction, contrariwise, aims to establish a general principle by observation of the natural world and seeks to confirm this principle through prediction and further observation. In contrast to deductive reasoning, inductive reasoning proceeds from the particular to the general. While there can be no doubt that much of modern science strives to make progress through inductive methods, the deductive principle has a firmer grounding in logic. As Hume pointed out, simply observing that one event follows another, no matter how many times it occurs, does not establish that one event *caused* the other.

The concept of what a cause is needs to be set in context with the knowledge of the time. In 1855 John Snow established the link between a 'morbid matter' carried in water and acute, often fatal, diarrhoea in London (Snow, 1855). Snow's evidence consisted of temporal statistical associations, geographical associations in relation to the water companies supplying the city and consideration of a plausible route of infection through ingestion of drinking water. It was the assembly of these various strands of evidence that led to the premise that the water source caused the diarrhoea and a subsequent outbreak in Central London gave Snow the chance to establish deductive proof, by removing the Broad Street water pump with the immediate effect of stopping the epidemic (see HISTORY OF MEDICAL STATISTICS). Snow postulated a cause of cholera 30 years before the bacterium was isolated. As science delves deeper into genetic and molecular mechanisms, we alter our level of definition of causal factors. In reality, few cause-effect associations are simple two-factor problems. Many of our prominent chronic diseases are multi-factorial in nature and many of the factors that contribute to causation are yet to be discovered.

Despite Snow's example, much scientific work progresses without deductive proof; empirical knowledge seems to accumulate through methods that may lend support to but do not actually guarantee correct conclusions. Statistical procedures are employed in observational sciences, where a host of unknown sources of error, including MEASUREMENT ERROR and random fluctuations, must be considered before even progressing toward consideration of causality. Formal 'proof' is generally not attainable in observational sciences and it may be fruitless to try to demonstrate causality in a formal way. More often, a number of associations must be considered together to assemble the totality of evidence. The BRADFORD HILL CRITERIA offer guidelines for considering the totality of evidence. Some of these criteria, such as establishing temporality and demonstrating reversibility, are powerful tools in determining causality, whereas others may depend on specific circumstances.

Bradford Hill's aim was primarily to provide a more structured approach to informing decisions for preventive action. Other writers have advocated decisions based on Popper's concept of refutation. Refutationists would suggest that science can advance more rapidly by formulating radical hypotheses and discarding erroneous theories than it can by fruitless accumulation of supporting evidence. We could make many statements in favour of a hypothesis and still fail to establish it, but we could take just *one* example that disproves the hypothesis to conclude it is false (e.g. one black swan is proof against the assertion that all swans are white). However, even the process of refutation depends on observation and is therefore itself not devoid of uncertainty. There remains a crucial role for statistics in any science based on observation: to set probabilistic limits on whether an observed association exists or should be ignored.

Many widely accepted statistical practices appear to adhere to deductive reasoning. The null hypothesis is a statement formulated prior to any knowledge of the data and therefore a test of the null is an inference from the hypothetical general population to the sample: 'If there is no association in the general population a result like the one seen in the sample would have probability P.' In the LIKELIHOOD approach to estimation, computations proceed from consideration of the hypothetical value for the parameter to support for that value in the particular data observed. However, frequentist theory would appear to be embedded in inductive reasoning: we imagine an experiment repeating an infinite number of times, under the assumption that given enough repetitions we will ultimately arrive at the truth. While this reasoning seems logical if conditions remain unaltered, some would argue that if conditions are likely to change in different populations or under the influence of additional variables, then a general principle cannot be asserted on this basis.

As with any discipline, our ability to determine meaningful results in statistical analysis depends on the approach we adopt. The discovery of a statistically significant result is grounds for rejecting a null hypothesis, but is not evidence for a previously unformulated hypothesis on the strength of the current data. Hence, dredging data for significant results takes us no nearer to establishing

causality and will at best raise possibilities for future investigation. Likewise, if we are seeking 'explanation' in a statistical model, the decision to include a term in the model, guided only by considerations of statistical significance (refutation of the null), would not respect deductive principles (Maclure, 1985). If scientific explanation relies on testing specified prior hypotheses, a more consistent modelling approach would be to include model terms, even if they were not significant in the current data. *JGW*

Maclure, M. 1985: Popperian refutation in epidemiology. *American Journal of Epidemiology* 121, 343. **Snow, J.** 1855: *On the mode of communication of cholera*, 2nd edn. London: Churchill. **Weed, D.L.** 1986: On the logic of causal inference. *American Journal of Epidemiology* 123, 965–79.

cause-specific death rate A death rate calculated for people dying from a particular disease. All-cause mortality rates provide a summary of the overall mortality of a population, but the distribution of causes of death can vary considerably between populations. Classically, mortality from infectious diseases is higher in countries that are less developed, whereas diseases that are chronic, and primarily affect the elderly, predominate in the developed world. In studying a population's mortality experience, it is therefore necessary to consider the specific causes of death rather than simply the all-cause death rate.

The table gives the cause-specific rates for a variety of diseases for different countries. The rates are calculated by dividing the number of deaths from the cause in question during the year by an estimate of the mid-year population. Thus, the Romanian rate for tuberculosis is derived from 2130 (the deaths from tuberculosis occurring in the year 2000), divided by 22,435,000 (the number in the population for that year). The result is then multiplied by 100,000 to give the rate of 9.5 per 100,000 population.

The table shows that accidents and violence are high in South Africa, whereas cardiovascular disease is of concern in Romania. It must be noted that these are crude rates and the different age structures of the populations have not been considered; the comparisons can therefore be misleading (see AGE-SPECIFIC RATES).

Cause-specific death rates are published by many countries and often are presented as age- and sex-specific rates for each cause. The rates are presented by cause of death as classified by the International Classification of Diseases (World Health Organisation, 1992). Regular updates to the classification are required to account for the changing definitions of disease and, in particular, to recognise new diseases. For example, Acquired Immunodeficiency

cause-specific death rate *Cause-specific death rates per 100,000 from selected causes from various countries (UN 2002)*

Country	Tuberculosis	HIV/AIDS	Lung cancer	Cardiovascular disease	Accidents and violence	All causes
Argentina (1996)	29.5	–	23.2	297.3	52.2	863.9
Australia (1999)	0.2	0.4	17.9	135.2	21.9	337.9
Bahamas (1997)	0.7	50.2	3.6	81.9	28.8	264.8
Japan (1999)	2.1	0.0	20.6	122.2	29.7	740.8
Panama (1997)	4.8	15.6	6.0	118.3	56.9	418.7
Romania (2000)	9.5	2.2	37.9	701.9	64.2	1140.3
South Africa (1995)	32.2	13.2	9.7	103.6	119.4	606.2
United Kingdom (1999)	0.9	0.3	58.3	426.2	33.4	1062.3
United States (1998)	0.5	5.0	57.1	349.3	55.6	863.9

Syndrome (AIDS) did not feature in the 9th revision but has been included in the 10th. For analysis of disease time trends, 'bridging' across the revisions can present some difficulties due to the changing definitions.

Cause-specific rates can also be obtained for new cases of specific diseases. Many countries now have cancer registries that publish national and/or regional cancer incidence rates. These are collated internationally by the International Agency for Research (Parkin *et al.*, 2003), which publishes age- and sex-specific incidence rates for various types of cancer from many countries across the world. Similarly, rates for over 200 conditions have been compiled by the World Health Organisation (Murray and Lopez, 1996). *HI*

[See also AGE-SPECIFIC RATES]

Murray, C.J.L. and Lopez, A.D. 1996: Global health statistics. A compendium of incidence, prevalence and mortality estimates for over 200 conditions. Harvard: World Health Organisation. Parkin, M., Whelan, S., Ferlay, J., Teppo, L. and Thomas, D.B. 2003: *Cancer incidence in five continents*. Vol. VIII. Lyon: IARC Scientific Publications. United Nations 2002: *2000 Demographic Yearbook*. New York: United Nations. World Health Organisation 1992: *International statistical classification of diseases and related health problems*. 10th revision. Geneva: World Health Organisation.

censored observations

A distinguishing characteristic of time-to-event data (see SURVIVAL ANALYSIS). Censored observations contain only partially observed information about the time to the event of interest. That is, the exact time of the event is unknown as it may not yet have occurred or be known to have occurred. For example, in a study of time to recurrence of a particular medical condition, say leukaemia after 'successful' bone marrow transplantation, some patients may not experience a recurrence at the end of the study, some may drop out or be lost to follow-up, some may experience the event of interest during successive medical visits, while yet others may experience a 'competing' event, say death, which prevents further follow-up of these subjects.

There are different forms of censoring. The most common in medical studies is *right censoring*. This occurs when by the end of a subject's follow-up the event of interest has not been observed. In this situation all that is known is that the true unobserved 'survival' time exceeds the observed censored time. Most of the examples already seen are of this form.

Left censoring occurs when the true survival time of a subject is less than the actual time observed. For example, in the leukaemia study just examined, subjects may relapse before their first medical visit. Thus, only the incomplete information that the true recurrence times are less than the times to their first medical visit is available. Both forms of censoring are special cases of *interval censoring*, where a subject is known only to have experienced the event within a specific time interval.

Furthermore, the censoring mechanism can be independent or dependent. In the former, the true survival time of a subject, whose observation has been censored, is independent of the mechanism that brought about this censoring. Alternatively, the survival prospects for a homogeneous group of subjects are the same in those censored and in those continued to be followed up. Dependent censoring can occur when subjects are withdrawn from a study because of their apparent high or low risk of experiencing the event. This type of censoring makes standard survival analysis techniques invalid. Thus it is important when censoring occurs to collect as much information as possible on those subjects with censored observations, in order to decide whether the mechanisms behind the censoring types encountered are independent or dependent.

Censoring should not be 'ignored' as valuable information is contained in those subjects with censored times. Therefore, any analysis performed must take account of censoring to make valid inferences. *BT*

Collett, D. 2003: *Modelling survival data in medical research*, 2nd edn. London: Chapman & Hall/CRC.

central limit theorem   See NORMAL DISTRIBUTION

Central Office for Research Ethics (COREC)
See ETHICAL REVIEW COMMITTEES

chi-square distribution

The PROBABILITY DISTRIBUTION of the sum of the squares of independent normally distributed random variables (sometimes referred to as chi-squared, and denoted χ^2). If we have a variable, X_1, that has a NORMAL DISTRIBUTION with MEAN 0, and VARIANCE 1, then the square of X_1 will have a chi-square distribution with one DEGREE OF FREEDOM, often denoted $\chi^2(1)$ or χ^2_1 depending on the text. Similarly, if we have n independent observations, each from a normal distribution with mean 0 and variance 1, say, $X_1, X_2 \ldots X_n$, then the sum $X_1^2 + X_2^2 + \ldots + X_n^2$ will have a chi-square distribution with n degrees of freedom, here denoted χ^2_n.

The chi-square distribution can arise from many other circumstances, but this definition makes it clear that since it is the distribution of a sum of squared numbers, the distribution's density function can only be positive for non-negative numbers. It can also be seen that a variable taking a chi-square distribution with, for example, seven degrees of freedom is the sum of seven independent variables each with a χ_1^2 distribution. Since the χ_1^2 distribution has a mean of 1 and variance of 2, this result tells us that the χ_n^2 distribution will have a mean of n and variance of $2n$.

In addition to these relationships, we note that the χ_2^2 distribution is identical to the EXPONENTIAL DISTRIBUTION with parameter 0.5 and that, in general, the χ_n^2 distribution is identical to the GAMMA DISTRIBUTION, with parameters $n/2$ and 2. As n becomes large, the χ_n^2 distribution is better approximated by a normal distribution (with mean n and variance $2n$). It has a slightly more complicated relationship with the F-DISTRIBUTION, for which it is the limiting distribution after scaling. The shapes that the distribution can take and some of these relationships are illustrated in the Figure on page 52. As can be seen, with one or two degrees of freedom the mode of the density function is at zero and it is strictly decreasing with the value of the random variable. With more degrees of freedom, the density function takes the 'whale' shape that is more usually associated with the chi-square distribution.

The chi-square distribution may be used when testing hypotheses about variances, when performing LIKELIHOOD RATIO tests, CHI-SQUARE TESTS and some NON-PARAMETRIC METHODS, e.g. KRUSKAL-WALLIS test.

Here the *central* chi-square distribution has been discussed. There is also a *non-central* chi-square distribution that arises when the normal random variables that define the distribution have a non-zero mean.   *AGL*

Altman, D.G. 1991: *Practical statistics for medical research.* Boca Raton: CRC Press/Chapman & Hall. **Leemis, L.M.** 1986: Relationships among common univariate distributions. *The American Statistician* 40, 2, 143–6.

chi-square test Statistical significance test used to assess a variety of hypotheses of categorical data, particularly when interest centres on the distribution of observations across categories. For example, a study might record the ethnic group of individuals and interest might centre on the proportion of individuals in each ethnic group.

Categorical data are often presented in FREQUENCY TABLES (or CONTINGENCY TABLES), where each cell of the table shows the number of observations (counts) for a particular combination of categories for the variables of interest.

Chi-square tests are a form of HYPOTHESIS TEST where the hypothesis specifies the expected distribution of observations across the cells of the frequency table (the expected number of individuals in each cell).

The chi-square test statistic, χ^2, provides a measure of how much the counts recorded in the study (the 'observed counts') deviate from counts predicted by the hypothesis (the 'expected counts'). A small P-VALUE is evidence that

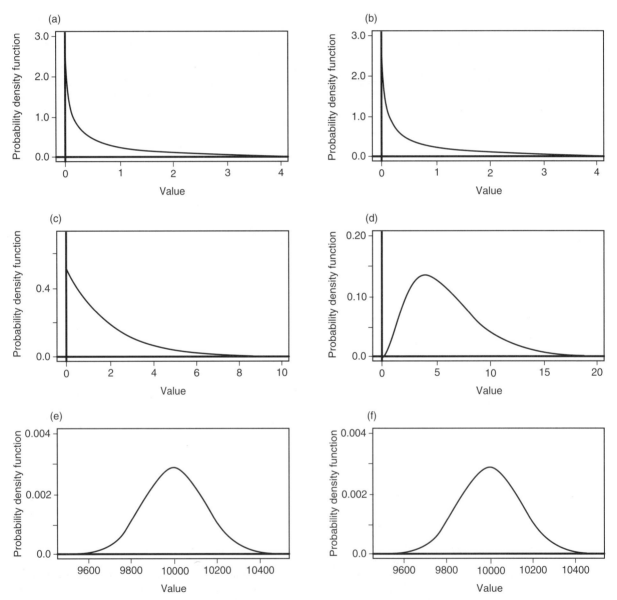

chi-square (χ^2) distribution *Illustrating the form of the chi-square probability density function and its relationships with other distributions: (a) chi-square distribution with one degree of freedom; (b) the F-distribution with one and one thousand degrees of freedom; (c) chi-square distribution with two degrees of freedom (equivalently the exponential distribution with a parameter of 0.5); (d) chi-square distribution with six degrees of freedom; (e) chi-square distribution with ten thousand degrees of freedom; (f) normal distribution with mean of ten thousand and variance of twenty thousand* the hypothesis is false. (The formula for the chi-square test statistic is given in the entry for CONTINGENCY TABLES.)

Freeman *et al.* (2002) provides an example of the use of chi-square tests. This re-audit of hip fracture in East Anglia involved 7 hospitals and analyses were performed to establish whether there were any differences between hospitals in terms of patient demographics. One of the variables tested was patient gender. In this case, the hypothesis to test was that the distribution of patients across male and female categories was the same at all of the hospitals. In other words, the hypothesis was that the proportion of hip fracture patients who were male was the same at all of the hospitals. The result of a chi-square test was $\chi^2 = 7.50$ and $P = 0.48$, indicating that there was no evidence of a difference between hospitals in the proportion of hip fracture patients who were male.

There are three common types of chi-square test: the goodness-of-fit test, the test for independence and the test for homogeneity.

The chi-square *goodness-of-fit* test is appropriate when there is a single group of subjects and a single variable of interest. The hypothesis in this sort of test specifies a precise distribution of subjects across categories. For example, this test could be used to determine whether the ethnic mix of a patient group from a study is different from the (known) ethnic mix in the general population.

The chi-square test for *independence* is appropriate when there is a single group of subjects and two variables of interest. In this case, the hypothesis is that the distribution of subjects across categories in one variable is the same for (i.e. independent of) the categories of the other variable. For example, this test could be used to determine whether the incidence of a disease is related to the ethnic mix of a patient group; in other words, whether the proportion of patients with a disease is the same for all ethnic groups.

The chi-square test for *homogeneity* is appropriate when there are several groups of subjects and a single variable of interest. This test is used to determine whether the distribution of a variable across categories is the same for all groups. The study by Freeman *et al.* (2002) provides an example of this sort of test where the groups are hospitals and interest centres on whether the distribution of male and female patients is the same at all hospitals.

Each of these tests is only appropriate when there is no natural ordering to the categories (i.e. the data are nominal). If the categories are ordered (i.e. the data are ordinal), for example when the variable of interest is age group, then other analyses should be used, such as the chi-square test for trend (see, for example, Altman, 1991).

The chi-square test is a parametric test; it is only a valid test when the expected number of observations in each cell is not too small. (A rough rule of thumb is that the expected number of observations in each cell should be at least 5. However, a less stringent criterion is commonly used and has been shown to yield satisfactory results, namely, no more than 25% of cells should have an expected cell count of less than 5, provided none is less than 1.) The test can become invalid when the expected number of observations in a cell is very small and/or when the total number of observations is small. In such cases it can be prudent to use a continuity correction (see YATES' CORRECTION) or, even better, employ a NON-PARAMETRIC or EXACT METHOD alternative (e.g. FISHER'S EXACT TEST).

The sampling method should be considered when determining what sort of chi-square test to use. It is only valid to test a hypothesis that makes sense in relation to the way in which the data were gathered. In the hospital example, there are several independent groups of patients (from the 7 hospitals) and a single variable of interest (gender). In this case, it is valid to perform a test for homogeneity, but it is not valid to perform a test for independence.

Chi-square tests only provide an overall test of a hypothesis. If a chi-square test is significant, it may be necessary to perform further post-hoc tests in order to determine in more detail where significant deviations from the hypothesis exist. In the example from Freeman *et al.* (2002), had the test been significant, this would have indicated that the proportion of hip fracture patients who were male was *not* the same at all of the hospitals in the audit. This does not specify precisely those hospitals that were significantly different from each other. In this case, a t-test of the difference between proportions for each pair of hospitals could be used, but it should be noted that such post-hoc tests would be subject to the usual problems of multiple comparisons (see MULTIPLE COMPARISON PROCEDURES).

When a variable has only two categories, e.g. gender, the data may be analysed in terms of proportions rather than frequencies. This situation may be analysed using LOGISTIC REGRESSION, which allows more complex hypotheses to be tested. An alternative and more flexible analysis for any number of variables with any number of categories is POISSON REGRESSION.

Chi-square tests are described in most introductory statistics texts (e.g. Agresti, 2002; Altman, 1991; Wild and Seber, 2000). *PM*

Agresti, A. 2002: *Categorical data analysis*, 2nd edn. New York: John Wiley & Sons. Altman, D.G. 1991: *Practical statistics for medical research*. London: Chapman & Hall. Freeman, C., Todd, C., Camilleri-Ferrante, C., Laxton, C., Murrell, P., Palmer, C.R., Parker, M., Payne, B. and Rushton, N. 2002: Quality improvement for patients with hip fracture: experience from a multi-site audit. *Quality & Safety in Health Care* 11, 3, 239–45. Wild, C. J. and Seber, G.A. 2000: *Chance encounters: a first course in data analysis and inference*. New York: John Wiley & Sons.

chi-square test for trend   See CASE-CONTROL STUDIES

Christmas tree adjustment   See INTERIM ANALYSIS

classification and regression trees (CART)   See TREE-STRUCTURED METHODS

classification function   See DISCRIMINANT FUNCTION ANALYSIS

clinical equipoise   See ETHICS AND CLINICAL TRIALS

clinical trial protocols   See PROTOCOLS FOR CLINICAL TRIALS

clinical trials   Also known as randomised controlled trials (RCTs), these are studies of a medical intervention in which the allocation of patients to the various experimental groups, at least one of which is a control group, occurs by an *aleatory*, or chance, mechanism. Such a study has a number of essential features in addition to randomisation. It is hypothesis-driven with an unambiguous

ENDPOINT assessed in a way that assures unbiased measurement; it has secondary endpoints that add credibility and interpretability to the primary outcome; it defines its study group in a way that allows logical inference to some definable population; it uses an ethically and scientifically defensible control group; and a clearly written protocol governs its procedures. Because the experimental units are humans, these trials require a formal process of informed consent as well as assurance that the safety of the participants is monitored during the course of the study.

Randomised controlled trials may enrol tens, hundreds or even thousands of participants. While the general structure of the design of such a trial is independent of its size, the number of participants enrolled affects many aspects of the conduct of a trial. Small single-centre trials tend to collect a lot of data. Multi-centre trials typically collect somewhat fewer data on each patient, but the methods of collection tend to be highly structured to ensure comparability across centres. A so-called 'large simple trial' recruits thousands of people and collects a parsimonious amount of data directed at a few pointed questions (Yusuf, Collins and Peto, 1984).

A classification of trials of drugs or biologics relevant in the regulatory setting categorises them according to their phase. PHASE I TRIALS, the first trials of the product in humans, aim to gain a preliminary understanding of the safety of the product and to select doses for further study. PHASE II TRIALS define the dose more precisely and perhaps collect data germane to a preliminary glimpse at efficacy, often through the use of surrogate endpoints or biologic markers. In many therapeutic areas, Phase I and II trials are not randomised, and sometimes not controlled, because their goals can be achieved with simpler designs. Confirmatory, or PHASE III TRIALS aim to test the efficacy of the product. Typically, a Phase III trial is randomised. Trials performed after the product has been approved for licensing, whether they are randomised or not, are sometimes called PHASE IV TRIALS.

This section touches on the early history of the modern randomised controlled trial, discusses its salient features and describes some of its limitations. Several textbooks provide thorough introduction to these trials (Friedman, Furberg and DeMets, 1998; Meinert, 1998; Pocock, 1997).

The earliest modern randomised clinical trial studied streptomycin, the first truly active drug for the treatment of tuberculosis. Streptomycin, discovered in 1944, had shown very promising results in uncontrolled pilot studies in the USA. At the end of the Second World War, limited supplies of the drug were made available in Great Britain for clinical use. Because of the belief that the drug had promising therapeutic activity, a portion of the available supply was reserved for patients with the two most lethal forms of tuberculosis – meningeal and miliary disease. The rest could be used for the large majority of patients, who had pulmonary disease. Since it was manifestly impossible to treat everyone with pulmonary tuberculosis, the Medical Research Council decided that the best use of the small amount available would be to study its effects in a controlled setting. The study that followed (Marshall, Blacklock, Cameron et al., 1948) was a multi-centre controlled trial comparing streptomycin to standard bed rest. Random numbers placed in sealed envelopes governed treatment assignment of the 109 patients entered. Patients were eligible if they had 'acute progressive bilateral pulmonary tuberculosis of presumably recent origin, bacteriologically proved, unsuitable for collapse therapy, age group 15 to 25 (later extended to 30)'. The narrow age group was chosen to limit the number of eligible patients. Physicians responsible for evaluating radiological change with treatment were unaware of the treatment assignment. Results showed a clear benefit of streptomycin; the published report refers to a few of the observed treatment differences as 'statistically significant'.

Two anonymous editorials accompanied the publication of this trial. One dealt with the implications of the results for tuberculosis therapy. The second, entitled 'The controlled therapeutic trial' (Anon, 1948) commented on the noteworthy aspects of this study, including the precise definition of the patient population, the advantages of multi-centre collaboration to assure adequate numbers of study subjects, the need for screening potential subjects so that they conform to the eligibility requirements and the value of the 'ingenious system of sealed envelopes' to ensure that advanced knowledge of the treatment assignment would not influence the decision about patient eligibility.

Within 6 years of publication of the streptomycin trial, another trial dramatically exhibited the unprecedented power of the new methodology. The field trial of the newly developed Salk vaccine for the prevention of poliomyelitis was an enormous effort. Centrally coordinated at the University of Michigan by a group convened for that purpose, it involved public health departments in 44 of the 48 states of the USA. Within about a 6-week period, from 26 April to 15 June 1954, 402,000 children received either Salk vaccine or placebo by random assignment. The very large numbers were required because of the relatively low attack rates of the poliovirus in normal populations of children.

The trial showed that the vaccine effectively reduced the incidence of polio and, by providing rough estimates of effectiveness for certain subgroups, suggested that the effectiveness of vaccination varied somewhat according to the primary manifestations of the disease (bulbospinal versus spinal) and according to the type of virus recovered. The comprehensive report describing this heroic effort and its results (Francis et al., 1955) was published less than 2 years after the National Foundation for Infantile Paralysis first announced its decision to sponsor a formal trial of the vaccine.

Since then, use of the randomised prospective methodology has burgeoned. Bolstered by subsequent developments in statistical methodology, the randomised clinical trial is widely acknowledged as the 'gold standard' of evidence for evaluating therapies. However, because the randomised trial can only be employed to address a small fraction of the unanswered questions relating to medical interventions, a variety of methodologies – experimental and observational, prospective and retrospective – have been and continue to be widely used.

The statistical framework of a randomised clinical trial involves two sets of basic notions: TYPE I ERROR rate, P-VALUE and validity; POWER and precision. The *Type I error rate* is the probability that if the treatments under study do not differ (that is, the null hypothesis is true), the study will show a statistically significant difference between them. The *P-value* is the probability under the null hypothesis that data would show by chance a difference as large as the difference observed. *Validity* in clinical trials refers not to the correctness of the answer in any particular trial, but to the expectation that, under the null hypothesis, the data would behave in a way consistent with the pre-specified Type I error rate and that if the sample size were large enough, the estimated treatment effect would be the true effect.

Power, by the same token, is the probability that the study will show a statistically significant effect of treatment if the true effect of treatment is not zero. Power is then a function of the true effect: the larger the effect, the higher the power. *Precision* is a measure of the variability of the estimated effect of treatment. The higher the sample size, and the lower the underlying variability of the measurements, the higher the precision.

Results from studies of interventions may help physicians decide on the best therapeutic option for particular patients. They permit regulatory agencies to approve products for marketing and widespread commercial distribution. Increasingly, governments, insurance companies, and managed-care organisations use such studies to help decide which therapies to reimburse. The use of formal clinical data as the basis for these decisions rests on two obvious assumptions. The first is that the studies that form the database have in fact yielded correct results; that is, any differences in outcome can with confidence be attributed to differences in the therapy administered. To the extent that studies possess this quality, they are said to have *internal validity*. The second is that the study results are, to some degree at least, generalisable to a population of subjects that is broader than the study population from which the data are derived. Studies having this property are said to have *external validity* and the broadness of a study's external validity is one critical measure of the study's overall importance.

A study lacking internal validity has no redeeming value. The mere presence of internal validity, however, does not guarantee its general usefulness if the study has very limited external validity. For example, selecting a very tightly defined a study population that does not represent the larger universe of patients with the same condition may render the results at best narrowly applicable. Or perhaps the intervention under study is of such technical complexity that it is only available in a few selected centres and cannot be applied broadly. Examples of such problems have occurred in virtually every field of medicine.

The major barriers to internal validity relate mainly to the extent to which three major sources of confusion are permitted to interfere with unambiguous inference – bias, confounding and chance (Hennekens, 1987).

Used in the context of analytic clinical studies, 'bias' does not connote moral opprobrium but simply refers to any systematic error in the design or execution of a study that distorts the true relationship between intervention and outcome. Bias can originate with either the investigators or the study subjects and is of several types. Sometimes the very manner of selecting a study's participants introduces bias (*selection bias*); this is a particular problem, for example, in CASE-CONTROL STUDIES when the selection of cases, or agreement of the patient to participate, is not independent of the chance that the patient will have been exposed to the intervention of interest. In retrospective studies, the ability of patients to recall interventions in the past may be influenced by whether or not they have experienced certain medical outcomes (RECALL BIAS). The history obtained from a patient in any study may be skewed by knowledge on the part of either the interviewer (*observer bias*) or the study subject (*subject bias*) of the nature of the study or what interventions have occurred or what outcomes they have experienced. In prospective studies, losses to follow-up often occur; non-random losses that occur differentially in one group or the other may introduce serious bias. By far the best insurance against the various types of bias in clinical studies is the use of a prospective, randomised study design that keeps both the investigators and the study subjects unaware of which intervention the individual subjects are receiving (the so-called *double-blind* or *double-masked* design). Certain study designs, such as those that compare a surgical to a medical intervention or those where the side-effects of treatment frequently reveal the nature of the therapy preclude blinding of either subjects or investigators. These cases require the most objective endpoints available (for example, death from any cause, if this is an appropriate measure of treatment effectiveness). Where less objective endpoints are the most meaningful medically, evaluators who are blind to the therapy received should assess them. In designs that are not prospective and randomised, minimisation of bias poses a major challenge because there are no good analytic tools to correct for it. Once bias is present, the extent to which it has been eliminated by sound design and conduct is always open to question. The primary advantage of a well-conducted randomised clinical trial is that it removes many sources of bias.

Confounding refers to the distortion of the association between intervention and outcome by the association of another factor (the *confounder*) with both. A factor A is a confounder of an intervention I and an effect E if A has an effect on E independently of I and the use of I depends in some way on A. For example, if one were to try to compare two regimens for leukaemia (say, a vigorous and a more gentle one) by reviewing past series of patients treated with each, one might find that the aggressive regimen performed much better than the other. A more detailed analysis, however, might reveal that the aggressive regimen was used preferentially in younger patients, while the gentle treatment was reserved for older patients. Age would confound any attempt to compare the two regimens in this simple manner, since it is well known that younger leukaemia patients have a better prognosis than elderly ones when treated with virtually any regimen.

Note that, in contrast to bias, confounding is nobody's fault. It does not represent errors of commission or omission, but rather is a natural consequence of the often complex relationships among the many factors that determine clinical outcome following an intervention (or, more generally, following exposures of any kind). In OBSERVATIONAL STUDIES, when a variable is suspected of being a source of confounding, one attempts to correct for the confounding in either the design or the analysis. A prospective randomised design provides the strongest protection against confounding because randomisation tends to equalise the distribution of potential or actual confounders among the various treatment arms. Randomisation does this with both known and unknown confounders. While statistical methods are available for adjusting for known confounders, nothing other than randomisation can even approach the control of unknown confounders.

The very nature of clinical investigation permits the play of chance to deal the investigator a misleading answer. The reliability of a result is in part a function of the number of patients studied; increasing the sample size of any randomised study, no matter what the design, will decrease the probability that the patients studied are peculiar in some identified or unidentified manner. Moreover, an inadequate sample size clearly increases the likelihood that chance alone can deal a false or misleading result. A trial that is too small may end up showing a difference where none really is present, or, more commonly, may fail to show a difference where a medically important one really does exist. The statistical procedure that evaluates the degree to which the observed result is consistent with chance is called a test of *statistical significance*.

The great virtue of randomisation is that it removes selection bias from the allocation of patients to therapy and that it tends to equalise baseline patient characteristics (actual or potential confounders) in the various arms of the study whether these characteristics are known or unknown. Thus, if the sample size is sufficiently large, any statistically significant differences in outcome can be attributed to the differences in therapy with much greater confidence than with other methodologies. Finally, randomised treatment assignment provides theoretical support for the inference that permits calculation of the probability that the observed differences might have arisen by chance (the p-value).

The conclusions of a clinical trial are usually stated in probabilistic terms; therefore, even when a trial has shown a statistically significant difference between two treatments, there remains the possibility that the results might have been due to chance. If, however, several independent trials show a consistent effect, the probability that the result can be ascribed to chance is enormously reduced. In such a case, chance plays a far smaller role in interfering with a strong conclusion that it does in most other aspects of daily life.

Various features of the randomised controlled trial, when taken together, form the most reliable route toward the documentation of a causal relation between an intervention and a clinical outcome. The prospective collection of data, with suitable measures to ensure correctness and completeness, serves to minimise MISSING, misclassified or erroneous DATA elements. The use of blinding, whenever feasible, minimises the presence of observer or subject bias; the use of a PLACEBO, when medically appropriate, allows isolation of the true effects of the test therapy from those attendant on the therapeutic setting in general. The contemporaneous relationship of test and control groups eliminates secular changes in patient selection or ancillary therapy that might affect results. Finally, as already described, the use of randomisation tends to equalise the distribution of confounding variables, known and unknown, among the intervention options and provides a formal basis for the application of statistical inference to the data.

Of course, a randomised controlled trial is not the only route to truth. Few would quibble with the claim that appendectomy cures acute appendicitis, that penicillin cures pneumococcal pneumonia, that radiotherapy cures early Hodgkin's disease or that the use of parachutes saves people who jump from planes (Smith and Pell, 2003),

although no randomised data exist to support any one of these claims. In the presence of striking clinical effects, formal testing of a clinical hypothesis with a randomised trial may be unnecessary. Neither does a randomised trial necessarily always give the right answer. Like any other scientific experiment, a clinical trial is fallible. Careless data collection, inaccurate observations, inadequate sample size, faulty techniques of inference or simply the play of chance can result in misleading or frankly erroneous conclusions.

Adherence to high standards of design, conduct and analysis, as best one can judge from the published report, tends to bolster the credibility of the trial. The larger the difference in outcomes between control and test therapies, the larger the sample size (or in trials that count events, the more events), the smaller the p-value of the comparison and the more precisely estimated the differences, the more credible the results.

In randomised controlled trials, as in other experiments, the design should address the question at hand. A clear medical question leads to a crisp design, while a fuzzy purpose may lead to an inadequate amount of data, concentration on irrelevant details and failure to answer useful questions. In practice, many trials have foundered because their vaguely articulated hypotheses have spawned inadequate designs. One should think the scientific hypothesis underlying the clinical experiment makes sense, for the more biologically plausible the hypotheses; the more likely the results will be believable. There is often much subjectivity here, however, and what makes eminent sense to some may be implausible to others. One may, from time to time, be faced with results in clinical trials that seem to have no plausible scientific support.

Many of the most important clinical trials have been founded on hypotheses about the putative mechanism of action of the intervention. It is gratifying when such trials turn out positive, since then the result is consistent with the proposed mechanism. In the real world, however, it is often extraordinarily difficult to use clinical trials productively as probes for underlying mechanism.

A randomised controlled clinical trial has a protocol that discusses the purpose of the trial, describes the procedures to be used and defines the endpoints as well as the criteria used to define 'success'. It justifies the sample size, the study group, the strata – if any – and plan for follow-up and the method to be used for monitoring safety during the course of the trial. Regulatory bodies often require that they review protocols for trials performed for the purpose of licensing a product or extending the indication in the label.

The complexity of the study and of the protocol depends on a number of factors. A small single-centre trial that is studying a short-term intervention for symptomatic relief may have a brief protocol, while a large, multi-centre study measuring a complicated endpoint in subjects followed for several years may require a much more detailed protocol. Whether the protocol is simple or complicated, it should be written clearly and essential parts should be easily identified. Other documents may provide further description of the study. For example, a data analysis plan may present the details of the statistical methods to be used. If the study has a data safety monitoring committee or an endpoint committee, their charters will describe them and their roles.

The International Conference on Harmonization, in its guidelines for Good Clinical Practice, describes elements of a well-constructed protocol.

While randomisation produces study groups with equal expected distributions of both measured and unmeasured characteristics at baseline, randomisation by itself cannot ensure that the results of a study will be unbiased. The unbiasedness conferred by randomisation requires a statistical analysis that classifies people according to the treatment to which they were randomised, not the treatment they actually received. Analysis that preserves the randomisation is called *intent-to-treat* analysis.

A perfectly conducted clinical trial would have no problem analysing the groups as they were randomised, for each person would receive the assigned therapy, each would adhere to the protocol and each would provide a measurement for the primary endpoint. Even rigorously executed clinical trials, however, rarely meet this ideal. Many participants in trials adhere incompletely or not at all with their assigned regimen. The primary endpoint may be missing for some participants. Thus, while the principle of performing statistical analysis according to the randomised assignment is central to producing an unbiased result, in practice one is often forced to violate those principles. One needs reasonable approaches to assigning outcomes when actual observations are unavailable.

Often investigators are tempted to analyse data from the subset of participants who complete the study according to the protocol. Such analyses can be subject to severe selection bias (Lamm *et al.*, 1981).

Sometimes an analysis other than the intent-to-treat analysis is appropriate. For example, in studies of infectious disease where treatment is given presumptively before determination of the infecting organism, the primary analysis may include only those patients who have an organism against which the agent being studied is likely to be effective. Such an analysis leads to an unbiased assessment of the effect of the intervention on people infected with the target organism.

A clear objective along with focused hypotheses will drive the choice of endpoints. When the endpoint is unambiguous, its definition and measurement is simple. The more subjective the endpoint, the more need for independent assessment. For example, in unblinded trials of cancer therapies where the endpoint is a measurement of change in tumour size as assessed by a CT scan, independent readers who do not know whether the subjects are in the treated or control group may be required to ensure unbiased measurement of size of the tumours. If the endpoint is a report by the subject (for example, a score on a scale measuring pain), the trial may use several outcomes to support and corroborate the primary endpoint.

Control groups are essential to the design of a randomised controlled trial and the inferences that can be drawn from them. The control can be a placebo, usual care, a different therapy or usual care plus a placebo. In selecting a control therapy, the investigators should choose one that is relevant to the question at hand and should attempt, insofar as possible, to choose a control that allows blinding.

The study group in a randomised controlled trial is necessarily heterogeneous. Sometimes, investigators want to ensure equal allocation of treatment and control in specific subgroups. In such cases, they define strata and randomise within strata. For example, in a study of prevention of heart attack, one might stratify by occurrence of a prior heart attack. The choice of whether or not to stratify should depend on the size of the study and the relationship of the particular variable to the outcome of interest. If a variable has the potential to be a strong confounder and the study is small, then stratification may be useful.

At the end of a study, one might want to analyse the data by subgroup, either those that defined the randomisation strata or others. The purpose of such analyses is sometimes to assess whether the treatment is effective within specific subgroups of the population and sometimes to assess whether the effect of treatment varies by subgroup. Such analyses should be undertaken and interpreted with great caution because trials are rarely large enough to support reliable inference within subgroups (Yusuf *et al.*, 1991).

While randomised controlled trials have great advantages over other designs in terms of producing validity inference about the effect of treatment, they have severe limitation in the actual setting of clinical investigation. A prospective trial is often large, complex and expensive, requiring the coordination of a small army of participants and many sites spread over counties, countries or continents. There is no realistic prospect, therefore, of employing the randomised clinical trial in more than a small proportion of the unresolved questions in therapy. Within specific disease categories, the restrictive ELIGIBILITY CRITERIA of many trials mean that the results of the study will be directly applicable only to a narrow segment of the total patient population with that disease. Sometimes, a trial would need to be very long to yield clinically meaningful results. The polio vaccine trial realised its scientific goals quickly because the effect of the vaccine could be determined over the few months following immunisation. It is another matter entirely to assess the impact of a screening intervention or preventive drug on the incidence of heart attacks or cancer; here the necessary follow-up time may be measured in decades. Even for trials that determine the endpoint of individual treatments quickly, slow accrual may make the study take so long to complete that the therapeutic question it poses is no longer of interest by the time the answer is available. Some subspecialties have particular problems with the use of the randomised controlled trials; for surgery, in particular, the acceptance and application of the randomised trial has been slow. And finally, a randomised controlled trial may not be usable at all if the competing interventions have been in use for enough time that the attitudes of physicians are fixed; physicians are understandably reluctant to randomise patients if they think they already know the answer. The decision to perform a randomised controlled trial requires a sizeable commitment in time, money and effort; the decision not to perform one entails some sacrifice in the quality of evidence provided to physicians when they are making choices for therapies for their patients. A combination of medical, societal and financial forces determines those questions that become the subject of randomised controlled trials.   *JW*

Anon 1948: The controlled therapeutic trial. *British Medical Journal* 2, 791–2. **Francis, T. Jr.** *et al.* 1955: An evaluation of the 1954 poliomyelitis vaccine trials. Summary report. *American Journal of Public Health* 45, 1–51. **Friedman, L.M., Furberg, C.D. and DeMets, D.L.** 1998: *Fundamentals of Clinical Trials,*

3rd edn. Heidelberg: Springer Verlag. **Hennekens, C.H. and Buring J.E.** 1987: *Epidemiology in medicine*. Boston and Toronto: Little, Brown and Co. **Lamm, G.** *et al.* 1981: Influence of treatment adherence in the coronary drug project. *New England Journal of Medicine* 304, 612–13. **Marshall, G., Blacklock, J.W.S., Cameron, C.** *et al.* 1948: Streptomycin treatment of pulmonary tuberculosis. A Medical Research Council investigation. *British Medical Journal* 2, 769–82. **Meinert, C.** 1998: *Clinical trials*. New York: Oxford University Press. **Pocock, S.** 1996: *Clinical trials: a practical approach*. New York: John Wiley & Sons. **Smith, G.C. and Pell, J.P.** 2003: Parachute use to prevent death and major trauma related to gravitational challenge: systematic review of randomised controlled trials. *British Medical Journal* 327, 1459–61. **Yusuf, S., Collins, R. and Peto, R.** 1984: Why do we need some large, simple randomized trials? *Statistics in Medicine* 3, 409–20. **Yusuf, S., Wittes, J., Probstfield, J. and Tyroler, H.** 1991: Analysis and interpretation of treatment effects in subgroups of patients in randomized clinical trials. *Journal of the American Medical Association* 266, 93–8.

clinical v. statistical significance

clinical v. statistical significance A pair of terms often confused, being mistakenly considered as interchangeable, when, in reality, neither implies the other necessarily. One of the unnecessary difficulties of statistics is that we are using ordinary English words, such as 'normal', 'confidence' and 'population' in a technical way. If only our founders had followed the example of the anatomists and named everything in Latin. It is too late now and we are stuck with our English terminology. Of all the words our predecessors appropriated, the one that must cause the greatest confusion is 'significant'.

The *Shorter Oxford English Dictionary* gives two definitions of 'significance': 'the meaning or import of something, meaning, suggestiveness' and 'importance, consequence'. The statistical usage relates to the first interpretation. If a difference is significant in a sample, there is evidence that the difference exists in the population that the sample represents. Hence the difference has meaning beyond the individuals who make up the sample. By clinical significance, we mean that the difference we have observed is important; that, for example, it implies that we should change clinical practice. Thus, this usage relates to the second interpretation, meaning that the significant difference is important.

If a difference or relationship is statistically significant, this implies that we have evidence that it is real, existing in the larger population, but not that it is important, having implications for clinical practice. Concluding that a difference or relationship is important depends on its magnitude, together with non-statistical factors, so that we can decide whether it is big enough to influence clinical decisions. For example, in a large clinical trial with 2000 subjects in each arm, a difference of 1mmHg in mean diastolic blood pressure would be statistically significant. As this was a trial, it would be reasonable to conclude that the difference was real and that the treatments had slightly different effects on blood pressure. Yet it is unlikely that such a difference would influence treatment decisions. It would not be important and so not clinically significant. Contrariwise, a small study might produce a non-significant difference that is quite large. We could not conclude that the difference was real, but we might think it important enough to carry out another trial.

Statisticians cannot expect to appropriate ordinary English words and then demand that their use be restricted. However, the use of 'significant' in research reports to mean something other than statistical significance can be potentially misleading and it makes sense to avoid it. In its instructions to authors, the *Lancet* asks that authors 'avoid non-technical uses of technical terms in statistics, such as . . . "significant"'. *JMB*

[See also CRITICAL APPRAISAL]

cluster analysis in medicine

cluster analysis in medicine The term cluster analysis covers a very wide range of methods for discovering groups in multivariate data. It is distinct from classification techniques such as DISCRIMINANT FUNCTION ANALYSIS or *classification and regression tree* (CART, see TREE-STRUCTURED METHODS) analysis. These classify individuals into groups that have already been identified whereas cluster analysis looks for groups within the data. General texts on cluster analysis are by Everitt, Landau and Leese (2001) and Gordon (1999) and technical developments are often published in the *Journal of Classification*. However, there is a vast literature dealing with cluster analysis in various guises and this is necessarily a very brief review of the more widely used methods. Many specialised methods dealing with particular subject matters have become separated from mainstream cluster analysis, often using their own terminology, and they may be classified under other headings such as pattern recognition, ARTIFICIAL INTELLIGENCE or DATA MINING IN MEDICINE.

In medicine, the cases to be clustered are generally people and the multivariate data describe various aspects of their clinical, psychological or service use status. However, other units of analysis can of course be clustered, for example hospitals or health authorities, and cluster analysis can also be used to group variables, although this is less common. The data may be in the form of attributes, such as ethnic group, or continuous measurements such as blood pressure, or a mixture of both types may be analysed (mixed mode data). The objective of the analysis is to find subgroups of people who are relatively homogenous with respect to these characteristics. The reason for performing the analysis might be administrative (for example, to define strata in a survey sample) or, more usually, it might be related to a research question (for example, to identify groups of people with a common gene structure). (A review of methods used in medicine is given by McLachlan, 1992.)

In the most widely used methods, one typically proceeds by choosing a measure of the proximity between cases in terms of the multivariate data (the term proximity covers both similarity and distance, either of which may be calculated). Next, an algorithm for forming clusters is applied to the matrix of proximities. The investigator usually has to decide on the number of clusters forming the 'solution', that is a partition of the data based on a particular choice of proximity measure, algorithm and number of clusters. The choice of number of clusters is particularly difficult, since there are few reliable formal tests and the investigator may have to consider a range of solutions that seems reasonable based on the subject matter. The ROBUSTNESS of the final solution can be tested in a number of ways. These include using alternative clustering methods, using *split-half* methods on the data, the detection and exclusion of outliers or influential cases and validation against external data. Formal hypothesis tests of the null hypothesis of absence of cluster structure are theoretically possible but are rarely applied.

The definition of proximity between individuals depends on the type of data and the relative weight to be placed on different variables (Everitt, Landau and Leese, 2001). For example binary attribute data may be coded as series of 1s and 0s, denoting presence or absence of an attribute. In the case where each category is of equal weight, such as gender or white/non-white ethnic group, a *simple matching coefficient* (the proportion of matches between two individuals) could be used. However, if the attributes were the presence of various symptoms, proximity might be more appropriately measured using the asymmetric *Jaccard coefficient*, based on the proportion of matches where there is a positive match (i.e. ignoring joint negative matches). For continuous data, the *Euclidean distance* between individuals i and j, $\left[\sum_{k=1}^{p}(x_{ik} - x_{jk})^2\right]^{1/2}$, where p is the number of variables, is often used (applied to binary data it is the same as the simple matching coefficient). For mixed mode data, *Gower's coefficient* can be used to combine components of distance from either attribute or continuous data, after first scaling the continuous data to a 0–1 range. Many alternative proximity measures have been proposed to deal with specialised types of data, for example in genetics binary matches may be assigned different weights depending on the part of the genetic sequence from which they arise.

Hierarchical algorithms are possibly the most widely used of general purpose clustering methods and are included in most STATISTICAL PACKAGES. They use a heuristic algorithm to successively join or divide clusters on the basis of their proximity (thus being referred to as agglomerative or divisive methods respectively). The methods differ in the way in which the inter-cluster proximities are calculated from the inter-individual distances. *Single linkage*, for example, uses the proximity between the closest individuals in two clusters to be joined, whereas *complete linkage* uses the most distant. *Ward's method* is another popular agglomerative method that joins clusters on the basis of an error sum-of-squares criterion; unlike the two linkage methods mentioned it requires the raw data (rather than just the proximity matrix) to be available during the clustering process. Divisive methods are less commonly used than agglomerative methods, except perhaps those specifically designed for attribute data. An example of the latter is the *monothetic divisive* method, which divides the sample according to the value of a single attribute at each stage, the attribute being chosen so as to create the most homogenous groups at that stage. *Polythetic divisive* methods divide according to a number of variables considered together.

Both agglomerative and polythetic divisive methods generally produce a tree diagram, or *dendrogram*, which shows the process by which cases have been joined or divided, and this can be used to suggest the number of clusters present (by examining the jumps in the proximity at which clusters are joined or divided). Here we can see that a small dendrogram is formed using single linkage from the following matrix of proximities (the proximity between case 1 and itself is, of course, 0.0, and between cases 1 and 2 it is 2.0, etc) (the Figure that follows shows the relationship in diagrammatic fashion):

Case
1	0.0				
2	2.0	0.0			
3	6.0	5.0	0.0		
4	10.0	9.0	4.0	0.0	
5	9.0	8.0	5.0	3.0	0.0

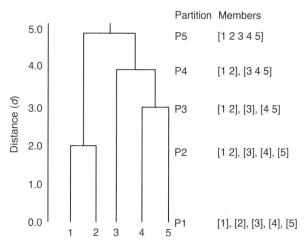

cluster analysis in medicine *A dendrogram produced using single linkage applied to a matrix of pairwise distances. A sequence of partitions P1–P5 is produced according to the minimum distance between cases in clusters to be joined. Cases 1 and 2 join first, then 4 and 5; case 3 joins the 4–5 cluster and finally all cases are joined*

A study of people with eating disorders made by Hay, Fairburn and Doll (1996) illustrates the use of two of the standard hierarchical methods mentioned and some of the robustness checks that can be made. The rationale for their study was that: 'Clinical experience, however, indicates that a substantial number of those who present for treatment of an eating disorder do not fulfil diagnostic criteria for either of these disorders ... The aim of the present study was to derive an empirically based scheme for classifying those with recurrent binge eating.' The data were the first 7 principal components based on 22 items from a QUESTIONNAIRE measuring eating disorder behaviours and attitudes. Ward's method was used, with complete linkage as a check. Clinical judgement, inspection of the dendrogram and formal tests were used to determine the number of clusters. The analysis was repeated without two OUTLIERS and robustness was examined using a 75% sub-sample. Tests of construct validity were performed using variables external to clustering and predictive validity was assessed in terms of its success in predicting the time course of the illness compared to using standard diagnostic criteria.

Partitioning methods divide the data into a single partition (rather than a series as in hierarchical methods), the number of clusters being specified in advance. They iteratively reassign cases to clusters and re-compute cluster centres, so as to optimise an objective function such as within-cluster variance. One popular method is *k-means*; a non-parametric method is *partitioning around medoids* (PAM). These methods usually need to have an initial partition from which to start the process and require the whole dataset to be available during the process. The *Kohonen* or *self-organising map* (SOM), a type of NEURAL NETWORK that successively reassigns cases to clusters, is an example of an 'online' method, i.e. one where cases are taken one at a time and 'presented' to cluster centres. The 'winning' (closest) centre is moved toward the case and the process continues with the next case, recycling cases until the system is stable. This method is quite similar k-means, but does not need all cases to be available and can therefore cope with much larger datasets.

In addition to methods using heuristic algorithms, a number of so-called *model-based* methods have been developed. The model that underlies such methods is usually that the data are a sample from a FINITE MIXTURE DISTRIBUTION (see McLachlan and Peel, 2000). For categorical data, the populations could be multinomial: a method based on this assumption is *latent class analysis* (see Everitt, Landau and Leese, 2001). For continuous data, a mixture of MULTIVARIATE NORMAL DISTRIBUTION may be appropriate. Estimating the multivariate normal parameters and the mixing proportions by MAXIMUM LIKELIHOOD ESTIMATION can be a difficult computational problem, especially with small samples. However, the use of classification likelihood methods (which involve estimating cluster memberships treated as indicator variables rather than estimating mixing proportions) have simplified this task and made clustering based on multivariate normal models more widely available in standard software packages. Implementation of this method requires a specification of how size and shape (spherical or ellipsoidal)

are assumed to vary. The second figure shows a three-component mixture identified by fitting a mixture of multivariate normals using classification likelihood and illustrates the results of making these choices for a particular dataset.

There are many methods that do not fall into the categories mentioned. For example, in *fuzzy* methods individuals have a grade or weight of cluster membership for different clusters as opposed to *crisp* methods, where cases are definitely assigned to one cluster. Model-based methods that produce probabilities of membership of the clusters for each case can be regarded as fuzzy, but there are also fuzzy methods that do not rely on a probabilistic model. Some methods can allow for *overlapping* clusters (overlap being a different concept to fuzziness, in that cases can belong to more than one cluster simultaneously).

Other methods can cluster cases and variables simultaneously. An example is *hierarchical classes* (not to be confused with the more general term 'hierarchical methods' as described earlier). This is a method appropriate for attribute data and relatively often used in psychological or psychiatric applications. Another method for clustering both cases and variables is *direct data clustering*, which involves rearranging the rows and columns of the data matrix so that cases that are similar in terms of variables (and vice versa) appear next to each other. Arabie, Hubert and De Soete (1996) give a general review of standard and non-standard methods and individual entries in this volume describe some of these in more detail.

Two types of medical data that may need special treatment, because of the size and complexity of their typical

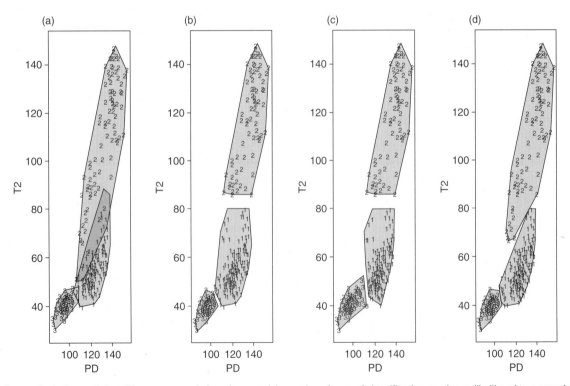

cluster analysis in medicine *Three-group solutions from applying various forms of classification maximum likelihood to a sample of 500 voxels from fMRI imaging data: (a) an* a priori *classification; (b) clusters assuming same-size spherical clusters; (c) clusters assuming same-size ellipsoidal clusters; (d) clusters allowing ellipsoidal clusters of different sizes*

datasets, are genetic and imaging data. Gene expression data produced by *microarrays* (solid surfaces containing many, often thousands, of target genes against which genetic samples are compared) are characterised by very large datasets and also include a temporal dimension if the samples from the same person are taken at different time points (see MICROARRAY EXPERIMENTS). The correlation that this induces is sometimes modelled by including an *autoregressive* component in the analysis. Medical images, for example from functional magnetic resonance imaging, are also often characterised by large datasets. Furthermore, in addition to a temporal dimension, they may also exhibit *spatial autocorrelation* due to the physical contiguity of the measurements (see STATISTICS IN IMAGING). Genetic and imaging datasets often require methods not available in standard software and a number of websites are devoted to this type of specialised analysis. *ML*

Arabie, P., Hubert, L.J. and De Soete, G. (eds) 1996: *Clustering and classification.* Singapore: World Scientific. **Everitt, B.S., Landau, S. and Leese, M.** 2001: *Cluster analysis,* 4th edn. London: Edward Arnold. **Gordon, A.E.** 1999: *Classification,* 2nd edn. New York: Chapman and Hall. **Hay, P.J., Fairburn, C.G. and Doll, H.A.** 1996: The classification of bulimic eating disorders: a community-based cluster analysis study. *Psychological Medicine* 26, 801–12. **McLachlan, G.J.** 1992: Cluster analysis and related techniques in medical research. *Statistical Methods in Medical Research* 1, 27–48. **McLachlan, G.J. and Peel, D.** 2000: *Finite mixture models.* New York: John Wiley & Sons.

cluster randomised trials

Trials in which groups or clusters of individuals are randomly allocated to treatments. The difference between cluster randomised trials and individually randomised trials is that in a cluster trial the main unit of randomisation is not the same as the unit on which the analysis is carried out. Thus the unit of randomisation may be as a group of people such as a town but the outcome will be the behaviour of people in the town. The intervention is often aimed at and delivered by healthcare professionals, such as education to modify their treatment of patients, but the effectiveness of the intervention is assessed in terms of the outcome for the patient. In contrast, in individually randomised trials, both intervention and outcome are aimed at the same person.

The main reason for using a cluster trial is fear of *contamination.* This occurs because subjects in the same unit or treated by the same healthcare professional are likely to receive the same intervention. Thus it can be very difficult to ensure that subjects in a control group do not receive at least some of the intervention if they are physically in the same unit as the treated subjects. It may be difficult for healthcare professionals to switch from one style of treatment to another or subjects may compare notes on the treatments they have received. There are many different features associated with cluster randomised trials and some of the statistical aspects were first discussed by Cornfield (1978). The main feature is that patients treated by one healthcare professional tend to be more similar than those treated by different healthcare professionals. If we know by which doctor a patient is being treated, we can predict slightly better than chance the performance of the patient and thus the observations for one doctor are not completely independent, which is the usual assumption for analysis.

What is surprising is how even a small correlation can greatly affect the design and analysis of such studies.

Cluster trials can be divided into those with a cohort design, in which patients are followed up over time, and cross-sectional design, in which the patients at baseline are not the same as those in the follow-up. A cohort design would follow up patients after treatment, but a public health campaign might adopt a cross-sectional design in which different individuals are questioned before and after the intervention, say a local radio campaign to reduce drink driving.

It is helpful, when planning and analysing a study, to have a model in mind from the start. We will consider a cohort design in general practice in which the same patients are followed up over time. For continuous outcomes y_{ij} for an individual j in practice i we assume that:

$$y_{ij} = \mu + z_i + \tau\delta_i + \beta x_{ij} + \varepsilon_{ij} \qquad (1)$$

where $j=1\ldots n_i$ is the number of patients per practice and $i=1\ldots N=$ total number of practices. Here z_i is assumed to be a random variable with $E(z_i)=0$, $Var(z_i)=\sigma_B^2$ and reflects the overall effect of being in practice i, τ is the additional effect of being in one of the treatment arms relative to the other where δ_i takes the value 1 for one treatment arm and zero otherwise and x_{ij} is a vector of the individual level (or practice level) covariates with regression coefficients β. We assume $Var(\varepsilon_{ij}) = \sigma^2$ and thus $Var(y_{ij}) = \sigma^2 + \sigma_B^2$. It can be shown that when a model is fitted which ignores z_i the STANDARD ERROR of the estimate of β is too small and thus in general one is likely to increase the Type I error rate.

One feature of the model as written is that both σ^2 and σ_B^2 are assumed constant and independent of the treatment effect, but clearly this can be investigated and the model modified if necessary.

For some models, we need to assume also that z_i and σ_{ij} are normally distributed.

The INTRACLUSTER CORRELATION (ICC) is given by:

$$\rho = \frac{\sigma_B^2}{\sigma^2 + \sigma_B^2}. \qquad (2)$$

With cluster trials there are two sample size issues: how many clusters and how many patients per cluster. The basic principles for a completely randomised design have been discussed by Donner and Klar (2000). The idea is to obtain the sample size for an individually randomised trial and inflate the sample size by the design effect (DE) where $DE = 1 + (\bar{n} - 1)\rho$ and $\bar{n}$ is the average cluster size.

Values of the ICC up to about 0.05 are found in practice in primary care. Even with this small ICC, with 20 patients per practice the sample size has to be doubled for a fixed POWER compared to an individual randomised trial.

Cornfield (1978) states that one should 'analyse as you randomise'. Since randomisation is at the level of the practice, a simple analysis would be to calculate 'summary measures', such as the mean value for each practice, and analyse these as the primary outcome variable.

Omitting the covariates from the model for simplicity it is easy to show that:

$$\bar{y}_i = \mu + \tau\delta_i + \bar{\varepsilon}_i \qquad (3)$$

where $\bar{y}_i$ is the mean value for y_{ij} for practice i and:

$$Var(\bar{y}_i) = \sigma_B^2 + \frac{\sigma^2}{n_i} \qquad (4)$$

Equation (3) is a simple model with independent errors, which are homogeneous if n_is are always of similar size. An ordinary least squares estimate at practice level of τ is unbiased and the standard error of estimate is valid provided the error term is independent of the treatment effect.

Thus a simple analysis at the cluster level would be the following: if n_is are the same or not too different, then carry out a two sample t-test on the practice level means; if the n_is are different, then carry out a weighted two-sample t-test using the estimated inverse of the variance for weight. It is worth noting that if σ^2 is zero (all values from a practice are the same) then practice size does not matter in the analysis and if σ_B^2 is zero, then the weight is equivalent to the number of patients per practice.

The advantage of a practice-level approach is that it is simple and intuitive. It works for both continuous and binary data; for the latter, one analyses the proportions in each cluster and treats the proportions as continuous measures (as, for example, using a paired t-test). Donner and Klar (2000) describe this method and other methods of adjusting the CHI-SQUARE TEST for clustering.

However, there are a number of problems with a cluster-level approach. The main one is how should patient level covariates be allowed for. It seems unsatisfactory to use cluster averaged values of the patient-level covariates. The method is also possibly inefficient since the number of DEGREES OF FREEDOM for any practice-level comparison is constrained by the number of practices and the method takes no account of the number of patients per practice. The precision of the estimate of τ is increased marginally by increasing the number of patients per practice.

The model given in equation (1) is termed a RANDOM EFFECTS MODEL or a two-stage multilevel model. The main method for fitting mixed models is by MAXIMUM LIKELIHOOD and this is available in a number of packages such as MlWin, SAS Proc Mixed, STATA and Splus. Some of the methods require some distributional assumptions such as normality of the between cluster random effect, which can be difficult to verify empirically. A further refinement to model fitting is to use a technique known as restricted maximum likelihood (REML). This method is useful for estimating variance components because the usual maximum likelihood estimates are biased (see COMPONENTS OF VARIANCE). This procedure is available in SAS Proc Mixed and MlWin. These methods estimate the parameters from a *cluster-specific* model and try to estimate the effect of the intervention *within* clusters.

A rather different method of estimating the parameters uses GENERALISED ESTIMATING EQUATIONS (GEE), which provide valid estimates of treatment effects even if the intracluster correlation is not precisely specified. Since it is an approximate method it requires more than 20 clusters to give valid estimates. GEE estimates parameters from a *population* or *marginal* model that tries to estimate the effects *on average* over clusters.

To explain this it is easier to select an example outside of clinical trials. Suppose we had patients, clustered in some way, for example in families, and we were interested in the risk of high blood pressure for stroke. A marginal model looks at the risk of intervention people with high blood pressure, compared to low blood pressure, *on average*. In contrast, a cluster specific looks at average of risk of people with high v. low pressure *within a cluster* such as a family. For a linear model, the marginal and cluster specific methods are estimating the same *population parameter*, although different methods of estimation may give differing *estimated* results. For a non-linear model such as a logistic regression, the population parameters are different, to a degree related to the difference in the mean levels of the clusters. (Further details are given by Neuhaus, Kalbfleisch and Hauck, 1991.)

Some packages have an option to estimate a 'robust' standard error for a large number of procedures such as multiple and LOGISTIC REGRESSION under clustering, also known as the Huber-White estimate, for which no distributional assumptions are required. The method to avoid is the FIXED EFFECTS approach in which one fits dummy variables to each cluster. This removes the cluster-level variability, but gives estimates that are biased (Murray, 1998). *MJC*

[See also CLINICAL TRIALS, CLUSTERED BINARY DATA]

Cornfield, J. 1978: Randomization by group: a formal analysis. *American Journal of Epidemiology* 108, 100–2. **Donner, A. and Klar, N.** 2000: *Design and analysis of cluster randomisation trials in health research.* London: Arnold. **Murray, D.M.** 1998: *Design and analysis of group randomized trials.* Oxford: Oxford University Press. **Neuhaus, J.M., Kalbfleisch, J.D. and Hauck, W.W.** 1991: A comparison of cluster-specific and population-averaged approaches for analysing correlated binary data. *ISI Review* 59, 25–35.

clustered binary data

clustered binary data   Binary responses on units that are nested in clusters. Examples include repeated responses where occasions are nested in subjects, twin data where twins are nested in twin pairs and responses on children nested in doctors. Here the units are said to be at level 1 and the clusters at level 2. In three-level data, the 'level-2' clusters are themselves nested in 'level-3' clusters. For instance, children may be nested in doctors who are nested in hospitals as shown in the Figure.

Units within a cluster are expected to be more similar to each other than to units in different clusters. Three types of statistical methods, accommodating the dependence induced by clustering, have been suggested for analysing clustered binary data.

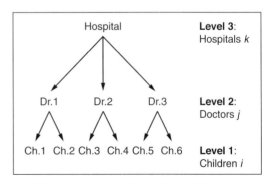

clustered binary data   *Three-level clustered data*

- *Cluster-specific models* where each cluster has its own effect(s).
  - RANDOM EFFECTS MODELS where dependence is explicitly modelled by including cluster-specific random intercepts (and possibly coefficients) that are drawn from a distribution and hence vary over clusters. These models are typically estimated using maximum marginal likelihood where the random effects are 'integrated out' (see RANDOM EFFECTS MODELS for discrete longitudinal data). The random effects are sometimes specified as categorical latent classes, leading to mixture regression.
  - Fixed intercept models where dependence is explicitly modelled by including fixed intercepts that vary over clusters. These models are typically estimated using maximum conditional likelihood where the cluster-specific intercepts are 'conditioned out'.
- *Marginal approaches* for marginal or population-averaged effects.
  - GENERALISED ESTIMATING EQUATIONS (GEE) where dependence is treated as a nuisance. GEE is an estimation algorithm that need not correspond to any statistical model.
  - Truly marginal models, for instance the Bahadur, Dale and George-Bowman models. These models are usually estimated using MAXIMUM LIKELIHOOD ESTIMATION.
- *Transition models* where effects are conditional on responses of other units in the cluster. These models require that the units within a cluster are not 'interchangeable', the canonical example being longitudinal data where responses are time ordered. In this case, autoregressive models are sometimes used.   *AS/SR-H*

[See Fahrmeir and Tutz (2002), Molenberghs (2002) and Skrondal and Rabe-Hesketh (2004) for further discussion.]

Fahrmeir, L. and Tutz, G. 2001: *Multivariate statistical modelling based on generalized linear models*. New York: Springer. **Molenberghs, G.** 2002: Model families. In Aerts, M., Geys, G., Molenberghs, G. and Ryan, L.M. (eds), *Topics in modelling of clustered data*. Boca Raton: Chapman & Hall/CRC, 47–75. **Skrondal, A. and Rabe-Hesketh, S.** 2004: *Generalized latent variable modelling: multilevel, longitudinal and structural equation models*. Boca Raton: Chapman & Hall/CRC.

Cochran Q-test

A test to see if the proportion of positive dichotomous outcomes varies between sets of matched data. Used for example to test whether there is heterogeneity between people rating subject data or to see if there is a difference between treatments for trials using matched patients.

Where MCNEMAR'S TEST is applied to two paired groups, the Cochran Q-test seeks to identify whether the proportions of positive responses vary among many matched groups. The Cochran Q-test can be viewed as an extension of McNemar's and they are equivalent when the number of groups is two.

To calculate Cochran's Q-statistic, one must identify for each of the N samples or subjects the number of groups in which its response is positive and denote these values $S_1, S_2, ..., S_N$. One must also identify for each of the c groups (e.g. raters or time points) the total number of samples or subjects that are given a positive response and denote these values $T_1, T_2, ..., T_c$. These two sets of values

will both sum to the total number of positive responses, which we denote T.

The Cochran Q-statistic is then calculated as:

$$Q = (c - 1) \times \frac{c\sum_{j=1}^{c} T_j^2 - T^2}{cT - \sum_{n=1}^{N} S_n^2}$$

and compared to the CHI-SQUARE DISTRIBUTION with $c-1$ DEGREES OF FREEDOM.

Cochran illustrates this with an example where 4 different media are investigated for effectiveness in growing a bacterium when 69 matched specimens were grown in each medium. Four of the specimens had S_n values of 4 (i.e. bacteria grew in all four media), five had S_n values of 3, one had an S_n value of 2 and the rest S_n values of 0, giving $\sum_{n=1}^{N} S_n^2 = 113$, $c = 4$, $T = 33$. The total numbers of successful specimens by medium (the T_j) were 6, 10, 7 and 10, giving $\sum_{j=1}^{c} T_j^2 = 285$, $Q = 8.052$.

When compared to the chi-square distribution with 3 degrees of freedom this gives a P-value of 0.045, indicating that there is evidence that the media do not all perform alike.

It may be apparent from these calculations that since only the sums of positive responses are used, any specimen (or row of matched data in the more general case) that contributed no positive responses can be ignored. By arguments of symmetry, one can see that specimens that give a positive response in every case are similarly uninformative and can be ignored. Note that this is akin to McNemar's test where the concordant pairs do not contribute to the test statistic.   *AGL*

Cochran, W.G. 1950: The comparison of percentages in matched samples. *Biometika* 37, 256–66. **Fleiss, J.L.** 1981: *Statistical methods for rates and proportions*. New York: John Wiley & Sons.

Cochrane Collaboration

The Cochrane Collaboration is an international organisation that aims to help people make well-informed decisions about healthcare by preparing, maintaining and promoting the accessibility of systematic reviews of the effects of healthcare interventions. Systematic reviews produced by the Collaboration are published in The Cochrane Database of Systematic Reviews as part of The Cochrane Library, available online and on CD-ROM on a subscription basis (Cochrane Database of Systematic Reviews, 2004). The Cochrane Collaboration is currently the largest organisation in the world engaged in the production and maintenance of systematic reviews. In 2003 more than 9000 contributors from 80 countries were involved and the second issue of the database in 2004 contained 1999 completed reviews and 1441 protocols for reviews.

The Cochrane Collaboration was named after Archie Cochrane, the British epidemiologist who, in his influential text, *Effectiveness and efficiency*, promoted the use of evidence from randomised controlled trials to inform the provision of healthcare services (Cochrane, 1972). He went on to emphasise the importance of systematic reviews, when in 1979 he wrote: 'It is surely a great criticism of our profession that we have not organised a critical summary, by specialty or subspecialty, adapted periodically, of all relevant randomised controlled trials' (Cochrane, 1979). This challenge led to the establishment during the 1980s of an international collaboration to develop the *Oxford database of perinatal trials* (Chalmers, 1989–1992). In 1987, the year before Cochrane died, he referred to a systematic review of randomised controlled trials (RCTs) of care during pregnancy and childbirth as 'a real milestone in the history of randomised trials and in the evaluation of care' and suggested that other specialties should copy the methods used (Cochrane, 1989). His encouragement, and the endorsement of his views by others, led to the opening of the first Cochrane Centre by Iain Chalmers (in Oxford, UK) in 1992 and the founding of the Cochrane Collaboration in 1993.

The Collaboration produces reviews through its Collaborative Review Groups, which are supported by fields, Cochrane centres and methods groups (Cochrane Collaboration website). There are currently 50 Cochrane collaborative review groups, each being responsible for reviews in a particular area of healthcare. The 12 regional Cochrane centres support review activity and dissemination of the library around the world, while the 9 fields provide links between the Collaboration and particular areas of healthcare (e.g. primary care), types of consumer (e.g. older people) or types of intervention (e.g. vaccines). The 10 methods groups undertake statistical and methodological research related to systematic reviews, advise the Collaboration on how systematic reviews should be undertaken and reported, monitor the quality of reviews and assist in the development of software and training materials.

Cochrane reviews aim to minimise bias and therefore reviews of healthcare interventions attempt to locate all randomised trials, whether or not they have been published. The Collaboration has worked to improve the identification of randomised controlled trials in the literature by systematically handsearching journals and conference proceedings and by working with the National Library of Medicine to improve indexing of randomised trials on Medline and PubMed. The resulting collection of citations, The Cochrane Central Register of Controlled Trials, is available as a second database on The Cochrane Library. In April 2004 it contained over 400,000 citations.

Publication of Cochrane reviews as electronic rather than paper documents has advantages that include the ability to update reviews when new trials are completed, full reporting of standardised details from all trials, including FOREST PLOTS and data, and the ability for users of the Cochrane Library to reanalyse reviews using alternative summary statistics and statistical models, as well as viewing the analyses chosen by the author. Comments and criticisms of reviews can also be made online and published alongside the original review.

In its second decade the Cochrane Collaboration is continuing to register and publish new reviews of healthcare interventions, as well as tackling the challenges of how to obtain better systematic evidence of the harmful effects of interventions and how to ensure that systematic reviews are updated in a timely manner. The Collaboration is also now developing plans for the publication of Cochrane

Reviews of diagnostic test accuracy.   *JD*

Chalmers, I. (ed.) 1989–1992: *The Oxford database of perinatal trials.* Oxford: Oxford University Press. (Contents subsequently transferred to and maintained in The Cochrane Database of Systematic Reviews.) **Cochrane, A.L.** 1972: *Effectiveness and efficiency. Random reflections on health services.* London: Nuffield Provincial Hospitals Trust. **Cochrane, A.L.** 1979: 1931–1971: a critical review, with particular reference to the medical profession. In *Medicines for the year 2000.* London: Office of Health Economics, 1–11. **Cochrane, A.L.** 1989: Foreword. In Chalmers, I., Enkin, M. and Keirse, M.J.N.C. (eds), *Effective care in pregnancy and childbirth.* Oxford: Oxford University Press. **The Cochrane Collaboration website**: www.thecochranelibrary.com and www.cochrane.org. **The Cochrane Database of Systematic Reviews** 2004: Issue 2. The Cochrane Library. Chichester: John Wiley & Sons.

coefficient of determination   See CORRELATION

cohort studies   Also called medical follow-up studies, cohort studies are considered to be any epidemiological study in which the study population is identified before the occurrence of the disease event of interest and then followed in time until the first occurrence of the disease event or the end of the study, whichever comes first. These may also be referred to as survival studies, in which the outcome is death. Typically, subjects are classified as exposed or not exposed to one or more putative risk factors at the beginning of the study or, alternatively, they may provide more detailed information on exposure.

Because exposure is determined prior to an illness, this study design avoids bias due to selective recall by patients who have been recently diagnosed as in a CASE-CONTROL STUDY, especially when there may be rumours or preconceptions regarding the association between disease and the putative risk factor. Nevertheless, the potential for bias always deserves considerable thought when designing a study, especially for an observational study (Kelsey, Thompson and Evans, 1986; Kleinbaum, Kupper and Morgenstern, 1982; Prentice, 1995; Rothman and Greenland, 1998). The strongest evidence of the effect of an exposure on a disease event or death is provided by a study in which the level of exposure is assigned at random, as in a randomised controlled clinical trial. However, for factors that may be harmful, this would not be feasible in a human population due to ethical concerns.

In a typical cohort study, subjects are recruited for a period of time and then followed until a specified date, when the status of subject is recorded and the results analysed. The Figure on page 65 presents a diagram showing a chronological representation for four hypothetical subjects. The date of enrolment is represented by a circle (●) and the date at which the disease is diagnosed or the subject dies is represented by a diamond (♦). A complete history from enrolment to the outcome is available for the first two subjects, but for the last two, only incomplete information is available because they are not observed until the outcome. In the third subject, follow-up continues until the study ends, when they are withdrawn alive. However, the fourth subject is lost to follow-up during the period represented by the dotted line and the fact that the outcome had actually occurred before the end of the study was not known to the investigators. The last two subjects are said to be *right censored* because only partial information on time to the outcome is avail-

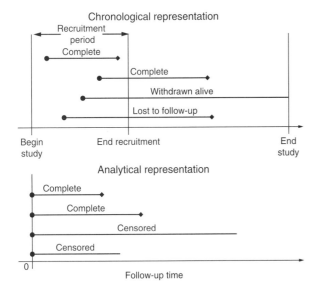

Chronological representation

Analytical representation

cohort studies *Chronological and analytical representations of a cohort study (● = start time, ♦ = time of outcome)*

able, i.e. it is known that outcome occurred sometime to the right of the last date of observation.

For analysis, the time of follow-up and an indicator of whether the outcome was observed are used, as shown in the analytical representation in the figure. The hazard function, which is also called the incidence rate for a disease outcome or a mortality rate for a death outcome, is the basic quantity of interest. A proportional hazards or Cox model is commonly employed:

$$\lambda(\mathbf{X};t) = \lambda_0(t)\exp[\mathbf{X}\boldsymbol{\beta}]$$

in which $\mathbf{X}$ is a row vector of covariates, $\boldsymbol{\beta}$ a column vector of corresponding parameters to be estimated and $\lambda_0(t)$ the underlying hazard that may depend on time (Holford, 2002; Prentice, 1995). Among the elements in the vector of covariates are indicators of the exposure level for each subject.

The number of disease cases or deaths usually exerts the greatest impact on the statistical power of a cohort study. Therefore, a rare disease will typically require a huge and expensive effort to accomplish. This may be due to the need to enrol a very large population that will be followed in time or it may be due the need for a long period of follow-up, especially if there is a long incubation period between the time when the exposure of interest occurs and the disease process begins. For example, in studies of cardiovascular disease, e.g. the Framingham Study and the MRFIT Study, a sample size of 5000 to 20,000 was used to obtain results of interest. However, for studies of diseases such as cancer, e.g. the Nurses' Health Study and the Iowa Women's Study, the outcome is less common, so sample sizes in the range of 50,000 to 100,000 or even larger may be used.

At one time, cohort studies were identified as prospective studies, but the current usage of retrospective and prospective refers to the temporal identification of the study population in relation to the study itself. Thus, a prospective cohort study would start by recruiting a study population

that would subsequently be followed in time. However, in some circumstances, a more efficient design strategy would be retrospectively to identify a population in which records are available that will allow an investigator to reconstruct the cohort experience that would have been observed had the study population been enrolled in the study for the entire time period. For example, in a study of factors affecting occupational safety, company records might allow an investigator to go back in time and thus reconstruct the disease history of cohorts exposed to different factors of interest, i.e. a retrospective cohort.   *TRH*

Holford, T.R. 2002: *Multivariate methods in epidemiology*. New York: Oxford University Press. **Kelsey, J.L., Thompson, W.D. and Evans, A.S.** 1986: *Methods in observational epidemiology*. New York: Oxford University Press. **Kleinbaum, D.G., Kupper, L.L. and Morgenstern, H.** 1982: *Epidemiologic research: principles and quantitative methods*. Belmont: Lifetime Learning Publications. **Prentice, R.L.** 1995: Design issues in cohort studies. *Statistical Methods in Medical Research* 4, 273–92. **Rothman, K.J. and Greenland, S.** 1998: *Modern epidemiology*. Philadelphia: Lippincott-Raven.

coefficient of determination   See CORRELATION

coincidences   Surprising concurrencies of events, perceived by some as meaningfully related, with no causal connection. Carl Jung was fascinated by coincidences and even introduced the term *synchronicity* for what he saw as an *acausal* connecting principle needed to explain the phenomenon, arguing that such events occur far more frequently than chance allows. But Jung gets very little support from Fisher who commented thus on coincidences: 'The one chance in a million will undoubtedly occur, with no more and no less than its appropriate frequency, however surprised we may be that it should occur to us.' Most statisticians would agree with Fisher and put down coincidences to the 'law' of truly large numbers: With a large enough sample, any outrageous thing is likely to happen. Some examples are given in Everitt (1999).

Those interpreting medical research studies should be aware of this when faced with an extremely small *P*-VALUE if such did not arrive from a pre-planned analysis, perhaps arriving from a data-dredging exercise (or 'fishing expedition').   *BSE*

[See also PITFALLS IN MEDICAL RESEARCH, POST-HOC ANALYSES]

Everitt, B.S. 1999: *Chance rules*. New York: Springer.

collective ethics   See ETHICS AND CLINICAL TRIALS

competing risks   A term used particularly in SURVIVAL ANALYSIS to indicate that the event of intent (e.g. death) may occur from more than one cause. Survival analysis is concerned with the time (T) to the occurrence of some event of interest such as remission, death due to a specific disease, discontinuation of use of a contraceptive device etc. For some individuals T may not be observable due to the occurrence of some competing event. For example, if death from prostate cancer is of interest, then death from cardiovascular disease is a competing risk, as is death from old age. There may be multiple competing failure types from which each subject is at risk. We assume that there is only one failure time per study subject. For more than one time observed for each subject multistate models as discussed by Kalbfleisch and Prentice (2002) are recommended. The survival function of any specific failure type of interest is typically estimated by the product-limit estimator (KAPLAN-MEIER ESTIMATOR (KM)), treating the observed times of the other failure types as CENSORED OBSERVATIONS. The complement of the Kaplan-Meier estimator (1-KM) is often used to estimate the probability of failure due to a specified failure cause even in the presence of COMPETING RISKS. The KM approach is only reasonable under the assumption that all competing risks are independent.

Independence can be considered to mean that the probability of the occurrence of some competing event is independent of the occurrence of any of the other competing events. In most situations this assumption is not valid. For example, patients with local relapse of breast cancer may have a higher probability of distance recurrence. In fact it has been argued that in the presence of competing risks a cause-specific survival function has no biological meaning since 'elimination' of some of the competing risks must influence the others. For example, Hougaard (2000) points out that treatment of stroke owing to thromboses by dissolving blood clots would increase the probability of haemorrhage. In order to avoid unrealistic assumptions on the relationships between the various competing risks the KM method should not be used but rather the cumulative incidence function needs to be estimated. The cumulative incidence function for a specific cause of interest (often called the sub-distribution function) is the probability of the event of interest occurring before time t from an individual subject to all of the competing causes. To illustrate, suppose that 10 patients, subject to two competing risks (A and B) die at the times shown in the Table.

Corresponding cumulative incidences for causes A and B are presented in the first Figure.

In order to illustrate the cumulative incidence computations consider time 5. The probability of death from cause A at time 5 or before is estimated by the number of cause A deaths occurring by time 5 divided by the total number of subjects in the study or 1/10; for cause B the corresponding probability is 3/10. Note that the sum of these two probabilities 4/10 is the overall probability of death at time 5 or before and is equivalent to 1-KM computed on all the deaths ignoring cause.

competing risks *Survival experience of 10 patients subject to two competing risks of death (A and B)*

Patients	Time to death	Cause of death
1	2	A
2	17	A
3	3	B
4	14	A
5	5	B
6	9	B
7	4	B
8	8	A
9	10	B
10	12	B

However, when computed for a specific cause 1-KM and the cumulative incidence estimate can differ substantially as illustrated for cause A in the second figure.

As the second Figure (see page 67) shows, 1-KM tends to overestimate the probability of interest. The presence of censoring and/or explanatory variables complicates the computations (Kalbfleisch and Prentice, 2002). Statistical inference, both for a single cumulative incidence function and for the comparison of several cumulative incidences can be quite complex.

Crowder (2001) discusses in detail parametric modelling for competing risks; an approach not often taken for biomedical research. Green, Benedetti and Crowley (2003) focus on applications in oncology, although their methods are more generally applicable. In many situations it may not be clear which of the possible competing causes resulted in death. Flehinger, Reiser and Yashchin (2001) review the analysis of such *masked* data.   *DF/BR*

Crowder, M. 2001: *Classical competing risks.* New York: Chapman and Hall. **Flehinger, B.J., Reiser, B. and Yashchin, E.** 2001: Statistical analysis for masked data. In Balakrishnan, N. and Rao, C.R. (eds), *Handbook of statistics.* Vol. 20: *Advances in reliability.* London: Chapman & Hall, 499–522. **Green, S., Benedetti, J. and Crowley, J.** 2003: *Clinical trials in oncology*, 2nd edn. New York: Chapman & Hall. **Hougaard, P.** 2000: *Analysis of multivariate survival data.* New York: Springer Verlag. **Kalbfleisch, J.D. and Prentice, R.L.** 2002: *The statistical analysis of failure time data*, 2nd edn. New York: John Wiley & Sons.

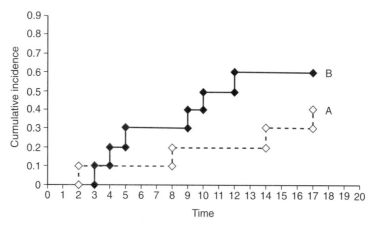

competing risks *Cumulative incidences of death for cause A and B for data in the competing risks table*

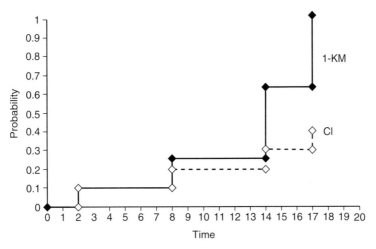

competing risks *Cumulative incidence and 1-KM estimates for probability of death by cause A*

complementary log-log model Another commonly used model, besides the LOGISTIC REGRESSION model and the PROBIT MODEL, for investigating the relationship between a binary (or binomial) response, Y say, and explanatory or predictor variables. It is used in a variety of settings, for example, in the analysis of data from toxicology studies (dose-response data) where interest lies in determining the effect on subjects' survival (e.g. mice mortality) of the exposure to different doses of a 'toxic' chemical compound. It is also used in serological studies in which serological tests are performed to detect the presence (i.e. the seropositivity) or absence of antibodies produced in response to an infectious disease such as malaria, so as to be able to calculate infection rates. Further examples are in dilution studies where an estimate of the number of infective organisms present in a solution is required but can only be obtained through applying different dilutions of the solution to a number of plates that contains a growth medium and recording whether any growth has occurred after a fixed incubation period; in ageing studies where interest lies in self-reported mobility disability; and in the analysis of grouped (or interval) survival data (see SURVIVAL ANALYSIS) where the presence or occurrence of an event is known only to within a specific time interval.

Mathematically, the model relates the probability, P say, of a 'positive' response ($Y = 1$), to a linear combination of the explanatory variables through the complementary log-log link function (see GENERALISED LINEAR MODELS). That is:

$$\log(-\log(1 - P)) = \beta_0 + \beta_1 x_1 + ... + \beta_k x_k,$$

where $x_1,...,x_k$ are the k explanatory variables, and the βs are the corresponding regression coefficients.

The Figure presents a plot of the complementary log-log transformation of the probability P against the probability P itself. Also included on the graph are plots of the logit and probit transformations of P against P. Each of these three transformations converts a probability in the unit interval $(0,1)$ to any value whatsoever, thus eliminating the need to impose any restrictions on the regression coefficients. However, unlike the logit and probit transformations that are both ($180°$ rotationally) symmetric about $P=1/2$, the complementary log-log transformation is asymmetric (see Figure). Thus this transformation is found more suitable where it is appropriate to deal with the probability of a positive response in an asymmetric manner. That is, when the probability increases from 0 fairly slowly but approaches 1 quite suddenly. Observe also that the complementary log-log transformation does not differ appreciably from the logit transformation when P is small, say less than 0.2.

The justification for using this type of model in the analysis of data from many studies comes from assuming that each subject has an underlying, continuous latent or unobservable tolerance or threshold variable, $Y^\star$, which is assumed to come from the Gumbel or extreme value distribution (see Davison, 1998). If a subject's tolerance variable, $Y^\star$, exceeds a certain threshold θ (i.e. $Y^\star > \theta$), then a positive response, $Y = 1$, is observed. For example, in a toxicological study investigating the effect of different doses of an experimental drug on mice, a mouse may die if the exposure dosage exceeds the underlying tolerance

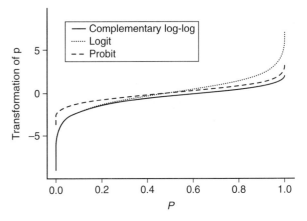

complementary log-log model *Three transformations of probability*

the mouse has for the drug. In studies concerning mobility disability in the elderly, the underlying latent response variable for self-reporting inability to walk a quarter of a mile may be the subject's true mobility level. Hence each individual's response to the question: 'Are you able to walk a quarter of a mile?' will depend on his or her cut-off point, which is the threshold level on this latent scale at which he or she will move from $Y = 0$ to $Y = 1$. Thus coefficients in the regression model above may be interpreted as the effects of the covariates on the latent variable, $Y^\star$.

The complementary log-log model can also be derived from noting the relationship between the probability of a positive response in a time interval of length T say (or an analogous measure, say volume), and the response rate, μ say, for this time interval, under the Poisson assumption (see POISSON DISTRIBUTION). For example, this relationship is utilised in the development of models for dilution and serological studies, where the probabilities of growth occurring on a plate at a particular dilution and of a person living in a particular disease endemic area being infected with this disease in one year, respectively, are of interest.

This model also follows naturally from the application of the proportional hazards assumption to grouped survival data. The regression coefficients in this case are interpreted as log hazard ratios (see SURVIVAL ANALYSIS) or log relative risks. However, if P is small ($P < 0.2$), the regression coefficients can also be interpreted as log odds.

BT

Collett, D. 2002: *Modelling binary data*, 2nd edn. London: Chapman & Hall/CRC. Davison, A.C. 1998: Extreme values. In Armitage, P. and Colton, T. (eds), *Encyclopedia of biostatistics*. Chichester: John Wiley & Sons.

complete case analysis

An analysis that uses only individuals who have a complete set of the intended measurements included in a study. An individual with a missing value on one or more variables will not be included in the analysis. When there are many individuals with missing values this approach can considerably reduce the effective sample size. In most circumstances complete case analysis is not to be recommended since other approaches such as MULTIPLE IMPUTATION can be used in order to retain as full a dataset as possible thereby improving efficiency and reducing bias.

BSE

[See also DROPOUTS]

complier average causal effect (CACE)

See ADJUSTMENT FOR NON-COMPLIANCE IN RANDOMISED CONTROLLED TRIALS

component bar chart

See BAR CHART

components of variance

Variance parameters that quantify the variation attributable to random effect terms included in a regression model. For example, a simple RANDOM EFFECTS MODEL for diastolic blood pressure measurements on patients recruited from a number of clinics includes random effects to represent the variability between clinics and random residual effects to represent the variability between patients. If no further random effect terms are added to this model, the model is said to include two components of variance. The VARIANCE of the random clinic effects in the model is the between-clinic

variance component and the variance of the random residual effects is the between-patient variance component in this example. Under this model, the total variance of the individual patient measurements is assumed to be equal to the sum of the variance components.

Suppose in this example of blood pressure measurements on patients within clinics that the overall mean value is estimated as 80mmHg, with the between-clinic variance component estimated as 7 and the between-patient variance component estimated as 135. The estimated between-clinic variance component allows construction of a 95% range for the mean blood pressure values at the different clinics, using the approach for calculating a reference interval. Here, values that are within approximately two (between-clinic) standard deviations of the overall mean are $80 - 1.96\sqrt{7} = 74.8$mmHg and $80 + 1.96\sqrt{7} = 85.2$mmHg. It is therefore estimated that the majority of mean blood pressure values for different clinics lie between 74.8mmHg and 85.2mmHg.

Estimation of variance components is relevant in a number of application areas. In HEALTH SERVICES RESEARCH, variance components can be used to describe the variability between administrative or geographical units such as clinics, hospitals or towns and, separately, the variability between patients within units. In LONGITUDINAL DATA, variance components can be used to describe the variability between patients and, separately, the variability between measurements within patients.

When the data of interest are from a balanced design, there is a standard approach for estimation of variance components that is based on ANALYSIS OF VARIANCE. As an example, consider some data representing six repeated measurements of peak expiratory flow rate (PEFR) for 10 patients with asthma. A simple random effects model for the PEFR measurements includes a between-patient variance component σ_b^2 and a within-patient variance component σ_w^2. Because the same number of observations is available for every patient, the dataset is balanced and the variance components can be estimated using an analysis of variance table for the data. The Table presents the observed sums of squares and mean squares, as in a conventional analysis of variance. Under the random effects model assumed here, the expected values for the mean squares can be expressed in terms of the variance components σ_w^2 and σ_b^2.

By equating the observed mean squares with their expected values, estimates for σ_w^2 and σ_b^2 are obtained as 191.41 for σ_w^2 and $(11903.83 - 191.41)/6 = 1952.07$ for σ_b^2.

Many study designs produce unbalanced data, for example health services research studies that include a number of hospitals or clinics commonly recruit varying numbers of patients from these and longitudinal studies need not

components of variance *Observed sums of squares and mean squares*

Source of variation	Degrees of freedom	Sums of squares	Mean squares	Expected mean squares
Between patients	9	107134.51	11903.83	$\sigma_w^2 + 6\sigma_b^2$
Within patients	50	9570.70	191.41	σ_w^2
Total	**59**	**116705.21**		

collect equal numbers of measurements from all subjects. Several methods are available for estimation of variance components in unbalanced datasets. Extensions of the analysis of variance approach to the unbalanced case have been proposed, but these are not now commonly used. Estimation of variance components using the method of MAXIMUM LIKELIHOOD ESTIMATION can be achieved within many statistical software packages. However, maximum likelihood estimates of variance components are biased downwards in general. The preferred method for estimation of variance components in unbalanced data is restricted maximum likelihood estimation (REML), which is also available within many software packages. In balanced datasets, REML estimation gives the same results as the analysis of variance approach as just described, whereas maximum likelihood estimation does not.

By definition, a component of variance is non-negative, since it corresponds to the variance of a set of random effects. However, the methods for estimation of variance components can produce negative values. Usually, this occurs when the true value of the variance component is small and non-negative. One approach to proceeding is to set the negative estimate to zero. Estimation and reporting should be handled with care for data in which a negative variance estimate has been obtained (Brown and Prescott, 1999). (For further accounts of variance components, see Goldstein (1995), Searle (1971) and Snijders and Bosker (1999).) *RT*

Brown, H. and Prescott, R. 1999: *Applied mixed models in medicine*. Chichester: John Wiley & Sons. **Goldstein, H.** 1995: *Multilevel statistical models*. London: Arnold. **Searle, S.R.** 1971: *Linear models*. New York: John Wiley & Sons. **Snijders, T. and Bosker, R.** 1999: *Multilevel analysis*. London: Sage.

composite endpoint See ENDPOINTS

compound symmetry

A term used to describe the structure of a covariance matrix that has all its diagonal elements equal to the same value (say σ_1^2) and all its off-diagonal elements equal to another value (say σ_{12}), i.e. a covariance matrix with the form:

$$\Sigma = \begin{bmatrix} \sigma_1^2 & \sigma_{12} & . & . & . & \sigma_{12} \\ \sigma_{12} & \sigma_1^2 & . & . & . & \sigma_{12} \\ . & . & & & & . \\ . & . & & & & . \\ . & . & & & & . \\ \sigma_{12} & \sigma_{12} & . & . & . & \sigma_1^2 \end{bmatrix}$$

Such a structure is assumed by some approaches to the analysis of longitudinal date, for example, the random intercept model, although it is generally unrealistic since, in practice, variances often increase with time and covariances frequently increase with the time interval between two measurements. *BSE*

[See also LINEAR MIXED EFFECTS MODELS]

conditional independence graphs See GRAPHICAL MODELS

conditional logistic regression

A form of logistic regression that can be applied to matched datasets, particularly data from matched CASE-CONTROL STUDIES (see MATCHED PAIRS ANALYSIS). For such data the usual logistic regression model cannot be used since the number of parameters increases at the same rate as the sample size with the consequence that MAXIMUM LIKELIHOOD ESTIMATION is no longer viable. The problem is overcome by regarding particular parameters as a 'nuisance' that do not need to be estimated (see NUISANCE PARAMETERS). A conditional likelihood function can then be created which will yield maximum likelihood estimators of the parameters of most interest, i.e. the regression coefficients of the EXPLANATORY VARIABLES involved. The mathematics of the procedure are described, for example, in Collett (2003). The conditional logistic regression models can be applied using standard logistic regression software as follows: first, set the sample size to the number of matched pairs; next, use as explanatory variables the differences between the values for each case and control; then, set the value of the response variable to one for all observations; and, finally, exclude the constant term from the model. *BSE*

Collett, D. 2003: *Modelling binary data*, 2nd edn. Boca Raton: Chapman & Hall/CRC Press.

conditional probability

A conditional probability is the probability of an event given that another event has occurred. For example consider two events a and b, the probability of both a and b occurring, denoted $P(a \wedge b)$, using the *multiplication rule* [see PROBABILITY] can be expressed as:

$$P(a \wedge b) = P(a|b) \times P(b) \tag{1}$$

Rearranging (1) yields the conditional probability of a given b as:

$$P(a|b) = \frac{P(a \wedge b)}{P(b)} \tag{2}$$

If a and b are independent, then $P(a \wedge b) = P(a) P(b)$ and hence from (2) $P(a|b) = P(a)$. Frequently, we wish to reverse the conditioning, i.e. rather than $P(a|b)$ we want $P(b|a)$ and this can be achieved using BAYES' THEOREM.

Conditional probabilities are frequently used in epidemiology (Clayton and Hills, 1993). The Figure shows a typical situation is which individuals can be develop a disease or not denoted D+ and D− respectively, having been exposed or not, denoted E+ and E− respectively. The conditional probability that individuals develop the disease given that they were exposed, i.e. $P(D+|E+)$, is 0.8. *KRA*

Clayton, D.G. and Hills, M. 1993: *Statistical models in epidemiology*. Oxford: Oxford University Press.

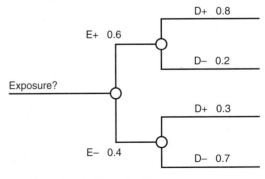

conditional probability *Decision tree*

confidence intervals A range of values calculated from a sample so that a given proportion of intervals thus calculated from such samples would contain the true population value. In research, we collect data on our research subjects so we can draw conclusions about some larger population. For example, in a randomised controlled trial comparing two obstetric regimes, the relative risk of Caesarean section for active management of labour compared to routine management was 0.97, with confidence interval 0.60 to 1.56 (Sadler, Davison and McCowan, 2000). This trial was carried out in one obstetric unit in New Zealand, but we are not specifically interested in this unit or in these patients. We are interested in what they can tell us about what would happen if we treated future patients with active management of labour rather than routine management. We want to know not the relative risk for these *particular* women but the relative risk for *all* women.

The trial subjects form a sample that we use to draw some conclusions about the population of such patients in other clinical centres in New Zealand and other countries, now and in the future. The observed relative risk of Caesarean section, 0.97, provides an estimate of the relative risk we would expect to see in this wider population. It is called a *point estimate* because it is a single number. If we were to repeat the trial, we would not get exactly the same point estimate. Other similar trials cited by Sadler, Davison and McCowan (2000) have reported different relative risks: 0.75, 1.01 and 0.64. Each of these trials represents a different sample of patients and clinicians and there is bound to be some variation between samples. Hence we cannot conclude that the relative risk in the population will be the same as that found in our particular trial sample. The relative risk that we get in any particular sample would be compatible with a range of possible differences in the population.

We estimate this range of possibilities in the population with the confidence interval. A 95% confidence interval is defined in such a way that if we were to repeat the trial many times and calculate a confidence interval for each, 95% of these intervals would include the relative risk for the population. Thus if we estimate that the population value is within the 95% confidence interval, we will be correct for 95% of samples.

This is a pretty difficult concept to get to grips with. The Figure shows a computer simulation of relative risks and confidence intervals for 100 studies where the relative risk in the population is 0.90 and the sample size and Caesarean rate similar to those in the New Zealand study (Sadler, Davison and McCowan, 2000). Of these 100 confidence intervals, 5 include the population value (chosen to be 0.90).

Many researchers misunderstand confidence intervals and think that 95% of samples will produce point estimates within this confidence interval. This is simply not true. In the simulation, the first sample confidence interval is 0.46 to 1.15, and only 83% of sample relative risks are within these limits.

Such intervals are not unique and indeed many intervals with this property could be chosen. We usually choose the interval so that, of those intervals that do not include the population value, half will be wholly greater than that value and half wholly less. This often leads to intervals that are symmetrical about the point estimate, although in the case of RELATIVE RISKS AND ODDS RATIOS this symmetry usually occurs on the logarithmic rather than the natural scale.

In principle, a confidence interval can be found for any quantity estimated from a sample. There are several different methods for doing this, some simple and some not. First, we shall show how confidence intervals can be found for two of the simplest statistics, MEAN and proportion for continuous and categorical data, respectively, and then see what they show about confidence intervals in general.

In the St George's Birthweight Study (Brooke *et al.*, 1989) data on birth weight and gestational age on 1749 pregnancies were obtained. For the 1603 births at 37 weeks' gestation or more the mean birth weight was 3384g

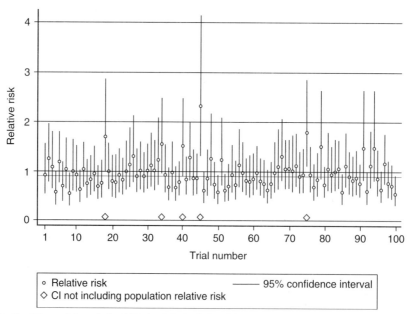

confidence intervals *Confidence intervals for 100 simulated relative risks*

and the STANDARD DEVIATION was 449g. This is a large sample and the sample mean will be an observation from a normal distribution whose mean is the unknown mean birth weight in the population and whose standard deviation is well estimated by the standard error $449/\sqrt{1603} = 11.2$. For a normal distribution, 95% of observations are less than 1.96 standard deviations from the mean, so 95% of sample means will be less than 1.96 standard errors from the population mean. The 95% confidence interval has as lower limit the sample mean minus 1.96 standard errors and as upper limit the sample mean plus 1.96 standard errors, $3384 - 1.96 \times 11.2$ to $3384 + 1.96 \times 11.2 = 3362$ to $3406g$.

Similar methods can be used for many large sample estimates. We need the estimate to be from an approximately normal distribution and the standard error to be well estimated.

We can estimate a confidence interval for a proportion p using the standard error formula for a BINOMIAL DISTRIBUTION $\sqrt{p(1-p)/n}$. For example, in the St George's Birthweight Study 146 of 1749 births occurred at less than 37 completed weeks' gestation. The proportion is thus $146/1749 = 0.08348$ or 8.3%. The standard error is estimated by $\sqrt{0.08348(1 - 0.08348)/1749} = 0.006614$. The 95% confidence interval is thus $0.08348 - 1.96 \times 0.006614 = 0.07052$ to $0.08348 + 1.96 \times 0.006614 = 0.09644$. Rounding this, we get 0.071 to 0.096, which is from 7.1% to 9.6%.

For small samples things get much more complicated. We cannot assume that the estimate follows a normal distribution or that the standard error is a good estimate of the standard deviation of whatever distribution it does follow. For means, we can use a method based on the standard error if we assume that the data themselves follow a normal distribution. If we make this assumption then for a sample of n observation the difference between the sample mean and the unknown population mean divided by the standard error follows a t distribution with $n - 1$ DEGREES OF FREEDOM. Rather than 95% of samples having means within 1.96 standard errors of the population mean, they have means within $t_{0.05}$ standard errors of the population mean, where $t_{0.05}$ is the two-sided 5% point of the t distribution with degrees of freedom. In the birth weight study there were 11 babies born at 34 weeks' gestation. Their mean birth weight was 2477g with standard deviation 531g, giving standard error $531/\sqrt{11} = 160.1g$. There were $11 - 1 = 10$ degrees of freedom and the 5% point of the t-DISTRIBUTION is 2.228. The 95% confidence interval for the mean birth weight of babies born at 34 weeks is therefore $2477 - 2.228 \times 160.1$ to $2477 + 2.228 \times 160.1$, namely from 2120 to 2834g.

For a proportion estimated from a small sample or small number of events, things do not work in the same way. The standard error estimate can go disastrously wrong. In a study of isolated intracardiac echogenic foci in foetuses, we found one trisomy-21 abnormality among 177 subjects (Prefumo *et al.*, 2001). The proportion was thus $1/177 = 0.00565$, or 5.65 per thousand. The usual 95% confidence interval using the normal approximation to the binomial distribution gives −5.4 to 16.6 per thousand, clearly impossible. The large sample assumption has broken down. Researchers will actually quote such impossible intervals and journals have been known to publish them! Sometimes, realising that the negative limit is

impossible researchers will replace it by zero, but this, too, though better, is still wrong. The lower limit of the confidence interval cannot actually be zero in this example. Since we have found a case in the sample, it is not possible that there are no cases in the population.

There are a number of different methods to improve this interval (Newcombe, 1998). One of these uses a procedure based on the exact individual probabilities of the binomial distribution. The binomial distribution has two parameters, the number of independent observations n we make (e.g. number of patients) and the probability P that any given observation will be a 'yes'. This probability is what we are trying to estimate. We find the lower confidence limit as the value of P so that the probability of obtaining the observed number of 'yes's or more will be 0.025 and the upper limit as the value of P so that the probability of the observed number of 'yes's or fewer will be 0.025. These probabilities are obtained by summing the exact binomial probabilities for all the possible numbers of 'yes's equal to and beyond that observed. The calculations for such methods are extremely tedious, but not to a computer. For the echogenic foci data the 95% confidence interval by this method is 0.00014 to 0.03107, or 0.014 to 31 per thousand. This is an example of an exact method calculation, because it uses the exact probabilities of the distribution (see EXACT METHODS FOR CATEGORICAL DATA). There are several other computer-intensive methods that can be used, such as the BOOTSTRAP and those based on rank tests.

The confidence interval allows for what is called sampling variation. This means that it reflects the difference between estimate and population value likely in random samples from that population. However, it does not take into account other sources of variation, termed non-sampling variation. The sample that we have is from geographical space, in that it contains one hospital, as in the active management trial (Sadler, Davison and McCowan, 2000). Even the largest clinical trial will contain at most only a few hospitals and their patients. The hospitals are not chosen randomly, so the sample will differ from the population in an unknown and inestimable way. It is also a sample in time, in that we want the sample of patients seen in the past to tell us about patients whom we will see in the future. The sample may not be as good at estimating quantities in this wider population as the confidence interval suggests.

The interval quoted in the active management trial was a 95% confidence interval and 95% of such intervals would contain the relative risk for the population. We could also calculate intervals for other percentages, for example a 99% interval, calculated so that 99% of possible intervals would contain the population estimate. For the Caesarean section relative risk the corresponding 99% confidence interval would be 0.52 to 1.81, wider than the 95% interval of 0.60 to 1.56 reported. In compensation, more of these intervals would contain the population value.

We could calculate a much narrower interval. A 50% confidence interval is calculated as estimate minus or plus 0.67 standard errors, compared to estimate minus or plus 1.96 standard errors for a 95% confidence interval. The 50% interval based on a large sample normal approximation is only 34% of the width of the 95% interval. This is not very useful as an estimate, as only 50% of such intervals contain the population value they are estimating.

However, it shows that if we calculate 95% confidence intervals, we can say that for about 50% of samples the middle third of the 95% confidence interval will contain the population parameter. Thus, 95% is chosen as a standard confidence level as a reasonable compromise between width (or precision) and coverage probability (accuracy).

Significance tests and confidence intervals are closely related. Many null hypotheses are about the value of something we can also estimate, such as the difference in mean between two groups. It will usually be the case that if the null hypothesis value (difference or regression coefficient = 0, odds ratio or relative risk = 1.0) is contained within a 95% confidence interval then the P-value will be greater than 0.05. For example, in the Birthweight Study, we might want to test the null hypothesis that mean birth weight in the population is 3400g. To test this, we subtract 3400 from the observed mean and divide by the standard error, 11.2. This ratio, $(3384 - 3400)/11.2 = -1.43$, would be an observation from the standard normal distribution if the null hypothesis were true, giving $P = 0.15$. Here the 95% confidence interval (3362 to 3406g) includes the null hypothesis value for the mean, 3400g, and $P > 0.05$. Contrariwise, we might want to test the null hypothesis that the population mean birth weight was 3500g. Now the test statistic is $(3384 - 3500)/11.2 = -10.36$, giving $P < 0.0001$. The null hypothesis value is not included in the confidence interval and the difference is significant. Thus the 95% confidence interval can be used to do a significance test at the 5% level.

For means and their differences there is an exact relationship between the usual confidence interval and the usual significance test, because the standard error is not related to the quantities being compared (means) and thus is not affected by the null hypothesis. It may not work for proportions, relative risks, odds ratios, etc. For example, let us test the null hypothesis that in the population the proportion of births at less than 37 weeks' gestation is 8%. Under the null hypothesis, the proportion is 0.08, and the standard error is $\sqrt{0.08(1 - 0.08)/1749} = 0.006487$, not the same as the 0.06614 used for the confidence interval. The test statistic is $(0.08348 - 0.08)/0.006487 = 0.54$, $P = 0.59$. The null hypothesis value of the proportion is within the confidence interval (0.071 to 0.096) and the difference is not significant. Now let us consider a null hypothesis value just outside the confidence interval, 0.97. The standard error, if the null hypothesis were true, would be $\sqrt{0.097(1 - 0.097)1749} = 0.007077$. The test statistic is $(0.08348 - 0.097)/0.007077 = -1.91$, $P = 0.056$, not significant. This effect of the null hypothesis on the standard error is why we sometimes see odds ratios, relative risks and standardised mortality ratios where the 95% confidence interval includes 1.0, but the ratio is reported as significant.

Researchers are now encouraged to present results as confidence intervals instead of, or in addition to, P-values (Gardner and Altman, 1986). This approach is more informative than the practice of giving a P-value or stating 'significant' or 'not significant', as it provides an estimate of the size of the possible difference or ratio between the groups in the population. This is particularly useful when differences are not statistically significant, as it enables the reader to judge whether a potentially important difference could have been missed. P-values and confidence intervals both have their role and if possible both should be given. Most major medical journals now include in their recommendations to authors that the main results of studies be presented using confidence intervals (or their equivalent) and that authors should avoid relying solely on hypothesis testing.

Finally, some comments on the Bayesian perspective, there being two differing statistical philosophies, the Bayesian and the frequentist. At present few Bayesian analyses appear in the medical literature, although we may expect to see more of them in future (see BAYESIAN METHODS).

People often talk about a 95% confidence interval as including the unknown population value with probability 0.95, saying, for instance, there is a 95% chance the true value lies within the computed 95% CI. Now, it is true that if we set out to collect a new sample, the probability that its confidence interval will include the population value is 0.95. But once the sample has been collected and the interval calculated, it either includes the population value or it does not, we just do not know which.

In strict frequentist terms, we cannot talk about the probability of the population parameter having any given value or range of values. It has a constant, albeit unknown, value with no probability distribution. A Bayesian is willing to think of the population value as a variable with a distribution, which represents the uncertainty in our estimate of it. Bayesians quote something called a CREDIBLE INTERVAL, which is a range of possible values that has a given probability of including the unknown population value. This probability is often set at 95%. Thus a 95% credible interval is a set of values that is estimated to include the population value with probability 95%, whereas a 95% confidence interval is a set of values chosen so that 95% of such sets would include the population value. For the proportion of births before 37 weeks, a Bayesian credible interval, assuming no prior knowledge, is 7.1% to 9.7%, virtually the same as the confidence interval (7.1% to 9.6%). The difference is academic, which is perhaps why academics have spent so much time arguing about it. *JMB*

Brooke, O.G., Anderson, H.R., Bland, J.M., Peacock, J.L. and Stewart, C.M. 1989: Effects on birth weight of smoking, alcohol, caffeine, socioeconomic factors, and psychosocial stress. *British Medical Journal* 298, 795–801. **Gardner, M.J. and Altman, D.G.** 1986: Confidence-intervals rather than p-values – estimation rather than hypothesis-testing. *British Medical Journal* 292, 746–50. **Newcombe, R.G.** 1998: Two-sided confidence intervals for the single proportion: comparison of seven methods. *Statistics in Medicine* 17, 857–72. **Prefumo, F., Presti, F., Mavrides, E., Sanusi, A.F., Bland, J.M., Campbell, S. and Carvalho, J.S.** 2001: Isolated echogenic foci in the fetal heart: do they increase the risk of trisomy 21 in a population previously screened by nuchal translucency? *Ultrasound in Obstetrics and Medicine* 18, 126–30. **Sadler, L.C., Davison, T. and McCowan, L.M.** 2000: A randomised controlled trial and meta-analysis of active management of labour. *British Journal of Obstetrics and Gynaecology* 107, 909–15.

confidence level See CONFIDENCE INTERVALS

confirmatory factor analysis A procedure for testing a hypothesised factor structure for a set of observed variables. The hypothesised structure will specify both the number of factors and which observed variables are related to which factors (Dunn, Everitt and Pickles, 1993). This contrasts with FACTOR ANALYSIS when used in its exploratory mode when the number of factors has to be determined in some ways from the data and no *a priori* constraints are placed on the factor structure. Confirmatory factor analysis is a theory-testing model as opposed to a theory-generating method like exploratory factor analysis. The first step in a confirmatory factor analysis involves the calculation of either a correlation or a COVARIANCE MATRIX for a set of observed variables. Then possibly a number of competing factor models are proposed, derived either from theory or previously performed exploratory factor analyses on other datasets. The models will differ in their specifications of 'free' and 'fixed' parameters. MAXIMUM LIKELIHOOD ESTIMATION is generally used to estimate the free parameters in a model. Confirmatory factor analysis models can be fitted using one of a number of available software packages (LISREL, EQS, MPLUS) and a variety of methods can be used to test the fit of a model and to compare the fit of two competing models.

As an example of where this approach might be applied, consider a psychiatrist who measures a number of variables on a sample of mentally ill patients. The psychiatrist believes that some of the observed variables are related to a patient's depression and others to anxiety and he or she is particularly interested in estimating the correlation between these two, essentially, LATENT VARIABLES. To make things specific suppose there are six observed variables with the first three indicating depression and the remaining three, anxiety. The correlated, two-factor model to be fitted is described graphically by the path diagram shown in the Figure. Apart from the error variances, the parameters to be estimated are the loadings of the first three variables on factor one (depression) – variables four, five and six are constrained to have zero loadings on this variable – and the loadings of the last three variables on factor two (anxiety) – now the first three variables are constrained to have zero loadings. The estimated correlation between the latent variables, depression and anxiety will be a disattenuated correlation, i.e. one in which the effects of measurement errors in the observed variables have been effectively removed.

Detailed examples of the application of confirmatory factor analysis are given in Huba, Wingard and Bentler (1981) and Dunn, Everitt and Pickles (1993). *BSE*

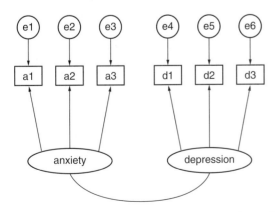

confirmatory factor analysis *Path diagram for depression and anxiety example*

Dunn, G., Everitt, B.S. and Pickles, A. 1993: *Modelling covariances and latent variables using EQS.* Boca Raton: CRC Press/Chapman & Hall. **Huba, G.J., Wingard, J.A. and Bentler, P.M.** 1981: A comparison of two latent variable causal models for adolescent drug use. *Journal of Personality and Serial Psychology* 40, 186–93.

Consolidation of Standards for Reporting Trials (CONSORT) statement
A research tool designed to improve the quality of reports of clinical trials (Begg *et al.*, 1996). The core contribution of the CONSORT statement consists of a flow diagram (see Figure on page 74) and a checklist. The flow diagram enables reviewers and readers to grasp quickly how many eligible participants were randomly assigned to each arm of the trial and whether any imbalances are apparent regarding numbers of patients withdrawing from or failing to comply with their assigned treatment (see DROPOUTS). Large discrepancies or imbalances suggest the need for conducting not only INTENTION-TO-TREAT analyses but also PER PROTOCOL analyses to seek corroboration. Such information is frequently difficult or impossible to ascertain from trial reports as they were reported in the past. The checklist identifies 21 items that should be incorporated in the title, abstract, introduction, methods, results or conclusion of every randomized clinical trial. More details can be found at www.consort-statement.org. *BSE*

[See also CRITICAL APPRAISAL, STATISTICAL REFEREEING]

Begg, C., Cho, M., Eastwood, S., Morton, R., Moher, D., Ohlein, I. *et al.* 1996: Improving the quality of reporting of randomized clinical trials; the CONSORT statement. *Journal of the American Medical Association* 276, 637–9.

consulting a statistician
'To consult the statistician after an experiment is finished is often merely to ask him to conduct a post-mortem examination. He can perhaps say what the experiment died of.' So said R.A. Fisher, later Sir Ronald, widely considered the founding father of modern statistics, and of RANDOMISATION in particular, as long ago as 1938. His tongue-in-cheek message remains sage advice, just as true today as a reminder of the single most important aspect of seeking statistical advice – seeking it early. Many novice researchers make the mistake of believing the statistician to be the numbers person to be approached, and then with trepidation, only once data have been collected. In actuality, a consultation with a statistician should be a positive experience and opportunity to assist planning all aspects of study design, meaning neither just the subsequent analysis nor the narrow matter of SAMPLE SIZE DETERMINATION.

Naturally, there are important differences in how statistical consulting takes place according to whether the setting is within a university, hospital, pharmaceutical company, government agency and so on, due to the obvious differences between public and private sector employers, not to mention geographical differences from one continent to another. Statistical consulting can also take place in a variety of ways: telephone, email, face to face or a mixture thereof.

This entry focuses on the most productive manner, namely face to face, since this maximises effective two-way communication. It also concentrates on those aspects of research projects that are reasonably consistent regardless of the particular environment, although the author's

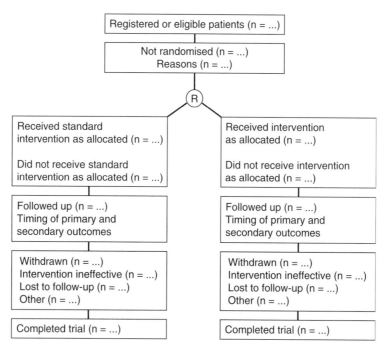

Consolidation of Standards for Reporting Trials statement *Flow diagram of CONSORT statement*

perspective is based on experience within academic settings. The remainder of the entry examines the sort of project-specific advice a statistician can give, including, notably, general guidance on preparing for a first meeting with a statistician and some observations on the interaction between statistician and clinical researcher. What cannot be included, necessarily, is local advice on where to find a nearby consulting statistician in the first place. In the event none is available one should consider using textbooks or WEB RESOURCES IN MEDICAL STATISTICS, or even travelling to attend a short course offering an introduction to the subject. For further details concerning technical content, in addition to the process, of statistical consultations, the reader is referred to the rest of this volume or to Hand and Everitt (1987), Derr (2000) or Cabera and McDougall (2001).

Broadly, research can be subdivided into a number of distinct stages as depicted in the Figure. The worst time to first approach a statistician is at the post-refereeing stage of a submitted journal article. Consultant statisticians may be able to offer some remedial help at this late stage, but only on matters of analysis, interpretation or presentation. The most common reasons why statistical referees recommend rejection of submitted manuscripts to biomedical journals pertain to design issues, which is hardly surprising when one realises that fundamental flaws in study design simply cannot be retrieved by sophisticated analyses (see STATISTICAL REFEREEING). Thus, if the paper has not been rejected outright on statistical grounds, there may be hope for the manuscript after suitable revision. A statistician approached at such a late stage is likely to drop more than a subtle hint that it would be altogether more satisfactory essentially to heed Fisher's advice and request that the researcher come along sooner in a project's life cycle the next time!

There is a temptation to think seeing a statistician is

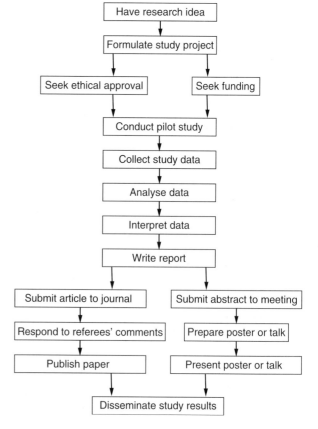

consulting a statistician *Schematic diagram of research process, from initial thoughts through to dissemination of study results. Statistical input should ideally be sought at study formulation stage*

unnecessary if one has confidence in one's own statistical knowledge and ability (and access to relevant software). This can be a dangerous policy for the novice researcher, especially if the confidence turns out to be misplaced, or handling the data more complex than envisaged. Even veterans of medical research with substantial statistical skills of their own can find consulting a statistician invaluable, despite the time and effort required in the midst of busy research agendas and clinical commitments. This is by no means just to delegate data-related tasks but to gain additional, independent input about the intended study from an altogether different perspective. Statisticians do not, after all, see the world of medicine and research in the same way as do those on the frontline dealing directly with patients or for that matter those working with test tubes in the laboratory.

What sort of help can a statistician offer? Clearly, this depends very much on the nature of the project itself and the extent of the statistician's involvement. For example, if in an academic environment, a student seeks advice on a research project forming a part of a degree then involvement will be necessarily less than in a full collaboration. In the former case, the student needs to own the analyses and be able to defend them single-handedly, so that the role of the statistical consultant is to point in the right direction by recommending an appropriate choice of study design and method for data analysis. To help avoid becoming a surrogate supervisor by default it can be useful if the student's project supervisor also attends the consultation. It is important to clarify early on in the consultation process if it is expected to become a full collaboration, for then issues of payment, if indicated, and co-authorship (or acknowledgement for lesser statistical involvement) need to be discussed and agreed.

Payment for statistical advice remains a delicate matter and local rules would dictate. It is sensible, so as not to discourage those who most need statistical help, to have a policy whereby the first meeting (of say about an hour) is provided free of any direct charge to the consultee. Parker and Berman (1998) provide some helpful criteria for suggesting when authorship may or may not be appropriate. As a rule, if the finished piece of work could not have attained its statistical quality without the assistance of the consultant statistician, and more than just elementary descriptive or inferential statistics are involved, then the default ought to be co-authorship for the statistician. There is at least anecdotal evidence that statistical co-authorship enhances chances of publication in first-choice journals. Equally, there is a danger that statisticians' names can be used against their wishes to lend perhaps more credence than is due to some submitted papers or grant applications!

What should be brought to a first meeting? In order to make the most use of the time available it is best for the consultee to have made some specific preparations. A checklist can assist, perhaps in the format of a QUESTION-NAIRE to be completed in advance of the initial meeting. Useful questions to address both 'housekeeping' matters as well as more substantive issues concerning the project, include the following: *1. What is the single main aim of the project?* (A brief answer to this fundamental question at least ensures the meeting can be focused.) *2. What stage is the project at right now?* (Options can be forming ideas/ designing protocol/collecting data/analysis of data/writing up/referee's comments.) *3. What area(s) do you think you need help with?* (Formulating ideas/sample size calculation/ designing protocol/making grant application/RANDOMISA-TION practicalities/carrying out the study/collecting data/ managing data/analysis you are doing/checking your analysis/checking written report/responding to referee.) *4. What role would you like statistician to play?* (Advisor/co-applicant/interpreter of results/co-author, although note that statistician would reserve right to decline the latter if authorship was felt to be inappropriate.) *5. Does this work form part of a dissertation or thesis?* (See comments already made on student work.) *6. What is the source of patients or subjects and the criteria for selecting them?* (Allows opportunity to discuss or review appropriate study design.) *7. How many subjects are required or available?* (If this is to be a topic for advice, need to know clinically relevant differences in proportions involved and/or standard deviations for continuous outcomes.) *8. What is the main outcome measure?* (Again to focus attention on primary as opposed to secondary ENDPOINTS or, in worst case, to ensure project does pre-specify at least one endpoint.) *9. What is the main comparison or relationship of interest?* (To encourage being as specific as possible and to check for suitable control group.) *10. What other quantities are being measured and when?* (For example, BASELINE MEASUREMENTS, covariates, secondary outcomes.) *11. What problems have been or are anticipated in data collection?* (To discuss e.g. accuracy, missingness, repeated measures, matching but essentially any potential bias.) *12. What are expected or hoped for results at study's end?* (Again to focus on real reason for performing the research.) *13. Are there any specific approaches to data analysis intended?* (For instance, same method as a previously published study, preferably with a hard copy to be handed over.) *14. Is there any further information you would like to give regarding the study?* (A suitable closing question to allow, one hopes, any pertinent facts to emerge.)

It is best if answers to this catalogue of questions can be sent in advance of the meeting, along with a brief description of the project and copies of related documents to assist the statistician's understanding (for example, protocol, grant application, ethics committee submission).

In terms of practicalities, the statistician may have some further expectations of the consultee to bring or transmit in advance of the first meeting at which data are to be analysed (recall, ideally, this is *not* at the first encounter!) Statisticians do not usually take on the more mundane data-entry tasks, so would not be prepared to type in the numbers. They may express preferences for how data are presented electronically in terms of file type (e.g. Excel being a common choice) and media (floppy disks are fine, although somewhat outmoded; email attachments generally work better for small-to-moderate sized datasets). In any event, it is always important to check for viruses to avoid spreading contaminated files. The layout of the data should ordinarily be as a spreadsheet, with well-labelled variable names, one column per variable and one row per subject. It is best to ask if there is a data-entry preference when handling repeated measures data, but if in doubt the spreadsheet works fine. In any case, data provided must be reasonably clean, free from data-entry errors, although the odd OUTLIER is excusable.

Due to confidentiality issues (e.g. the Data Protection Act 1998 in the UK) there should not be any uncoded individual patient identifiers, that is, names and addresses and other information that could be used to trace individuals must have been removed. Obviously, the anonymisation process must generate unique patient IDs in order to be fully reversible so that queries with data can be checked from original records that are stored elsewhere. While it is not a serious problem, it is better to code data numerically rather than alphanumerically. For example '1' and '2' for 'male' and 'female', respectively is better than use of 'M', 'm', 'male', 'Male', 'MALE', etc., especially as accidental leading or trailing blanks can add to potential confusion possibly creating a needless missing data point on subsequent conversion to numeric format. In general, categorical variables should have a different number representing each group, with an accompanying description, or internal labelling, of how the categories are coded. Equally, missing data are better handled by inserting an obviously impossible value (e.g. '–99' when all other values are positive) rather than just leaving a spreadsheet cell blank. The statistician would rather be told about any such embedded code, however, to avoid unnecessary runs of software routines after noticing e.g. strange residuals in regression analyses.

An altogether less tangible item to bring along, but arguably the most important for a successful meeting, can be summarised as the *right attitude*. Statistical consultation involves a high degree of communication and mutual respect. Since areas of expertise are different, jargon is to be avoided – by both the statistician and the consultee. (Medics are not alone in having big words or abbreviations and acronyms, to describe things that are obvious only to themselves!) Punctuality is important but it is understood that medical emergencies can and do occur that necessitate being late, in which case arranging for a telephone message is a simple courtesy, or cutting short an ongoing meeting at a bleeper's notice. However, there is no such thing as a statistical emergency, so there is little excuse for the consultee who demands an immediate appointment with a statistician or expects results to be turned around within, say, 24 hours to meet his or her deadline for a grant, ethics or conference submission, particularly as such deadlines are typically known months in advance. Also bear in mind some consulting statisticians are new to their jobs. Just as some training of junior doctors occurs 'on the job', so too do junior statisticians have to learn, ideally under supervision from someone more experienced, by interacting with real clients in real consultations. The transition from a university degree course to practising statistical consultant is never automatic. An attitude of patience is helpful in these circumstances, much as required by drivers stuck behind a learner struggling with hill starts (we were all learner drivers once!)

To close, and in keeping with the spirit of Fisher's advice quoted earlier, it can be instructive to consider ways of having an *unhelpful* meeting between medical researcher and statistician. So long as both parties can avoid making these mistakes, there is scope for real progress and genuine collaboration.

First, what are some of the ways a statistican can upset medical colleagues? 1. Being too nit-picky, precise, detail oriented and fail to see the big picture. 2. Being slow to respond to requests for appointments or to analyse data. 3. Being overly critical of genuine-but-flawed attempts to analyse data themselves. 4. Using unnecessary jargon. 5.

Using unnecessarily complicated methods when simpler ones suffice. 6. Spending too much or too little time during the consultation. 7. Embarking on a mathematical lecture within a consultation. 8. Expecting to meet only on your home turf (despite owning a laptop). 9. Believing there is such a thing as an average patient. 10. Thinking EVIDENCE-BASED MEDICINE (EBM) means clinical experience counts for nothing compared to having a few well-honed CRITICAL APPRAISAL skills and a recently published META-ANALYSIS to hand.

Finally, how to upset your statistician? 1. Saying 'This will only take 5 minutes of your time', for it will not. 2. Arriving unannounced, late or not at all (genuine emergencies notwithstanding). 3. Waiting until the grant or ethics application deadline is tomorrow and leaving no time for review of statistical input before sending the document off. 4. Dripfeeding data or hypotheses or telling half the story ('Oh, actually it's the same patient seen five times') or shifting between study aims. 5. Taking for granted – not considering acknowledgement or co-authorship or bothering to inform if that application or journal submission was ever successful or not. 6. Saying, in earshot, 'I just need the statto to crunch the numbers' and generally regarding statistician as a technical service provider. 7. Expecting knowledge of specialist medical terminology. 8. Expecting poorly entered data to be cleaned or forgetting to run a virus check on your floppy disk. 9. Demanding 'What's the p-value?' or 'Can't you find one that *is* significant?' 10. Coming too late in research process and complaining about a statistical post-mortem!   *CRP*

Cabera, J. and McDougall, A. 2001: *Statistical consulting.* New York: Springer. **Derr, J.** 2000: *Statistical consulting: a guide to effective communication.* Pacific Grove: Duxbury Press. **Hand, D.J. and Everitt, B.S.** (eds) 1987: *The statistical consultant in action.* Cambridge: Cambridge University Press. **Parker, R.A. and Berman, N.G.** 1998: Criteria for authorship for statisticians in medical papers. *Statistics in Medicine* 17, 2289–99.

contingency coefficient A measure of the strength of an association between two categorical variables. While the CHI-SQUARE TEST can detect an association between two variables, it is not a good measure of the strength of that association. This is because it is also dependent on the sample size and the number of categories into which the variables are classed. Typically, contingency coefficients are adjustments of the chi-square statistic, intended to remove the dependence on those factors. Because they are based on the chi-square statistic, any attempt to test the contingency coefficient for significance will merely resolve into repeating the chi-square test of independence.

The two most common contingency coefficients are Cramér's contingency coefficient (also known as Cramér's C, Cramér's V and occasionally Cramér's v) and Pearson's contingency coefficient (often just referred to as the contingency coefficient or as Pearson's coefficient of mean square contingency). For a table with r rows and c columns, with k being set as equal to the smaller of r and c, that produces a chi-square statistic of X^2 from n observations, the formulae for Cramér's and Pearson's coefficients are:

$$\text{Cramér's coefficient} = \sqrt{\frac{X^2}{n(k-1)}}$$

and

$$\text{Pearson's coefficient} = \sqrt{\frac{X^2}{X^2+n}}$$

While Cramér's coefficient can take values from zero to one, Pearson's coefficient can never reach one (the denominator is clearly always larger than the numerator). In fact, Pearson's coefficient has a known maximum of $\sqrt{(k-1)/k}$ so it is possible to rescale this coefficient to lie in the range 0 to 1.

While the use of these measures is popular in some fields, more so if we consider that the phi coefficient for a 2×2 table (see CORRELATION) is a special case of Cramér's coefficient, interpretation is not straightforward. Clearly, in some sense, the larger the coefficient is, the greater the association. However, the absolute value does not have any clear meaning and comparing correlation coefficients from two tables (especially tables of different dimensions) is not straightforward.

Contingency coefficients are widely used as a result of their convenience and in spite of their limitations. For 2×2 tables, odds ratios are possibly a better measure as it is easy to produce confidence intervals and they have a familiar interpretation. For larger tables with at least one ordered categorical variable a measure based on the Spearman rank correlation might be more appropriate. *AGL*

Conover, W.J. 1999: *Practical nonparametric statistics*. New York: John Wiley & Sons. Fleiss, J.L. 1981: *Statistical methods for rates and proportions*, 2nd edn. New York: John Wiley & Sons. Goodman, L.A. and Kruskal, W.H. 1954: Measures of association for cross-classifications. *Journal of the American Statistical Association* 49, 732–64. Siegel, S. and Castellan, N.J. Jr 1988: *Nonparametric statistics for the behavioural sciences*, 2nd edn. New York: McGraw-Hill.

contingency tables Cross-tabulations that arise when a sample from some population is classified with respect to two or more qualitative variables. The first Table shows a simple example involving two such variables each with three categories. A more complex contingency table that involves a classification with respect to three variables is shown in the second Table.

Contingency tables such as these two can be used to test various hypotheses about the variables from which they are formed. To begin with, we shall illustrate this using tables formed from just two variables (two-dimensional contingency tables), since these are the ones encountered most commonly in practice. The hypothesis of interest for two-dimensional tables is whether or not the two variables are independent.

contingency tables *Incidence of cerebral tumours*

		Type			
		A	B	C	Total
	I	23	9	6	38
Site	II	21	4	3	28
	III	34	24	17	75
Total		78	37	26	141

I: frontal lobe; II: temporal lobes; III: other cerebral areas. A: benign tumours; B: malignant tumours; C: other cerebral tumours

contingency tables *Coronary heart disease*

		Serum cholesterol			
	Blood pressure	1	2	3	4
	1	2	3	3	4
CHD	2	3	2	1	3
(yes)	3	8	11	6	6
	4	7	12	11	11
	1	117	121	47	22
CHD	2	85	98	43	20
(no)	3	119	209	68	43
	4	67	99	46	33

Blood pressure: 1 <127mm Hg; 2 127–146mm Hg; 3 147–166mm Hg; 4 >167mm Hg.
Serum cholesterol: 1 <200mg/100cc; 2 200–219mg/100cc; 3 220–259mg/100cc; 4 >260mg/100cc

This may be formulated more formally in terms of p_{ij}, the PROBABILITY of an observation being in the ijth cell of the table, $p_{i.}$ the probability of being in the ith row of the table and $p_{.j}$ the probability of being in the jth column of the table. The hypothesis of independence can now be written:

$$H_0 : p_{ij} = p_{i.} \times p_{.j}$$

Estimated values of $p_{i.}$ and $p_{.j}$ can be found from the relevant marginal totals $(n_{i.}, n_{.j})$ and overall sample size (n) as:

$$\hat{p}_{i.} = \frac{n_{i.}}{n}, \ \hat{p}_{.j} = \frac{n_{.j}}{n}$$

These can then be combined to give the estimated probability of being in the ijth cell of the table under independence, $\hat{p}_{i.} \times \hat{p}_{.j}$. The frequencies to be expected under independence, E_{ij}, can then be obtained simply as:

$$E_{ij} = n \times \hat{p}_{i.} \times \hat{p}_{.j} = \frac{n_{i.} \times n_{.j}}{n}$$

The hypothesis of independence can now be assessed by comparing the observed (O_{ij}) and estimated (E_{ij}) expected frequencies using the familiar CHI-SQUARE TEST statistic:

$$X^2 = \sum_{i=1}^{r} \sum_{j=1}^{c} \frac{(O_{ij} - E_{ij})^2}{E_{ij}}$$

where r is the number of rows and c the number of columns in the table. If H_0 is true X^2 has, asymptotically, a CHI-SQUARE DISTRIBUTION with $(r - 1) (c - 1)$ DEGREES OF FREEDOM. For our first Table, the estimated expected values under independence are given in the third Table (page 78). Here $X^2 = 7.84$ which with 4 degrees of freedom gives an associated P-VALUE of 0.098. There is no evidence against the independence of site and type of tumour.

Since the distribution of the test statistic is only a chi-square asymptotically there has been considerable work on trying to find when the sample size is sufficient for the P-values derived in this way to be valid and alternative procedures have been derived that do not rely on the asymptotic assumption (see EXACT METHODS FOR CATEGORICAL DATA).

contingency tables *Estimated expected values under the hypothesis of independence for data in the cerebral tumour table*

		Type			
		A	B	C	**Total**
	I	21.02	9.97	7.01	**38**
Site	II	15.49	7.35	5.16	**28**
	III	41.49	19.68	13.83	**75**
Total		**78**	**37**	**26**	**141**

When the contingency table is formed from more than two variables more than a single hypothesis may be of interest. We may, for example, wish to test the mutual independence of the variables forming the table or the conditional independence of two of the variables given a third and so on. For some hypotheses, estimated expected values can be found from particular marginal totals but for others an iterative scheme is needed (see Everitt, 1992, for details). In general the analysis of three-dimensional and higher contingency tables is best undertaken with the use of LOG-LINEAR MODELS. *BSE*

[See also CORRESPONDENCE ANALYSIS]

Everitt, B.S. 1992: *The analysis of categorical tables*, 2nd edn. Boca Raton: Chapman & Hall/CRC.

convenience sample

A convenience sample is a non-random sample chosen due to its easy access. A convenience sample is unlikely to be representative of the population, the main disadvantage being that it is unclear how representative the sample is of the population of interest. One example is surveying people who walk by on the street. Another would be selecting patients who attend a clinic or doctors in a particular hospital. The main advantage is that the sample is simple to obtain and may save money.

A classic example is the use of medical students as study subjects when conducting medical research. If the study involves seeking opinions or, for that matter, measuring certain characteristics, such as height, one needs to bear in mind the sample is atypical of the population as a whole and, hence, limit conclusions to the population of all medical students perhaps, to ensure valid inference. *SLV*

Crawshaw, J. and Chambers, J.A. 1994: *Concise course in A level statistics*, 3d edn. Cheltenham: Stanley Thornes Publishers Ltd.

Cook's distance

Cook's distance (Cook, 1977; Cook and Weisberg, 1999) is a measure of the influence of a case on the estimated parameters $\hat{\beta}$ of a linear regression. It measures the global impact of deleting the case on all the parameter estimates taken together and is the distance from $\hat{\beta}$ to $\hat{\beta}_{(i)}$, expressed in terms of confidence ellipsoids about $\hat{\beta}$, where $\hat{\beta}_{(i)}$ is the vector of parameters estimated with the ith case omitted.

For a dependent variable y_i, D_i is given by:

$$D_i = \frac{(y_i - \hat{y}_i)^2}{s^2(p + 1)}\left[\frac{h_i}{(1 - h_i)^2}\right],$$

where p is the number of independent variables, s^2 is the variance of the estimate and h_i is the leverage of the ith

observation, given by the ith diagonal element of the so-called 'hat' matrix $H = X (X^\mathrm{T} X)^{-1} X^\mathrm{T}$, where X is the data matrix of independent values (see Cook and Weisberg, 1999).

For a point to be influential it must be both an OUTLIER, i.e. have a high residual, and it must also have high leverage, i.e. be far from the centre of gravity of the points (see Figure). A general rule of thumb is to examine cases for which $D_i > 1$; alternatively Hamilton (1992) has suggested examining cases for which $D_i > 4/n$. An informal approach is to sort the distances in order and examine the few cases with the highest distances. A large jump between these and the rest can suggest points worth investigating. Cases thus identified might be considered for removal or at least further investigation (subject to the caution that removal of outliers always requires). Analogous quantities for other models are available, e.g. for LOGISTIC REGRESSION (see Pregibon, 1981). If the interest is in one or more particular parameters in the regression, rather than the complete set taken as whole, 'dfbetas' can be computed: these estimate the changes in the individual parameters after deleting each case. *ML*

Cook, R.D. 1977: Detection of influential observations in linear regression. *Technometrics* 19, 15–18. **Cook, R.D. and Weisberg, S.** 1999: *Applied regression including computing and graphics*. New York: John Wiley & Sons. **Hamilton, L.C.** 1992: *Regression with graphics*. Belmont: Duxbury. **Pregibon, D.** 1981: Logistic regression diagnostics. *Annals of Statistics* 9, 705–24.

coplots

See TRELLIS GRAPHS

COREC

See ETHICAL REVIEW COMMITTEES

correlation

Correlation is used to measure the strength of the linear relationship between two random variables. If we plot two variables on a SCATTERPLOT, their correlation is a measure of how closely the points lie to a straight line. We measure correlation by a correlation coefficient. The simplest of these is PEARSON'S CORRELATION COEFFICIENT, also known as the *product-moment*

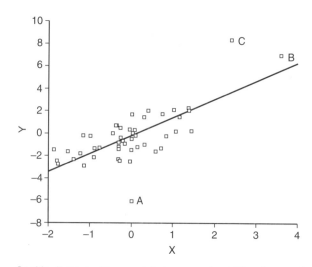

Cook's distance *Three points in a sample of 50, only one of which (C) has a high Cook's distance. Point A has a high residual but low leverage and B has a low residual but high leverage*

correlation coefficient or simply as the correlation coefficient. This is the ratio of the sum of products of differences from the mean divided by the square roots of the two sums of squares about the mean and is usually denoted by r:

$$r = \frac{\sum (y_i - \bar{y})(x_i - \bar{x})}{\sqrt{\sum (y_i - \bar{y})^2 \sum (x_i - \bar{x})^2}}$$

The confusing symbol 'r' (rather than 'c') is for historical reasons; it appears to have indicated 'regression' originally. It is now well established and if a medical paper uses '$r = \ldots$' without explanation, it usually means the correlation coefficient. When we want to distinguish between the correlation coefficient in a sample, r, and the correlation coefficient in the population from which the sample was drawn, we use 'ρ', the Greek letter 'rho', to denote the latter.

The Figure shows some sample correlation coefficients. The coefficient is positive when large values of y are associated with large values of x, the variables being said to be positively correlated, as in (a), (b) and (c) in the Figure. The majority of observations will have either both observations greater than the mean or both less than the mean. In either case, observation minus mean will have the same sign, either positive or negative, for both variables and the product of these differences will be positive. Hence the sum of products will be positive and the correlation coefficient will be positive. The correlation coefficient is negative when small values of y are associated with large values of x, the variables being negatively correlated as in (g), (h) and (i) in the Figure. The majority of observations will have one observation greater than the mean and the other less than the mean. Observation minus mean will have different signs for the two variables and the product of these differences will be negative. Hence the sum of products will be negative and the correlation coefficient will be negative. The correlation coefficient has a maximum value of +1 when the points all lie exactly on a straight line and the variables are positively correlated and a minimum of –1 when the points all lie exactly on a straight line and the variables are negatively correlated. When there is no linear relationship at all the coefficient is zero and the variables are said to be uncorrelated, as in (d) in the figure.

Correlation only measures the strength of the linear (i.e. straight line) relationship. Non-linear relationships may be missed or underestimated by it. In the Figure, (e) shows a strong relationship yet the correlation coefficient is zero and (f) shows an exact mathematical relationship, without any random variation, yet the correlation coefficient is less than one because the relationship is not a straight line.

We can test the null hypothesis that the population correlation is zero, i.e. that there is no linear relationship between the two variables, using a simple t-test. At least one of the two variables must follow a normal distribution and the observations must be independent. If we can assume this, we require only the value of r and the sample size n. Then, if the null hypothesis were true:

$$t = r \sqrt{\frac{n - 2}{1 - r^2}}$$

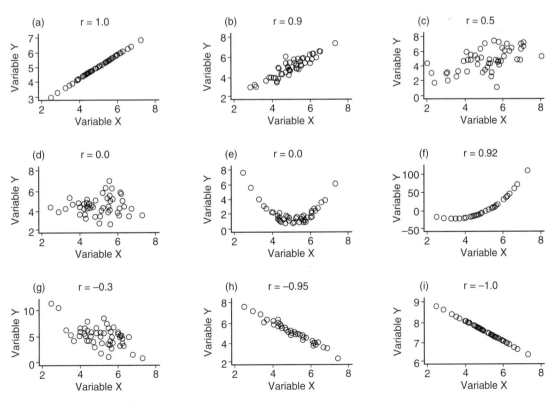

correlation *Nine correlation coefficients*

would follow a t-distribution with $n-2$ DEGREES OF FREE-DOM. There are tables of this test in many books and almost all programs that calculate r also give the P-VALUE. As a result, correlation coefficients in medical papers are almost invariably followed by P-values, e.g. '$r = 0.57$, $P < 0.01$', whether the null hypothesis of zero correlation is plausible or not.

The distribution of the sample correlation coefficient is not a simple one, but it can be converted to the normal using a TRANSFORMATION known as Fisher's z-transformation:

$$z = \frac{1}{2} \log_e \left(\frac{1 + r}{1 - r} \right)$$

This works provided observations are independent and both variables follow normal distributions, a stronger assumption than that required for the test of significance. Provided it is met, the z-transformation can be used to find a confidence interval for r, the standard error on the transformed scale being $\sqrt{1/(n-3)}$. We can calculate the confidence interval for z and transform back. Curiously, many programs do not perform this. The standard error can also be used in a power calculation to estimate the sample size required to detect a relationship between two continuous variables. Bland (2000) and Machin et al. (1998) give formulae and tables.

We can still calculate correlation coefficients when normal assumptions are not met, but cannot use P-values or confidence intervals found by these methods. The assumption of independence is very important. It could be seriously misleading to take several observations from each subject and treat them as a simple sample for the calculation of correlation coefficients and their P-values and confidence intervals (Bland and Altman, 1994).

The correlation coefficient and regression equations between two variables are closely related. The proportion of variation explained by the regression is r^2, whether we have the regression of Y on X or of X on Y. There is only one correlation coefficient although there are two possible regression lines; correlation has no choice of dependent and independent (or outcome and predictor or explanatory) variables. The product of the two regression slopes will also be equal to r^2, which is sometimes called the *coefficient of determination*.

The tests of the null hypotheses of zero correlation and zero slope for the regression line give the same P-value. The two methods provide the same test for a linear relationship.

The product-moment correlation is only one of several correlation coefficients in use. There are two non-parametric rank correlation coefficients, SPEARMAN'S RHO and *Kendall's tau*, useful when the assumptions of normal distribution necessary for confidence intervals and significance tests are not tenable. The intra-class or INTRA-CLUSTER CORRELATION COEFFICIENT is used when, rather than two variables, we have two or more observations of the same variable on each subject. The *tetrachoric correlation coefficient*, seldom seen in practice in the modern literature, can be used when we have two underlying continuous variables but can only observe whether the subject is above or below some cut-off value for each, making both dichotomous. The *biserial correlation coefficient* can be used when one variable is continuous and the other

dichotomous. These are not the same as the correlation coefficients found by simply making the dichotomous variable zero or one and calculating r, called the phi coefficient and point-biserial correlation coefficient respectively.

We can adjust the correlation between two variables for their mutual relationship with a third variable using a partial correlation coefficient. This is an estimate of the correlation between the two variables of interest for subjects who all have the same value of the third variable. Partial correlation is seldom seen now, multiple regression being preferred. There is also a partial rank correlation, using Kendall's approach. We can calculate a *multiple correlation coefficient*, usually denoted by R, which expresses the strength of the relationship between a chosen variable and several others. Time series (see TIME SERIES IN MEDICINE), where observations are measured successively over time, may show serial correlation or autocorrelation, where adjoining observations are correlated. A correlation matrix is the set of all the correlations between each pair of a set of variables and is the starting point for several multivariate techniques (see, for example, PRINCIPAL COMPONENT ANALYSIS). *JMB*

[See also SPEARMAN'S RHO (ρ)]

Bland, M. 2000: *An introduction to medical statistics*, 3rd edn. Oxford: Oxford University Press. **Bland, J.M. and Altman, D.G.** 1994: Correlation, regression and repeated data. *British Medical Journal* 308, 896. **Machin, D., Campbell, M.J., Fayers, P. and Pinol, A.** 1998: *Statistical tables for the design of clinical studies*, 2nd edn. Oxford: Blackwell.

correspondence analysis

A technique for graphically displaying the associations among the categorical variables forming a CONTINGENCY TABLE in the form of a SCATTERPLOT. A correspondence analysis should ideally be seen as an extremely useful supplement to, rather than a replacement for, more formal inferential analysis such as a CHI-SQUARE TEST of the independence of the variables. Correspondence analysis provides a 'window' onto the data that may allow researchers easier access to the associated numerical results, facilitate discussion of the data and possibly generate interesting hypotheses about the data. The mathematics behind correspondence analysis (Everitt, 1997; Greenacre, 1992) leads to two sets of multidimensional coordinate values, one of which represents the categories of the row variable and the other the categories of the column variable. In general, the first two coordinate values representing each row and column category are used to provide a single scatterplot of the data. In the resulting diagram, the distance between a plotted row point and column point represents as accurately as possi-

correspondence analysis *Age and boyfriends contingency table*

	Age[a]				
	1	2	3	4	5
No boyfriend	21	21	14	13	8
Boyfriend/no sexual intercourse	8	9	6	8	2
Boyfriend/sexual intercourse	2	3	4	10	10
Totals	31	33	24	31	20

[a] Age groups: 1 = <16 years; 2 = 16–17 years; 3 = 17–18 years; 4 = 18–19 years

$\chi^2 = 20.6$, $df = 8$, $p = 0.008$

correspondence analysis *Two-dimensional correspondence analysis coordinates for the row and column categories in the first table*

Category	x	y
No boyfriend	0.193	0.061
Boyfriend/no sexual intercourse	0.192	−0.143
Boyfriend/sexual intercourse	−0.732	0.000
Age group 1	0.355	0.055
Age group 2	0.290	0.000
Age group 3	0.103	0.000
Age group 4	−0.281	−0.134
Age group 5	−0.717	0.123

ble how the corresponding cell of the contingency table departs from independence, as we shall illustrate using the data on age and boyfriends shown on page 80. The coordinates resulting from a correspondence analysis of these data are shown in the table above.

These coordinates can be plotted to give the scatterplot shown in the Figure. Of most interest in correspondence analysis solutions is the joint interpretation of the points representing the row and column categories. It can be shown that row and column coordinates that are large and of the same sign correspond to a cell with considerably more observations than if independence held. Row and column coordinates that are large, but of opposite signs, imply a cell in the table with far fewer observations than required under the assumption of independence. Finally, small coordinate values close to the origin correspond to cells where the observed frequency is close to the expected frequency under independence. In the figure, for example, age group 5 and boyfriend/sexual intercourse both have

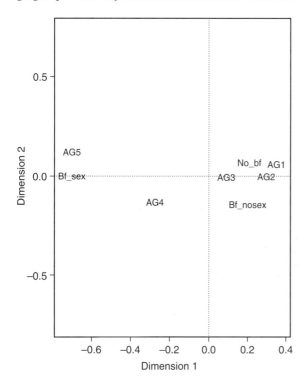

correspondence analysis *Two-dimensional correspondence analysis solution for age and boyfriends data*

large negative coordinate values on the first dimension; consequently the corresponding cell in the table contains more observations than would be the case under independence. Again, age group 5 and boyfriend/no sexual intercourse have coordinate values with opposite signs on both dimensions, implying that the corresponding cell in the table has fewer observations than expected under independence.

BSE

Everitt, B.S. 1997: Annotation: correspondence analysis. *Journal of Child Psychology and Psychiatry* 38, 737–45. **Greenacre, M.** 1992: Correspondence analysis in medical research. *Statistical Methods in Medical Research* 1, 97–117.

cost benefit analysis (CBA) See COST-EFFECTIVE-NESS ANALYSIS

cost-effectiveness analysis A tool for comparing costs and benefits in terms of patient outcomes (changes in health and welfare), so that the value for money of a proposed healthcare intervention can be judged. Cost-utility analysis (CUA) is a specific form of CEA, the main difference being that benefit is expressed in the form of patient preferences and converted to a measure such as the number of quality-of-life adjusted life-years (QALYs). CUA thus allows the comparison of competing health programmes that have very different sorts of outcome. CEA, and to a lesser extent CUA, now appear in many health services research studies, unlike cost-benefit analysis (CBA), in which benefits are expressed in purely monetary terms. Because of time limitations on clinical and health service trials, cost-effectiveness can often only be established for intermediate outcomes and it may be necessary to apply techniques such as SURVIVAL ANALYSIS to extrapolate values into the future (for example, to predict mortality from risk factors). Drummond and McGuire (2001) discuss this point and other key methodological principles involved in CEA.

The incremental cost-effectiveness ratio (ICER) is a key measure in cost-effectiveness analysis and is defined (for a comparison of two treatments) as $\Delta C/\Delta E$, where ΔC is the mean difference in the costs of the treatments and ΔE is the mean difference in effectiveness. A treatment is considered cost-effective if $\Delta C/\Delta E < \lambda$, where λ is the maximum amount that the decision maker is willing to pay or the 'ceiling ratio'. Note that the term 'incremental' stresses the comparison of the treatments with each other: the less useful 'average' cost-effectiveness ratio is often estimated separately for each treatment under study and compared without testing the differences statistically.

Many trials of new therapies collect data on the costs for individual patients, as well as the effectiveness in terms of changes in clinical status or quality of life, and can thus calculate ICERs as part of an economic evaluation. Indeed regulatory bodies in most countries insist on such evaluation before considering drug licensing and provide guidelines as to acceptable methodology. Kobelt (2002) describes the workflow of an economic evaluation in relation to the typical drug development process, from preclinical studies to PHASE III TRIALS and marketing, and discusses the typical resource items that might be included and the economic perspectives from which such studies are performed.

In an economic evaluation, the term 'perspective' refers

to the level at which the costs are to be considered. For example, the societal perspective would treat all costs as relevant, including loss to production due to illness, whereas a health service perspective might consider only direct treatment costs. As well as influencing the type of data collected, the perspective has a bearing on the summary statistics and type of analysis that might be considered appropriate. For example, where the perspective is that of a healthcare provider, it can be argued that it is the mean cost and the mean effectiveness that are relevant, rather than some other summary measure such as the MEDIAN. This is because the total cost aggregated over all patients (which is the important quantity for planning or budgeting purposes) is obtained by multiplying the mean cost by the number of patients.

Various types of uncertainty apply to economic data and all may need to be considered in CEA. For example, the amount of a service used by a patient will need to be multiplied by a unit cost (for example, the cost per hour of employing a therapist) to obtain the total cost per patient for that service. The true unit costs may be available only as point estimates, for example in the form of approximate published values. Furthermore, costs and benefits may have to be discounted to take account of the preference for earlier benefits and/or later costs and this involves the application of discount rates, which are generally estimated. The impact of such deterministic sources of uncertainty is generally assessed through sensitivity analyses, in which ranges of plausible values are considered. Contrariwise, data that have been obtained from a random sample, for example on the service use of individual patients, are subject to stochastic rather than deterministic uncertainty, and this is generally expressed in the form of statistical quantities such as CONFIDENCE INTERVALS and P-VALUES.

Costs often have very skewed distributions and for this reason normal distribution theory may not be appropriate.

Furthermore, if the emphasis is on the estimation of means as suggested here, simple TRANSFORMATIONS (for example log transformation) may not be appropriate since the quantity about which inferences are to be made would no longer be the mean (see Thompson and Barber, 2000). The use of GENERALISED LINEAR MODELS is one solution since these can model mean values directly while also allowing for skewed distributions such as the GAMMA DISTRIBUTION. An alternative is to use nonparametric bootstrapping (see BOOTSTRAP) in which a large number of re-samples is generated, with individuals replicated by sampling with replacement. However, while widely used, there is a potential problem with bootstrapping applied to the ICER, as discussed later, and it has been criticised in more general terms by O'Hagan and Stevens (2002), who argue for a Bayesian framework (see BAYESIAN METHODS) for analysing cost-effectiveness data.

The ICER and some related quantities are illustrated and discussed by O'Brien and Briggs (2002), using an example relating to the costs of treatment and life-years gained in the Canadian Implantable Defibrillator Study (CIDS). The incremental cost-effectiveness plane for interpreting ICERs is shown at (a) in the first Figure. Each quadrant can be labelled according to the interpretation of an ICER falling within it and typically new treatments are more effective but also more costly and would appear in the NE quadrant. If the new treatment is both more effective and less costly than the control or comparison treatment (quadrant SE) then it is said to dominate. In this diagram the point denoted 'CIDS data' represents the observed $(\Delta C, \Delta E)$ pair. The point estimate of the ICER is the slope of the line joining this point to zero (in this case the ICER is 49.115k/0.23, or \$213.5k per additional life-year gained).

The decision as to cost-effectiveness can be made for all $\Delta C, \Delta E$ pairs consistent with the observed data, as represented by the bootstrapped values, a set of 1000 pairs for

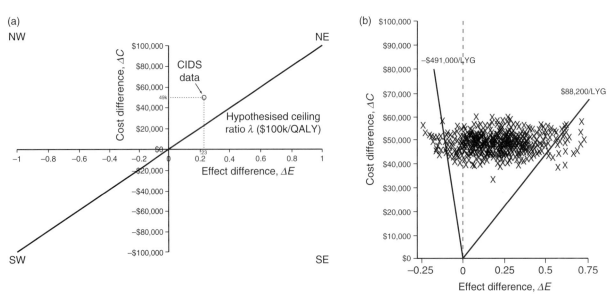

cost-effectiveness analysis *Incremental cost-effectiveness plane for Canadian Implantable Defibrillator Study data showing (a) the four quadrants, point estimates of ΔE and ΔC, from which the ICER is obtained and a ceiling ratio line; (b) bootstrapped values for ΔE and ΔC and confidence limits for the ICER derived from these values* the CIDS data being shown at (b) in the first Figure. Also shown are 95% confidence limits derived from the lines corresponding to the 26th and 975th replicates (ordered from smallest to largest ratio).

Ratios, even of normally distributed quantities, tend to be unstable and have discontinuities since both numerator and denominator could be 0. This can give rise to anomalies since the same ratio can arise from two opposing sets of results, one where the new treatment is less effective and more costly (quadrant NW) and the other more effective and less costly (quadrant SE). When the ratios are ordered and used to estimate confidence limits there is no way to distinguish these cases. Thus it is usually recommended to plot the bootstrapped points in addition to calculating numerical confidence limits so that this situation can be detected.

One way around difficulties arising from using ratios is to cast the problem in a slightly different way, based on plotting the willingness-to-pay line on the cost-effectiveness plane. The region below this line (also called the *ceiling ratio line*) is the *acceptability* region. In this example the willingness-to-pay is $100k per QALY and the point estimate of the ICER is $214k per QALY, so the treatment would not be considered cost-effective. The proportion of the bootstrapped values falling in the acceptability region can then be plotted against a range of hypothetical values for the ceiling ratio to give a *cost-effectiveness acceptability curve*. This approach is useful where no fixed willingness-to-pay has been established since it indicates how probable it is that a treatment will be cost-effective at any given hypothetical willingness-to-pay.

The second Figure illustrates an acceptability curve for the CIDS data. For example, given that a healthcare provider considers $214k as an acceptable upper limit, one might be able to claim that a new treatment is, say, 50% likely to be cost-effective. At $87k it would only be about 2.5% likely to be cost-effective. This latter Figure can be used as a lower 95% confidence limit, the upper 95% confidence limit being infinity in this case.

Another approach, mathematically equivalent to the cost acceptability curve technique, is to calculate the *net monetary benefit* (NMB), which re-expresses the ICER decision rule to give the quantity NMB = $\lambda \Delta E - \Delta C$. This

is now expressed in monetary terms and because it is linear in ΔE and ΔC, parametric confidence limits are simple to calculate, given variances for ΔE and ΔC. The value of NMB can be plotted against λ, for a range of hypothetical values, and the value of λ for which the NMB is zero is a breakeven point, at which the likelihood of being cost-effective is 50%. Of course, the value $214k is obtained as before.   *ML*

Drummond, M. and McGuire, A. 2001: *Economic evaluation in health care – merging theory with practice*. Oxford: Oxford University Press. **Kobelt, G.** 2002: *Health economics: an introduction to economic evaluation*, 2nd edn. London: Office of Health Economics. **O'Brien, B.J. and Briggs, A.H.** 2002: Analysis of uncertainty in health care cost-effectiveness studies: and introduction to statistical issues and methods. *Statistical Methods in Medical Research* 11, 455–68. **O'Hagan, A. and Stevens, J.W.** 2002: Bayesian methods for design and analysis of cost-effectiveness trials in the evaluation of health care technologies. *Statistical Methods in Medical Research* 11, 469–90. **Thompson, S.G. and Barber, J.A.** 2000: How should cost data in pragmatic randomised trials be analysed? *British Medical Journal* 320, 1197–200.

cost utility analysis (CUA) See COST-EFFECTIVENESS ANALYSIS

counterfactual model See CAUSAL MODELS

covariance See COVARIANCE MATRIX

covariance matrix A symmetric matrix in which the off-diagonal elements are the covariances of pairs of variables and the elements on the main diagonal are the variances of the variables. The sample covariance of two variables with sample values (x_1, y_1), (x_2, y_2),...,(x_n, y_n) is defined as:

$$\text{Cov}(x, y) = \frac{1}{n} \sum_{i=1}^{n} (x_i - \bar{x})(y_i - \bar{y})$$

where $\bar{x}$ is the arithmetic mean of the x variable and $\bar{y}$ the arithmetic mean of the y variable. The covariance matrix is often a better basis for the application of STRUCTURAL EQUATION MODELS than the correlation matrix.   *BSE*

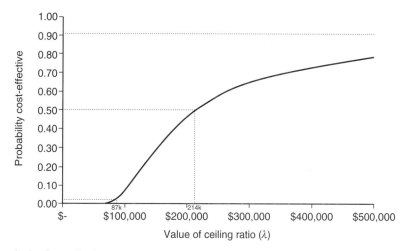

cost-effectiveness analysis *Cost-effectiveness acceptability curve for the Canadian Implantable Defibrillator Study data*

Cox's proportional hazards model See Cox's
REGRESSION MODEL, PROPORTIONAL HAZARDS

Cox's regression model
In 1972 David Cox developed the Cox (or proportional hazards) regression model. Since that time it has become probably the most widely used method of analysing time-to-event (survival) data. This model allows us to link three of the main components of such data for the first time: (i) an indicator variable reflecting whether the individual has experienced an event or not (i.e. has/has not been censored); (ii) the length of time from entry in a study to the event or to the censoring time; (iii) one or more explanatory variables such as age, sex, treatment received, and usually collected at the time of entry of an individual into a study. The popularity of the model is due to its relative computational simplicity, its interpretability, its ability/appearance to perform well in many situations and its incorporation into most major STATISTICAL PACKAGES.

The approach used was novel because it modelled the hazard function over time – made up from components (i) and (ii) above – and related it to the explanatory variables – component (iii). The hazard function can be thought of as the probability that someone now event-free will experience an event in the next small unit of time. The model makes no assumptions about the underlying distribution of hazards in the different groups and, indeed, this is left unestimated in the process of estimating the parameters in the model. The basic model relies on the assumption that the hazard functions are proportional across the groups being studied, i.e. the relative hazards experienced by any two groups of patients are constant over time.

The Cox model can be used to perform a number of different analyses for time-to-event data including: estimating a treatment effect in a study while adjusting for a number of explanatory or baseline variables, such as age, sex; assessing which of a number of explanatory variables are most important and consequently developing a prognostic index; performing stratified analyses; and assessing interactions between variables. It has also been extended to deal with situation where the relative hazard function changes over time, the so-called time-dependent Cox model and for situations when there are deviations from proportional hazards for the hazard functions in different groups.

The Cox model can be written as

$$h_1(t) = h_0(t).\ \exp(\beta_1 x_1 + \beta_2 x_2 + \ldots + \beta_k x_k)$$

where $h_1(t)$ is the hazard function in a given group, $h_0(t)$ is the hazard function in a baseline group (which remains unspecified), β_i are the regression coefficients and x_i are the explanatory variables (from $i=1$ to k). Therefore, the hazard ratio (HR) between groups is

$$h_1(t)/h_0(t) = \exp(\beta_1 x_1 + \beta_2 x_2 + \ldots + \beta_k x_k).$$

One should note the independence from time (t) of the hazard ratio on the right-hand side of this equation. Hazard ratios are relatively simple to interpret; they are the relative risk of one group experiencing the event to another group experiencing the event. Note that, as the baseline hazard is not estimated, only relative measures such as the hazard ratio are provided by the Cox model

and thus no estimates are given in absolute terms using this method. Such estimates have to be calculated indirectly.

A variety of data types can be used in the model, including binary, categorical, ordered categorical and continuous variables. The number of variables one may include in a Cox model is theoretically limitless, but in practice it is limited by number of events in the analysis. One guide is not to use more variables than the fourth root of the number of events. A more lenient guide is to have at least 15–20 events for each category combination.

For each variable being considered in a Cox model we test the null hypothesis that the variable is not important to the model, i.e. that the parameter value associated with the variable, β, is zero; this is equivalent to the hazard ratio for that variable, HR$=\exp(\beta)=e^0=1$. This can tested with a z-statistic where $z=b/\text{SE}(b)$, where b is the estimate of the parameter and $\text{SE}(b)$ is its standard error. Under the null hypothesis this should follow a normal distribution and thus P-VALUES can be calculated in the usual way.

We may assess models and the addition or removal of variables to models using a variety of different tests including the Wald test, LIKELIHOOD RATIO test and score test. The score test is the most complex and less commonly used test. The Wald test looks at the change in the overall χ^2 value between two models where the DEGREES OF FREEDOM is the number of variables different between the models. The likelihood ratio test compares the 'likelihoods' of the two models and takes a more general approach than the Wald test: it looks at how the included variables explain the variation in the model. This is, therefore, the preferred method for reasons of consistency and stability.

The time of each outcome event (failure time) is not actually relevant in a Cox model, but the ordering of these failures is. Therefore, consideration needs to be given to the order of failures in the event of failures with tied event times. These can be dealt with in a series of methods including marginal calculation, partial calculation, Efron approximation and Breslow approximation (see Kalbfleish and Prentice, 2002). The last of these is the simplest and is an adequate approximation if there are relatively few tied failures. Care should be taken when using the Cox model if there are too many tied event times.

As for normal linear regression, it is possible to assess the fit of the Cox model by calculating residuals. However, there are no unique residuals for the Cox model. Commonly used residuals are Schoenfield and Martingale residuals, although it can be difficult to interpret whichever are used. It is also possible to assess whether individual explanatory variables violate the proportional hazards assumption (see proportional hazards) and therefore assess whether a variable should be included in the model. *MS/MP*

Cleves, M.A., Gould, W.W. and Gutierrez, R.G. 2003: *An introduction to survival analysis using Stata®*, rev. edn. Texas: Stata Press. **Cox, D.R.** 1972: Regression models and life tables (with discussion). *Journal of the Royal Statistical Society* B34, 187–220. **Kalbfleisch, J.D. and Prentice, R.L.** 2002: *The statistical analysis of failure time data*, 2nd edn. New York: John Wiley & Sons. **Machin, D. and Parmar, M.K.B.** 1995: *Survival analysis: a practical approach*. London: John Wiley & Sons.

Cramér's contingency coefficient See CONTINGENCY COEFFICIENT

credible interval When the aim of a Bayesian analysis is to provide a scientific inference about an unknown parameter all the required information about the uncertainties involved are contained in the POSTERIOR DISTRIBUTION. There is a sense in which the only true satisfactory inference summary is the complete 'picture' represented by the posterior distribution. Alternatively, a range of posterior distributions corresponding to a range of prior specifications allows a display of the sensitivity of 'conclusions' to 'assumptions'. Sometimes, however, providing a complete picture of the uncertainty in estimation by a posterior distribution is less convenient than providing a low-level summary of the message contained within it. Credible intervals are to Bayesian statistics as CONFIDENCE INTERVALS are to frequentist statistics; they provide a simple summary of the uncertainty associated with the estimate of an unknown parameter.

If we suppose that the posterior distribution for an unknown parameter δ, is denoted by the posterior distribution $p(\delta)$ then an interval (δ_L, δ_U) is said to form a

$100(1 - \alpha)\%$ posterior credible for δ if $\int_{\delta_L}^{\delta_U} p(\delta)d\delta = 1 - \alpha$.

There are infinitely many ways to determine a credible interval, some of which are illustrated in the first Figure. Credible interval (1) is determined so that it excludes regions of equal posterior probability, each tail corresponding to a probability of $1 - \alpha/2$. Credible interval (2) excludes a region of exactly α on the lower side extending to infinity on the right. In contrast, credible interval (3) excludes a region of exactly α content on the right beginning at zero. The final credible interval (4) is termed the highest posterior density (HPD) interval and is constructed so that every parameter value within the interval has a higher density than every value outside the interval and hence they are more likely values. It can be demonstrated that the HPD interval in any particular case determines the shortest credible interval. If the posterior distribution is symmetric then the equal-tailed and HPD intervals coincide. The concept of a credible interval generalises to more than a single parameter.

The second Figure illustrates a bivariate (two-parameter) HPD region constructed in exactly the same way as the univariate case every point within the region having a higher density than every point outside it. The specific

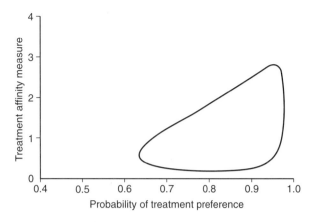

credible interval *Bivariate HPD region*

example is taken from an extension of the Bradley-Terry paired-comparison model (see, for example, Imrey, 1998), accounting for ties. For a given probability content such a credible region has the smallest area. *AG*

Imrey, P.B. 1998: Bradley-Terry model. In Armitage, P. and Colton, T. (eds) *Encyclopedia of biostatistics.* Chichester: John Wiley & Sons.

critical appraisal The process of evaluating research reports and assessing their contribution to scientific knowledge; typically this process is applied to research papers in medical journals. A careful evaluation of the medical literature is important because the quality of research is variable, and often very poor. It is imprudent to assume that a paper is error free just because it has been published: even papers in well-respected journals contain faults that cast doubt on the conclusions. Altman has researched the extent and implications of errors in the medical literature, estimating that reviews have found statistical errors in about half of published papers (Altman, 1991a).

The problem of poor-quality research is set in the context of the increasing use of statistics in the medical literature. Altman (1991a) describes two surveys of research papers published in the *New England Journal of Medicine*, in 1978–9 and 1990. In this time the proportion of papers containing nothing more than descriptive statistics fell from 27% to 11%, while the proportion using more complex statistical methods, such as SURVIVAL ANALYSIS, increased dramatically. A good understanding of statistical analysis, alongside an awareness of statistical issues surrounding research design and execution, therefore, is essential to effective appraisal of the medical literature.

Altman (1994) argued, in an editorial entitled 'The scandal of poor medical research', that research in the medical arena is often done with the aim of furthering a curriculum vitae, rather than promoting scientific knowledge. He suggests that: 'Much poor research arises because researchers feel compelled for career reasons to carry out research that they are ill equipped to perform, and nobody stops them.' The situation is compounded because the individual is 'expected to carry out some research with the aim of publishing several papers', the number of publications being 'a dubious indicator of ability to do good research; its relevance to the ability to be a good doctor is even more obscure'.

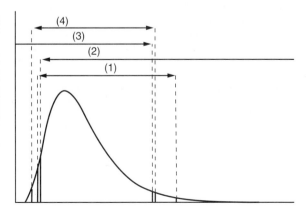

credible interval *Credible intervals for an unknown parameter*

This culture, Altman argues, leads to poor-quality research. An additional difficulty arises because junior doctors typically move jobs frequently, but are nevertheless often expected to conduct research during their short tenures. This may lead to small sample sizes as well as inadequate time for training, planning, analysis and formulation of conclusions. Further problems may occur when investigators are expected to complete research initiated by their predecessors. Altman (1991b) suggests that easy access to computers and statistical packages unaccompanied by corresponding technical understanding, as well as inadequate statistical education, also contribute to the errors.

Elsewhere, Altman (1980) describes the grave ethical implications of poor-quality research. He argues that it is unethical to carry out bad scientific experiments since patients may be subject to unnecessary risk, discomfort and inconvenience, while other resources, including the researcher's time, are diverted from more valuable functions. The publication of erroneous results is also unethical since it may lead directly to patients receiving an inferior treatment. More subtle consequences are the encouragement to other researchers to replicate flawed methods or to do further research based on erroneous premises, as well as the difficulty in getting ethics committees to permit further research when it is thought that the 'correct' answer is known.

Many medical journals employ statistical reviewers in an attempt to improve the quality of research design, statistical analysis and presentation of results (see STATISTICAL REFEREEING). Goodman, Altman and George (1998) report that in a 1993–1995 study 37% of journals surveyed had a policy that guaranteed a statistical review before an acceptance decision.

Direct evidence of the effect of statistical reviewing is limited. However, Schor and Karten (1966) studied the implementation of a programme of statistical review at a leading medical journal. Of the 514 original contributions considered, 26% were judged statistically acceptable; this increased to 74% once these manuscripts had been published after statistical review. Gardner and Bond (1990) performed a similar study on 45 papers submitted to the *British Medical Journal*. They found that only 11% were initially considered suitable for publication, but after statistical review 84% were regarded to be of an acceptable statistical standard.

However, there is much research that has not undergone statistical review and reviewing itself is a subjective process. It is thus essential to read papers in the medical literature cautiously; the reputation of a journal is not a guarantee of the quality of research reported. Errors in research vary in their magnitude and impact and a major element of critical appraisal is therefore to evaluate their potential effects on conclusions.

The following describes some common errors in the design, analysis, presentation and interpretation of medical research. The comments are not comprehensive, but represent some of the more widespread and important errors made in the research process (see also PITFALLS IN MEDICAL RESEARCH). Andersen's (1990) book, *Methodological errors in medical research*, contains a more complete description of errors illustrated by examples from the medical literature, although the author nevertheless describes it as an incomplete catalogue.

Medical research can be broadly divided into CLINICAL TRIALS, COHORT STUDIES, CASE-CONTROL STUDIES and CROSS-SECTIONAL STUDIES. Clinical trials are experimental studies where the investigator assigns participants to different interventions, preferably randomly. The well-conducted randomised controlled double-blind clinical trial comes the closest to establishing cause and effect between intervention and outcome in a single study.

Cohort studies, case-control studies and cross-sectional studies are all observational studies. Here the investigator observes participants without making any intervention. Conclusions are not considered as robust as those from experimental studies because factors controlling exposure may also be related to the outcome. However, observational studies are common because it is often impractical or unethical to assign participants to interventions; for example, it would not be possible to assign subjects to be smokers or non-smokers. Each study design has advantages and disadvantages for specific research questions and an important initial consideration in critical appraisal is whether an appropriate experimental design has been employed. Several of the following criteria relate to clinical trials where rigorous design and conduct of studies is imperative if results are to be conclusive.

The vast majority of research studies cannot consider the whole population of interest and therefore a sample is selected. Results from this sample are then applied to the population of interest. If this inference is to be valid it is vital that the sample is representative of the population. A key concept is that of random selection; if the participants are randomly selected from the population then there is the best chance of the sample's being truly representative. The research setting is often a pertinent consideration here; a study of childbirth in a maternity hospital receiving a high proportion of referrals for complications may not be representative of childbirths throughout the country. DROPOUT or refusal rates are also important issues because there is a strong possibility that those who do not take part in a study are systematically different from those who do. Although dropouts and refusals should be minimised, they are usually inevitable and a good research paper will describe the representative nature of a sample by reporting clearly the number originally selected, as well as the number completing the study. Reasons for dropout should be given, if possible, and any available characteristics of those who do not complete the study compared with those that do. All research papers must describe features of the study sample so that comparisons with the relevant population can be made.

A very common problem in experimental design is the lack of a pre-study sample size calculation. This indicates the number of participants required to be reasonably likely to detect a clinically significant effect. It is considered unethical to undertake a study with insufficient numbers to detect such an effect. Therefore it is important that a pre-study sample size calculation is performed and described in the research report, providing sufficient detail about the assumptions made, so that the calculation can be verified. Sample size considerations should be based on the primary outcome variable in a study, and should also allow for dropout or refusal rates.

In clinical trials the concepts of blinding and random allocation to intervention are essential aspects of experimental design. Blinding is necessary because BIAS may enter a study through a participant or observer knowing the intervention allocation. In a double-blind clinical trial neither the participant nor the observer is aware of the allocation. Blinding is clearly not always feasible, for example in a trial comparing an intervention of physiotherapy to no physiotherapy among a sample of elderly patients who have had a fall. In some trials, it may only be possible to blind the participant and not the observer (known as single-blind trials), but it is important that the maximum level of blindness possible is used.

Random allocation to intervention is a further desirable feature of clinical trials. It is necessary that groups of participants receiving different interventions are as similar as possible so that any effects at the end of the trial are attributable only to differences in the intervention. RANDOMISATION optimises the chance that the groups will be as similar as possible. Unfortunately, many 'trials' are not planned, but instead are based on existing routinely collected data. Allocation to intervention in these instances is never truly random and is often particularly defective. For example, two surgeons in a hospital performed many operations to reduce snoring, each surgeon using a different technique. Analysis of several years of routine outcome data attempted to compare the two techniques. Here the surgeon was a confounder and it is not possible to deduce whether differences in outcome were due to the effects of the surgical technique or of the surgeons who operated.

The double-blind randomised controlled trial (see CLINICAL TRIALS) is considered the gold standard of medical research. If a research report states that blinding and random allocation have been used then it is important that the procedures employed in implementing each are described; it is insufficient to assume that authors understand the meaning of these terms.

Errors in research design would be reduced if statisticians were consulted more often in the early stages of the research process so that statistical issues could be considered throughout (see CONSULTING A STATISTICIAN). Unfortunately, errors in the design of experiments are nearly always impossible to correct and therefore the research may be fatally flawed.

Errors in statistical analysis are also widespread. Many statistical techniques make assumptions about the data to which they are applied, but a mistake often observed in research papers is that these assumptions have not been met. A common assumption is that of data conforming to a NORMAL DISTRIBUTION. It is, unfortunately, not always possible to tell whether a variable is normally distributed when the raw data cannot be inspected. However, summary statistics may be provided and for measurements that cannot be negative, which is often the case in medical research, it can be inferred that the data have a skewed distribution if the standard deviation is more than half the mean, although the converse is not necessarily true. When data do not conform to the assumption of normality they should either be transformed (see TRANSFORMATION) or NON-PARAMETRIC METHODS used instead.

It may be clear from graphs or ranges that OUTLIERS are present in data. These can have a considerable effect on statistical analyses. Generally, however, values should not be altered or deleted if there is no evidence of a mistake. Instead if outliers are present a research paper should indicate that steps were taken to investigate their effects.

Again, transformations, or non-parametric methods may be appropriate.

A common assumption of statistical tests is that all the observations are independent. However, multiple observations on one subject are not independent and should therefore not be analysed as such. For example, the results of hearing tests in the right and left ears of a group of study participants should not all be entered into an analysis where observations are assumed to be independent. Instead the average of the right and left measurements could be taken, or the results from just the left or right ear might be chosen. It is also erroneous to analyse paired data ignoring the pairing. Paired data can arise when a one-to-one matched design has been used or when two measurements are made on the same subject, for example before and after treatment.

METHOD COMPARISON STUDIES are common in medical research and CORRELATION is often misused to assess agreement between the two. Correlation measures linear association, rather than agreement, so if one method always gives a value of exactly twice the other method a perfect correlation would be found although agreement is clearly lacking. Instead agreement between two continuous variables should be assessed using the technique described by Bland and Altman (1986).

A major problem encountered in the analysis of medical research is that of multiple testing (see MULTIPLE COMPARISON PROCEDURES). Choosing the conventional significance level of 0.05 means that if 20 statistical tests were performed we would expect one to be significant purely by chance. Therefore the conclusions of a paper reporting one significant result among 20 tests performed should be tempered by this fact. It may be that an adjustment for multiple comparisons, such as a BONFERRONI CORRECTION, is appropriate. A distinction should always be made between prior hypotheses and those resulting from exploration of the data, so that the same data are not used for testing a hypothesis as for generating it (see POST-HOC ANALYSIS).

Other errors in analysis abound, including the use of correlation to relate change to initial value, failure to take account of ordered categories or the evaluation of a diagnostic test only by means of SENSITIVITY and SPECIFICITY when the POSITIVE and NEGATIVE PREDICTIVE VALUES would be more informative. Whatever method of analysis is used, an important requirement of the research report is that all techniques employed are clearly specified for each analysis. Unusual or obscure methods should be referenced and methods that exist in more than one form, such as Pearson's or Spearman's correlation coefficient, must be identified unambiguously.

Errors can also be made in presentation, although these may have more trivial implications for the conclusions of a paper than the errors described earlier. Nevertheless, good presentation is important to ensure that the reader is not misled or confused. It is worth noting that a poor-quality paper may not necessarily describe poor-quality research, but if insufficient detail is provided in a report it is unsatisfactory to assume that the research has been performed acceptably.

P-values are often used in the medical literature to indicate statistical significance. However, it is preferable that CONFIDENCE INTERVALS are used in the presentation of results to give an immediate idea of the clinical significance of an effect. If a 95% confidence interval does not include zero (or more generally, the value specified in the null hypothesis) then the P-VALUE will be less than 0.05. Thus there is a close relation between confidence intervals and P-values (see TESTS AS CONFIDENCE INTERVALS), but confidence intervals additionally demonstrate the magnitude of the effect of interest.

MEASURES OF SPREAD should be quoted alongside MEASURES OF LOCATION to indicate variability around the average measurement. However, the ± notation is discouraged because its use to denote the STANDARD DEVIATION, the standard error and the half-width of a confidence interval has led to some ambiguity. Thus, rather than describing mothers in a study of pregnancy by saying 'the mean age of mothers was 28 ± 4.6 years', the data are better summarised as 'the mean age of mothers was 28 years (SD 4.6)'.

Since the vast majority of statistical analysis is now performed using computers, research papers should present exact P-values which are far more informative, such as $P = 0.014$, rather than ranges, such as $P < 0.05$. The notation 'NS' for non-significant is even less revealing. However, there is no need to be specific below 0.0001. Authors must justify the appropriateness of a one-sided P-value quoted in a research paper. A one-sided P-value should only be used in the very rare situation that an observed difference could only have occurred in one direction. The decision to use a one-sided P-value should be made prior to the data analysis and hence not be dependent on the results.

Spurious precision is another common error in the medical literature that impairs the readability and credibility of a paper. When presenting results the precision of the original data must be borne in mind. Altman (1991b) suggests that means should not be quoted to more than one decimal place than the original data and standard deviations or standard errors to no more than two. Likewise, percentages need not be given to more than one decimal place and P-values need not have more than two significant figures.

Errors also arise in graphical presentation (see GRAPHICAL DECEPTION). Graphs that do not include a true zero on the vertical axis or that change scale in the middle of an axis can be misleading, as can the unnecessary use of three-dimensional effects. Other errors include the plotting of means without any indication of variability and the failure to show coincident points on a SCATTERPLOT.

Misinterpretation is common when P-values are presented. It must be remembered that the conventional cut-off of 0.05 is purely arbitrary. A frequent mistake is to interpret a value of, say, 0.045 as significant, but a value of 0.055 as not significant, when in reality there is very little difference between the two. There is also a prevailing belief that significant P-values are indicative of more successful research than non-significant P-values. This attitude is reflected in studies being described as 'positive' or 'negative', depending on the significance of the findings. Results should not be evaluated solely on the statistical significance of the findings, but also on their clinical significance (see CLINICAL V. STATISTICAL SIGNIFICANCE). The use of confidence intervals is a helpful antidote to this problem.

A further serious error of interpretation is to interpret ASSOCIATION as causation. The only type of study where CAUSALITY can be inferred is a well-conducted randomised controlled trial. Otherwise, great care should be taken in the interpretation of results; in particular, the likely effect of confounders must be considered.

A final area where conclusions are often not treated with sufficient caution is that of inference from a sample to a population. Although a sample should theoretically be random, in practice this may not be realistic. Therefore a research paper should attempt to report any likely biases in the selection process and implications this may have for the findings reported.

When critically appraising a research paper it is helpful to have a checklist of issues to consider. A checklist is particularly useful because it is easier to spot errors than omissions and, as already noted, it is inappropriate to infer that a correct procedure was employed when the relevant information is not included. The *British Medical Journal* provides two checklists for use by its statistical reviewers that can be used when critically appraising a paper; these are published in Gardner, Machin and Campbell (1986) or can be found on the *British Medical Journal* website. One checklist is intended specifically for clinical trials and so includes questions relevant only to this study design, the other is for use with all other study types.

In conclusion, critical appraisal is an essential skill for users of the medical literature; it is important that readers have the confidence to question conclusions stated by the authors and the statistical knowledge to assess the methods used. The consequences of the range of errors described in this section can vary between reducing the readability of a paper to reversing the direction of the results. An important part of the critical appraisal process, therefore, is to make a judgement about the implications of any issues raised. A study should not be discarded because a single flaw is found, but, instead, a subjective assessment of the impact on the findings must be made.

SRC

Altman, D.G. 1980: Statistics and ethics in medical research. *British Medical Journal* 281, 1182–4. **Altman, D.G.** 1991a: Statistics in medical journals: developments in the 1980s. *Statistics in Medicine* 10, 1897–913. **Altman, D.G.** 1991b: *Practical statistics for medical research.* London: Chapman and Hall. **Altman, D.G.** 1994: The scandal of poor medical research. *British Medical Journal* 308, 283–4. **Andersen, B.** 1990: *Methodological errors in medical research.* Oxford: Blackwell. **Bland, J.M. and Altman, D.G.** 1986: Statistical methods for assessing agreement between two methods of clinical measurement. *Lancet* 1, 307–10. **Gardner, M.J. and Bond, J.** 1990: An exploratory study of statistical assessment of papers published in the *British Medical Journal*. *Journal of the American Medical Association* 263, 1355–7. **Gardner, M.J., Machin, D. and Campbell, M.J.** 1986: Use of check lists in assessing the statistical content of medical studies. *British Medical Journal* 292, 810–12. **Goodman, S.N., Altman, D.G. and George, S.L.** 1998: Statistical reviewing policies of medical journals: caveat lector? *Journal of General Internal Medicine* 13, 753–6. **Schor, A. and Karten, I.** 1966: Statistical evaluation of medical journal manuscripts. *Journal of the American Medical Association* 195, 1123–8.

cross-over trials Trials in which patients are allocated to sequences of treatments with the object of studying differences between individual treatments or sub-sequences of treatments (Senn, 2002). That is to say that each patient is treated more than once and the responses under different treatments for the same patient can then be compared. This is best explained by considering some examples.

Suppose we are interested in general in comparing treatments A, B, C etc. and that patients will be allocated to sequences of treatment of the form ABC, CBA etc. where, for example, ABC means that the patient will receive A in a first period, B in a second and C in a third. When only two treatments are being compared, a very popular type of cross-over design is one in which patients are allocated at random and usually in equal numbers to one of two sequences AB or BA. Such a trial was run by Graff-Lonnevig and Browaldh comparing the effects of single doses of inhaled formoterol (12μg) and salbutamol (200μg) in 14 moderately or severely asthmatic treatment (Graff-Lonnevig and Browaldh, 1990). If we give the label A to formoterol and B to salbutamol, then children were allocated at random to one of the two sequences AB or BA. Where three treatments are being compared, patients may be allocated in equal numbers to one of three sequences forming a Latin square, either ABC, BCA and CAB or ACB, BAC and CBA, or it may be that both Latin squares would be employed, so that patients would be allocated in equal numbers to each of the six possible sequences involving each of the three treatments. For example, Dahlof and Bjorkman compared two doses of the potassium salt of diclofenac (50mg or 100mg) to PLACEBO in the treatment of migraine in 72 patients (Dahlof and Bjorkman, 1993). If A is placebo, B is the lower dose of diclofenac and C the higher one, then their design involved allocating patients to one of the six sequences ABC, ACB, etc.

More complex designs than this are possible. For example, it may sometimes be the case that the number of treatment that one wishes to study is greater than the number of periods in which it is considered realistic to treat patients. So-called *incomplete block designs*, in which patients receive suitable chosen subsets of the treatments to be investigated are then popular. At the other extreme, it may be that it is possible to treat patients in more periods than there are treatments, leading to so-called *replicate designs*. As we shall discuss, these are extremely useful for the purpose of studying individual response.

Because cross-over trials permit comparisons on a within-patient basis, they are efficient compared to parallel group trials and considerable savings in patient numbers are possible. However, cross-over trials are clearly unsuitable for any condition in which death or cure is the outcome and their appropriate use is restricted to chronic diseases and treatments whose effects are reversible. Suitable conditions include asthma, rheumatism and migraine. However, it is not just the condition but the treatment and the ENDPOINT that determine the suitability of cross-over trials. For example, they can be used to study blood pressure itself in short-term trials in hypertension but not the long-term sequelae of hypertension, such as, for example, stroke or kidney or eye damage. In asthma they are more suitable for studying the effects of beta-agonists, which are relatively short term and reversible than those of steroids, which have longer term effects.

In such conditions where cross-over trials may be employed, it is nearly always the case that the sample size required to prove efficacy, even if a parallel group trial is used, is considerably less than that required to demonstrate safety of the drug. Hence, in Phase III, where safety

considerations are extremely important, there is no point in reducing the sample size by employing cross-over trials anyway (see PHASE III TRIALS, PHARMACOVIGILANCE). Consequently, some discussions of the comparative merits of cross-over trials and parallel group trials that appear in the scientific literature are rather misleading. In practice, cross-over trials are never an alternative for the major parallel group trials carried out in Phase III. They can, however, be extremely useful in Phases I and II for pharmacokinetic and pharmacodynamic modelling, for dose finding for tolerability in healthy volunteers and for efficacy using pharmacodynamic outcomes in patients (see PHASE I TRIALS, PHASE II TRIALS). They can also be useful elsewhere for answering certain specialist questions such as, for example, demonstrating equivalence (see EQUIVALENCE STUDIES: DESIGN) of generic and brand name products using so-called bioequivalence studies (Senn and Ezzet, 1999).

Unlike the parallel group trial, the basic unit of replication in a cross-over design is not the patient but an episode of treatment. Since a general necessary assumption in standard analyses of experiments is that there is no interference between units, this is clearly potentially more problematic for cross-over trials than for parallel group trials. It is inherently more plausible that the treatment given to a patient in an earlier period may affect the response for the same patient when being given a further treatment in a subsequent period, a phenomenon known as *carry-over*, than that the treatment given to one patient may affect another. (There are some cases where even parallel group trials may suffer from interference between units, in particular if infectious diseases are involved or if group therapy takes place and this may lead to cluster randomisation being necessary but this is plausibly an infrequent problem.) In fact, carry-over is regarded as being the central (potential) difficulty of cross-over trials and much of the considerable literature devoted to the design and analysis of these trials is concerned with matters to do with controlling for carry-over.

The phenomenon of carry-over means that it is prudent, indeed necessary, to employ a so-called *washout period*. This is a period between the measurement of the effect of one treatment and the next in which the effect of the previous treatment is allowed to dissipate. Washout treatments can be *passive*, if washout is allowed to occur without any treatment being given (Senn, 2002). This may seem the natural approach from the experimental point of view. It has, however, the disadvantage that the patient is expected to tolerate a period in which no therapy is offered. An alternative strategy is that of employing an *active* washout period (Senn, 2002). This might involve a near immediate switch of the patient's therapy but a delay of measurement until a suitable period has taken place during which the effects of the previous treatment have disappeared. (For further details, see Senn, 2002.)

It seems plausible that cross-over trials will be more vulnerable to dropouts than parallel group trials because of the greater demands on patient time that the former make, because dropout in one period will lead to loss of data from subsequent period also and because incomplete data will unbalance designs and lead to disproportionate losses in information.

It should be noted that in nearly all cross-over trials,

subjects are not recruited simultaneously. The exception is some designs in which healthy volunteers are used. For designs involving patients they must, of course, be treated when they present. Consequently, 'period' has a *relative* meaning in the context of cross-over trials. For example, in an AB/BA cross-over some patients will usually have completed both periods of treatment before others have even started in the trial.

A popular linear model for responses for cross-over trial with I patients in periods J with T treatments giving rise to L forms of carry-over may be expressed as follows (Jones and Kenward, 1989). We let the response in period $j, j = 1...J$ on patient $i, i = 1...I$ be Y_{ij}, the treatment given to that patient in that period be $t(i, j) = 1...T$ and the form of carry-over be $l(i, j)$. Then we write:

$$Y_{ij} = \mu + \phi_i + \pi_j + \tau_{t(i,j)} + \lambda_{t(i,j)} + \varepsilon_{ij}.$$

Here μ is a grand mean, ϕ_i is an effect due to patient i, π_j is an effect due to period j, $\tau_{t(i,j)}$ is the effect of treatment $t(i,j)$, $\lambda_{l(i,j)}$ is the carry-over effect of type $l(i,j)$ and the ε_{ij} are within-patient error terms usually assumed identically and independently distributed with variance σ^2 (say). The following points may be noted in connection with this model.

The model is severely over-parameterised. However, interest centres on contrasts between the various τ terms and, given various restrictive assumptions about the carry-over terms, these will usually be estimable.

Since there can be no carry-over in period 1, for each patient $\lambda_{l(i,1)} = 0$ for all i. In practice, to make progress in estimation, further restrictive assumptions are introduced about the carry-over terms. There are two very popular choices. The first is to assume that any washout strategy has been successful and that all carry-over terms are zero. The second is to assume that 'simple' carry-over applies and that carry-over depends only on the treatment given in the previous period so that we may write $l(i,j) = t(i,j-1), j \geq 2$.

This last assumption may seem more reasonable than the first but in practice there are very few imaginable circumstances under which the second assumption would apply if the first did not, as it seems plausible that if carry-over occurred the effect of the engendering treatment would be modified by the perturbed treatment (Senn, 2002).

In practice, although designs can easily be found in which patient, period and treatment effects are orthogonal to each other, if carry-over effects are included, the design matrix will usually be non-orthogonal and there will be a loss in efficiency.

For certain designs, for most purposes it makes no difference whether the patient effects ϕ_i are taken as FIXED EFFECTS or RANDOM EFFECTS. However, for incomplete block designs in which $T > J$, inter-patient information will usually be recoverable by taking the patient effects as random and this will also usually be the case if carry-over effects are included in the model (Senn, 2002).

The following are a number of controversies and issues that are relevant to cross-over designs. The most notorious controversy concerning carry-over has been in connection with the AB/BA design. For many years a popular approach to dealing with carry-over was the so-called two-stage procedure originally proposed by Grizzle (1965). He

noted that in the presence of carry-over the treatment effect was not estimable and hence proposed that a preliminary test of carry-over be made. If carry-over were detected, the second period data should be ignored and a between-patient test using first-period data only should be employed. However, a subsequent paper by Freeman (1989) showed that this strategy was extremely biased as a whole and did not maintain nominal Type I error rates.

It is possible to adjust the two-stage procedure so that it maintains the overall Type 1 error rate (Senn, 1997; Wang and Hung, 1997) but it has less POWER than the strategy of simply ignoring carry-over and is not recommended (Senn, 1997).

Various extremely complicated designs and analysis strategies have been proposed for dealing with carry-over. They all make restrictive and unrealistic assumptions about the nature of carry-over, however, and they nearly all involve a penalty in terms of increased variances of estimators of the treatment effect (Senn, 2002).

This would seem to leave washout as the only reasonable strategy for dealing with carry-over. However, this approach is bound to leave some investigators unhappy because of the reliance it makes on judgement based on biology and pharmacology rather than strategies of design or analysis based on purely statistical principles.

More general error structures than those considered here are possible. In particular, one could allow for a true random effect, that is to say the possibility that different patients react differently to treatment. From one point of view we would then have ϕ_i as a random intercept parameter for each patient but then add a slope parameter for a given treatment for a given patient. For a given treatment these would then be assumed to be randomly distributed with unknown variance to be estimated. It is also possible, although this appears to be rarely attempted, to allow for an autocorrelation of the within-patient errors.

Baseline values at the beginning of each treatment period are sometimes collected in cross-over trials but extreme care is required in their use. For many designs it is quite plausible that the outcome values may be unaffected by carry-over but that the baseline values would be. In that case, incorporating the baseline values in the analysis might introduce a bias due to carry-over that would not otherwise be present.

There have been various attempts to produce Bayesian analyses of cross-over trials (Grieve, 1985). In theory this is attractive in that it permits compromise positions to be adopted between that of assuming that carry-over is absent to allowing that it may have any value at all. In practice, it is difficult to capture in the model the dependence that must inevitably exist between belief in the magnitude of the treatment effect and that of the carry-over effect.

Ironically, despite the considerable potential of cross-over trials to measure individual response to treatment, especially if replicate designs are employed whereby the number of periods exceeds the number of treatments so that $J > T$ and hence make a genuine contribution to the currently fashionable field of pharmacogenomics, this possibility has received most attention where it is least important, namely, in investigating individual response to different formulations in the context of bioequivalence.

Despite some limitations of application and some difficulties in their use it would be wrong to conclude, however, that cross-over trials have no place in drug development. They can be extremely efficient compared to parallel group trials and are far superior for the purpose of investigating true random effects. They are extremely valuable on occasion, in particular in pharmacokinetic studies and in dose finding in Phase II. *SS*

Dahlof, C. and Bjorkman, R. 1993: Diclofenac-K (50 and 100 mg) and placebo in the acute treatment of migraine. *Cephalalgia* 13, 2, 117–23. **Freeman, P.** 1989: The performance of the two-stage analysis of two-treatment, two-period cross-over trials. *Statistics in Medicine* 8, 1421–32. **Graff-Lonnevig, V. and Browaldh, L.** 1990: Twelve hours bronchodilating effect of inhaled formoterol in children with asthma: a double-blind cross-over study versus salbutamol. *Clinical and Experimental Allergy* 20, 429–32. **Grieve, A.P.** 1985: A Bayesian analysis of the two-period crossover design for clinical trials. *Biometrics* 41, 4, 979–90. **Grizzle, J.E.** 1965: The two-period change over design and its use in clinical trials. *Biometrics* 21, 467–80. **Jones, B. and Kenward, M.G.** 1989: *Design and analysis of cross-over trials.* London: Chapman & Hall. **Senn, S.J.** 1997: The case for cross-over trials in Phase III [letter; comment]. *Statistics in Medicine* 16, 17, 2021–2. **Senn, S.J.** 2002: *Cross-over trials in clinical research,* 2nd edn. Chichester: John Wiley & Sons. **Senn, S.J. and Ezzet, F.** 1999: Clinical cross-over trials in Phase I. *Statistical Methods in Medical Research* 8, 3, 263–78. **Wang, S.J. and Hung, H.M.** 1997: Use of two-stage test statistic in the two-period crossover trials. *Biometrics* 53, 3, 1081–91.

cross-sectional studies The objective of a cross-sectional study is to determine the distribution of a variable or the joint distribution of more than one variable in a population. This may be accomplished by obtaining a representative sample of the population of interest through the use of a SIMPLE RANDOM SAMPLE, a *stratified random sample* or a complex survey design. Such a study is characterised by the fact that subjects are only observed at a single point in time even though the phenomena associated with the variables of interest may have evolved through a dynamic process that develops over time (Kleinbaum, Kupper and Morgenstern, 1982; Rothman and Greenland, 1998). However, because the study subjects are only observed at a single point in time, essential features in the temporal patterns will be missing, which renders it impossible to conduct a thorough longitudinal analysis of the phenomenon of interest. This approach is also sometimes used when conducting an epidemiologic study in which subjects are recruited without regard to their exposure or disease status, so that the information on each corresponds to the status of subjects at the time of the interview only.

In order to appreciate the inherent limitation that exists when observations are only observed at a single point in time, consider the hypothetical example illustrated by the SCATTERPLOT in the Figure, at (a). Subjects are observed at different ages and the scatterplot suggests that the outcome tends to decrease as age increases. In contrasts, a *longitudinal study* would observe subjects at multiple time points, thus enabling the investigator to track the development of the outcome over time. It is apparent, that the

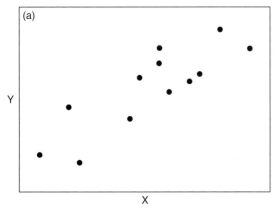

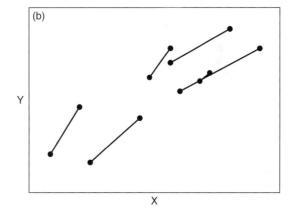

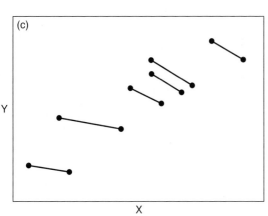

cross-sectional studies *Result from a hypothetical cross-sectional study (a) and corresponding longitudinal studies with increasing (b) and decreasing (c) time trends*

tracking of individual subjects in our hypothetical example may have arisen either from an increase in the response as the subject ages (Figure at (b)) or a decrease (Figure at (c)). By only observing subjects at a single point in time, it is impossible to distinguish between age trends associated with enrolment into the study and those that evolve as each individual subject ages (Diggle, Liang and Zeger, 1994). This limitation is not resolved by conducting repeated cross-sectional studies carried out at different points in time, unless the studies are designed so as to obtain repeated assessments of the same individuals.

In epidemiology, a cross-sectional study contrasts with a COHORT STUDY and a CASE-CONTROL STUDY. In a cohort study, subjects are selected on the basis of their exposure status and then followed until the disease develops so that an investigator can directly assess the association with disease development. In a typical case-control study, incident cases are recruited near the time at which the disease is diagnosed and exposure is assessed by recall. In either case, an investigator would be studying incident cases while a cross-sectional study would be studying prevalent cases, i.e. cases that may have occurred at some time in the past. This would confound effects on disease incidence with effects on prognosis or survival. A cross-sectional study is especially prone to LENGTH-BIASED SAMPLING because the prevalent cases with a long period of illness before by death would be more likely to enter the study than would a subject who died shortly after diagnosis.

Therefore, the design is primarily used in the study of diseases with relatively short-term effects. One example of such a study would be an attempt to discover causes of a food poisoning outbreak in a school, by identifying all students and assessing the specific food they had consumed and whether they had become ill.

Another concern in a cross-sectional study of disease is whether there is a systematic BIAS or inaccuracy in the reporting of exposure by disease status. In some cases this can be avoided by using exposure measures that are not affected by disease, e.g. the determination of a particular genotype through the use of genomic analyses. However, if this cannot be avoided, then this potential source of bias may limit the strength or the association, as well as the strength of the evidence that the exposure of interest affects the aetiology of disease.   *TRH*

Diggle, P.J., Liang, K.-Y. and Zeger, S.L. 1994: *Analysis of longitudinal data.* Oxford: Clarendon Press. **Kleinbaum, D.G., Kupper, L.L. and Morgenstern, H.** 1982: *Epidemiologic research: principles and quantitative methods.* Belmont: Lifetime Learning Publications. **Rothman, K.J. and Greenland, S.** 1998: *Modern epidemiology.* Philadelphia: Lippincott-Raven.

cross-validation See DISCRIMINANT FUNCTION ANALYSIS

crude birth/death rate See DEMOGRAPHY

cubic spline See SCATTERPLOT SMOOTHERS

cure models A cure model can be used in survival analysis when there are 'immunes' or 'long-term survivors' present in the data (Maller and Zhou, 1996). In such a setting, immune or cured subjects are censored since cure can never be observed, while susceptible subjects would eventually develop the event if followed for long enough. A

typical example where a cure model might be appropriate would exhibit a Kaplan-Meier estimate of the marginal time-to-event distribution that levelled off at long follow-up times to a non-zero value (see KAPLAN-MEIER ESTIMATOR). An example is in studies of cancer for which a significant proportion of patients may be cured by the treatment.

A mixture model formulation is one approach to analysing such data (see FINITE MIXTURE DISTRIBUTIONS). Assume that a fraction p of the population are susceptibles and the remaining are not, then the survival function $S(t)$ for the population is given by:

$$S(t) = pS_1(t) + (1 - p)$$

where $S_1(t)$ is the survival function for the susceptible group and where covariates can affect both p and $S_1(t)$. Let (t_i, δ_i, Z_i) be the observations, where Z_i is a vector of covariates, t_i the observed or censored time and δ_i the censoring indicator. Let D_i indicate cure status for each subject denoted by $D_i = 1$ for a susceptible subject and $D_i = 2$ for cured. Thus each censored subject has either $D_i = 1$ and the event has not yet occurred or has $D_i = 2$. The incidence model is typically given by:

$$p(Z_i) = P(D_1 = 1 | b, Z_1) = \frac{e^{b'Z_i}}{1 + e^{b'Z_i}}$$

Among susceptible individuals, the time to event has a distribution, such as a Weibull (Farewell, 1982):

$$S_1(t_i | D_i) = \exp\left[- \exp(\gamma' Z_i) t_i^{\alpha}\right]$$

An attractive feature of this model is the two separate components. The parameters **b** measure the effect of covariates on whether the event will occur and the parameters γ measure the effect of the covariates on when the event will occur given that the subject is susceptible. These two components are sometimes called incidence and latency and can have nice interpretations in given applications.

Different formulations can be used. Li and Taylor (2002) and Yamaguchi (1992) considered parametric and semi-parametric accelerated failure time models for the latency model. Kuk and Chen (1992), Peng and Dear (2000) and Sy and Taylor (2000) considered a semi-parametric PROPORTIONAL HAZARDS model for the latency model.

One problem associated with the cure model is near non-identifiability (Farewell, 1986; Li, Taylor and Sy, 2001). This arises due to the lack of information at the end of the follow-up period, resulting in difficulties in distinguishing models with high incidence of susceptibles and long tails of $S_1(t)$ from low incidence of susceptibles and short tails of $S_1(t)$. The incorporation of LONGITUDINAL DATA into the cure model is one way to reduce the problem (Law, Taylor and Sandler, 2002).

While the parameters in p and $S_1(t)$ have nice interpretations, in some applications the marginal survival distribution $S(t)$ and its dependence on Z may be of most interest. This distribution is easily obtained from the estimates of p and $S_1(t)$. Predicting the cure status of a censored subject may also be of interest. The formula to estimate the probability that a censored subject is in the susceptible group is given by:

$$P(D_i = 1|T_i > t_i) = \frac{pS_1(t_i)}{pS_1(t_i) + 1 - p}$$

The mixture cure model $S(t)$ does not in general have a proportional hazards structure. In order to keep this, however, non-mixture cure models have been proposed (Chen, Ibrahim and Sinha, 1999; Tsodikov, 1998). In these models, a bounded cumulative hazard is assumed $\lim_{t\to\infty}\Lambda(t) = \theta$. One way to enforce this property is to write $\Lambda(t) = \theta F(t)$, where $F(t)$ is the distribution function of a nonnegative random variable. Then the survival distribution $S(t)$ for the population can be written as $S(t) = e^{-\theta F(t)}$, which has cure rate $e^{-\theta}$. Covariates can be incorporated into the non-mixture cure model by assuming $\theta(Z_i) = \exp(\beta'Z_i)$.

Cure models are worthy of considering for analysing data for which there is a strong scientific rationale for the existence of a cured group and empirical evidence of a non-zero limiting survival fraction, together with a substantial number of censored observations with long follow-up times.

An example where the cure model was applied arose from a study of 672 tonsil cancer patients treated with radiation therapy (Sy and Taylor, 2000). The radiation can eliminate all the cancer cells in the tonsil of some patients and thus the cancer will not reappear in the tonsil and the patient is regarded as being cured. If the radiation is not successful at eliminating all the cancer cells in the tonsil, those that remain will re-grow and become detectable, as a local recurrence, within about 3 years. This is a good situation where a cure model could be appropriate, because there is a scientific rationale for a cured group and because a Kaplan-Meier estimate of time of local recurrence will exhibit a long plateau region if there is sufficient follow-up in the data. For these data, there were 206 events of local recurrence and most patients had more than 3 years follow-up.

The main interest was in understanding the effect of the total dose of radiation and the overall treatment time between the start and the end of radiation on local recurrence. Other covariates, such as stage of the tumour and age of the patient were included in the analysis. A mixture cure model was used, with a logistic model for the incidence and a semi-parametric proportional hazards model for the latency. The results suggested that stage, dose and treatment time were strongly associated with whether the tumour recurred, as indicated by the parameters in the logistic model. Age, however, was not associated with the incidence. The estimates of the relative hazards parameters in the latency part of the model suggested that stage, dose and overall treatment time were not associated with when the recurrence would occur. The patient's age, however, was *strongly* associated with when recurrence would happen, given that the patient was not cured. The direction of the association was that younger patients would recur earlier. One possible interpretation of this is that young patients tend to have the same susceptibility to treatment as older patients but they tend to have faster growing cancers that will recur earlier if not cured. The initial size or stage of the tumour and how it is treated are important factors in determining whether a patient is cured, but are not important in determining how fast the tumour grows back after treatment if not cured.   *JMGT*

Chen, M.H., Ibrahim, J.G. and Sinha, D. 1999: A new Bayesian model for survival data with a survival fraction. *Journal of the American Statistical Association* 94, 909–19. **Farewell, V.T.** 1982: The use of mixture models for the analysis of survival data with long-term survivors. *Biometrics* 83. 1041–6. **Farewell, V.T.** 1986: Mixture models in survival analysis: are they worth the risk? *The Canadian Journal of Statistics* 14, 257–62. **Kuk, A.Y.C. and Chen. C.H.** 1992: A mixture model combining logistic regression with proportional hazards regression. *Biometrika* 79, 531–41. **Law, N.J., Taylor, J.M.G. and Sandler, H.** 2002: The joint modelling of a longitudinal disease progression marker and the failure time process in the presence of cure. *Biostatics* 3, 547– 63. **Li, C.S. and Taylor, J.M.G.** 2002: A semi-parametric accelerated failure time cure model. *Statistics in Medicine* 21, 3235–47. **Li, C.S., Taylor, J.M.G. and Sy, J.P.** 2001: Identifiability of cure models. *Statistics & Probability Letters* 54, 389–95. **Maller, R.A. and Zhou, X.** 1996: *Survival analysis with long-term survivors.* New York: John Wiley & Sons. **Peng, Y. and Dear, K.B.G.** 2000: A nonparametric mixture model for cure rate estimation. *Biometrics* 56, 237–43. **Sy, J.P. and Taylor, J.M.G.** 2000: Estimation in a Cox proportional hazards cure model. *Biometrics* 56, 227–36. **Tsodikov, A.** 1998: A proportional hazard model taking account of long-term survivors. *Biometrics* 54, 1508–15. **Yamaguchi, K.** 1992: Accelerated failure time regression models with a regression time model of surviving fraction: an application to the analysis of 'permanent employment'. *Journal of the American Statistical Association* 87, 284–92.

curtailment sampling   See INTERIM ANALYSIS

D

data and safety monitoring boards Committees of experts set up to monitor the safety of participants and validity and integrity of data in CLINICAL TRIALS. Some form of data and safety monitoring is called for in any trial to ensure minimal acceptable risks to trial participants and to continually reassess the risks versus benefits of trial interventions during the conduct to make sure that there is an *equipoise* in continuing the trial.

The International Conference on Harmonization defines good clinical practice (GCP) as 'an international ethical and scientific quality standard for designing, conducting, recording and reporting of trials that involve participation of human subjects'. Monitoring of trials for safety of participants, integrity of data leading to valid conclusions, adequate trial conduct and considerations for early termination to avoid unnecessary experimentation on human subjects is thus necessary to meet the stated GCP requirements.

The trial sponsor, the investigators and the institutional review board (IRB), also known as the ethics committee (EC), are at the frontline of safety monitoring for trial participants and they assume and share the responsibilities. However, the sponsor may elect to establish a data and safety monitoring board (DSMB), also known as an independent data monitoring committee (IDMC), and delegate part of its responsibilities to the DSMB. The establishment of a DSMB is recommended based on the recognition that monitoring of safety at regular intervals is essential to ensure safety of trial participants and that individuals directly involved in the conduct and management of a trial may not be suited for objective review of emerging interim data.

All clinical trials require monitoring of safety and efficacy data, but not all require monitoring by a DSMB independent of the sponsor and investigators. The degree and extent of such monitoring should depend on the potential risks associated with interventions, the severity of disease and endpoints of the trial and the method of monitoring on the size, scope and complexity. A DSMB is generally required for large, randomised controlled trials comparing mortality or major irreversible morbidity as a primary endpoint or pivotal trials for regulatory approval of marketing.

A DSMB is a body of experts who review accumulating data, both safety and efficacy, from an ongoing trial at regular intervals and advise the sponsor about the risks versus benefits and the scientific merit of continuing the trial. A typical DSMB is made up of people with pertinent expertise, including clinicians and scientists knowledgeable about the disease and interventions under investigation, a statistician knowledgeable about clinical trials methodology including methods for INTERIM ANALYSIS, to interpret the emerging data appropriately. A DSMB may also include a patient advocate or an ethicist. A DSMB is a separate entity from an institutional review board and its members should not be involved with the trial they monitor and have no conflict of interest, either scientific or financial.

A DSMB is primarily responsible for the appropriate oversight and monitoring of the conduct of trials for safety of participants and validity and integrity of the data. More specifically, the primary responsibilities of a DSMB include review of the study protocol and the plans for data and safety monitoring; evaluation of the progress of the study, including recruitment of trial participants, timeliness and completeness of follow-up, compliance with protocol procedures, performance of participating sites and other factors that may affect study outcome; assessments of risks versus benefits; making recommendations to the sponsor and the investigators concerning continuation, modifications to the protocol or termination of the trial; and communicating the findings from data and safety monitoring to the local IRBs.

A DSMB will allow difficult, mid-study decisions about the trials. DSMB members are provided unblinded data on the important outcome measurements at regular intervals or at intervals specified in the protocol. These unblinded data should be kept confidential from the sponsor and the investigators. A DSMB is responsible for making recommendations to the sponsor whether the trial should continue as originally planned or with modifications to the design, be temporarily suspended of enrolment or trial interventions until some uncertainty is adequately addressed or be terminated either because there is no longer equipoise among trial interventions or because it is highly unlikely that the trial can be successfully completed or meet its scientific goals.

The independence of the DSMB is intended to control the sharing of important comparative information and to protect the integrity of the trial from adverse impact resulting from premature knowledge about the emerging data. While small differences may be well accepted as non-definitive, awareness of such differences may make investigators reluctant to enter patients on the trial, to limit entry to a certain subset of patients or to encourage patients to withdraw if they are assigned what they perceive as the inferior intervention. Such tendencies will introduce biases and diminish the reliability of the trial's eventual results or even preclude the completion of the trial. Limiting the access to unblinded interim data to a DSMB relieves the sponsor of the burden of deciding whether it is ethical to continue to randomise patients and helps protect the trial from biases in patient entry or evaluation.

A DSMB should have standard operating procedures and maintain records of all its meetings and deliberations, including interim results, and these should be available for review when the trial is completed. The DSMB standard operating procedures should specify meeting quorum, schedule and procedures, its decision-making rules and meeting follow-up. A DSMB should be consulted about the contents of interim reports that serve as a basis for the DSMB deliberations. A practical perspective on DSMBs and the recommendations for the operation and management of DSMBs can be found in Ellenberg, Fleming and

DeMets (2002), reflecting a recent guidance for clinical trial sponsors on the establishment and operation of clinical trial data monitoring committee by the Food and Drug Administration of the US Department of Health and Human Services (www.fda.gov/cber/gdlns/clindatmon.htm).

Interim analyses of comparative trials are necessary to ensure that large differences between interventions do not go unnoticed, as well as to detect excess toxicity or unanticipated flaws in study designs. Routine reporting of toxicities or information about intervention administration helps ensure that interventions are being given safely and properly and improves trial quality. Routine reporting of outcome results, however, can harm study quality.

In general a DSMB would examine not only the trial data but also relevant external evidence from other sources. Its recommendation to the sponsor should be based on the interpretation of the results of the ongoing trial in the context of existing outside scientific data relevant to such interpretation. A final decision, as to whether or not to continue the trial, should not rely solely on a formal test of statistical significance.

The DSMB meetings provide a setting in which the clinical significance of early differences or lack thereof can be discussed openly with interim data and the complex statistical issues involved in sequential monitoring of a trial can be discussed at length. Focused discussions of the progress towards the scientific goals of a study are facilitated by a DSMB with access to unblinded data. Since intervention effects will be examined by a small group, the danger will be reduced that a promising trial will be informally stopped early with reduced accrual because of over-interpretation of interim results by the sponsor or the investigators. In addition, sequential monitoring rules are at best guidelines for complex decisions involving many aspects of a trial.

Deliberations and conclusions of the monitoring should be communicated to the sponsor and the IRBs without compromising the integrity of the trial. Recommendations resulting from monitoring activities should be reviewed by the study team and adequately addressed. Local IRBs should be provided feedback on a regular basis, including findings from adverse events and recommendations derived from data and safety monitoring.   *KK*

[See also INTERIM ANALYSIS]

Ellenberg, S., Fleming, T.R. and DeMets, D.L. 2002: *Data monitoring committees.* Boca Raton: Chapman & Hall/CRC.

data entry The process of putting observations into electronic format for computer analysis. No successful statistical investigation takes place without the reliable and accurate collection of data and its conversion into a suitable electronic form for computerised analysis. While ostensibly a simple clerical process, it often suffers neglect in planning and execution that can jeopardise the smooth running of a research project.

The reliability of data collection is not specifically an issue for data entry, but we will see later how technological changes in data entry can encroach on the process. Most important for the majority of investigators is the accurate entry of data. In a formal research project such as a CLINICAL TRIAL there will be established and inviolable

clerical procedures for data collection and entry that will help to ensure accuracy. But in many academic studies the researchers themselves will take responsibility for the complete collection and entry process.

With modern statistical packages and moderate IT literacy on behalf of the user, this is a perfectly feasible and economic process for studies up to a few hundred variables and a few hundred cases. The spreadsheet data entry facilities of SPSS or Excel provide an easy way of entering data and, given that the researcher is entering the data, she can make checks as she goes along.

Two problems occur with this approach. One is simple clerical error or absent-mindedness in typing data, the other is a lack of an audit trail for changes in the spreadsheet. Dual entry is typically used to correct the first. Programs such as SPSS Data Entry or a program written in MS-Access or similar permit one user to enter data and then another to re-enter it from scratch. Any inconsistency is flagged and the appropriate variable checked. Such programs can also incorporate range checking. While taking extra effort, it is well worth the initial investment in design. Some argue against the administrative burden of double data entry, however, on the grounds that range checks etc. will detect most clerical errors, yet it remains a sensible precaution, especially if temporary or external staff are to be used for data entry.

The audit of change is important, particularly if several researchers are reviewing the data. An individual correcting a variable may unwittingly invalidate another's previous analysis. It is good practice in these circumstances to set up a core dataset and then use a program to change individual data elements if they need revision. So, for example, a file with SPSS syntax language data transformation commands can be used to compute changes to an SPSS data file. It is then available for review by all in the team.

There is much interest in using personal digital assistants (PDAs), or internet browsers, for data entry, sometimes directly by the subject themselves. The superficial attractiveness of these procedures can be misleading. Transferring and merging data from a PDA is not necessarily simple and will usually require significant manual intervention. This can be a source of error and care needs to be taken in design to prevent this.

The use of a web page for data entry potentially gives access to many thousands of respondents. Setting up a reliable data-entry page is not so simple. Browsing sessions often terminate for communications reasons mid-session and therefore program logic needs to identify successful completion. Care needs to be taken to identify unique data entry sessions by, for example, originating IP address of the client browser. Data security is needed so a user cannot accidentally see other entries. A reasonable amount of programming effort is required to do this and will certainly require database, programming and HTML design skills to achieve it successfully. This does not mean it is not possible to design a simple web page to acquire data; it is just more complicated to acquire data both reliably and accurately.

Planning is the key to successful data entry. Before any data are collected the process flow for entering data into the computer package and its checking should be described and adhered to rigidly by the research team.

Such discipline will pay off in smoothing the path to analysis. *CS*

[See also DATA MANAGEMENT]

data management The systematic management of a large structured collection of information. 'Data management' is always a component of data analysis, but is usually a more significant issue in large or multi-centre studies where the data management features of software packages such as SPSS or Excel are inadequate. This will also be the case when the 'data model' of the study – the entities for which data are collected and the relationships between them – does not fit the standard rectangular data model or spreadsheet of the classical statistical package. So, for example, a study comparing treatment in hospitals may have three entities – hospital, ward and patient – that need data recording at each level. Longitudinal or repeated measurement studies also generate data that does not so easily fit the rectangular model.

Nonetheless, very many complicated studies are managed and analysed entirely in packages such as SPSS or SAS (see STATISTICAL PACKAGES). SAS in particular has very strong data management features. Several data files for each entity can be created, and the data merge features of these programs used to prepare specific analyses. Because this merging of files is manual, more skill and experience on behalf of the researcher is needed and thorough documentation and understanding of merge procedures is essential to prevent error. Nonetheless, because only one programming language is used, the procedures are consistent and easier to learn. Although such an approach seems 'low-tech', there is much to recommend it for many studies.

The main weakness of this approach is the manual management of transaction updates and production of an audit trail. If, in the example above, more patients are recruited in a particular ward, then derivative files which include hospital or ward variables need to be recreated manually. In a very dynamic data environment this is tedious and also error prone. Equally the correction of values in one file similarly requires the recreation of all the derivative files.

An alternative is to consider using a formal data management tool, and this usually implies a database. With a fast modern PC, desktop database packages such as MS-Access are capable of managing datasets with some tens of thousands of cases and several hundred variables. Only the very largest studies will require a full SQL compliant database, although there may be sound reasons for using the latter for security and access control.

Almost inevitably deployment of a database will require the production of data entry and update screens, a process that requires some programming ability. This is particularly the case if transaction control and an audit trail of changes are needed. Secondly, the database query statements needed to provide the appropriate rectangular matrix datasets for analysis can be complicated, and can require subtle understanding of SQL. Such in-depth expertise is not normally easily accessible in a research team and may be expensive to provide. Before deciding to use a database for data storage the research team should plan and budget for such skills to be available throughout the life of the project. Employing a programmer who then gets another job just before the end of the study can leave a research team without the support they need when wanting finally to analyse the data.

For this reason alone, it is often sensible to consider the acquisition of specialised clinical data management packages. These often include all the extra checks and forms necessary for formal clinical trials. Entering the appropriate terms in any web search engine will bring up several hundred companies offering products that are suitable – the difficulty will be selecting one. Although there may be a seemingly significant initial cost (perhaps several thousand euros or dollars) the saving on development time, as well as the predictability and security of software operation, give a rapid payback.

At project conception it is usually possible to outline the extent of data management requirements dependent on the complexity of the problem. It is sensible for prior specification and budgeting of the software needed to take place, rather than awaiting project start and then developing ad hoc solutions. This will give the research team the security of control of the data over the project lifetime. *CS*

[See also DATA ENTRY]

data mining in medicine A branch of both computer science and statistics devoted to extracting useful knowledge from databases (also known as KDD, knowledge discovery in databases). In general, such knowledge is obtained by detecting various types of regularity and relation among the data, most often: association rules; classification rules (see DISCRIMINANT FUNCTION ANALYSIS); linear and nonlinear dependencies; clusters (see CLUSTER ANALYSIS).

Depending on the context in which it is performed, data-mining research may emphasise computational scalability of the algorithms or statistical significance of the results. The field benefits from a major injection of ideas and tools from general MACHINE LEARNING and pattern recognition and, as such, it is often considered also part of ARTIFICIAL INTELLIGENCE.

Data mining is often described as an interactive process that involves both the computer and the human component. This is also why data visualisation is considered an essential part of the process. DM is more general than traditional statistical analysis, in the type of regularities that can be found (for example, decision trees); in the size of the datasets (often in the range of millions of data items); and in the strong emphasis on visualisation of the data and automation of the analysis.

The application of DM to medicine has a long tradition. Automatic data collection in modern medicine is increasingly pushing towards the development and deployment of tools able to handle and analyse data in a computer-supported fashion.

Being able to detect sets of symptoms that are often simultaneously present (association analysis) can help predict which other symptoms may be observed (association rules). Observing many patient descriptions as well as their diagnoses may help find a rule to predict the diagnosis given a new patient (classification analysis). Spotting groups of similar patients can help customise the therapy (cluster analysis). And, finally, being able to predict the expected cost of a patient based on his or her history can help insurance companies optimise their services (regression analysis – see MULTIPLE REGRESSION).

An early application of data mining in medicine is the decision tree learner ASSISTANT (Cestnik, Kononenko and Bratko, 1987; Witten and Frank, 1999). It was developed specifically to deal with the particular characteristics of medical datasets.

A whole new chapter in the application of DM techniques to biomedical data is being written with the introduction of genome-wide datasets. Genomic sequences for several organisms are now available online and the availability of high-throughput gene expression and proteomic data highlight the urgent need for efficient and flexible algorithms to extract the wealth of medical information contained in them. Datasets recording human genetic variability (SNPs) are soon expected and, with them, the possibility of correlating genotypic with phenotypic information (see GENETIC EPIDEMIOLOGY).

Classic examples of modern data-mining methods are systems such as BLAST (Altschul *et al.*, 1990), which allows researchers to find related genetic sequences efficiently, together with a statistical assessment of the degree of similarity.

Significant biological discoveries are now routinely being made by combining DM methods with traditional laboratory techniques. For example, the discovery of novel regulatory regions for heat shock genes in *C. elegans* (Thakurta *et al.*, 2002) was made by mining vast amounts of gene expression and sequence data for significant patterns. *NC/TDB*

Altschul, S.F., Gish, W., Miller, W., Myers, E.W. and Lipman, D.J. 1990: Basic local alignment search tool. *Journal of Molecular Biology* 215, 403–10. **Bratko, I. and Kononenko, I.** 1987: Learning diagnostic rules from incomplete and noisy data. In Phelps, B. (ed.), *AI methods in statistics*. London: Gower Technical Press. **Cestnik, B., Kononenko, I. and Bratko, I.** 1987: ASSISTANT 86: a knowledge elicitation tool for sophisticated users. In Bratko, I. and Lavrac, N. (eds.), *Progress in machine learning*. Wilmslow: Sigma Press. **Hand, D.J., Mannila, H. and Smyth, P.** 2001: *Principles of data mining (adaptive computation and machine learning)*. Cambridge, MA: MIT Press. **Lavrac, N.** 1999: Selected techniques for data mining in medicine. *Artificial Intelligence in Medicine* 16, 1, 3–23. **Thakurta, D.G., Palomar, L., Stormo, G.D., Tedesco, P., Johnson, T.E., Walker, D.W., Lithgow, G., Kim, S. and Link, C.D.** 2002: Identification of a novel *cis*-regulatory element involved in the heat shock response in *Caenorhabditis elegans* using microarray gene expression and computational methods. *Genome Research* 12, 5, 701–12. **Witten, I.H. and Frank, E.** 1999: *Data mining: practical machine learning tools and techniques with Java implementations*. London: Morgan Kauffmann.

data-dependent designs Methods for allocating treatments to patients in clinical trials that make constructive use of the emerging responses. Compared with traditional trial designs using pre-determined sample sizes, data-dependent designs aim to impart some advantage to trial participants, reaching a conclusion sooner and/or exposing fewer to inferior therapy during the course of the trial. Such designs have been around in theory for at least as long as modern clinical trials, although their practical applications have hitherto been very limited. Other terms in use for similar methodological approaches for such trials include *flexible designs, dynamic designs, adaptive designs* and *learn-as-you-go designs*, although there is no apparent consensus on the nomenclature.

There are four broad categories of data-dependent design, all of which share the same spirit of learning from the accumulating data within the trial, as opposed to ignoring intermediate results until completion of the trial. These categories are: sequential, Bayesian, decision theoretic and adaptive. Descriptions given later in this section deliberately avoid too much mathematical detail. Also, a distinction is drawn here from two other related types of clinical trial design not discussed further. First, there are designs that use minimisation to incorporate knowledge of covariates of patients already entered into a trial (and hence self-modify according to treatment allocation but not treatment *response*) and, second, there are trial designs intended to have an internal pilot study (see PILOT STUDIES).

Initially, however, it is worth considering briefly some historical background to help understand why modern CLINICAL TRIALS have emerged in the way in which they have. Typically, they feature fixed sample sizes dictated by error probability considerations (see TYPE I ERROR and TYPE II ERROR rates), treatments being allocated equally (usually, to maximise POWER of a test) and results are kept hidden (to all but a DATA AND SAFETY MONITORING BOARD (DSMB), if appointed) until the final analysis, which is conducted well after the final patient has been enrolled.

Interestingly, and tellingly, the roots of today's trials lie not in medicine, but in agriculture. In the UK in the 1920s, R.A. Fisher began conducting crop field trials to try to determine which type of fertiliser produced higher yields of wheat. Realising there were more factors than could be listed (soil composition, aspect, slope, water and so on) that might influence total yield, Fisher pioneered RANDOMISATION to cope with the problem of balancing all the known and unknown variables as far as possible (Fisher, 1926). It was a statistical masterstroke, for such use of an external chance mechanism alone could ensure that the comparison between fertilisers was fair and unbiased. Specifically, any difference observed in crop yield at harvest time could be attributed to the one factor that was known to be different between the groups, namely the fertiliser, all other factors being expected to be equal. Hence, inference from any observed differences between groups would link cause and effect (here, fertiliser and yield) as strongly as possible (see CAUSALITY).

The first medical application of randomisation came in the late 1940s, when A.B. Hill used Fisher's technique in a clinical trial testing streptomycin for the treatment of pulmonary tuberculosis. This was not without some controversy at the time, but Hill convinced sceptics by arguing that randomisation was also a fair way of allocating the scarce resource involved, given that the treatment was in strictly limited supply. This Medical Research Council-sponsored trial became the first randomised controlled clinical trial to be published (MRC, 1948).

However, trials of today are fundamentally quite similar to those of 50 or more years ago, in that they typically involve equal allocation of treatments to patients, generally after performing a power calculation to determine a target number to be recruited. So, in a two-treatment comparative trial, half the patients customarily receive the standard, half the experimental treatment. As already mentioned, with the possible exception of DSMB committee members and a statistician conducting an INTERIM ANALYSIS, no one looks at the results until all the patients have been randomised and followed up. At the end of the trial it is possible that the experimental treatment is declared a statistically significant improvement and heralded as a clinical success. It is an ethical problem, however, if statistical 'failure' means the patient died and one can look back with some remorse, wondering: 'If only we had come to this conclusion sooner perhaps we could have saved some lives' (see ETHICS AND CLINICAL TRIALS). Even if the outcome is not as serious as death, the argument persists: could fewer patients in the study have suffered on the way to reaching a valid conclusion?

This last question has motivated much research by ethically-minded statisticians. Ironically, this work dates back at least as far as the first modern clinical trial, for the whole area of sequential analysis traces its history to the 1940s, the Second World War and US government-contracted statistician Abraham Wald (see Wald, 1943). His work, like Fisher's was not in the medical area of application, but in ammunition testing, an altogether different example of seeking to cope with precious and limited resources. Medical application of sequential methods does seem entirely appropriate, after all, patients arrive to be treated sequentially (they are not all waiting in line outside the doctor's office, or hospital clinic, at the start of a trial) and, similarly, results from some are available sooner than from others.

The rationale for sequential trials involves looking carefully at data *as they accrue* with a view to stopping just in time. Hence, the number of experimental units required is not fixed in advance but is a random variable. Theory shows that the expected numbers involved in a sequentially analysed randomised controlled trial is less than the corresponding fixed sample size trial, for any given power and level of significance. It is possible, when treatment groups fare broadly equally well, for a sequential trial to need slightly more patients overall compared with a trial using traditional design, but this would be quite unusual.

For better or worse, the clinical trial as conducted and analysed today is not in Wald's style of testing ammunition but rather in Fisher's application of fertiliser to fields of wheat. These two metaphors illustrate the fundamental difference between the statistics behind clinical trials that strive to learn-as-they-go and those that wait, literally, until harvest time before beginning to make scientific inferences. The reader may decide whether it is right that normative practice sees clinical trial volunteers afforded the same respect as the fertiliser rather than the ammunition.

Following Wald's pioneering research, sequential designs have evolved as sophisticated tools to assist those on DSMBs and hence can be considered mainstream, in contrast to the remaining design types, discussed now. It should be said, however, that these methods are not routinely implemented as primary analytical tools for driving trials. Instead, they are used at best as 'back seat drivers' to exert indirect influence on trial conduct. How do they do this? Essentially, as data accumulate, a test statistic can be plotted on a graph of treatment difference versus time and trial recruitment can be recommended to terminate just as soon as a predetermined boundary is crossed (see SEQUENTIAL ANALYSIS).

This boundary may take on various shapes, the simplest being triangular with two possible options, either treatment A or B is declared better depending on which side of the triangle is crossed first. To allow for a third, non-conclusive option with a predetermined maximum trial sample size, the boundary outline is modified to include a vertical line at a given point on the time (strictly 'information') axis. The idea is to stop the trial in favour of treatment A, say, if the upper line of the boundary is crossed first; B if the lower line; or else, conclude no clinically relevant difference between A and B if the vertical line is reached first.

There are variations on this theme with rules such as that derived by Pocock (1983) being a popular example. Thus it is not necessary to update the graph after every single observation. One can apply rules, called *group sequential methods*, which update after small batches of results become available. (For more details, refer to Jennison and Turnbull, 2001). Statistical software for implementing these rules is readily available in several commercial packages (e.g. EaSt, PEST, S+SeqTrial).

One disadvantage with sequentially designed experiments is that their usefulness, namely their potential to learn while in progress, is self-limiting to trials having relatively rapid ENDPOINTS. Thus a sequential trial offers little benefit over a traditional, fixed sample size trial if the outcome remains unknown until years after randomisation. This may be so in breast cancer for example, but is no limitation for instance in emergency medicine or in rapidly fatal diseases.

Turning to Bayesian designs, investigators start by eliciting a PRIOR DISTRIBUTION, either from a panel of clinical experts or from a reasonable selection of available theoretical distributions thought to mimic reality in terms of treatment success distributions (see BAYESIAN METHODS). For example, a beta distribution with suitably chosen parameters can represent initial beliefs about a treatment's efficacy ranging from negatively skewed to uniformly distributed to positively skewed. In practice, there is virtue in choosing a prior that makes the experimental treatment appear initially a weak contender, so that positive results in favour of the treatment are not too dependent on initial choice of prior. As the patients' results accumulate, the conditional distribution given the data thus far is evaluated – the so-called POSTERIOR DISTRIBUTION, amalgamating the prior and the LIKELIHOOD. Inference is based on the posterior, including the evaluation of CREDIBLE INTERVALS, analogous to CONFIDENCE INTERVALS in the frequentist context.

One advantage is the ease of interpretation of these intervals for they have more intuitive meaning to clinicians and patients. A disadvantage is the general lack of awareness of Bayesian methods since these are less often encountered than those from the frequentist school. This is reflected in the comparative lack of statistical textbooks, courses and software aligned to the Bayesian paradigm. (Spiegelhalter, Freedman and Parmar, 1994, provide an excellent overview of Bayesian methodology applied to clinical trials.) Some see the subjective or arbitrary nature of the prior distribution involved as a weakness; others regard it as a positive opportunity to incorporate provisional information about the potential new treatment.

The third broad category of data-dependent designs involves the use of DECISION THEORY. Some experimental studies can be conducted with the resulting inference, in terms of how the information will be used to reach a practical decision concerning which treatment to recommend, as the driving force. For example, one can specify a criterion such as minimising expected successes lost or maximising successes gained, over the course of a predetermined number of future patients, called the horizon, within and outside a comparative trial. Another criterion could be maximising the probability of correct selection of superior treatment. Either way, the focus is on the pragmatic need to make a decision and use one of the treatments or not once the trial is over in a direct attempt to balance the needs of current and future patients.

It is possible to discount future patients by putting more weight on present results, although this whole area can become mathematically quite intricate, especially when modelling with unconstrained so-called 'multi-armed bandits' in the context of deciding among several treatments. Nevertheless, practical simplifications can be incorporated such as limiting allocation among remaining treatments. In the case of just two treatments this amounts to allocating pairs of treatments until such time it is optimal, by whatever criterion, to cease the comparative stage. After that one can switch all remaining patients within the horizon to the preferred treatment, or maybe enter them into a brand new randomised trial comparing this 'winner' with another novel treatment that is ready for a comparative trial. That is, one is not constrained in actuality to put all remaining patients onto the indicated treatment, but one can act safely in the knowledge that the selection of the winner is working to the best available information, where 'best' is guaranteed until the original horizon is reached. (Note, in practice, the choice of horizon in absolute terms is not critical, for one only need specify an approximate size.)

Objections to the subjective nature of prior distributions involved in this type of decision-theoretic framework can be alleviated, for example, by appealing to minimax criteria. This means implementing a design that has good theoretical properties across a broad range of priors. Development of computer software to allow such designs to be implemented has been slower than for sequential methods, contributing to the current lack of use of decision-theoretic methods in practice.

The fourth category considered here, (response-)adaptive designs, is the most extreme type of data-dependent design. It incorporates the accruing information from the data to modify the treatment allocation probabilities away from 50:50 in the case of two treatments. Thus, for example, whereas the trial would start with equal allocation, as the data begin to favour one treatment even slightly then it affects the odds of the next allocation being accordingly fractionally higher. In practice, it works like this (see ADAPTIVE DESIGNS). Imagine a bag containing an equal number of red and blue balls. A red ball drawn indicates the next allocation is to treatment A; a blue ball, treatment B. If a success occurs a ball of the appropriate colour is added to the bag before the next drawing, and hence treatment allocation, takes place.

Adaptive designs were set back by a rather poor prototypical example of a mid-1980s' trial (Bartlett, Roloff, Cornell et al., 1985), involving extra-corporeal membrane oxygenation (ECMO) therapy and which has received much attention in the statistical and medical literature. Ethicists, clinicians and statisticians have all contributed to the debate about this particular trial. It involved critically ill newborn babies and the relevant outcome in question really was a matter of life and death. In retrospect, it was clearly a mistake to begin this trial with precisely one ball of each colour in the bag instead of, say, 10 of each. What ensued was a highly unbalanced distribution of

treatment allocation (for ECMO babies generally lived, unlike many of those not on ECMO therapy) rendering sensible inference difficult, if not impossible. By the same token, it can be said that since the ECMO trial, computing power and mobile technology, two prerequisites for successfully conducting an adaptive design, have taken huge leaps forward, making this design far more feasible to implement successfully than ever before.

These adaptive designs are the most controversial in the family of data-dependent designs. This is because they appear to react too quickly to early data, which may be subject to systematic bias, or time trends, and if not careful can begin to adapt too swiftly to chance results. There is also the criticism that if one treatment happens to be a PLACEBO, why should anything change after a success or a failure on such an inert substance? Nevertheless, with suitable cautions and awareness of the issues involved, adaptive designs can be a highly effective and ethically appealing design, despite once again the relative dearth of positive examples of their use so far.

A growing number of statisticians believe the 21st century will be characterised by more use of computer-intensive, data-dependent methods, so long as those responsible for conducting clinical trials are open to receiving suggestions on how to advance trial methodology. For further details, including when data-dependent methods are considered most suitable and a proposed strategy for their introduction, see Palmer (2002).

In closing, it is worth remembering why one should consider using data-dependent designs. The primary reason is for their ethical advantage in terms of how patients within trials are regarded, without compromising the scientific rigour or usefulness of studies for the sake of future patients. There are, in addition, secondary reasons, with benefits derived from the side-effect of expecting fewer patients to be involved in learn-as-you-go trials compared with traditional trials. These benefits pertain to trial sponsors (notably the pharmaceutical industry), doctors, patients and ultimately the science of medicine itself. *CRP*

Bartlett, R.H., Roloff, D.W., Cornell, R.G. *et al.* 1985: Extracorporeal circulation in neonatal respiratory failure: a prospective randomised study. *Pediatrics* 76, 479–87. Fisher, R.A. 1926: The arrangement of field experiments. *Journal of the Ministry of Agriculture, Great Britain*, 503–13. Jennison, C. and Turnbull, B.W. 2001: *Group sequential methods with applications to clinical trials.* London: Chapman & Hall/CRC. MRC Streptomycin in Tuberculosis Trials Committee 1948: Streptomycin treatment for pulmonary tuberculosis. *British Medical Journal*, 769–82. Palmer, C.R. 2002: Ethics, data-dependent designs and the strategy of clinical trials: time to start learning-as-we-go? *Statistical Methods in Medical Research* 11, 381–402. Pocock, S.J. 1983: *Clinical trials: a practical approach.* Chichester: John Wiley & Sons. Spiegelhalter, D.J., Freedman, L.S. and Parmar, M.K.B. 1994: Bayesian approaches to randomised trials. *Journal of the Royal Statistical Society, Series A* 157, 357–416. Wald, A. 1943: Sequential analysis of statistical data: report submitted to Applied Mathematics Panel National Defense Research Committee (declassified in Wald, A. 1947: *Sequential analysis.* New York: John Wiley & Sons).

data dredging See POST-HOC ANALYSES

decision theory An approach to the analysis of data that leads to choice between a number of alternative actions by consideration of the likely consequences. This is in contrast to the commonest form of analysis of data from a CLINICAL TRIAL that is based on hypothesis testing. The decision-theoretic approach is most suitable for decisions in which the possible actions are entirely within control of the decision maker. In a clinical trials setting, most suggestions for the use of decision theory have been in early-phase trials, the final outcome of which is usually a decision as to whether or not to continue with the clinical development programme.

In a decision theoretic framework, the actions that will be taken as a result of the analysis are explicitly identified and a utility, or gain, assigned to each expressing the desirability of the action as a function of some unknown parameter. For example, in an early-phase drug trial, possible actions might be either conducting further clinical trials with the drug or abandoning the clinical development programme. The desirability of each of these actions depends on the true unknown efficacy. Information on the unknown parameter is summarised by a Bayesian posterior distribution (see BAYESIAN METHODS), indicating those values that are plausible given the observed data and this can be used to obtain an expected value for the utility for each action. The action with the largest posterior expected utility may then be identified. This is the action that will be chosen by a rational decision maker whose preferences are accurately represented by the utility function.

A simple example based on that considered by Sylvester (1988) (see also the correction by Hilden, 1990) illustrates decision making in a PHASE II TRIAL. At the end of the trial a decision will be made as to whether or not to continue with Phase III development. The desirability of each of these two options is summarised by a utility function, which, if the observed data are binary (success/failure), depends on the true success rate, which will be denoted by p. Suppose that the success probability for the existing standard treatment is known, for example it may be known to be 0.5. Suppose also that if the Phase II trial is successful, some known number, denoted m, of patients will be treated with the new treatment in PHASE III TRIALS and that if it is found to be effective in the Phase III trial a total of t additional patients will be treated with the new treatment. Patients treated with the standard treatment in the Phase III trial will receive the same treatment, regardless of the outcome of the Phase II trial, so need not be considered.

Suppose that the utility of each action can be measured by the number of future successes expected if that action is taken. If the Phase III trial is not conducted, the $m + t$ future patients will all receive the standard treatment. The success rate for these patients will then be 0.5, so that the expected number of future successes is $0.5(m + t)$. This does not depend on the success rate for the new drug since this will not be used for any further patients. If the Phase III trial is conducted, m patients will receive the new treatment in the trial, so that the expected number of successes for the patients in this trial is pm. If the Phase III trial is unsuccessful, the t further patients will receive the standard treatment, and the expected number of successes for these patients will be $0.5t$. If the Phase III trial is successful, these patients will receive the new treatment so that the expected number of successes will be pt. We will assume that the Phase III trial will give the correct answer, so that it will be successful whenever $p > 0.5$, in which case the number of extra successes from treating the t future patients with the new rather than the standard treatment is the difference between pt and $0.5t$, that is $(p - 0.5)t$. The

total expected number of successes if the Phase III trial is conducted will be $mp + 0.5t + (p - 0.5)tI(p > 0.5)$, where the indicator function $I(p > 0.5)$ is equal to 1 if $p > 0.5$ and 0 if $p \leq 0.5$. If p is large, this utility is large, reflecting the fact that continuation to Phase III is desirable, and if p is small, the utility is smaller as continuation to Phase III is undesirable.

If the value of p were known, we would take the action corresponding to the larger of the two utilities, that is we would continue to Phase III if the expected number of successes from doing so, that is $mp + 0.5t + (p - 0.5)tI(p > 0.5)$ was greater than the expected number from abandoning development of the experimental treatment, that is $0.5(m + t)$. In practice, of course, p is not known, but instead the information on p given by the observed data is summarised by its posterior distribution and the expected number of future successes from each action must be averaged over this distribution. The optimal action corresponding to the larger expected number of successes can then be selected.

In addition to making decisions at the end of a clinical trial as illustrated here, decision theory can be used to make decisions before the study starts regarding the study design for clinical trials, as discussed by Sylvester (1988), and it is in this context that the approach is most often proposed. Design decisions considered might be those taken before the study starts regarding the sample size for a fixed sample size study or those taken during a sequential trial (see SEQUENTIAL ANALYSIS) about the future conduct of the trial. In the latter case, a method known as 'dynamic programming' may be used to obtain a sequence of optimal decisions by working backwards through the trial considering each decision point in turn. Examples are given by Berry and Stangl (1996), who consider the problems of when to stop a sequential trial involving a single experimental treatment and of deciding which treatment to use for each patient in a sequential trial comparing an experimental treatment with a control.

Although the suggestion to use decision theory in clinical trials has a long history (see, for example, Colton, 1963), there has been little practical application (see DATA-DEPENDENT DESIGNS). The use of the approach has probably been limited by the difficulties associated with specification of appropriate utility functions. The detailed specification of the gain function also means that designs must be obtained with a particular type of trial in mind. One possible solution is to use what has been called a stylised Bayesian approach, as illustrated, for example, by Stallard, Thall and Whitehead (1999) in which parameters in the utility function are selected so as to lead to a design with attractive frequentist properties. *NS*

Berry, D.A. and Stangl, D.K. 1996: Bayesian methods in health-related research. In Berry, D.A. and Stangl, D.K. (eds), *Bayesian biostatistics*. New York: Marcel Dekker. **Colton, T.** 1963: A model for selecting one of two medical treatments. *Journal of the American Statistical Association* 58, 388–400. **Hilden, J.** 1990: Corrected loss calculation for Phase II trials. *Biometrics* 46, 535–8. **Stallard, N., Thall, P.F. and Whitehead, J.** 1999: Decision theoretic designs for Phase II clinical trials with multiple outcomes. *Biometrics* 55, 971–7. **Sylvester, R.J.** 1988: A Bayesian approach to the design of Phase II clinical trials. *Biometrics* 44, 823–36.

degrees of freedom An elusive concept that occurs throughout statistics. Essentially, the term degrees of freedom (df) means the number of independent units of information in a sample relevant to the estimation of a parameter or the calculation of a statistic. For example, in a 2×2 CONTINGENCY TABLE with a given set of marginal totals, only one of the four cell frequencies is free and the table is therefore said to have one degree of freedom. In many cases the term corresponds to the number of parameters in a model and in others to the number of parameters in a statistical distribution such as the t-DISTRIBUTION, the f-DISTRIBUTION and the CHI-SQUARE DISTRIBUTION. *BSE*

demography The study of population processes (Preston, Heuveline and Guillot, 2001). This entry provides a brief survey of the following topics: measures of fertility, measures of mortality, age standardisation, sources of data, historical demography and the demographic transition, population projection, population ageing and summary measures of population health.

Note that many demographic measures that are defined as 'rates' are not true rates in the sense that they are not measures of events per unit of person-time. These measures are identified by placing the 'rate' of their title in quotes.

We begin by discussing measures of fertility. Fertility refers to actual childbearing *performance*, not childbearing potential, which is called *fecundity*. The *crude birth rate* is the number of births per conventional unit of person-time. The person-time denominator is typically based on estimates of population size at mid-period multiplied by the length of the period. Where the period is a single calendar year (the usual circumstance) then this equals 1. For example, in England and Wales in 2001 there were 594,634 live births registered and the mid-year population was estimated at 52,084,500, giving a crude birth rate of 11.4 births per 1000 population per year.

The analogously calculated *crude death rate* may be subtracted from it to give the *rate of natural increase*. More specific measures of fertility are desirable because population age structure affects the childbearing potential of the population and because, at an individual level, births (unlike deaths) can be repeated and the likelihood of this happening depends on reproductive experience to that point. Thus cumulative measures of individual fertility are also desirable.

The *general fertility 'rate'* (GFR) is calculated as the number of live births per conventional unit of female person-years in the age range 15 to 49, while the *total fertility 'rate'* (TFR) estimates the average number of babies that would be born per full reproductive lifetime – given current age-specific fertility rates. It equals the sum of the probabilities of giving birth in each of the years of life in which a birth could occur, conventionally from 15 to 49.

The *gross reproduction 'rate'* (GRR) is the 'rate' at which mothers are reproducing themselves. It is an estimate of the average number of daughters that would be born to a woman during her lifetime if she passed through the childbearing ages experiencing the age-specific fertility rates of the population of interest. It can be estimated on the assumption that the proportion of female births is (approximately) $100/(100+105) = 0.488$. The GRR is then $0.488 \times$ TFR.

The *net reproduction 'rate'* (NRR) takes into account the prevailing mortality among women and thus estimates the extent to which each generation of mothers actually repro-

duce themselves, allowing for the proportion who die before reproducing. It can be calculated from a hypothetical birth cohort (e.g. of 1000 females) who are aged through the reproductive lifespan and exposed to the given death rates using lifetable methods. This yields an expected number of person years lived by the cohort of potential mothers in each of the age intervals in which births could occur. Thus, formulaically (with Σ denoting 'sum of') the NRR = {0.488 × Σ (probabilities of giving birth in each of the years of life in which such a birth could occur × the person years lived by the cohort at each age)}/ number in the cohort.

By definition, a NRR of 1.0 equals 'replacement level fertility'. 'Zero population growth' will not typically be approached until several decades after the attainment of replacement level fertility because (previously) increasing populations typically have a higher proportion in the pre-reproductive ages than would obtain in the corresponding stationary population. This excess reproductive potential creates substantial momentum that is not slowed until the age structure approaches that of a stationary population. (See discussion of stable population to follow.)

Turning to measures of mortality, the most basic is the *crude death rate*, analogous to crude birth rate, giving the number of deaths per conventional unit of population time. Thus in 1999 in the USA, 2,391,399 deaths were reported and the estimated mid-year population was 272,691,000 giving a crude death rate of 8.77 per 1000 population per year.

Death rates may be specific for sex, age group and cause: for example 8337 men aged 55–64 had their cause of death entered as heart attack (acute myocardial infarction) on their death certificates in England and Wales in 1990 – out of an estimated mean population at risk of 25.26×10^5, giving a rate specific for age, sex and cause of 330 per 10^5 per year.

Among other specific death 'rates' and ratios, an important one is the *infant mortality 'rate'*, conceptually, the probability of dying between birth and exact age 1 ($_1q_0$ in lifetable notation). It is operationally defined, in relation, for example, to events occurring in a given calendar year, as:

$$\frac{\text{number of deaths of liveborn infants who have not reached their first birthday}}{\text{number of live births}} \times 1000$$

Note that this operational definition requires accurate counts of births and infant deaths and is therefore difficult to implement in the absence of a national vital statistics system with complete (e.g. greater than 95%) coverage. Only 75 of 191 member states of WHO met this criterion in 2000. Thus the infant mortality rate is most difficult to measure in those populations where infant mortality tends to be highest and of greatest public health importance. In such populations it is usually estimated using model life-tables starting from estimates of the *child mortality 'rate'*, which tend to be more robustly estimated.

Another important 'rate' is the *child (or under 5) mortality 'rate'*, conceptually, the probability of dying between birth and exact age 5 ($_5q_0$ in lifetable notation), conventionally multiplied by 1000. It is the most robustly estimated measure of mortality in early life in low and middle income countries without comprehensive vital statistical systems. In such countries, it can be measured operationally (in demographic and health surveys and in censuses) by asking women of reproductive age about all the babies they have had and which of these have since died. There are standard demographic methods for using answers to these questions to estimate $_5q_0$. If details of dates of birth and death are available then mortality rates can be estimated directly. If only the numbers ever born and numbers alive (or dead) are known then the indirect method (also known as the 'Brass' method) is used. The WHO estimates that each year about 22% of global deaths occur in populations for which estimates of this type provide the only available evidence on mortality levels (at any age).

The *adult mortality 'rate'* is the probability of dying between exact age 15 and exact age 60 ($_{45}q_{15}$). It is typically used by international agencies as a summary measure of adult mortality levels in low and middle income countries. High income countries with comprehensive vital statistical systems tend not to use this measure for their own purposes.

Maternal mortality is a topic of great policy interest globally but its measurement is fraught with difficulty. The WHO defines maternal death as the 'death of a woman while pregnant or within 42 days of termination of pregnancy, irrespective of the duration and the site of the pregnancy, from any cause related to or aggravated by the pregnancy or its management but not from accidental or incidental causes'. The *maternal mortality ratio* is the ratio of maternal deaths to live births $\times$ 100,000. Even in countries with the best vital statistical systems it is estimated that around one-third of maternal deaths are not identified as such by the ICD code assigned for the underlying cause of death. Elsewhere the ratio is subject to even greater uncertainty – making it unsuitable for comparisons between countries or over time. The global maternal mortality ratio for 1995 was estimated at 397/100,000 births with an uncertainty interval extending from 234 to 635 – emphasising the magnitude of the uncertainty associated with this measure.

In order to make fair comparisons, especially internationally, in demography it is necessary to standardise vital (birth and death) rates. Crude (unstandardised) death rates are poor guides for comparing the force of mortality in different populations: a retirement town, with many of its population in the older (dying) age ranges, will, purely as a function of its age structure, tend to have a very high crude death rate. The processes used to age standardise can be conveniently described by distinguishing between the *'population of interest'*, i.e. the population whose vital rates are being characterised, and the *'reference' or 'standard' population*, i.e. either an artificial or a real population, used for standardisation.

Direct standardisation is one method requiring relatively precise estimates of the age-specific death rates in the population of interest. The standard population provides a standard age structure. The age-specific death rates of the population of interest are applied to the component age strata (of standardised size) of the standard population. In this way, each age stratum of the standard population is made to experience the same force of mortality as the corresponding age stratum in the population of interest. The resulting sum of deaths (in the standard population) is no longer influenced by the age structure of the population of interest and, when this sum is divided by the appropriate denominator (100,000 in this case), it yields a directly age-standardised death rate. A directly age-standardised death rate is, in effect, a weighted mean of the age-specific rates using a standard set of weights – with the weight for each age stratum being the standardised proportion it comprises of the total standard population.

The second method is called *indirect age standardisation*. If the population of interest is small or the deaths of interest are from an uncommon cause, the number of deaths occurring in some age strata may be too small to produce the stable estimates of the age-specific death rates that the direct method requires. In the indirect method, the age-specific death rates of a standard population are projected onto the age strata of the population of interest to give the number of deaths that would be expected in each age stratum on the basis of the standard rates. The ratio of the total observed deaths to the total 'expected deaths' is usually called the standardised mortality ratio (or SMR). Because SMRs are still influenced by the age structure of the populations of interest, each should, strictly only be compared with the value for the standard population, i.e. with 1.00 (or 100 depending on which base is chosen).

Sources of data used for demographic measures can be illustrated for mortality. Around one-quarter of the 57 million deaths estimated to occur each year occur in countries where the vital statistical system has been judged to be at least 95% complete. Around 13% occur in populations whose vital statistical systems are less than 95% complete. For India, China and several smaller countries, vital rates are estimated using data from sample registration and surveillance systems. In these systems some 1% or so of the national population is covered by intensive surveillance for vital events. For populations in which around 22% of global deaths occur, child mortality can be estimated from survey and census returns on the numbers of children born and numbers still alive, even though there is little or no direct evidence on adult mortality levels. These are typically estimated using model lifetables to match plausible adult mortality levels to estimated child mortality. This leaves around 5% of deaths occurring in populations with no recent data on child or adult mortality.

Estimates of mortality in this last category of populations are entirely 'model based': that is, they are predicted from other known or estimated characteristics of the population. The calculation of death rates also requires estimates of populations at risk of dying. A minority of countries have regular censuses with coverage deemed complete. These countries estimate populations in intercensal years using adjacent censuses. At the other end of the data availability spectrum are populations with no recent censuses. For this group, bodies such as the Population Division of the UN have a long experience in preparing 'model-based' estimates of the size and age and sex distribution of the population, albeit with substantial levels of uncertainty. Thus, while mortality estimates are now prepared by international bodies such as the WHO for all components of the human population, many of these are subject to substantial uncertainty. The evolving philosophy of the WHO has been to make the best use of all available evidence and then to seek to quantify the level of uncertainty attaching to the resulting estimates. Life expectancy estimates published by WHO are now presented with uncertainty intervals. These intervals aim to quantify all sources of uncertainty, not just that associated with sampling error – hence their description as *uncertainty* rather than CONFIDENCE INTERVALS.

Historical demography is the branch of demography that studies how and why the force of mortality has changed through historical time, informing our understanding of the main determinants of human health and is therefore of considerable interest. Historical demographers typically work their way backwards in time from more recent periods, with data that are readily available and of good reliability, to earlier periods where there are problems with either the availability or the quality of the available evidence. Mortality estimates based on a formalised system of data collection by parishes are available for Sweden from the mid-18th century. For England and Wales an official system of vital registration began in 1837. Before such systems were in place, parishes in England, for example, kept records of baptisms, burials and marriages. Historical demographers have used these records to 'reconstitute' families and from these geneaologies have obtained both numerators (vital events) and denominators (estimates of person-time lived) for the estimation of vital rates. Family reconstitution has yielded estimates of fertility and mortality levels for England that now extend back to the 16th century. These constitute the longest such series for a North Atlantic society.

There have been two main findings from these data. First, it has been shown that the main means by which the English population adjusted to cyclic variation in economic fortunes, in the early modern period, was via the regulation of marriage. When economic conditions became difficult, age at marriage increased and the proportion never marrying also increased. These departures from the pattern of universal early marriage as seen elsewhere have been characterised as the European marriage pattern. As nuptiality varied, so did fertility and with it the rate of population increase. Second, a high level of adult mortality in England in the early modern period has been observed. While somewhat more than 50% of those born survived to adulthood, among English males, for example only around 30% of 15 year olds could expect to survive to 65. It is of interest to note here that high levels of adult mortality were also typical of the poor agrarian society of India on the eve of its demographic transition. Around 1900, only 1 in 6 of 15-year-old Indian males could expect to survive to 65.

The overall transition from a 'pre-modern' to a 'late-modern' pattern of vital rates is described as the *demographic transition*. It begins with high mortality and fertility rates, followed by a period in which mortality declines in advance of the decline in fertility – a phase of the transition in which population growth accelerates. Fertility then declines – in an idealised form to reach replacement level (NRR=1.0), with a new equilibrium being finally established with high survivorship. As has already been implied, the starting point for this demographic transition was more favourable in northwest Europe (in say the 17th century, when birth and death rates were 'submaximal') than in poor agrarian societies such as India (around say 1900, when birth and death rates were exceptionally high).

Turning from the past to the future, another important aspect of demography is making *population projections* and forecasts. Population projections, as the name implies, project existing populations forward in time under stated

assumptions and in accord with established relationships between demographic parameters. Some projections may be known to be unrealistic but be carried out to explore 'what if' scenarios. Forecasts are those projections that are believed most likely to predict the future.

The standard method for projecting populations is known as the *cohort component* method. Typically, each 5-year age group in the population of interest is projected forward 5 calendar years at a time. It is depleted by expected losses to death and emigration and augmented by expected levels of immigration. At the beginning of life, births (to existing residents and to immigrants) are predicted. For these purposes, attention focuses on females to whom assumed fertility schedules are applied. A parallel exercise for males makes up the numbers. This exercise is repeated, starting again with the expected population in 5 years' time. The migration component usually introduces the largest levels of uncertainty into the calculations. Realistic assumptions entail non-linear trends in fertility and perhaps also mortality so that the assumed rates need to be adjusted for each 5-year calendar period. Both the United Nations Population Division and the US Bureau of the Census prepare projections on 'high', 'medium' and 'low' assumptions for key inputs.

Thus, estimates for the size of the US population in 2050 vary by 102 million between low and high fertility assumptions, by 48 million between low and high mortality assumptions and 87 million between low and high migration assumptions. There is a general recognition that this scenario-based approach needs to be replaced by a more systematic approach to the quantification of uncertainty and its representation in probability distributions.

Understanding of the determination of age structure rests on the theory of *stable populations*. Stable populations emerge when the growth rate in the number of births is constant (or the schedule of age-specific fertility rates is constant), the schedule of age-specific death rates (i.e. the lifetable) is constant and there is no migration. In such populations, to which many historical populations approximate, various mathematical relationships hold between key parameters. The age distribution, the birth rate, the death rate and the growth rate are entirely determined by the fertility and mortality schedules. Populations that are not themselves currently approximating the stable model can nonetheless be said to have a 'stable equivalent', i.e. the population that would emerge if the birth and death schedules were allowed to act continuously. From this equivalence an 'intrinsic growth rate' may be determined.

One of the most striking and counterintuitive findings from stable population theory is that population age structure is very much more sensitive to changes in the fertility schedule than to changes in the mortality schedule. Thus with a gross reproductive rate of 2, increases in life expectancy from 40 to 60 years are associated with *reductions* in the mean age of the population. This is because increases in survival are proportionally greatest at each end of the lifespan. The increases in survival in the early years of life lead to larger cohorts of parents who in turn produce more children, keeping the base of the population pyramid extended. However as fertility falls and life expectancy extends, proportions aged over 65 do increase.

Finally, as populations approach stationarity (sustained equality of birth and death rates), increases in survival are reflected in increased proportions of aged persons. On the way to such equilibrium, substantial perturbations may arise due to the passage of cohorts that are 'large' relative to those that immediately follow. These may have arisen from short periods of increased fertility, e.g. 'post-war baby boomers' in western countries or from the last 'large' birth cohorts before subsequent substantial and rapid falls in fertility, for example, in such countries as Japan, China and Italy. In the next half-century these presumptively transitional phenomena will result in periods of marked 'population ageing' when the relevant 'large' cohorts pass age 65. According to the UN Population Division's 'medium' variant projections, proportions aged over 65 will increase over the period 2000 to 2020 from 6.8% to 11.7% in China, from 18.1% to 23.7% in Italy and from 17.2% to an extraordinary 28.1% in Japan. By contrast, increases in the USA are expected to be more modest: from 12.3% to 15.9%.

As populations approach stationarity, assumptions about limits to life expectancy become increasingly relevant. Oeppen and Vaupel (2002) have shown how demographers have repeatedly underestimated such limits. Mortality decline at high ages has continued in low mortality countries and has so far shown little evidence of slowing down at the highest ages.

Demography has played an important role in the development of methods for measuring the burden of disease and injury. For example, the health-adjusted life expectancy (HALE) measure seeks to estimate the expectation of life in 'full health'. Time expected to be spent in less than full health is subtracted from total life expectancy, after weighting by the severity of the departure from full health. 'Health gap' measures, such as the disability-adjusted life year (DALY) lost, estimate the hypothetical flows of 'lost healthy lifetime' arising from deaths and from onsets of disease and injury during the period of interest. For the 'years of life lost' component (and for long-term non-fatal health losses), gaps are estimated relative to a standard life table with a female life expectancy at birth of 82.5 years and a male life expectancy at birth of 80.0 years. Unlike health expectancy-type measures (such as HALE), health gap measures can be decomposed by allocating DALYs lost to the diseases and injuries responsible and also into the determinants of the diseases and injuries.   *JP*

Coale, A.J. 1955: How the age distribution of a human population is determined. In *Proceedings Cold Spring Harbour symposia on quantitative biology*, 83–9. Murray, C.J.L., Salomon, J.A., Mathers, C.D. and Lopez, A.D. 2002: *Summary measures of population health: concepts, ethics, measurement and applications.* Geneva: World Health Organization (www.who.int/pub/smph/en/index.html). Oeppen, J. and Vaupel, J.W. 2002: Broken limits to life expectancy. *Science* 296, 1029–31. Preston, S.H., Heuveline, P. and Guillot, M. 2001: *Demography: measuring and modeling population processes.* Oxford: Blackwell. UN Fund for Population annual: *State of world population.* UN Fund for Population (www.unfpa.org/swp/swpmain.htm). United Nations. *World population prospects* (http://esa.un.org/unpp/). Wrigley, E.A., Davies, R.S., Oeppen, J.E. and Schofield, R.S. 1997: *English population history from family reconstitution, 1580–1837.* Cambridge: Cambridge University Press.

dendogram   See CLUSTER ANALYSIS IN MEDICINE

density estimation   The estimates of a probability distribution from a sample of observations. In many situations

in medical research we may wish to use a sample of observation to estimate the frequency distribution or probability density of a variable of interest. Commonly this estimation problem is approached by simply plotting a HISTOGRAM of the data. But the histogram may not be the most effective way of displaying the distribution of a variable, because of its dependence on the number of classes chosen. The problem becomes even more acute if two-dimensional histograms are used to estimate BIVARIATE DISTRIBUTIONS.

The density estimates provided by one- and two- dimensional histograms can be improved on in a number of ways. If, of course, we were willing to assume a particular form for the distribution, for example, normal, then density estimation would be reduced to estimating the parameters of the chosen density function. More commonly, however, we would like the data to 'speak for themselves' as it were, in which case we might choose one of a variety of the nonparametric density estimation procedures available. Perhaps the most common are the kernel density estimators which are essentially smoothed estimates of the proportion of observations falling in intervals of some size. The essential components of such estimators are the kernel function and bandwidth or smoothing parameter. The kernel estimator is a sum of 'bumps' placed at the observations. The kernel function determines the shape of the bumps while the window width determines their width. Details of the mathematics involved are given in Silverman (1986) and Wand and Jones (1995), but the essence of the procedure can be gleaned from the first Figure. Here the kernel function is Gaussian, and the diagram shows the individual bumps at each observation as well as the density estimate obtained from adding them up.

The kernel density estimator considered as a series of bumps centred at the observations has a simple extension to two dimensions as described in, for example, Silverman (1986). Here we content ourselves with an example. The second Figure (see page 105) shows a plot of birth and death rates for 69 countries. The third Figure then shows a two-dimensional histogram of the data and the fourth Figure (at (a) and (b)) shows perspective plots of density estimates given by using different kernel functions.   *BSE*

Silverman, B.W. 1986: *Density estimates for statistics and data analysis.* London: CRC/Chapman & Hall. **Wand, M.P. and Jones, M.C.** 1995: *Kernel smoothing.* London: CRC/Chapman & Hall.

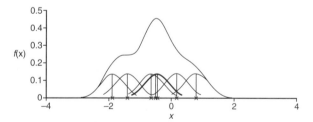

density estimation *Kernel estimate showing individual kernals. (Source: Silverman, 1986.)*

dental statistics   Dentistry is concerned with the provision of care for the teeth, supporting tissues and the gums, and the treatment of diseases affecting these areas of the mouth. In the United Kingdom, an Adult Dental

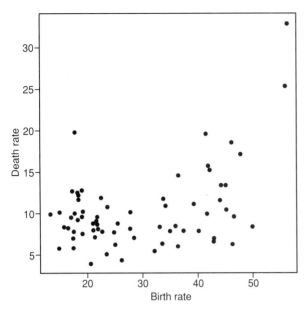

density estimation *Scatterplot of birth and death rates for 69 countries.*

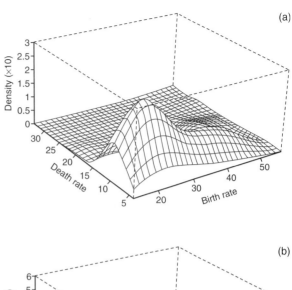

(a)

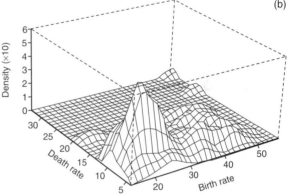

(b)

density estimation *Perspective plots of two density estimates for the birth and death rate date: (a) bivariate normal kernal; (b) Epanechnikov kernel.*

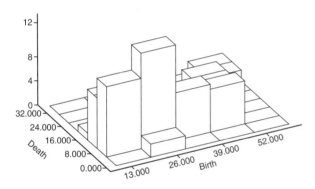

density estimation *Two-dimensional histogram of birth and death rates.*

Health Survey is carried out every 10 years (see, for example, the report on the 1998 survey (Kelly, Walker and Cooper, 2000)). Participants are interviewed face to face and in addition those with natural teeth are asked to undergo a home dental examination. Using a random sample of several thousand individuals aged 16 years and over, this survey yields information on issues that include the number and condition of teeth, dental hygiene behaviour, patterns of dental visits and attitudes towards the provision of dental healthcare. In a similar manner, the Child Dental Health Survey, involving schoolchildren aged between 5 and 15 years, has been conducted on a 10-yearly basis since 1973. Statistical analyses are provided in detailed official reports of these surveys.

For all dental specialties, current evidence is advanced through the conduct of suitably designed research studies that use statistical methods for data analysis. Developments in dental public health, particularly that of

children, have attracted the most attention in the media. Worldwide, important public health themes have included the impact of the fluoridation of public water supplies on dental caries, the effect of the introduction of fluoride toothpaste on dental health, the decline in dental caries experienced by schoolchildren since the 1960s and the influence of socioeconomic factors and ethnicity on the provision and uptake of dental services.

In dental studies, possibly more so than for those of other types of healthcare, data from consecutive patients should not be treated as independent observations. In routine dental appointments, a significant number of patients are examined as part of a family group, with members being seen consecutively. Correlation between observations occurs because, within a household, individuals tend to eat similarly and engage in the same type of routine dental care. Gulliford, Okoumunne and Chinn (1999) reported a household level INTRACLASS CORRELATION COEFFICIENT for the consumption of fruit, an important determinant in the level of sugar intake, of 0.33. Other types of cluster encountered include school classes in the study of adolescents and nursing homes in surveys of the elderly. CLUSTER RANDOMISED TRIALS can be used to address this problem (see also CLINICAL TRIALS) (Frenkel, Harvey and Newcombe, 2001).

Similarly, data from an individual's teeth cannot be treated as independent observations; an individual might, for example, have similar patterns of fillings on the left and right sides of the jaw. Consequently, in nearly all studies of teeth the unit of observation is taken as the individual rather than the tooth. Recently, with the development of more sophisticated statistical methods, studies that analyse individual teeth as correlated observations have started to appear, for instance that by Chuang *et al.* (2002) into possible factors influencing the survival time of dental implants. This paper also contains a useful review of survival analysis techniques that have been applied in the modelling of dental implant failure.

Continuous and near-continuous dental data rarely follow a NORMAL DISTRIBUTION. For instance, salivary counts of bacteria generally show an extremely high positive skew between individuals. Consequently, nonparametric techniques have played an important role in data analysis; even at a basic level the use of the MANN-WHITNEY RANK SUM TEST is commonplace. Alternatively, taking logarithms of the observations can produce a much more symmetrical distribution and allow methods that require an assumption of normality to be considered.

In studies that involve clinicians performing a dental examination, a fraction of the participants might be reassessed in order to gauge examiner reproducibility. For instance, in a study of the dental heath of pre-school children, 10% of the participants were examined on a second occasion for this purpose (Godson and Williams, 1996). Generally, a form of the kappa statistic (see KAPPA AND WEIGHTED KAPPA) is used as the measure of agreement. SENSITIVITY, SPECIFICITY and the measurement of agreement are important in the comparison of results from screening with those from definitive findings. Bell *et al.* (2003) compared apparent characteristics of third molar ('wisdom') teeth from a radiological assessment with the actual features seen at surgery.

Populations may consist of two or more distinct groups representing different levels of dental care. One group of individuals might exercise a high level of care including the use of dental floss and disclosing tablets, another group might rely solely on the brushing of teeth with a further group undertaking no regular dental care. For data consisting of counts, the Poisson model is therefore rarely appropriate. With the DMF score (sum of the numbers of decayed, missing and filled teeth) there is generally a higher proportion of individuals with a zero score (representing a perfect set of teeth – more than likely from the group exercising a high level of care) than this model would predict. Models that allow for over-dispersion, such as the zero-inflated Poisson, have been found to provide a better fit for this type of data (Böhning *et al.*, 1999).

As with medical studies, data can consist of repeated measurements, for which appropriate methods of analysis are required. For instance, in a study of xerostomia (self-reported dryness of the mouth) and reduced production of saliva in individuals over a period of 4 years, Navazesh *et al.* (2003) applied repeated measures regression to data from 6-monthly assessments.

META-ANALYSIS is increasingly being used as a tool in the review of specific issues in dental research. For example, Ismail and Bandekar (1999) described a meta-analysis of the studies published between 1966 and 1997 into the association between fluoride supplements and fluorosis, a dental condition that is characterised by staining of the teeth. Brief summaries of critical reviews can be found in the journal *Evidence-Based Dentistry*.   *NCS*

Bell, G.W., Rodgers, J.A., Grime, R.J., Edwards, K.L., Hahn, M.R., Dorman, M.L., Keen, W.D., Stewart, D.J.C. and Hampton, N. 2003: The accuracy of dental panoramic tomographs in determining the root morphology of mandibular third molar teeth before surgery. *Oral Surgery Oral Medicine Oral Pathology Oral Radiology and Endodontics* 95, 119–25. **Böhning, D., Dietz, E., Schlattmann, P., Mendonça, L. and Kirchner, U.** 1999: The zero-inflated Poisson model and the decayed, missing and filled teeth index in dental epidemiology. *Journal of the Royal Statistical Society A* 162, 195–209. **Chuang, S.K., Wei, L.J., Douglass, C.W. and Dodson, T.B.** 2002: Risk factors for dental implant failure: a strategy for the analysis of clustered failure-time observations. *Journal of Dental Research* 81, 572–7. **Frenkel, H., Harvey, I. and Newcombe, R.G.** 2001: Improving oral health in institutionalised elderly people by educating caregivers: a randomised controlled trial. *Community Dentistry and Oral Epidemiology* 29, 289–97. **Godson, J.H. and Williams, S.A.** 1996: Oral health and health related behaviours among three-year-old children born to first and second generation Pakistani mothers in Bradford, UK. *Community Dental Health* 13, 27–33. **Gulliford, M.C., Ukoumunne, O.C. and Chinn, S.** 1999: Components of variance and intraclass correlations for the design of community-based surveys and intervention studies: data from the Health Survey for England 1994. *American Journal of Epidemiology* 149, 876–83. **Ismail, A.I. and Bandekar, R.R.** 1999: Fluoride supplements and fluorosis: a meta-analysis. *Community Dentistry and Oral Epidemiology* 27, 48–56. **Kelly, M., Walker, A. and Cooper, I.** 2000: *Adult dental health survey: oral health in the United Kingdom 1998.* London: Stationery Office. **Navazesh, M., Mulligan, R., Barron, Y., Redford, M., Greenspan, D., Alves, M. and Phelan, J.** 2003: A 4-year longitudinal evaluation of xerostomia and salivary gland hypofunction in the Women's Interagency HIV Study participants. *Oral Surgery Oral Medicine Oral Pathology Oral Radiology and Endodontics* 95, 693–8.

descriptive statistics Summaries designed to encapsulate meaningful aspects of datasets. Here we focus on numerical descriptive statistics, GRAPHICAL DISPLAYS being considered separately. Individual observations are the basis of statistical analysis. However, when describing data it is rarely feasible to present all observations, and it is not always possible to illustrate the distribution using a graph. Therefore descriptive statistics are required to provide a numerical summary of the distribution.

MEASURES OF LOCATION are used to describe in a single figure the typical or representative level of all observations. The measures of location most often employed are the MEAN, MEDIAN, GEOMETRIC MEAN and MODE.

Variability around this central point is summarised by means of a MEASURE OF SPREAD. The RANGE, STANDARD DEVIATION and INTERQUARTILE RANGE are used as measures of spread.

Other aspects of a distribution are encapsulated by SKEWNESS, which measures how asymmetric the distribution is, and KURTOSIS, which quantifies its 'peakedness'.

It is important that descriptive statistics chosen are appropriate to the distribution of the data. Data that have an approximately symmetric distribution are usually summarised using the mean and standard deviation. On the other hand, the presence of skewness or OUTLIERS implies that the median and interquartile range are more appropriate. This is because they are based on ranks, and therefore make no assumptions about the distribution of the data. *SRC*

deviance A measure of the extent to which a particular model differs from the saturated model for a dataset. Defined explicitly in terms of the difference in the LIKELI-HOODS of the two models as deviance $= -2[\ln L_c - \ln L_s]$ where L_c and L_s are the likelihoods of the current model and the saturated model respectively. Large values of the deviance are encountered when L_c is small relative to L_s, indicating that the current model is poor. Small values of the deviance are obtained in the reverse case. Asymptotically, the deviance has a CHI-SQUARE DISTRIBU-TION with DEGREES OF FREEDOM equal to the difference in the number of parameters in the two models. *BSE*

[See also GENERALISED LINEAR MODELS, LOG-LINEAR MODELS]

digit preference The personal and often subconscious bias that frequently occurs in the recording of observations. For example, a person may round the terminal digit of a number (i.e the 5 in 624.75) systematically to a particular digit or set of digits that they prefer. Most frequently people will want to round to zero or five, although other numbers are of course possible. This is a problem when recording data from an analogue source, i.e. a clock or sphygmomanometer and when recall or estimation is required, i.e. recalling age at which menopause began or one's weight in kilos. It can also be a problem when using visual analogue scales or similar devices to garner information. In medicine the digit preference phenomenon is particularly troublesome in the recording of blood pressure where it has been estimated that clinicians have up to a 12-fold bias in favour of the terminal digit zero (see Figure). This type of bias may have grave implications for

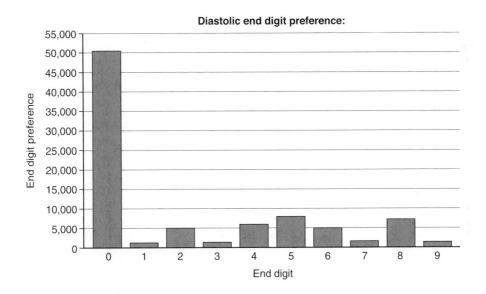

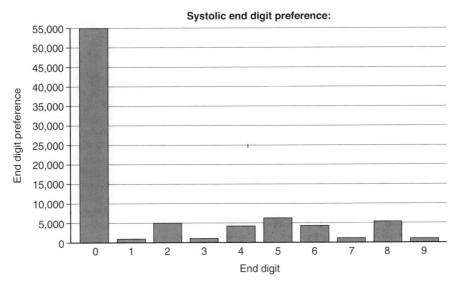

digit preference *Diastolic and systolic end digit preference*

diagnosis and treatment, but its greatest effect is perhaps in epidemiological and other research studies where it can distort frequency distributions and reduce the POWER of statistical tests (see Hessel, 1986). Johnstone (2001) identifies a study in which digit preference may have led the authors to the wrong conclusion about the effect of a drug in the treatment of hypertension (Persson, Vitols and Yue, 2000).

There are times when it is appropriate to compare the distribution of terminal digits to a discrete uniform distribution in order to detect digit preference. However, one should not lose sight of the fact that, as demonstrated in Crawford, Johannes and Stellato (2002), it is possible for the distribution of terminal digits to be non-uniform, but still not the result of digit preference.   *BSE/AGL*

[See also FRAUD DETECTION IN BIOMEDICAL RESEARCH]

Crawford, S.L., Johannes, C.B. and Stellato, R.K. 2002: Assessment of digit preference in self-reported year at menopause: choice of an appropriate reference distribution. *American Journal of Epidemiology* 156, 676. **Hessel, P.A.** 1986: Terminal digit preference in blood pressure measurement: effects on epidemiological associations. *International Journal of Epidemiology* 15, 122–5. **Johnstone, G.D.** 2001: Letter. *British Medical Journal* 322, 110. **Persson, M., Vitols, S. and Yue, Q.Y.** 2000: Orlistat associated with hypertension. *British Medical Journal* 321, 87.

direct standardisation   See DEMOGRAPHY

disability-adjusted life-year   See DEMOGRAPHY

disattenuated correlation   See CONFIRMATORY FACTOR ANALYSIS

discriminant function analysis

A collection of methods aimed at optimally distinguishing between *a priori* groups of individuals, so that future unassigned individuals can be classified to one of the groups.

To illustrate the problem in medical contexts, consider the following three situations.

First, patients entering hospital with jaundice could be suffering from one of a number of diseases. Some of these diseases require surgery, while others can be treated completely by medical means. Exact determination of disease may itself require surgery, which is to be avoided if at all possible, so it is hoped that diagnosis might be achieved via a battery of observations (signs, symptoms and laboratory measurements) taken on the patient. Such data are available on a sample of patients for whom either a biopsy or a *post-mortem* examination has established the underlying disease, and hence the medical or surgical status, with certainty. Can we use these data to formulate a rule for predicting the status of a future patient from the battery of observations made on him/her?

Second, a retrospective study is conducted on patients undergoing surgery and the appearance or otherwise of postoperative pulmonary embolism is recorded for each patient alongside a range of other variables (e.g. age, obesity measure, number of cigarettes smoked per day, nature of disease etc). Can the data be used to develop a screening index for predicting patients at high risk of appearance of postoperative pulmonary embolism?

Third, consider a prospective study being conducted on patients with thrombo-phlebitis. Each patient is monitored on a range of laboratory measurements; some

patients develop embolic thrombosis, while others do not. Can those who develop it be predicted from the measurements monitored in the study?

These situations share some common characteristics and objectives. In each of them there are two distinct *groups* of individuals and observations have been recorded on a set of *features* (*variables* or *attributes*) for each individual. The hope is that these features are able to distinguish the two groups from each other well enough for the measurements taken on them to be capable of predicting the group membership of a future individual. The process of distinguishing between groups is known as *discrimination*, while the prediction of group membership of future individuals is termed *classification* or *allocation*. Typically, the best way of utilising the features is to combine them in some way, i.e. to form a *function* of them.

Discriminant function analysis then aims to find the best function for distinguishing between the groups, while formulating a *classification rule* will provide a means of predicting group membership. Frequently, the best function for discriminating between two groups also directly provides the best classification rule, but this is not always the case. There are many different potential discriminant functions and classification rules in any practical situation, so we need to be able to judge their performances in order to choose the best ones. The worth of a discriminant function can be assessed by any measure that estimates the separation between the groups using this function, while the worth of a classification rule is generally determined by estimating the probabilities of misclassifying future individuals with this rule.

The ideas and problems can be readily generalised to situations where there are more than two groups. For example, in the earlier jaundice case, we may be interested in discriminating between the actual *diseases* causing the condition rather than just between the group that require surgery and the group that can be cured by medicine. The underlying principles remain the same, but the details become more complicated. For example, in discrimination we have to be able to assess the extent of separation among all groups (or all pairs of groups simultaneously), while in classification there are now many more potential mistakes that can be made in predicting an individual's group membership. For the purpose of this section, therefore, we will describe the methodology for the case of two groups and later merely indicate how the methods generalise to multiple group situations.

The first attempt at formulating and tackling the problem was made by Fisher (1936), who looked for the linear combination of features that maximally separates the two groups. He tackled this by maximising, over all linear combinations, the ratio of the squared difference between the group means to the pooled within-group variance of the observations, which is equivalent to maximising the squared t-statistic that tests for a difference between the two groups. The coefficients of the features in this linear combination are given by the elements of the vector formed on multiplying the vector of mean differences of the features by the inverse of their pooled covariance matrix. This very simple function has become known as *Fisher's linear discriminant function* (LDF).

Fisher derived his result in a purely practical setting, using actual data rather than statistical or probability models. Welch (1939) took a theoretical approach and showed that the classification rule maximising the *a posteriori* probability of correct group membership is given by comparing the ratio of probability density functions of observations in the two populations against a given threshold value. This threshold, or cut-off, value depends on the prior probabilities of observations in each of the two populations; an individual is allocated to one group if the threshold is exceeded and otherwise to the other group. Welch also showed that if the two populations were characterised by MULTIVARIATE NORMAL DISTRIBUTIONS that had a common dispersion matrix then the resultant classification rule was a linear combination of the observed features, while if the dispersion matrices differed then a quadratic function was necessary. Subsequently, the theory was extended to encompass differential costs incurred in making classification errors and applied to practical datasets. It transpires that Fisher's LDF provides the best classification rule in the case of populations having multivariate normal distributions with a common dispersion matrix and that the cut-off value for classification is a simple ratio of costs of misclassification as well as prior probabilities in the two populations (see McLachlan, 1992, for details).

Fisher's derivation shows that his linear discriminant function will provide a good separation between groups for many practical situations, but the subsequent theoretical developments warn that this function may not provide good classification performance if populations are not multivariate normal with equal dispersion matrices. Alternative functions are necessary in such cases. Data arising in different contexts may have aspects that can readily be modelled by parametric distributions other than the normal, so various functions have been derived for specific types of data. Examples include functions based on the MULTINOMIAL DISTRIBUTION for discrete feature data, on the location model for mixed discrete and continuous feature data and on distributions such as the EXPONENTIAL DISTRIBUTION, the STUDENT'S t-DISTRIBUTION and the inverse normal for continuous non-normal feature data (see McLachlan, 1992, for details).

An extreme assumption is that all features are independent, whence the class-conditional distributions can be simply estimated by products of marginal distributions. Although seemingly a totally inappropriate assumption in most practical situations, this method has had surprisingly good results on occasion (see Hand and Yu, 2001). However, approaches other than the parametric need to be sought if the resultant method is to be widely applicable.

Fix and Hodges (see Agrawala, 1977, 261–322) therefore initiated a stream of research into non-parametric methods. Here the data alone determine the classification rule without imposition of any distributional assumptions, so that the methods can be applied in almost any context. Two of their ideas which have undergone refinement but which retain their popularity are nearest-neighbour and kernel methods. The *k-nearest-neighbour (kNN)* rule simply allocates an individual to the group that is in the majority among that individual's k nearest neighbours. Although simple in concept, this approach has several obvious questions that do not have easy answers: how do we measure the 'distance' between individuals in order to determine the nearest neighbours and how do we choose an optimal value of k in a given situation? These questions

have been addressed in a number of contributions to the literature. The kernel method, by contrast, is a non-parametric method of estimating the probability densities in each group via the average of a so-called kernel function evaluated at each data point (see DENSITY ESTIMATION). Once the density functions have been estimated then computing their ratio at the point to be classified leads directly to an allocation rule. Fix and Hodges proposed a crude 'kernel' based on the empirical histograms of the data. Hand (1997) contains a good overview of both the kNN and the kernel methods, while McLachlan (1992) provides more technical detail.

A method intermediate between fully parametric models of the populations, in which the data are required to satisfy fairly strict assumptions, and the non-parametric approaches just described, is the idea of *logistic discrimination* (LD). This was introduced in the early 1960s by Cox, Day, Kerridge and others, but was mainly developed in a series of papers well summarised by Anderson (1982). The idea is to estimate directly the posterior probability of group membership for an individual by a simple function of its observed features. Since this probability has to lie between zero and one, the simplest such function is logistic with argument given by a linear combination of the observed features. It can be shown that this form of posterior probability is either exhibited, or approximately exhibited, by a range of different parametric models including some of those already mentioned, so that the approach potentially has wide applicability. Moreover, it only requires estimation of a small number of parameters, as opposed to some of the parametric methods that involve many parameters, so it should be simpler to apply. Once some technical difficulties had been overcome the method proved both popular and useful and can now be found alongside Fisher's LDF in many software implementations.

Dramatic increases in computer power achieved towards the end of the 20th century led to an explosion of interest in computationally intensive methods. One of the first ideas in this vein was regularised discriminant analysis, where an optimal mixture of different types of discriminant function (such as linear and quadratic, for example) is sought by computationally optimising a criterion such as cross-validated error rate (see later). This was followed by TREE-STRUCTURED METHODS such as classification and regression trees (CART), multivariate adaptive regression splines (MARS), and flexible discriminant analysis, while overshadowing all these approaches has been the development of NEURAL NETWORKS and SUPPORT VECTOR MACHINES among the computer science community. Unfortunately, the increasing reliance on computational power in these methods has turned each process into something of a 'black box', with results simply being produced at the end of a long series of computer operations and little chance being provided for either intervention in the process or interpretation of the underlying discriminant functions. More recently, therefore, attention has been given to computer-intensive enhancements of traditional methods. One general approach is *model averaging*, in which rather than seeking a single 'optimal' discriminant function of a given form many different such functions are derived and their average (in some sense) is used for future predictions. MARKOV CHAIN MONTE CARLO methods fall under this heading and much research is currently under way in their applications to discriminant functions. A good account of this work is given by Denison *et al.* (2002). The second general approach is in the use of *local models*, where instead of estimating parameters just once for all regions of the sample space, they are estimated separately for many sub-regions. Thus, for example, the optimal number k of nearest neighbours to use in kNN classification is estimated separately for all potential points to be classified.

Whichever method of discrimination or classification is chosen, a paramount consideration in practice is to obtain a reliable assessment of its performance. There are many possible measures that can be used for such assessment (see, e.g. Hand, 1997, Chapter 6), but overwhelmingly the most prevalent in practice is the misclassification rate. Again, there are many possible ways of defining such a rate, but here we will just consider the one relevant to most practitioners: given a particular classification rule formed from some sample data, what is the probability of misclassifying a future individual when using this rule?

It is possible to tackle this question theoretically, by postulating a probability model for the data and then following through with a sequence of probability calculations on implied SAMPLING DISTRIBUTIONS to arrive at a final value. Such calculations, however, frequently involve heavy simplifications to achieve tractability and stand or fall according to the appropriateness of the initial assumptions about the data. They have, therefore, long since been abandoned as genuine methods to use in practice and now usually serve only as benchmarks in simulation studies of properties of new methods. Attention instead has focused on purely data-based methods of assessment of performance, using the data from which the classification rule itself is constructed.

Given that the aim is to assess how often mistakes will be made in classifying *future* individuals and that in order to assess the accuracy of the classification we need to know the true group membership of each individual, an obvious method is to split the available sample data randomly into two portions. One portion, the *training* set, is used to form the classification rule, while the other, the *test* set, is used to assess its performance. Typically, the two sets are then combined and used to form the classification rule for actual use on future data. Such a process is known as *cross-validation*. Of course, it assumes that future samples are 'similar' in composition to the present ones and that the classification rule is stable over the different datasets. The former assumption is implicit in the classification procedure itself, but for the latter assumption to hold we really need large datasets. Problems arise when available samples are not large. Either the training set will be very small, so the training set classification rule may differ markedly from the final rule and the wrong rule will be assessed or the test set will be very small, so the assessment of the rule will be poor, or both drawbacks will occur.

An early attempt to solve this problem was by simply forming a classification rule from all available data and then reapplying it to the same data to assess its performance (re-substitution). However, it was soon realised that this method will provide a grossly overoptimistic assessment for small to medium samples. This is because most classification rules operate by optimising the group separation on the given data, so such a 're-substitution' error rate represents the best achievable for the data and

performance on genuinely future data will be much poorer. One possible solution is to conduct n distinct random training/test set divisions and to average the n resulting error rates as the final assessment of performance. This is known as *n-fold cross-validation*. Taking this process to the limit means removing each single observation in turn from the data, forming the classification rule using all the other observations and classifying the one that has been left out. The proportion of observations misclassified in this way then provides an estimate of the error rate of the rule. This is usually known as the *leave-one-out cross-validation* estimate.

The leave-one-out approach satisfactorily corrects for the known bias of the re-substitution error rate, but it has been shown to have the unsatisfactory property of a high variance. Thus, although it will give (approximately) the correct estimate *on average* over many replicates of equivalent datasets, any single application may yield an estimate far from the true value. An alternative line of attack was therefore developed in the 1980s using the idea of *bootstrapping*. Here the available data values are sampled with replacement to give a BOOTSTRAP sample, which is intended to mimic the drawing of a future sample from the populations under study, and relevant measures (such as error rate) of the bootstrap sample are computed. This process is repeated for a large number of bootstrap samples and this enables distributions of the measures to be studied. In the context of classification error rates, many potential bootstrap corrections to the re-substitution error rate have been considered. The most popular appears to be the '632 bootstrap' estimate. A large number of bootstrap samples are generated, the classification rule is computed for each bootstrap sample and the observations *not* represented in that bootstrap sample are classified by the rule. If *ea* represents the error rate obtained in this way and *eb* represents the re-substitution error rate of the original data, then the 632 bootstrap error rate is given by $0.632ea + 0.368eb$. This appears satisfactorily to correct the optimistic bias of *eb*.

These data-based methods are applicable for assessment of any classification rule. However, the derivation of some rules itself requires assessment of error rates as part of the procedure. For example, estimation of the number k of nearest neighbours to use in kNN classification can be effected by trying all possible values of k in a given range and picking the one that produces the fewest misclassification errors. Simply quoting the resultant misclassification error rate again gives an overoptimistic assessment of performance of the method, because a parameter has been chosen to optimise such performance on the given data. The correct procedure here is to randomly divide the data into *three* portions: a training set, a validation set and a test set. The classification rule is formed from the training set and parameters are optimised by calculating error rates over the validation set. Having thus settled on all parameter values, final assessment of performance is conducted on the (truly independent) test set. The corresponding correction in the leave-one-out process is a *nested* leave-one-out: one observation is omitted, then the classification rule is formed *and optimised* using the remaining observations, nesting a second leave-one-out process within the first for the optimisation. The omitted observation is thus only classified once all parameters of the rule have been estimated.

Many of the above ideas were applied by Asparoukhov and Krzanowski (2001) in an empirical investigation of a range of different discriminant functions on binary data. Five datasets were used, of which the following four were medical: *pulmonary data* – 15 features to discriminate 144 patients who suffered postoperative pulmonary embolism and 246 who did not; *thrombosis data* – 15 features to discriminate 34 patients with embolic thrombosis from 68 patients without the condition; *epilepsy data* – 15 features to discriminate 81 children with craniocerebral trauma epilepsy from 48 without the condition; and *aneurysm data* – 17 features to discriminate 102 patients with dissecting aneurysm from 140 patients diagnosed with other similar diseases.

All features were already either binary in nature or were converted to binary form, the two categories in each case being scored 0 and 1. Each dataset was subjected to a number of different discriminant functions, but the Table shows the error rates using those functions mentioned earlier. Each method was assessed exclusively using its leave-one-out error rates, so the best method on each dataset is the one with the lowest error rate.

discriminant function analysis *Error rates from 7 methods applied to 4 datasets*

Discriminant procedure	Pulmonary data	Thrombosis data	Epilepsy data	Aneurysm data
Independence	0.146	0.265	0.209	0.021
Fisher LDF	0.159	0.294	0.163	0.041
Logistic	0.159	0.255	0.217	0.050
kNN	0.208	0.245	0.202	0.103
Kernel	0.172	0.265	0.217	0.054
Neural net	0.156	0.245	0.186	0.070
Vector support	0.213	0.245	0.209	0.058

These results demonstrate a typical empirical finding, namely that no single method is dominant in all cases and that each method performs well on at least some if not all datasets. The independence assumption works well on the pulmonary and aneurysm sets, but badly on the epilepsy data. Fisher's LDF is the best method on the epilepsy data, but the worst on the thrombosis data. NEURAL NETWORKS, SUPPORT VECTORS and kNN classifiers are the joint 'winners' on the thrombosis data, but have mixed results on the other datasets. So the message for practical applications is to try a range of potential methods before classifying individuals.

Extensions of all methods to the situation of multiple groups is straightforward in principle, although may need careful computational implementation in practice. Fisher's LDF approach extends directly, by seeking the linear combination of features that maximises the ratio of between-group to within-group sums of squares. This is equivalent to maximising the F-ratio in standard ONE-WAY ANALYSIS OF VARIANCE, which is the multi-group extension of the two-group t-test for differences between the groups. The extra facet here is that more than one function results from this process; indeed, the number of functions will be the smaller of two values: the number of features present and one less than the number of groups. The resulting

functions are known as *canonical variates* or *discriminant coordinates*, and plotting the original data against these functions as axes will highlight group differences pictorially (see CANONICAL CORRELATION ANALYSIS).

Welch's theoretical approach leads to classification being done via a series of pairwise comparisons, where ratios of each pair of population densities are in turn compared against cut-off thresholds until unique classification is achieved. This can be a somewhat protracted process, so recourse is usually made to one of the other methods. Logistic discrimination gives an estimated probability of group membership for each available group and allocation is made to the group with highest probability. The kNN process gives allocation directly without any change in its definition. Kernel discrimination requires densities to be estimated separately for each group and allocation then follows directly from these densities, while all 'black box' routines deliver allocations for any number of groups. Likewise, all methods for estimating error rates naturally extend to the multigroup case.   *WK*

[See also CANONICAL CORRELATION ANALYSIS]

Agrawala, A.K. (ed.) 1977: *Machine recognition of patterns.* New York: IEEE Press. **Anderson, J.A.** 1982: Logistic discrimination. In Krishnaiah, P.R. and Kanal, L.N. (eds), *Handbook of statistics.* Vol. 2. Amsterdam: North Holland, 169–91. **Asparoukhov, O.K. and Krzanowski, W.J.** 2001: A comparison of discriminant procedures for binary variables. *Computational Statistics and Data Analysis* 38, 139–60. **Denison, D.G.T., Holmes, C.C., Mallick, B.K. and Smith, A.F.M.** 2002: *Bayesian methods for nonlinear classification and regression.* Chichester: John Wiley & Sons. **Fisher, R.A.** 1936: The use of multiple measurements in taxonomic problems. *Annals of Eugenics* 7, 179–88. **Hand, D.J.** 1997: *Construction and assessment of classification rules.* Chichester: John Wiley & Sons. **Hand, D.J. and Yu, K.** 2001: Idiot's Bayes – not so stupid after all? *International Statistical Review* 69, 385–98. **McLachlan, G.J.** 1992: *Discriminant analysis and statistical pattern recognition.* New York: John Wiley & Sons. **Welch, B.L.** 1939: Note on discriminant functions. *Biometrika* 31, 218–20.

disease clustering
Unusual aggregations of disease which appear on maps of disease incidence (Lawson, 2001; Elliott, Wakefield *et al.*, 2000). These are areas of such elevated risk that they could not have arisen by chance alone. For example, concerns about the influence of industrial installations on the health of surrounding populations have given rise to the development of methods that seek to evaluate clusters of disease around such installations. These clusters are regarded as representing local adverse health risk conditions, possibly ascribable to environmental causes. However, it is also true that for many diseases the geographical incidence of disease will naturally display clustering at some spatial scale, even after the 'at risk' population effects are taken into account.

The reasons for such clustering of disease are various. First, it is possible that for some apparently non-infectious diseases there may be a viral agent, which could induce clustering. This has been hypothesised for childhood leukaemia. Second, other common but unobserved factors or variables could lead to observed clustering in maps. For example, localised pollution sources could produce elevated incidence of disease (e.g. road junctions could yield high carbon monoxide levels and hence elevated respiratory disease incidence), or a common treatment of disease can lead to clustering of disease side effects. The prescription of a drug by a particular medical practice could lead to elevated incidence of side-effects within that practice area.

Hence, there are many situations where diseases may be found to cluster, even when the aetiology does not suggest it should be observed. Because of this, it is important to be aware of the role of clustering methods, even when clustering per se is not the main focus of interest. In this case, it may be important to consider clustering as a background effect and to employ appropriate methods to detect such effects.

Two extreme forms of clustering can be defined. These represent the spectrum of modelling from nonparametric to parametric forms and associated with these forms are appropriate statistical models and estimation procedures. First, as many researchers may not wish to specify *a priori* the exact form/extent of clusters to be studied, then a nonparametric definition is often the basis adopted. Without any assumptions about shape or form of the cluster, the most basic definition would be: 'any area within the study region of significantly elevated risk' (Lawson, 2001: 104).

This definition is often referred to as *hot spot clustering*. In essence, any area of elevated risk, regardless of shape or extent, could qualify as a cluster, provided the area meets some statistical criteria. Note that it is not usual to regard areas of significantly low risk to be of interest, although these may have some importance in further studies of the aetiology of a particular disease.

Second, at the other extreme, we can define a parametric cluster form: namely, that *the study region displays a prespecified cluster structure*. This definition describes a parameterised cluster form that would be thought to apply across the study region. Usually, this implies some stronger restriction on the cluster form and also some region-wide parameters that control the shape and size of clusters.

Non-specific clustering concerns the analysis of the overall clustering tendency of the disease incidence in a study region. This is also known as *general clustering*. As such, the assessment of general clustering is closely akin to the assessment of spatial autocorrelation. Hence, any model or test relating to general clustering will assess some overall/global aspect of the clustering tendency of the disease of interest. This could be summarised by a model parameter (e.g., an autocorrelation parameter in an appropriate model) or by a test that assesses the aggregation of cases of disease. For example, the correlated prior distributions used in the Basag, York and Mollié (BYM) model (see SPATIAL EPIDEMIOLOGY) provide an example of the former. It should be noted at this point that the general clustering methods discussed earlier can be regarded as *non-specific* in that they do not seek to estimate the spatial locations of clusters but simply to assess whether clustering is apparent in the study region. Any method that seeks to assess the locational structure of clusters is defined to be *specific*.

An alternative non-specific effect has also been proposed in models for tract-count or case-event data. This effect is conventionally known as uncorrelated heterogeneity (or OVERDISPERSION/extra-Poisson variation in the Poisson likelihood case).

Specific clustering concerns the analysis of the locations of clusters. This approach seeks to estimate the location, size and shape of clusters within a study region. For example, it is straightforward to formulate a non-specific

Bayesian model (see BAYESIAN METHODS) for case events or tract counts that includes heterogeneity. However, specific models or testing procedures are less often reported. Nevertheless, it is possible to formulate specific clustering models for the case-event and tract-count situation.

Another definition of clustering seeks to classify the methods based on whether the location or locations of clusters are known or not. Focused clustering is *specific* and usually seeks to analyse the clustering tendency of a disease or diseases around a known location. Often this location could be a *putative pollution source* or health hazard. Non-focused clustering does not assume knowledge of a location of a cluster but seeks to either assess the locations of clustering within a map or to assess the overall clustering tendency. Hence, non-focused clustering could be specific or non-specific.

The literature of spatial epidemiology has developed considerably in the area of hypothesis testing and, more specifically, in the sphere of hypothesis testing for clusters (see, for example, Lawson and Kulldorff, 1999). Early developments in this area arose from the application of statistical tests to spatio-temporal clustering, a particularly strong indicator of the importance of a spatial clustering phenomenon. As noted already, distinction should be made between tests for general (non-specific) clustering, which assess the overall clustering pattern of the disease and the *specific* clustering tests where cluster locations are estimated.

For case events, a few tests have been developed for non-specific clustering. Specific non-focused cluster tests address the issue of the location of putative clusters. These tests produce results in the form of locational probabilities or significances associated with specific groups of tract counts or cases. Openshaw and co-workers (Openshaw, Charlton *et al.*, 1987) first developed a general method that allowed the assessment of the location of clusters of cases within large disease maps. The method was based on repeated testing of counts of disease within circular regions of different sizes. The statistical foundation of this method has been criticised and an improvement to the method was proposed by Besag and Newell (1991). An alternative statistic has been proposed by Kulldorff and Nagarwalla (1995) (the scan statistic). The test can be applied to both case events and tract counts. Focused tests have also developed and there is now a range of possible testing procedures. Cluster modelling has seen some development but has not developed as fully as testing procedures. Usually the successful models are Bayesian with PRIOR DISTRIBUTIONS describing the clustering behaviour (see, for example, Lawson and Denison, 2002).

AL

Besag, J. and Newell, J. 1991: The detection of clusters in rare diseases. *Journal of the Royal Statistical Society, Series A* 154, 143. **Elliott, P., Wakefield, J.** *et al.* (eds) 2000: *Spatial epidemiology: methods and applications.* London: Oxford University Press. **Kulldorff, M. and Nagarwalla, N.** 1995: Spatial disease clusters: detection and inference. *Statistics in Medicine* 14, 799. **Lawson, A.B.** 2001: *Statistical Methods in Spatial Epidemiology.* Chichester: John Wiley & Sons. **Lawson, A.B. and Denison, D.** (eds) 2002: *Spatial cluster modelling.* London: Chapman & Hall. **Lawson, A.B. and Kulldorff, M.** 1999: A review of cluster detection methods. In *Disease mapping and risk assessment for public health.* Chichester: John Wiley & Sons. **Openshaw, S., Charlton, M.G.** *et al.* 1987: A mark 1 geographical analysis machine for the automated analysis of point data sets. *International Journal on Geographical Information Systems* 1, 335.

disease mapping See DISEASE CLUSTERING, SPATIAL EPIDEMIOLOGY

DMF score See DENTAL STATISTICS

dot plot A useful graphical display for data on some continuous variable recorded within the categories of a particular categorical variable. An example is shown in the Figure. A dot plot is generally far more effective in communicating the pattern in the data than either a PIE CHART or a BAR CHART, particularly if the number of categories is reasonably large.   *BSE*

dropout at random (DAR) See DROPOUTS

dropout completely at random (DCAR) See DROPOUTS

dropouts Patients in a study, commonly a CLINICAL TRIAL, who fail to attend protocol-scheduled visits or assessments of a response variable taken after some particular time point in the study. Dropping out of a study implies that once an observation at a particular time point is missing so are all the remaining planned observations. Such missing observations are a nuisance and the very best way to avoid problems with missing values is not to

have any! If only a small proportion of the patients in the trial drop out it is unlikely that these will cause any major difficulties for analysis and so on. If, however, a substantial number of dropouts occur there is potential for making incorrect inferences and/or producing biased estimates if a valid analysis procedure is not used. In such cases consideration needs to be given to the reasons why individuals drop out and how the probability of dropping out depends on the response variable, since this has implications for which forms of analysis are suitable and which are not (Little, 1995). Three dropout mechanisms are usually differentiated based on the classification of missing values originally suggested by Rubin (1976).

Dropout at random (DAR). The dropout at random mechanism occurs when the dropout process depends on the outcome measures that have been observed in the past, but given this information is conditionally independent of all the future (unrecorded) values of the outcome variable following dropout. Here 'missingness' depends only on the observed data with the distribution of future values for a subject who drops out at time t being the same as the distribution of the future values of a subject who remains in at time t, if they have the same covariates and the same past history of outcome up to and including time t. Murray and Findlay (1988) provide an example of this

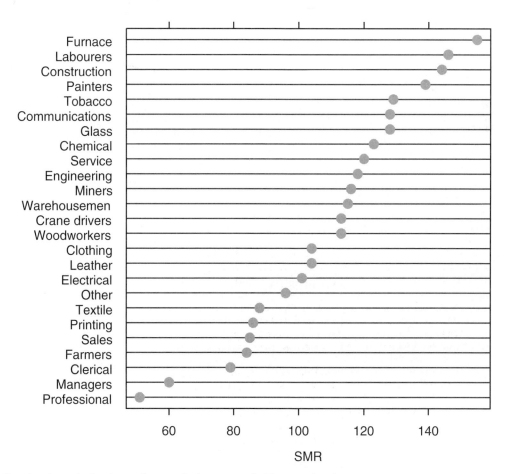

dot plot *Dot plot of standardised mortality rates for lung cancer in 25 occupational groups*

type of missing value from a study of hypertensive drugs in which the outcome measure was diastolic blood pressure. The protocol of the study specified that the participant should to be removed from the study when his/her blood pressure got too high. Here blood pressure at the time of dropout was observed before the participant dropped out, so although the missing value mechanism is not DCAR since it depends on the values of blood pressure, it is DAR, because dropout depends only on the observed part of the data.

Dropout completely at random (DCAR). Here the probability that a patient drops out does not depend on either the observed or missing values of the response. The observed (non-missing) values effectively constitute a simple random sample of the values for all subjects. Possible examples include missing laboratory measurements because of a dropped test tube (if it was not dropped because of the knowledge of any measurement), the accidental death of a participant in a study or a participant moving to another area. Completely random dropout causes least problem for data analysis, but it is a strong assumption.

Non-ignorable (sometimes referred to as *informative*) *dropout*. For this final type of dropout mechanism, missingness depends on the unrecorded missing values – observations are likely to be missing when the true values are systematically higher or lower than usual. A non-medical example is when individuals with lower income levels or very high incomes are less likely to provide their personal income in an interview. In a medical setting, possible examples are a participant dropping out of a longitudinal study when his/her blood pressure became too high and this value was not observed or when their pain became intolerable and the associated pain value was not recorded. Dealing with data containing missing values of this type is not routine.

Simple methods of analysis for longitudinal data, for example, COMPLETE CASE ANALYSIS or SUMMARY MEASURE ANALYSIS rely on the DCAR assumption, others such as LINEAR MIXED-EFFECTS MODELS, involve only the weaker DAR restriction. Identifying the type of dropout mechanism for a particular dataset is rarely straightforward, although some useful informal procedures are described in Carpenter, Pocock and Lamm (2002). When informative dropouts are suspected the methods suggested by Rabe-Hesketh, Pickles and Skrondal (2001) may be useful.   *BSE*

Carpenter, J., Pocock, S. and Lamm, C.J. 2002: Coping with missing data in clinical trials: a model based approach applied to asthma trials. *Statistics in Medicine* 21, 1043–66. **Little, R.J.A.** 1995: Modeling the dropout mechanism in repeated measure studies. *Journal of the American Statistical Association* 90, 1112–21. **Murray, G.D. and Findlay, J.G.** 1988: Correcting for the bias caused by dropouts in hypertension trials. *Statistics in Medicine* 7, 941–6. **Rabe-Hesketh, S., Pickles, A. and Skrondal, A.** 2001: GLAMM: a class of models and a STATA program. *Multilevel Modelling Newsletter* 13, 17–23. **Rubin, D.B.** 1976: Inference and missing data. *Biometrika* 63, 581–92.

dummy variables   A set of variables, each with only two possible outcomes, that are used to represent a categorical explanatory variable in a statistical model that is designed to handle quantitative variables. Usually, the two outcomes allowed for each dummy variable are taken to be zero and unity. Each dummy variable takes the value zero when the parent categorical variable attains its predefined reference, or base, level. When the categorical variable attains any other level, one unique dummy variable takes the value unity; the rest take the value zero. A categorical variable with k outcomes will require $k-1$ dummy variables to represent it.

For example, consider a situation where the hypothesis is that blood pressure is different between those who currently smoke, used to smoke (but have since quit) and have never smoked. Assuming that suitable data have been collected, the hypothesis could be tested by fitting an ANALYSIS OF VARIANCE model with smoking group as the explanatory variable and blood pressure as the dependent variable. This explanatory variable would have three levels (current/ex/never) and thus two DEGREES OF FREEDOM. An alternative approach would be to define two dummy variables to represent smoking group, say:

$$x_1 = \begin{cases} 1 \text{ for ex-smokers} \\ 0 \text{ for never smokers} \end{cases} \quad x_2 = \begin{cases} 1 \text{ for current smokers} \\ 0 \text{ for never smokers} \end{cases}$$

(see Table) and then fit a MULTIPLE REGRESSION model with x_1 and x_2 as the explanatory variables. The regression sum of squares (with two degrees of freedom) in this regression model would be the same as that for the variable 'smoking group' in the earlier analysis of variance model. Both x_1 and x_2 are contrasts between, respectively, ex- and never smokers and between current and never smokers. In this sense, never smokers are the reference group for analyses of smoking status.

Dummy variables are useful in that they remove the necessity to develop separate statistical models for categorical and continuous explanatory variables. They also allow variables of mixed type to be handled within the same, single methodology.

Some computer software requires the user to define dummy variables for themselves, whereas others do the computation automatically once the particular variable for which dummy variables are required has been declared as a categorical variable.   *MW*

dummy variables   *Dummy variables (x_1 and x_2) used to represent smoking status for 14 people*

Smoking status	x_1	x_2
Current smoker	0	1
Ex-smoker	1	0
Ex-smoker	1	0
Current smoker	0	1
Never smoker	0	0
Never smoker	0	0
Never smoker	0	0
Current smoker	0	1
Never smoker	0	0
Current smoker	0	1
Ex-smoker	1	0
Ex-smoker	1	0
Never smoker	0	0
Ex-smoker	1	0

dynamic designs   See DATA-DEPENDENT DESIGNS

E

EaSt A software package that allows the design and analysis of sequential trials. The name 'East' is derived from 'Early stopping'. As an alternative to standard, fixed-sample CLINICAL TRIALS, flexible clinical trials utilise group-sequential and adaptive methodologies to permit interim looks at accruing data with a view to making early stopping or sample size readjustment decisions, while preserving Type 1 error and POWER. Jennison and Turnbull (2001) provide a thorough treatment of sequential design and analysis. These methods have been incorporated into the East software package developed by Cytel Software Corporation (www.cytel.com).

East has three basic components: a design module, a simulation module and an interim monitoring module. The design module can be used to design two-arm superiority or non-inferiority trials of normal, binomial or time-to-event ENDPOINTS. Extensions to more general endpoints are available through the use of an inflation factor that increases the sample size of a fixed-sample design by the appropriate amount so as to preserve POWER. A special design worksheet is provided for designing studies on the basis of maximum information rather than maximum sample size. Such designs provide the flexibility to adjust the sample size during the interim monitoring phase, to accommodate adjustments to important design parameters, such as patient-to-patient variability, that might have been misspecified at the design stage. Many families of stopping boundaries and spending functions are available, thus providing great flexibility for making early stopping decisions either for efficacy or futility or both.

Trials created by the design module can be simulated in the simulation module. Since the statistical theory underlying East utilises large-sample assumptions, the simulation module is a useful tool for verifying that the operating characteristics of the design are preserved for small or unbalanced studies. A special feature of the simulation module is the capability to simulate adaptive designs.

The interim monitoring module includes a worksheet that accepts the current value of the test statistic and the current sample size of information. It then re-computes the stopping boundaries based on the specified spending functions, determines if the boundary has been crossed and provides important interim results such as conditional power and repeated CONFIDENCE INTERVALS.

East additionally provides tables, graphs and reports that allow investigators to visualise and clearly demonstrate the features and results of the planned design. For example, one can plot stopping boundaries as a function of time or present power calculations in graphical or tabular form. *CM*

Jennison, C. and Turnbull, B. 2001: *Group sequential methods with applications to clinical trials.* New York: Chapman & Hall/CRC.

EBM See EVIDENCE-BASED MEDICINE

ecological fallacy See EPIDEMIOLOGY

ecological studies See EPIDEMIOLOGY

eligibility criteria See INCLUSION AND EXCLUSION CRITERIA

EM algorithm A general computational method for calculating MAXIMUM LIKELIHOOD ESTIMATIONS with incomplete data, for example, MISSING DATA or data containing CENSORED OBSERVATIONS. The algorithm is based on the notion that if we had the missing or censored observations we could estimate parameters of interest in the usual way and that if we knew the parameters we could impute the missing observations by setting them to their predicted values under the model. Consequently, given some initial values for the parameters we can proceed iteratively between computing predicted values, filling in the missing observations and then estimating the parameters using new 'complete data'. The algorithm is widely used in statistics and a detailed technical account is given in Laird (1998). *BSE*

Laird, N. 1998: EM algorithms. In Armitage, P. and Colton, T. (eds), *Encyclopedia of biostatistics.* Chichester: John Wiley & Sons.

endpoints A measurement or discrete event, related to the disease under investigation, which measures the effectiveness of an intervention. The definition of suitable endpoints depends on the disease under study. In serious diseases, such as coronary heart disease, endpoints such as 'mortality' provide a reliable measure of disease progression, while after curative surgery for cancer, 'recurrent cancer' would be an example of such a measure. These examples are 'binary' in nature (that is, subjects have either had the event or not), but in some diseases it is more appropriate to measure disease progression in terms of a continuous outcome measure (e.g. blood pressure), or an ordinal scale (e.g. a measure of the quality of life, such as the SF-36).

When designing a randomised trial (see CLINICAL TRIALS), it is usual to define primary and secondary endpoints on which judgements about the overall benefits and harms of treatment are to be made. The 'primary endpoint' (or 'target variable') is chosen as the chief measure of the effects of an intervention, on which analyses are to be conducted in order to assess the primary hypothesis originally stated in the study protocol (see PROTOCOLS IN CLINICAL TRIALS). Generally, the primary endpoint is a measure that is expected to be influenced favourably by the intervention, i.e. it is a measure of clinical efficacy. For example, based on long-term randomised trials of aspirin conducted among patients who had survived a heart attack, it was anticipated that aspirin would reduce the clinically important endpoint 'vascular mortality' in the first few weeks after suspected acute heart attack, so this was the choice of primary endpoint in the Second International Study of Infarct Survival (ISIS-2, 1988). Occasionally it may be appropriate for a primary endpoint to measure safety: for example, if we were to compare a higher versus a lower dose of aspirin, the known pharmacology of aspirin might lead us to hypothesise that both regimens would have similar clinical efficacy, but that serious bleeding might be less frequent with the lower aspirin dose (Antithrombotic Trialists' Collaboration (ATC), 2002). In these circumstances, we might be advised to choose 'bleeding requiring transfusion' as a primary safety endpoint.

As well as defining a primary endpoint in the study protocol, together with the planned method of statistical analysis of that primary endpoint, it is usual to define a number of 'secondary endpoints'. These are measures that, when considered with the primary endpoint, provide helpful additional information about the clinical efficacy and safety of the intervention. In the ISIS-2 trial, for example, an assessment of the overall benefits and harms of aspirin (and of streptokinase) was facilitated by assessing the effects of these treatments on secondary endpoints such as re-infarction, haemorrhagic stroke, and bleeds requiring transfusion (ISIS-2, 1988). In view of the fact that the aim of assessing effects on secondary endpoints is to make sound clinical judgements about the balance of benefit and harm, it is imperative to limit the number of the secondary endpoints. If too many are chosen, the likelihood that an ineffective treatment might appear to influence the risk of one or more such endpoints (that is, a Type I error) increases and it is difficult to interpret any data that result.

In circumstances where a number of clinically important endpoints are likely to be influenced favourably by a treatment, it may be useful to define a 'composite' (or 'combined') endpoint, where a subject is considered to have reached this endpoint if they experience one (or more) of the component endpoints. When a treatment has similar effects on each of the components of a composite endpoint, use of that composite endpoint increases the statistical power not only of the primary analysis, but more especially of subgroup analyses aiming to assess whether the effects of treatment differ importantly among selected categories of patients of clinical interest. For example, to assess anti-platelet therapy for the prevention of occlusive vascular disease, which is a systemic disease affecting both cardiac and cerebral arteries, the composite endpoint 'myocardial infarction, stroke or vascular death' has been found to be useful, particularly when assessing effects in particular groups of patients (such as men and women, young and old etc.) (ATC, 2002; CAPRIE, 1996). Several problems arise, however, when a composite endpoint is designed to assess a 'global effect' of treatment by grouping together the major anticipated benefits and harms. In these circumstances, an estimated effect on the global composite outcome which is not statistically significant could reflect a worthwhile benefit masked by a harm and this would be entirely missed unless the benefits and harms are considered separately in a trial or meta-analysis which is large enough to assess the effects on both.

In circumstances when it is not practical to assess the effects of treatment on clinical endpoints, it is possible to consider the use of a 'surrogate endpoint' for assessing treatment effects. For an endpoint to be a surrogate for a clinical endpoint it must be a measure of disease such that: (i) the size (or frequency) correlates strongly with that clinical endpoint (for example, blood pressure is positively correlated with the risk of stroke); and (ii) treatments pro-

ducing a change in the surrogate endpoint also modify the risk of that particular clinical endpoint (for example, reducing blood pressure reduces the risk of stroke). In the past, however, many promising surrogate endpoints have proved unreliable. For example, cardiac arrhythmia was believed to be a good surrogate endpoint for mortality after acute heart attack, since in these circumstances patients with a higher risk of such an arrhythmia have a greater risk of death. But several drugs (e.g. lignocaine, flecainide) that prevent arrhythmias after a heart attack actually increase mortality (Echt et al., 1991). Similarly, there are blood pressure-lowering drugs (such as angiotensin-converting enzyme inhibitors) that have much larger effects on vascular mortality than might be predicted from their effects on blood pressure (Heart Outcomes Prevention Evaluation Study Investigators, 2000). For this reason, it is likely to be inappropriate to rely on a surrogate endpoint to assess the effects of a drug which is to be used for a common and serious disease.

The choice of endpoints and the method by which they are to be analysed should be set out clearly in the study protocol. It is important that this choice is given careful thought, since it may often determine whether a trial succeeds in answering a clinically useful question and it is difficult to change the choice of endpoints after the trial has closed without the risk of introducing serious bias.   *CB*

Antithrombotic Trialists' Collaboration (ATC) 2002: Collaborative meta-analysis of randomised trials for prevention of death, myocardial infarction, and stroke in high-risk patients. *British Medial Journal* 324, 71–86. **CAPRIE Steering Committee (CAPRIE)** 1996: A randomised, blinded, trial of clopidogrel versus aspirin in patients at risk of ischaemic events. *The Lancet* 348, 1329–39. **Echt, D.S., Liabson, P.R., Mitchell, L.B.** *et al.* **and the Cardiac Arrhythmia Suppression Trial (CAST) Investigators** 1991: Mortality and morbidity in patients receiving encainide, flecainide, or placebo: the cardiac arrhythmia suppression trial. *New England Journal of Medicine* 324, 781–8. **Heart Outcomes Prevention Evaluation Study Investigators** 2000: Effects of an angiotensin-converting enzyme inhibitor, ramipril, on death from cardiovascular causes, myocardial infarction, and stroke in high-risk patients. *New England Journal of Medicine* 342, 145–53. **ISIS-2 (Second International Study of Infarct Survival) Collaborative Group** 1988: Randomised trial of intravenous streptokinase, oral aspirin, both, or neither among 17,187 cases of suspected acute myocardial infarction: ISIS-2. *The Lancet* 2(8607), 349–60.

entry criteria   See INCLUSION AND EXCLUSION CRITERIA

EPIINFO   See CASE-CONTROL STUDIES

epidemiology   The study of disease and its risk factors. Originally used to describe the study of epidemics, it now encompasses non-communicable as well as infectious diseases. Simple examples would be an analysis of the trends over time in the number of cases of AIDS recorded in a certain country and a comparison of the age-specific death rates due to AIDS between countries. More complex examples would be an evaluation of the proximity of nuclear power stations to the homes of people diagnosed with leukaemia and an investigation into possible association between regular consumption of fast food and subsequent development of cardiovascular disease.

Many of the major public health issues of the day have been the subject of scrutiny by epidemiologists, whose careful amassing of facts and figures, and subsequent statistical analyses, have formulated hypotheses and sometimes demonstrated strong cases for causal explanations of disease. An early example is the work of John Snow, who plotted the locations of around 500 deaths due to cholera that occurred in the same area of London within a 10-day period in 1854 (see first Figure). This map demonstrated that the cholera deaths were clustered around the Broad Street water pump that served as the source of drinking water for many residents. His data fitted in with the theory, not generally accepted at the time, of the disease being carried by polluted water and with the practice of emptying sewerage into water that made its way to the well feeding the Broad Street pump (Chave, 1958). Snow had the handle of the pump removed and the epidemic ceased. (Another account of this study can be found in HISTORY OF MEDICAL STATISTICS.)

When there is a new, unexplained, health problem, epidemiologists will usually be charged with plotting the course of the problem, sifting the available information so as to uncover the natural history and likely cause and helping to devise plans for avoidance of the problem in future. Examples would be the so-called 'Gulf War Syndrome' attributed to surviving soldiers from the Gulf War of 1990/1 and the outbreak of Severe Acute Respiratory Syndrome (SARS) in 2002/3, which was particularly prevalent in Asia and Canada (second Figure). Epidemiologists tend to make considerable use of statistical methodology, but the profession requires a substantial level of medical knowledge also. In recent years, specialist areas of epidemiology have emerged, such as GENETIC EPIDEMIOLOGY where epidemiological tools are applied to genetic data.

Epidemiological studies form one of the two major types of study design in medical research, the other being CLINICAL TRIALS. The distinction between the two is that epidemiological investigations are observational whereas clinical trials involve *interventions*. For example, a large group of middle-aged women who use hormone replacement therapy (HRT) may be monitored for several years and the proportions of women who develop venous thrombosis compared between those women who typically used

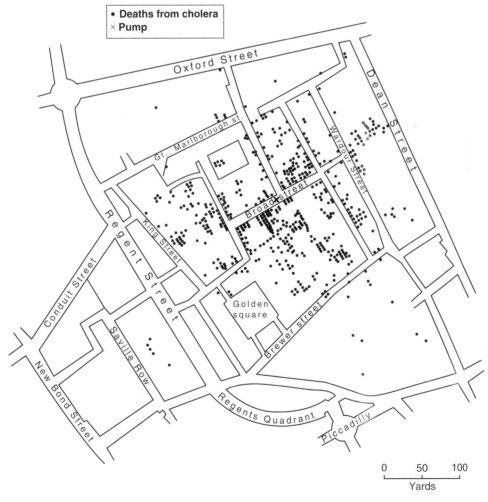

epidemiology *Cholera deaths in the Golden Square area of London in September 1854. Dots show location of cholera deaths and a cross marks the position of the water pump in Broad Street (redrawn from Tufte, 1983)*

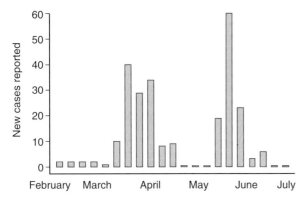

epidemiology *Number of new SARS cases, by week, in Canada in 2003 (WHO daily reports, with interpolation and extrapolation)*

different types of HRT. This would be an epidemiological study. A corresponding clinical trial might involve recruiting a number of post-menopausal women who have never used HRT, but who are medically eligible to do so. Some women would be allocated to receive a certain type of HRT and some to receive another; both groups would be followed over time to make the same comparison as above. The great advantage of the epidemiological approach would be that results are obtained in real-life circumstances. Furthermore, there are ethical advantages compared with the approach of deciding who is required to do what, even when the decision is made using some chance mechanism, as should be the case, whenever possible, in clinical trials. For example, no clinical trial would be allowed to randomise people to smoke cigarettes or not, since it would be unethical. In contrast, some of the classic epidemiological studies have compared smokers and non-smokers for their chance of disease. Contrariwise, clinical trials (when feasible) generally offer more reliable results because they can be designed to minimise the effect of *confounding*, which is a common source of bias in epidemiological studies.

In making the distinction between epidemiological studies and clinical trials, it should be understood that the practising epidemiologist will make use of information from clinical trials wherever it contributes to their subject of interest. Indeed, many intervention studies are conducted by people who would consider themselves to be epidemiologists, who are, quite sensibly, using the best tools available for the job at hand. Furthermore, a randomised clinical trial will often be considered as the ultimate test of the epidemiological theory. For example, many epidemiological studies have found that consumption of foods rich in certain vitamins, specifically fruit and vegetables, protects against heart disease. This has given rise to the epidemiological hypothesis that these vitamins protect the heart, and thus to several clinical trials of vitamin supplementation. At the time of writing, the combined evidence from these trials is that such supplementation has no beneficial effect, leaving open the question of whether the findings in epidemiological studies are simply due to confounding.

Epidemiological investigations might simply be examinations of routinely collected data, such as registrations of

death by cause, to search for seasonal patterns (as in the second Figure), or of registers of disease incidence, to look for differences by regions of the country or clusters of cases in time and space (as in the first figure). Such investigations identify specific health problems and help to formulate theories about the aetiology of the particular medical condition. The latter issue is sometimes addressed, using routine data, in a formal way through *ecological studies*. These are studies of data on average values of disease outcome and risk factor status from groups of people, typically those who live in different geographical regions. For example, St Leger, Cochrane and Moore (1979) plotted mortality from coronary heart disease (CHD) among men aged 55–64 in 18 countries against wine consumption (derived from industry sources) in the same countries (third Figure). The data seemed to suggest an inverse relationship: for example, France had the highest wine consumption and the lowest rate of CHD.

Routine, or other types of pre-existing (secondary), data are clearly relatively cheap and easy to collect and will often be considered authoritative when derived from government sources or from international organisations, such as WHO. However, they often are incomplete (such as when death registrations alone are used to examine morbidity), inadequate (such as when total numbers are recorded but not numbers within important demographic subgroups) and/or out of date. Ecological studies, used to investigate associations, often suffer from mis-matching of the groups in the two data series, those for disease and risk factor. For instance, in the St Leger, Cochrane and Moore (1979) study, deaths were for a particular age/sex group whereas wine consumption was for the entire population. In most cases, they offer little or no opportunity to control for confounding. Furthermore, there is no reason why relationships observed for groups should hold when individuals are observed, the so-called *ecological fallacy*. Thus,

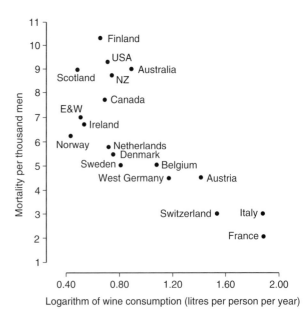

epidemiology *Death rates for men aged 55–64 years old in 1970 against the logarithm of wine consumption in 18 countries (St Leger, Cochrane and Moore, 1979)*

it *could* be that, while France generally does have a low rate of heart disease and a high consumption of wine, those Frenchmen who drink relatively large amounts suffer most CHD.

Ecological studies should be seen as hypothesis-generating tools rather than ways of deriving definitive information on relationships between risk factors and disease. Although many ecological studies may well give fallacious results, they may also be the first clue to an association that was not previously discussed. St Leger, Cochrane and Moore (1979) is a nice example of this: their demonstration that moderate wine consumption might be protective against heart attack was initially met with scorn and was usually assumed to be the result of bias or confounding. However, subsequent research, using more reliable epidemiological study designs (see later), has shown the benefit of moderate wine consumption to the heart, which is now commonly accepted. Even so, the apparent relationship could have been spurious – for instance, variations in the way heart disease is diagnosed across countries and confounding with other aspects of the diet besides wine might have explained away the inverse association between wine and heart disease. The ecological design generally cannot delve deeply enough to uncover such subtleties; collection of data from individuals is required.

There are three main types of epidemiological study that involve collection of new information from individual people: CROSS-SECTIONAL (surveys), CASE-CONTROL and COHORT STUDIES. Surveys are called cross-sectional because they occur at a single point in time (see fourth Figure). Generally, they involve the drawing of a sample of the entire population, although very occasionally the entire population is included, in which case a census has been conducted. Surveys have the advantage, over using routine data, that the investigator can collect precisely the information required for the subsequent analysis, within practical constraints. They are particularly useful for descriptive purposes.

Epidemiological surveys typically include questions about disease states and levels of risk factors for these diseases. The answers can be used to estimate prevalence of disease and the distribution of the risk factors. For instance, Tunstall-Pedoe *et al.* (1989) describe a national population survey in Scotland, which included taking blood samples from all participants, from which serum cholesterol (among many other things) was measured. The results gave a picture of the distribution of cholesterol

in Scotland at that time, allowing (for instance) an estimate of the number and percentage of Scots whose cholesterol was above the level that was considered 'safe' and thus were likely to benefit greatly from cholesterol-lowering treatment. Surveys can be made more accurate by using random sampling (to reduce BIAS), using sensible stratification (to increase precision) and taking a larger sample size (also to increase precision). This last point needs some qualification: there may be no benefit from increasing sample size if this leads to increased bias error, for instance through taking less time, per subject, to ensure that accurate responses are solicited from questioning. Cluster sampling is often used for convenience, or simply to reduce costs, but does have the unfortunate effect of decreasing precision, measured, for example, by the length of the CONFIDENCE INTERVAL associated with the estimate obtained from the survey (e.g. the mean cholesterol). Surveys have limited use in investigating CAUSALITY in associations because they are prone to the 'chicken and egg' effect – it is difficult, and often impossible, to ascertain whether the observed value of the risk factor was attained prior, or subsequent to, the onset of disease. For instance, the Scottish survey described earlier included the question: 'Have you ever been told by a doctor that you suffered from a heart attack?' Comparing average cholesterol levels between those who did and did not report having had a heart attack, gives a simple indication of whether cholesterol is associated with having had a heart attack. However, a high cholesterol reading today could be the consequence of a recent heart attack instead of the hypothesised effect of relatively high cholesterol increasing the risk of a heart attack. Even if we know, from other studies, that this is unlikely, we cannot rule it out using only the given survey data. Another example would be a survey where a particular chronic disease is found to be less common among those who smoke. This may not mean that smoking tends to protect people against the disease; instead it may be that smokers, having developed the disease, give up the habit, thus leading to a predominance of the disease among those not smoking at the time of the survey. Although it may be possible to discover when the risk factor was first encountered (e.g. when smoking was taken up), the reliability of such information, often requiring long-term recall, may be poor. In any case, it is rare to be able to fix a time for the onset of the disease. Thus surveys are not suited for investigations of causality, which are commonly the primary purpose of epidemiological investigations.

More reliable information on causality can be gleaned from a case-control study. A set of cases, those with the disease of interest, are identified, for example through hospital records, and the putative risk factor(s) of interest are recorded for each. In parallel, a contrasting set of controls, those without the disease, are selected and submitted to the same investigations as the cases. Comparison of the risk factor levels between cases and controls enables the risk factor-disease association to be assessed, usually measured by the odds ratio. In principle, case-control studies compare disease status now with risk factor levels in the past, which is why they are often called retrospective studies (see fourth Figure). However, this is only really true if incident (new) cases are used and even then certain potential risk factors (for instance, markers of inflammation) might be elevated so soon after

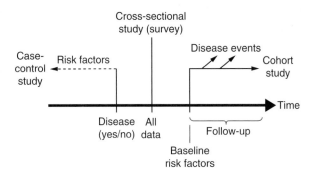

epidemiology *Schematic comparison of the three major study designs in epidemiology*

the disease hits that the 'chicken and egg' problem may occur. Even if this type of bias is not an issue, case-control studies are very susceptible to other kinds of bias, such as that caused by differential quality of information from cases (who are more interesting and thus may have been observed or researched more thoroughly) and controls. BERKSON'S FALLACY may also be an issue. Careful matching of controls to cases offers greater control over confounding and may increase precision, but still leaves the potential for several important sources of bias. NESTED CASE-CONTROL STUDIES are, by way of contrast, much less prone to bias error, as is the related case-cohort design. These are really no longer retrospective studies and are more usefully thought of as prospective. Although case-control studies are not the most reliable sources of information on causality for most epidemiological relationships, the case-control design is the design of choice in two situations. One is where the disease is so rare that any other kind of design is unlikely to produce enough cases of disease to obtain reliable estimates of association. The other is where the risk factor is transient, such as an outbreak of food poisoning.

In other situations the epidemiological design of choice is the cohort study. In the typical situation, a large group of people are surveyed at a point in time, or at least over a limited number of months and several putative risk factors recorded. Over succeeding years (the follow-up) instances of disease and death are recorded and related to the levels of the risk factors at initiation (baseline). Thus, cohort studies are said to be prospective (see fourth figure). For example, after the initial cross-sectional study of the Scottish population mentioned earlier, Tunstall-Pedoe et al. arranged for any hospital admissions for coronary disease and deaths experienced by any of their sample (now called the study cohort) to be recorded. Tunstall-Pedoe et al. (1997) describe the relationship between coronary disease and 27 different risk factors for this study over a 7-year period. The advantage of the cohort study over the case-control study is that the time sequence of risk factor preceding disease can be established, strengthening the argument for causality. For instance, Tunstall-Pedoe et al. were able to conclude that high cholesterol levels tended to be followed by heart attacks, rather than the other way round.

Another advantage is that the cohort study can be used to investigate both several risk factors and several diseases, whereas a case-control study is restricted to a single disease, that which defined the cases. Furthermore, unlike case-control studies, cohort studies can estimate the risk of disease in any recorded subgroup of the population. Provided that pre-existing cases of disease at baseline are excluded, incident disease is measured in a cohort study. The disadvantages of cohort studies are that they are time consuming, since it may take many years for enough cases of disease or death to occur to enable reliable estimation, and the problem of withdrawals. Although withdrawals (censoring) can be dealt with mathematically, at the analysis stage, by using survival models, there may still be a bias when withdrawal is related, in some unobserved fashion, to the disease under study. Cohort studies can be made more informative by re-measuring the cohort after baseline. The repeat measurements may be used to obtain a more accurate picture of the true association between the risk factor and the disease outcome, for instance through elimination of REGRESSION DILUTION BIAS.

A major question in many epidemiological investigations is whether it is reasonable to conclude that the hypothesised risk factor causes the disease in question. This issue was addressed by one of the pioneers of medical statistics and modern epidemiology, Sir Austin Bradford Hill. In 1965 he proposed a set of criteria that describe ideal conditions for verifying a risk factor hypothesis (Bradford Hill and Hill, 1991). These conditions include, there being: a strong association between the factor and the disease (e.g. a large relative risk); consistency of the association in different settings (e.g. time and place); specificity of the association (risk factor and disease usually occurring together); evidence of the risk factor preceding the disease (rather than vice versa); evidence of a biological gradient: the more the risk factor, the more the (chance of) disease; biological plausibility for the hypothesis; coherence of all the available evidence, including general knowledge of the disease.

If all these conditions are satisfied, most epidemiologists would accept that there is truly good evidence to conclude causality. In real life, the situation is often less clear cut, especially regarding specificity, since many diseases seem to have several risk factors. Nevertheless, anyone undertaking an epidemiological investigation would do well to judge their work against these general criteria before being tempted to ascribe causality. Two important features of the BRADFORD HILL CRITERIA are the acknowledgement that data alone are insufficient (medical or other biological interpretation is crucial) and that final conclusions can only be drawn with comprehensive meta-analyses. Single epidemiological studies may fail to find a significant relationship due to small numbers, confounding effects or other biases. It is only by considering a range of studies that sensible conclusions may be drawn, not only because of the reliability of estimation afforded by large numbers, but also because variations in results might be explained by comparing results from studies with different characteristics, such as by using META-REGRESSION. When epidemiological results are combined in meta-analysis it is usual to restrict to case-control and cohort studies, because of myriad biases inherent in ecological and cross-sectional designs. Even then, when there is a sufficient number of cohort studies, the tendency is to draw final 'best evidence' conclusions from the cohort studies alone.   *MW*

Ashton, J. (ed.) 1994: *The epidemiological imagination.* Buckingham: Open University Press. **Bradford Hill, A. and Hill, I.D.** 1991: *Principles of medical statistics*, 12th edn. London: Edward Arnold. **Chave, S.P.W.** 1958: John Snow, the Broad Street pump and after. *The Medical Officer* 99, 347–9. **Clayton, D. and Hills, M.** 1993: *Statistical models in epidemiology.* Oxford: Oxford University Press. **St Leger, A.S., Cochrane, A.L. and Moore, F.** 1979: Factors associated with cardiac mortality in developed countries with particular reference to the consumption of wine. *The Lancet* i, 1017–20. **Stolley, P.D. and Lasky, T.** 1995: *Investigating disease patterns. The science of epidemiology.* New York: WH Freeman. **Tufte, E.R.** 1983: *The visual display of quantitative information.* Cheshire, CT: Graphics Press. **Tunstall-Pedoe, H., Smith, W.C.S., Crombie, I.K. and Tavendale, R.** 1989: Coronary risk factor and lifestyle variation across Scotland: results from the Scottish Heart Health Study. *Scottish Medical Journal* 34, 556–60. **Tunstall-Pedoe, H., Woodward, M., Tavendale, R., A'Brook, R. and McCluskey, M.K.** 1997: Comparison of the prediction by 27 different factors of coronary heart disease and death in men and women of the Scottish heart health study: cohort study. *British Medical Journal* 315, 722–9. **Woodward, M.** 2005: *Epidemiology: study design and data analysis*, 2nd edn. Boca Raton: Chapman & Hall/CRC Press.

EQS See STRUCTURAL EQUATION MODELLING SOFTWARE

equivalence studies See ACTIVE CONTROL EQUIVALENCE STUDIES

errors in hypothesis tests Neyman and Pearson (1933) proposed that the subjective view of the strength of evidence against the null hypothesis inherent in Fisher's significance tests be replaced with an objective, decision-theoretic approach to the results of experiments. In this approach, the investigator decides, in advance, a rule that states when the null hypothesis (for example that there is no association between a risk factor and a disease outcome, or no effect of a treatment) will be rejected or not rejected (accepted).

The null hypothesis may be rejected when it is in fact true, or alternatively we may fail to reject it when it is false. These are called TYPE I ERRORS and TYPE II ERRORS respectively (see Table). Neyman and Pearson suggested that by fixing, in advance, the type I (α) and type II (β) error rates, investigators would limit the number of mistakes made over many different experiments.

The Figure shows the probabilities of occurrence of these two types of error, for a test at the 5% level, in the context of a normally distributed statistic such as the difference between two means. The *P*-VALUE (significance level) equals the probability of occurrence of a result as extreme as or more extreme than that observed if the null hypothesis were true. For example, panel (a) shows that there is a 5% probability that sampling variation alone will lead to a result significant at the 5% level ($P < 0.05$).

The second type of error is that the null hypothesis is not rejected when it is false. This occurs because of overlap between the real sampling distribution of the sample difference about the population difference, d ($\neq 0$) and the acceptance region for the null hypothesis based on the hypothesised sampling distribution about the incorrect difference, 0. This is illustrated in (b). The shaded area shows the proportion (β%) of the real sampling distribution that would fall within the acceptance region for the null hypothesis, i.e. that would appear consistent with the null hypothesis at the 5% level. The probability that we *do not* make a Type II error ($100 - b$%) equals the POWER of the test.

In the Figure the following holds. Panel (a) shows a Type I error: null hypothesis (NH) is *true*. Population difference = 0. The curve shows the sampling distribution of the sample difference. The shaded areas (total 5%) give

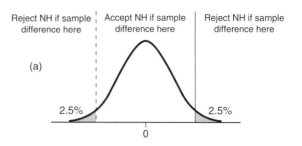

(a)

2.5%   2.5%

0

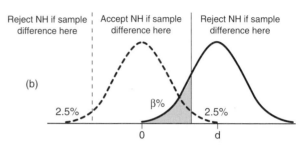

(b)

β%

2.5%   2.5%

0   d

errors in hypothesis tests *Probabilities of occurrence of Type I and Type II errors, for a test at the 5% level*

the probability that the null hypothesis is wrongly rejected. Panel (b) shows a Type II error: null hypothesis is *false*. Population difference = $d \neq 0$. The continuous curve shows the real sampling distribution of the sample difference, while the dashed curve shows the sampling distribution under the null hypothesis. The shaded area is the probability (b%) that the null hypothesis fails to be rejected. *JS*

Neyman, J. and Pearson, E. 1933: On the problem of the most efficient tests of statistical hypotheses. *Philosophical Transactions of the Royal Society, Series A* 231, 289–337.

ethical review committees Formally constituted and empowered groups charged with vetting and approving research protocols prior to study initiation to ensure sound ethics. The Declaration of Helsinki (2002) requires that experimental protocols be submitted to an 'ethical review committee, which must be independent of the investigator, the sponsor or any other kind of undue influence'. Such committees are variously known as institutional review boards (IRB), research ethics boards (REB) and human research ethics committees (HREC). In the UK, research ethics committees (REC) fall under the auspices of health authorities, ensuring independence from universities and teaching hospitals. A central office

errors in hypothesis tests *Types of error in hypothesis tests*

Conclusion of significance test	Reality	
	Null hypothesis is true	Null hypothesis is false
Reject null hypothesis	Type I error (probability = significance level)	Correct conclusion (probability = power)
Do not reject null hypothesis	Correct conclusion (probability = 1– significance level)	Type II error (probability = 1 – power)

(COREC) oversees the activities of multi-centre (MREC) and local (LREC) committees.

The perceived role of ethical review committees in practice varies both between and within countries. The Declaration of Helsinki requires that medical research 'conform to generally accepted scientific principles'. It is therefore the responsibility of the committee either to assess the scientific merit of each study or to satisfy itself that sufficient assessment has been undertaken.

Altman (1980) argued that poor use of statistics in medical research is unethical. First, if results cannot be trusted then the process is at best a waste of participants' time and may entail risk to participants without any possible benefit. Second, the process has also wasted scarce research resources. Finally, publication of incorrect conclusions may block or mislead future research, resulting in substandard patient care in the long term.

Statisticians on ethical review committees pay particular attention to the design of proposed studies: is the design appropriate to the aims; are there reasonable safeguards to limit potential confounding and BIAS? Unlike many errors of analysis and interpretation, fundamental errors in design cannot be remedied at a later stage. Vail (1998) described several issues arising in practice for both experimental and observational studies.

In therapeutic intervention studies, the unbiased allocation of participants to groups is essential to avoid selection bias. The statistician should ensure the use of RANDOMISATION or minimisation and the concealment of the randomisation process so that the next allocation cannot be reliably guessed. Blinding of clinicians, patients and outcome assessment, including the use of PLACEBO therapies where appropriate, should be explained, or absence of blinding justified explicitly. It is also the statistician's role to ensure that, where intervention studies differ from the standard two-group parallel trial, justification is given and results will be valid. For example, misuse of CROSS-OVER TRIALS and failure to recognise clustering (see CLUSTER ANALYSIS IN MEDICINE) are common.

In observational studies the definition and selection of study groups is key and must be appropriate to the study aims. Use of individual-level matching should be explained. The statistician should also ensure that common sources of bias, such as REGRESSION TO THE MEAN and the HAWTHORNE EFFECT, have been adequately addressed.

In all quantitative studies the proposed sample size is a statistical issue. An excessively large (overpowered) study would waste resources and unnecessarily delay dissemination of potentially useful findings. In practice, such studies are rare. More commonly, a study that is too small (underpowered) risks patient involvement and resources with little chance of finding useful results. Newell (1978) argues that underpowered studies involving additional discomfort or risk to the patient are unethical. Whereas many statisticians consider all underpowered studies to be unethical, this view is not universally held (Edwards et al., 1998) even for experimental studies. In general, statistical power calculations require several 'guesstimates' and there is no consensus on appropriate power, although 80% is often considered a minimum (see SAMPLE SIZE DISTRIBUTION).

The ethical review committee's statistical role in assessing analysis of studies is not easily defined. Occasionally it will be clear from a proposal that the planned analysis will be invalid or will be misinterpreted. For example, the investigators may propose to conclude equivalence of treatments from an underpowered, non-significant comparison, may confuse association with causation, may not recognise a need for case-mix adjustment or may simply propose a mathematically inappropriate analysis. In such cases, it may be considered unethical to allow the project to proceed without an undertaking to use appropriate statistical analyses. More usually, proposed analyses are sufficiently vague to cover valid as well as inappropriate analyses and individual committees vary in the extent to which they require detailed analysis plans.

Although there are good reasons for including a statistician in the membership of ethical review committees, and, indeed, MRECs in the UK are required to include a statistician, Williamson et al. (2000) found low representation in a survey of UK LRECs. Possible reasons for this include a shortage of statisticians who are qualified, available and willing to become involved. It may also reflect a lack of awareness of the benefits of statistical input: only 43 (29%) of 148 respondents without a statistician on their committee considered that they needed one. In the UK, official guidance since this survey requires each National Health Service REC to include expertise in 'statistics relevant to research', but falls short of requiring a professional statistician. *AV*

[See also ETHICS AND CLINICAL TRIALS, SAMPLE SIZE DETERMINATION IN CLINICAL TRIALS, SAMPLE SIZE DETERMINATION IN CLUSTER RANDOMISED TRIALS, SAMPLE SIZE DETERMINATION IN OBSERVATIONAL STUDIES]

Altman, D.G. 1980: Statistics and ethics in medical research: misuse of statistics is unethical. *British Medical Journal* 281, 1182–4. **Central Office for Research Ethics Committees:** www.corec.org.uk/. **Edwards, S.J.L., Lilford, R.J., Braunholtz, D.A., Jackson, J.C., Hewison, J. and Thornton, J.** 1998: Ethical issues in the design and conduct of randomised clinical trials. *Health Technology Assessment* 2, 15. **Newell, D.J.** 1978: Type II errors and ethics. *British Medical Journal* 2, 1789. **Vail, A.** 1998: Experiences of a biostatistician on a UK research ethics committee. *Statistics in Medicine* 17, 2811–14. **Williamson, P., Hutton, J.L., Bliss, J., Blunt, J., Campbell, M.J. and Nicholson, R.** 2000: Statistical review by research ethics committees. *Journal of the Royal Statistical Society Series A* 163, 5–13. **World Medical Association Declaration of Helsinki** 2002: Ethical principles for medical research involving human subjects. Edinburgh: 52nd WMA General Assembly.

ethics and clinical trials

Ethics and statistics meet one another head on, not exclusively but most acutely, in CLINICAL TRIALS. At first glance, one would think that this pair of disciplines are poles apart, linked at best tenuously by their common, albeit misplaced, perception as being necessary but peripheral topics within a medical course curriculum. However, while their differences may be obvious, there are surprising similarities linking the two diverse subjects. They are concerned, respectively, with the noble pursuits of what is true (at least numeric-based truth) and what is right, both amid uncertainty. For if there were no uncertainty, there would be nothing to pursue. One discipline appeals to probability to describe what might, may or could happen; the other appeals to morality to describe what ought, must or should happen. Clinical trials are experiments incorporating a delicate, three-part mixture of theory, practice and ethics, with the utmost importance attached to matters of ethics, in view of the priceless nature of the experimental units involved. They raise ethical questions before they start, while still in progress, when they end and, often, long after they are finished too, whereas theoretical and practical aspects tend to be more limited in their scope.

In an agricultural trial, it does not really matter if a field of wheat perishes under, say, Fertiliser A. One may actually be quite happy to gain a clear-cut result that Fertiliser B is superior to A, with happiness inversely proportional to the magnitude of the P-VALUE. However, when comparing Drug A and Drug B in a clinical setting, one must consider the people involved, not forgetting that statistical 'success' and 'failure' outcomes could be euphemisms for a patient's life and death. One may be happy to demonstrate a statistically significant difference between treatment groups and hence declare a positive result. Then again, one might think, 'Could not this conclusion have been reached sooner, with similar confidence, yet sparing the lives of some of those randomised to the inferior treatment?' This line of reasoning has motivated many statisticians to conduct research into DATA-DEPENDENT DESIGNS for clinical trials, including ADAPTIVE DESIGNS, sequential methods (see SEQUENTIAL ANALYSIS), Bayesian and decision-theoretic approaches to the design and analysis of trials (see BAYESIAN METHODS, DECISION THEORY).

Ethical concerns have, of course, been around for a longer time than statistics and the modern controlled clinical trial. A number of attempts to codify ethics for medical research in general (not just trials) have been made. The most famous such code is the World Medical Association's (WMA) Declaration of Helsinki, first adopted in 1964 and updated periodically (1975, 1983, 1989, 1996, 2000 and 2002). An online version can be found, for instance, at www.wma.net/e/policy/b3.htm. As a forerunner to this Declaration, in the aftermath of wartime atrocities in Nazi-occupied states, another set of international guidelines applicable to all types of medical research, the Nuremberg Convention was established. This has primary focus on the desire to protect defenceless subjects from unwilling participation in 'research'. See, for example, www.ohsr.od.nih.gov/guidelines/nuremberg.html for details.

Clearly, however, no set of regulations can be sufficient to guide researchers conducting any particular clinical trial and to protect its volunteers. Hence, recent decades have seen the emergence and growth of institutional review boards or more generally, ETHICAL REVIEW COMMITTEES. Their remit is to scrutinise study proposals, on a case-by-case basis, prior to granting study approval and to monitor ongoing research once underway. In the UK, for example, research is vetted by a network of local research ethics committees (LRECs) and, for larger studies, by multi-centre research ethics committees (MRECs). These committees work virtually independently of one another yet under the auspices of a central office for research ethics committees (COREC).

The remainder of this section will describe some general ethical principles, then outline important applications to clinical trials, emphasising statistical aspects, so that aspiring researchers may become familiar with these main areas for consideration when designing future clinical trials. Further details and discussion can be found in Edwards *et al.* (1998).

Bioethicists have developed various sets of principles by which to evaluate moral aspects of research. One such set, the 'four pillars of morality', are discussed at length by Gillon (1985) and by Beauchamp and Childress (2001). These pillars are *autonomy* (respecting a patient's right to self-govern), *beneficence* (doing good), *non-malificence* (avoiding harm) and *justice* (being fair). An alternative set of three principles seeks to solve ethical decision-making problems by appealing to utilitarianism (a consequentialist approach asking 'What maximises total good minus total harm?') and duty-based and rights-based deontological principles. In brief, duty-based deontology argues for doing that which is intrinsically right (asking 'Is it right or wrong?') whereas a rights-based deontological approach bases decision making on whether people are treated appropriately (asking 'Is he or she wronged?'). Thoughtful application of these sets of principles can help when faced with ethical quandaries, not limited to the conduct of clinical research. They serve useful purposes for those involved in trials, for they can be appealed to for justifying numerous research-related concepts. Among these are the role of RANDOMISATION, the need for obtaining informed consent, acceptability of blinding and use of PLACEBOS and, indeed, the rationale behind trials in the first place.

Statisticians, by contrast, tend to believe a set of two ethical principles to be preferable to three or four and make the simpler dichotomy into *collective ethics* and *individual ethics* (terms coined by Schwartz, Flamant and Lellouch, 1980). Applied to clinical trials, these concepts equate to doing what is right and best for future patients (those who stand to benefit from the results of a trial) and doing what is right and best for current patients (the volunteers in the trial), respectively. Indeed, a clinical trial can be thought of as a balance in delicate equilibrium between these two types of ethics (Pocock, 1983).

Collective ethics, also known as research ethics, and individual ethics tend to be in direct competition with one another. If one adhered purely to collective ethics, there would be unacceptable human sacrifices, but equally, if one adhered purely to individual ethics, there would be little scope for making medical progress.

According to individual ethics, each patient in a trial should receive the best possible treatment, whereas according to collective ethics, each trial should yield the best scientific result possible. The tension is clear. A doctor rightly has to pay greatest attention to the needs of his or her patients. This is the essence of the Hippocratic oath and fully supported by the Declaration of Helsinki. Among its precepts: 'In research on man, the interests of science and society should never take precedence over considerations related to the well-being of the subject.' In other words, that collective ethics can never be allowed to usurp individual ethics for the sake of scientific endeavour.

Turning to applications of ethics in clinical trials, it is convenient to categorise according to whether primarily affecting the period before, during or after the trial's recruitment phase. Chronologically, then, the first ethical consideration is whether a proposed trial should be conducted at all. Quite often there is only a limited window of opportunity (meaning in calendar time) in which to conduct a randomised controlled trial, assuming of course the situation is one wherein randomisation is itself acceptable.

Why is there only a limited time window? Ethicists have

coined the phrase, and notion, of *clinical equipoise*. It is a precondition for initiating a clinical trial and refers to the balance of clinical opinion among all doctors that needs to exist before it is ethical for a trial to begin. Thus, while it may not be possible for any one doctor to be perfectly balanced in their own mind concerning the relative merits of two or more treatments, perhaps including investigational new ones, it is quite possible that other doctors have preferences for the different treatments involved. Hence, a planned trial can be considered ethical on the basis of divergence of opinions, even if one has a slight personal preference, but not any firm evidence, in favour of one particular treatment. If, however, the weight of clinical opinion is too heavily in favour of a given treatment it can become too late to seize the opportunity to undertake a rigorous clinical trial. In turn, this means, the chance to secure best quality evidence to confirm, or overturn, such clinical (mere) opinion may be lost. EVIDENCE-BASED MEDICINE seeks to convert opinions (experience-based hunches, beliefs or gut feelings) into more objectively held evidence, based on sound data collection, gathered supremely through randomised controlled trials.

One certain point for debate at meetings of ethics committees relates to the process for obtaining each patient's informed consent to participate. This is not just because of the Nuremberg Convention, but a (happy) consequence of the composition of ethics committees being mandated to include a number of laypeople. Those nonmedically trained may or may not understand the intricacies of treatments involved in a research proposal, but they will definitely be able to identify with prospective participants. Hence, committees will include discussion on the all-important patient information sheet, or its equivalent, that outlines in everyday language the risks and benefits involved in trial participation.

Informed consent from participants is one of the most important safeguards built into clinical trials. It means that subjects never take part in a trial against their will (and for this reason it can be helpful to refer to participants as 'volunteers'). Ideally consent should mean written, fully informed consent although there are circumstances, usually emergencies, when witnessed verbal consent has to suffice. There are complications when the subjects of research include children, or those who are mentally ill, or comatose, or otherwise unable to understand the full implications of agreeing to enter a trial. In such cases, a proxy has to be appointed to serve as a spokesperson.

Ethical matters in general are heightened when dealing with special populations such as those just mentioned. In addition, one can add prisoners and medical students as special populations when undertaking research. Admittedly, it is unusual to put such groups together in the same breath, but in both cases, albeit for different reasons, there is a possible sense of coercion involved, meaning that one has to be extra careful when going about obtaining individuals' consent. Similarly, trials sponsored by developed nations that are to be conducted in developing nations are another major source of ethical conflict. This is especially true if wealthier nations stand to benefit more than the participating populations from the results of such foreign-based trials.

Another matter is exactly how much information is necessary to impart to the subjects at the time of trial recruitment. It surely includes relaying the uncertainty about which course of treatment is truly the best (for otherwise why perform a trial?) and that by volunteering they would be helping in the pursuit of medical progress to try and remove some of that uncertainty.

The act of giving informed consent is a statement from or on behalf of the trial participant that allows researchers to seek entry into the trial. Being randomised is not yet guaranteed, however, as there are strict eligibility requirements (see INCLUSION AND EXCLUSION CRITERIA) that may need to be checked after obtaining consent. Obviously, no subject should be forced into participating but from the scientific viewpoint it is preferable to have as high a proportion as possible of those invited going on to participate. This is analogous to seeking a high response rate in a sample survey – it reduces selection bias and enhances the generalisability of the trial's results (see BIAS, QUESTIONNAIRES). Part of the informed consent process should include a brief justification of the need for randomisation within the trial as a general principle. In addition, patients must be informed of specific details of what will be expected of them, the likely risks involved together with reassurance that they can withdraw from the trial at any time without compromising their future treatment or care.

So far informed consent has been discussed with regard to the prospective patient. It is their opportunity to decline to take part in the research. Next, consider the related decision that an investigator conducting research may have to make prior to involvement in a trial. Sometimes doctors or others are approached to become collaborators with someone else's research project. There is no formal equivalent to securing consent among investigators, but there are ethical considerations to be borne in mind. Chiefly, there is what is amusingly known as the *uncle test for randomisation*. It calls for the trial's investigators to answer affirmatively the question: 'Would you be willing to randomise either yourself or a close relative of yours (parent, spouse, sibling, child, uncle, etc.) into this trial?' That is, it seeks assurance that one's individual preferences are not so heavily biased towards one of the treatments that there would be a reluctance to take the risk of receiving the least favoured treatment for themselves or someone close to them. If investigators cannot honestly answer 'yes' to the uncle test then they simply should not enrol any patients into the trial (and certainly not succumb to financial inducements or other temptations to do so if the trial happens to be sponsored by deep-pocketed sources).

The use of placebos (inert substances made to mimic appearance of active treatments) and of PLACEBO RUN-IN periods (to assess a patient's compliance with treatment schedules, possibly involving the withholding of their usual medication), within trials is a controversial area, attracting much attention from those with ethical viewpoints. Note that a footnote to the most recent version of the Declaration of Helsinki addresses the use of placebos in clinical trials, arguing in their favour in the right circumstances. The choice of active treatment control or placebo control group is an example of how trials are an amalgamation of theory, practice and ethics. Statistically, one needs fewer subjects to demonstrate a difference in efficacy between a new drug and a placebo than between two active drugs. However, the decision whether to use placebo or not must not be dictated solely by sample size considerations, but primarily by whether it is ethically acceptable to put patients deliberately onto inactive treatment regimens. This further exemplifies the tension between individual and collective ethics. Similarly, the use of placebo run-ins prior to randomisation, while not necessarily completely unjustifiable, is harder to defend on ethical grounds (Senn, 1997).

The actual conduct of a clinical trial must be to highest scientific standards, for without such rigour the trial is compromised and the results unable to contribute meaningfully to medical progress. More positively, the well-conducted randomised controlled trial is rightly reckoned to be the most reliable source of evidence for or against any treatment. Note this includes adhering to the clinical trial's protocol, using a proper method for randomisation and, if blinded, employing suitable means to conceal treatment allocation effectively. The protocol, among other things, must include the hypotheses being investigated along with the primary and secondary outcomes. It is unethical to look first at one's data, then decide to promote in importance a non-primary outcome and demote the primary outcome, based on the actual findings. The excuse that unforeseen results may be more interesting does not justify departing from the protocol when publishing the study. (See POST-HOC ANALYSES for further discussion.)

A matter not always given full consideration is what to do with samples that are collected during the course of the clinical trial. Ideally, the protocol would specify not only where and for how long sensitive information, or equally blood, or DNA samples etc. are stored, but who has access to them in the future and under what conditions. For this ethical reason of protecting patient confidentiality, it is important that data and samples are stored securely and suitably coded or even anonymised altogether. For the benefit of future researchers, however, it is preferable whenever possible to have a system that allows access to individual patient information. This is a matter that should be included within the patient informed consent process if longer term research use of patients' data, or samples, is envisaged.

Another issue is whether a trial should be allowed the chance to stop earlier than planned. That is, can patient recruitment cease before the originally anticipated recruitment levels have been reached? Scientifically, there is a penalty for stopping a trial unexpectedly once initiated, so only in extreme cases are trials interrupted. There can be pressure, e.g. from disease-specific patient support groups, to expedite a drug development process. This arises in part from the long timespan involved before a promising treatment can be safely marketed. The statistical implication of planning possibly to stop early is best described by analogy with making multiple comparisons (see MULTIPLE COMPARISON PROCEDURES). Testing a dataset according to many different subsets will yield many false positive statistically significant findings. Similarly, multiple looks at the data at several interim analyses, each with the opportunity to stop the trial, make it more likely that an apparent treatment difference would emerge when in fact there is none. The penalty for unplanned early stopping is on the collective ethical side of the balance with individual ethics, for it is future patients who are denied the opportunity to learn more about the treatments under investigation. Then again, one

has to consider the needs and rights of patients entered towards the end of the trial too, so it is never a simple choice.

The accurate and timely reporting of clinical trials is yet a further matter with ethical implications. Choosing not to report a trial because results show sponsors' products unfavourably is without excuse and a clear abuse of ethics. For the vast majority for which publication in journals is sought, then conforming to the CONSOLIDATION OF STANDARDS FOR REPORTING TRIALS guidelines is helpful, if not mandatory, as it is becoming for a growing number of biomedical journals. An online version of the latest statement can be accessed at www.consort-statement.org. Authors failing to declare relevant conflicts of interest, financial or otherwise, or bulk-ordering expensive reprints of an article from a journal's office prior to formal acceptance are further examples of inexcusable behaviour at the pre-publication stage.

In an editorial in the *British Medical Journal*, Altman (1994) suggested there was rather too much research happening, not all of the highest quality and not always undertaken for the right reasons. If a clinical trial can be conducted, then it should be, in preference to an observational study, in order to gain the best quality evidence. It must first pass ethical review and be conducted properly, with suitable sample size, randomisation, analysis plans etc. detailed in the protocol and it should also be reported according to highest standards. All this is a tall order, hence another reason for CONSULTING A STATISTICIAN early in the trial's life, for it is notoriously easy to fall into PITFALLS OF MEDICAL RESEARCH. Finally, recalling the link between those not-so-disparate disciplines, forget not that bad statistics is bad ethics. *CRP*

Altman, D.G. 1994: The scandal of poor medical research. *British Medical Journal* 308, 283–4. **Beauchamp, T. and Childress, J.** 2001: *Principles of biomedical ethics*, 5th edn. New York: Oxford University Press. **Edwards, S.J.L., Lilford, R.J., Braunholtz, D.A., Jackson, J.C., Hewison, J. and Thornton, J.** 1998: Ethical issues in the design and conduct of randomised controlled trials. *Health Technology Assessment* 2, 15; www.hta.nhsweb.nhs.uk/execsumm/summ215.htm. **Gillon, R.** 1985: *Philosophical medical ethics*. Chichester: John Wiley & Sons. **Pocock, S.J.** 1983: *Clinical trials: a practical approach*. Chichester: John Wiley & Sons. **Schwartz, D., Flamant, R. and Lellouch, J.** 1980: *Clinical trials* (trans. Healy, M.J.R.). London: Academic Press. **Senn, S.J.** 1997: Are placebo run-ins justified? *British Medical Journal* 314, 1191–3. **World Medical Association** 2002: Declaration of Helsinki. Ethical principles for medical research involving human subjects. Edinburgh: 52nd WMA General Assembly.

evidence-based medicine (EBM) The conscientious, explicit and judicious use of current best evidence in making diseases about the care of individual patients. This is the definition of EBM given by one of its foremost proponents (Sackett *et al.*, 1996).

Alternative definitions that have appeared are very similar stressing the aim of assessing and applying relevant evidence for better healthcare decision making and allowing clinicians to practise better medicine by being aware of the evidence in support of clinical practice and the strength of that evidence. The primary tools used to drive evidence-based medicine are RANDOMISED CLINICAL TRIALS and SYSTEMATIC REVIEWS AND META-ANALYSIS. But as Sackett *et al.* (1996) make clear, evidence-based medicine is not restricted to these tools and, in particular circumstances, the best external evidence with which to answer a clinical question may involve CROSS-SECTIONAL STUDIES, genetic studies or immunological investigations. *BSE*

Sackett, D.L., Rosenberg, M.C., Gray, J.A., Haynes, R.B. and Richardson, W. 1996: Evidence-based medicine: what it is and what it isn't. *British Medical Journal* 312, 71–2.

exact methods for categorical data

A collective term for analytical methods that require no distributional approximations in order to validate the resulting inference. The 'exact' label applies when the probability distribution of the appropriate test statistic is fully determined, requiring no assumptions about unknown population characteristics and no large-sample distributional justifications (for example, using approximate normality). For expository reasons we illustrate the exact approach by focusing primarily on the P-VALUE yielded by a hypothesis test. It should be noted, however, that exact methods can also be used for estimation and computing exact CONFIDENCE INTERVALS.

A fundamental problem in statistical inference is summarising observed data in terms of a *P*-value. The *P*-value forms part of the theory of hypothesis testing and may be regarded as an index for judging whether to accept or reject the null hypothesis. A very small *P*-value is indicative of evidence against the null hypothesis, while a large *P*-value implies that the observed data are compatible with the null hypothesis. There is a long tradition of using the value 0.05 as the cut-off for rejection or acceptance of the null hypothesis. While this may appear arbitrary in some contexts, its almost universal adoption for testing scientific hypotheses has the merit of limiting the number of false-positive conclusions to at most 5%. At any rate, no matter what cut-off one chooses, the *P*-value provides an important objective input for judging if the observed data are statistically significant. Therefore it is crucial that this number be computed accurately.

Since data may be gathered under diverse, often nonverifiable, conditions, it is desirable, for *P*-value calculations, to make as few assumptions as possible about the underlying data-generation process. In particular one wishes to avoid making distributional assumptions, such as that the data came from a normal distribution. This goal has spawned an entire field of statistics known as nonparametric statistics. In the preface to his book, *Nonparametrics: Statistical Methods Based on Ranks*, Lehmann (1975) traces the earliest development of a nonparametric test to Arbuthnot (1710), who came up with the remarkably simple yet popular sign test. In the 20th century, nonparametric methods received a major impetus from a seminal paper by Frank Wilcoxon (1945) in which he developed the now universally adopted WILCOXON SIGNED RANK TEST and the Wilcoxon rank sum test. The contributions of many researchers advanced this field – an excellent survey of these developments is given in Agresti (1992).

The research just mentioned, and the numerous papers, monographs and textbooks that followed in its wake, deal primarily with hypothesis tests involving continuous distributions. The data usually consisted of several independent samples of real numbers (possibly containing ties) drawn from different populations with the objective of making distribution-free one, two or K-sample

comparisons, performing goodness-of-fit tests and computing measures of association. Much earlier, Karl Pearson (1900) demonstrated that the large-sample distribution of a test statistic, based on the difference between the observed and expected counts of categorical data generated from multinomial, hyper-geometric or POISSON DISTRIBUTIONS, is chi-square. This work was found to be applicable to a whole class of discrete data problems. It was followed by many significant contributions and eventually evolved into the field of categorical data analysis. An excellent up-to-date textbook dealing with this continually growing field is Agresti (2002).

The techniques of nonparametric and categorical data inference are popular mainly because they make only minimal assumptions about how the data were generated; assumptions such as independent sampling or randomised treatment assignment. For continuous data one does not have to know the underlying distribution giving rise to the data. For categorical data mathematical models like the multinomial, Poisson or hyper-geometric arise naturally from the independence assumptions of the sampled observations. Nevertheless, for both the continuous and categorical cases, these methods do require one assumption that is sometimes hard to verify.

They assume that the dataset is large enough for the test statistic to converge to an appropriate limiting normal or chi-square distribution. *P*-values are then obtained by evaluating the tail area of the limiting distribution, instead of actually deriving the true distribution of the test statistic and then evaluating its tail area. *P*-values based on the large-sample assumption are known as *asymptotic P-values*, while *P*-values based on deriving the true distribution of the test statistic are termed *exact P-values*. While one would prefer to use exact *P*-values for scientific inference they often pose formidable computational problems and so, as a practical matter, asymptotic *P*-values are used in their place. For large and well-balanced datasets this makes very little difference since the exact and asymptotic *P*-values are very similar. But for small, sparse, unbalanced and heavily tied data, the exact and asymptotic *P*-values can be quite different and may lead to opposite conclusions concerning the hypothesis of interest. This was a major concern of Fisher, who stated in the preface to the first edition of *Statistical Methods for Research Workers* (1925): 'The traditional machinery of statistical processes is wholly unsuited to the needs of practical research. Not only does it take a cannon to shoot a sparrow, but it misses the sparrow! The elaborate mechanism built on the theory of infinitely large samples is not accurate enough for simple laboratory data. Only by systematically tackling small problems on their merits does it seem possible to apply accurate tests to practical data.'

That Fisher's concern was justified, is seen from the following example of a 3×9 sparse contingency table:

```
0 7 0 0 0 0 0 1 1
1 1 1 1 1 1 1 0 0
0 8 0 0 0 0 0 0 0
```

The Pearson CHI-SQUARE TEST is commonly used to test for row and column interaction. For our contingency table, the observed value of Pearson's statistic is 22.29 and the asymptotic P-value is the tail area to the right of 22.29

from a chi-square distribution with 16 DEGREES OF FREE-DOM. This *P*-value is 0.1342 implying that there is no row and column interaction. However, we can also compute the tail area to the right of 22.29 from the exact distribution of Pearson's statistic. The exact *P*-value so obtained is 0.0013, implying that there is a strong row and column interaction.

We will conceptually describe further on how to compute an exact *P*-value for the chi-square statistic. However, even without knowing the technical details behind such a computation, an investigator comparing the asymptotic and exact *P*-values for this example might wonder at the disparity and not know which result is reliable. This example highlights the need to compute the exact *P*-value, rather than relying on asymptotic results, whenever the dataset is small, sparse, unbalanced or heavily tied. The trouble is that it is difficult to identify, *a priori*, that a given dataset suffers from these obstacles to asymptotic inference.

The concerns expressed by Fisher and others can be resolved if we directly compute exact *P*-values instead of replacing them by their asymptotic versions and hoping that these will be accurate. Fisher himself suggested the use of exact *P*-values for 2 × 2 tables (1925) as well as for data from randomised experiments (1956) (see FISHER'S EXACT TEST). For the 2 × 2 table, Fisher proposed permuting the observed data in all possible ways and comparing what was actually observed to what might have been observed. Thus exact *P*-values are also known as permutational *P*-values.

We demonstrate here how this approach can be used to obtain the exact distribution for the commonly used Pearson χ^2-test. The Table shows results from an entrance examination for fire fighters in a small US town.

All five white applicants received a pass result, whereas the results for the other groups are mixed. Is this evidence that entrance exam results are related to race? Note that while there is some evidence of a pattern, the total number of observations is only 20. A statistically inclined researcher might proceed as follows:

Null hypothesis: Exam results and race of examinee are independent.

Alternative hypothesis: Exam results and race of examinee are not independent.

To test the hypothesis of independence, one would ordinarily use the Pearson chi-squared test. The test statistic has the form:

$$\sum_{\text{Table cells}} \frac{(\text{Observed count} - \text{Expected count})^2}{\text{Expected count}}$$

exact methods for categorical data *Entrance examination results for fire fighters in a small US town*

Test results	Race				Row total
	White	Black	Asian	Hispanic	
Pass	5	2	2	0	9
No show	0	1	0	1	2
Fail	0	2	3	4	9
Col total	5	5	5	5	20

The distribution of this test statistic is *asymptotically* chi-square. Suppose we would like to conduct the test at the 0.05 level of significance for these data. Running this test, we obtain the following results:

Pearson chi-square 11.55556
Degrees of freedom 6
Significance 0.07265

Because the observed significance of 0.07265 is larger than 0.05, the researcher would conclude that exam results are independent of race of examinee. However, for this table the minimum expected cell frequency is 0.5, and all 12 cells in this table expected frequencies under the null hypothesis less than 5. That is, since all the cells in the table have small expected counts, what does this mean? Does it matter? The term 'asymptotically' means 'given a sufficient sample size', although it is not easy to describe the sample size needed for the chi-square distribution to approximate well the exact distribution of the Pearson statistic. Two widely used rules of thumb are given by:

(1) The minimum expected cell count for all cells should be at least 5.
(2) For tables larger than 2 × 2, a minimum expected count of 1 is permissible as long as no more than about 20% of the cells have expected values below 5.

While these and other rules have been proposed and studied, in the end no simple rule covers all cases (see Agresti, 2002, for further discussion). In our case, in terms of sample size, number of cells relative to sample size or small expected counts, it appears that relying on an asymptotic result to compute a *P*-value might be problematic.

What if, instead of relying on the χ^2-distribution to approximate the *P*-value, it were possible to use the true sampling distribution of the test statistic and thereby produce an exact *P*-value? Here we explain in an intuitive way how this *P*-value is computed and why it is exact. (For a more technical discussion, see Mehta, 1994.) The main idea is to evaluate our 3 × 4 cross-tabulation, relative to a 'reference set' of other 3 × 4 tables that are like it in every possible respect, except in terms of their reasonableness under the null hypothesis. It is generally accepted that this reference set consists of all 3 × 4 tables in the form of the observed table that have the same row and column margins as the observed table. This is a reasonable choice for a reference set, even when these margins are not naturally fixed in the original dataset, because they do not contain any information about the null hypothesis being tested. We refer to this as a *conditional exact approach*.

The exact *P*-value is then obtained by identifying all the tables in this reference set whose Pearson statistics equal or exceed 11.55556, the observed statistic, and summing their probabilities. This is an exact *P*-value because the probability of any table in the reference set of tables with fixed margins can be computed exactly under the null hypothesis.

For instance the table:

5 2 2 0	9
0 0 0 2	2
0 3 3 3	9
5 5 5 5	20

is a member of the reference set. The Pearson statistic for this table yields a value of 14.67. Since this value is greater than the observed value 11.55556, we regard this member of the reference set as 'more extreme' than the observed table. Its exact probability is 0.000108 and will contribute to the exact P-value. In principle we can repeat this analysis for every single table in the reference set, identify all those that are at least as extreme as the original table and sum their exact probabilities. The exact P-value is this sum.

In fact, the exact P-value based on Pearson's statistic is 0.0398. At the 0.05 level of significance, a researcher would reject the null hypothesis and conclude that there is evidence that the exam results and race of examinee are related. This conclusion is the opposite of what would be concluded using the asymptotic approach, since the latter produced a P-value of 0.07625. The asymptotic P-value, however, is only an approximate estimate of the exact P-value. As the sample size goes to infinity the exact P-value converges to the chi-square-based P-value. Of course, the sample size for the current dataset is not infinite and we observe that this asymptotic result has fared rather poorly.

This conditional approach to exact inference is currently the most widely used method for exact inference. However, conditional methods have their drawbacks. They can be computationally intensive. Until the advent of modern computing, exact tests were generally infeasible for any dataset that was not relatively very small. Over the past two or three decades, progress in computing technology along with the development of efficient algorithms have made conditional exact methods available to more practitioners for solving an increasingly larger class of applied problems. Virtually all commercial statistical software packages now contain at least some exact options for analysing categorical data.

More fundamentally, conditional exact methods are sometimes criticised for their conservatism. By construction exact conditional tests are guaranteed to control the Type 1 error rate at any desired level. (A Type 1 error occurs when we erroneously reject a null hypothesis.) This means, for example, that if you consistently use an exact P-value of 0.05 as your cut-off for deciding whether your results are statistically significant, this decision rule will limit your rate of declaring 'false positives' to at most 5%. However, since the exact distribution of the test statistic is discrete, you may not be able to achieve a Type 1 error rate of exactly 5%. Instead, the actual error rate of your decision rule will typically be smaller. This conservatism, which is entirely attributable to the discreteness of the test statistic, is the price you pay for exactness. The extent of the conservatism is not easy to determine. It does not manifest itself through exact P-values that are always larger than corresponding asymptotic P-values. On the contrary, there are plenty of examples (including the fire fighter data shown earlier) wherein the exact P-values are substantially smaller than the asymptotic P-values. Conservatism is a statement about a long-term error rate, rather than an individual P-value.

How serious is the conservatism? Not many empirical studies have been conducted to answer this question in general. For 2×2 tables, the extent of the conservatism has been investigated extensively and many alternatives have been proposed over the years to counter it. None of these other approaches has so far managed to dislodge

conditional exact tests as the methods of choice, for reasons discussed in Yates (1984) and Barnard (1949, 1989). In fact, it has been demonstrated that the conservatism of both types of tests is negligible in this setting, indicating that conservatism is also likely to be a negligible factor in the more general $r \times c$ setting.

Conservatism is still an issue for the single 2×2 contingency table. One way of reducing conservatism that has recently received greater attention is to use an unconditional approach.

Much of the blame for conservatism is attributed to the reference set having fixed row and column margins. In the single 2×2 table especially, such conditioning makes the distribution of the test statistic rather discrete in small samples. On the other hand eliminating NUISANCE PARA-METERS (for example, the odds ratio for a 2×2 table) by conditioning on their sufficient statistics, i.e. the row and column margins, is at the heart of exact conditional inference. Unconditional tests usually rely on large sample theory to eliminate nuisance parameters from the distribution of the test statistic. This is acceptable for large datasets, but may not be accurate for small, sparse or unbalanced data. There does exist an alternative unconditional exact approach, however, that is valid in small samples.

Barnard (1947) proposed an unconditional exact test based on a minimax elimination of the nuisance parameter. The reference set was defined to be the set of all 2×2 tables with fixed row margins and all possible column margins. Since the reference set for Barnard's test does not fix the column margins, the distribution of the test statistic is less discrete than would be obtained by permuting the conditional reference set in which both margins are fixed. However, Barnard was not satisfied with his test and disavowed it two years later (Barnard, 1949).

Barnard was invoking Fisher's principle of *ancillarity*, whereby inference should be based on hypothetical repetitions of the original experiment, fixing those aspects of the experiment that are unrelated to the hypothesis under test. In more recent publications Barnard (1989) provides additional arguments against the test.

Some prominent statisticians have expressed regret at Barnard's disavowal. Others continue to favour inference based on the conditional reference set. At any rate most statisticians agree that the case for conditioning is especially persuasive with RANDOMISED CLINICAL TRIALS, for then one can argue that the sum of the responses from the two treatment groups is fixed in advance under the null hypothesis; i.e. subjects predisposed to respond will respond regardless of the treatment received, since the two treatments are identical under the null hypothesis. Permuting the reference set merely amounts to assigning the treatments to the patients in all possible ways.

Even if Barnard's method were accepted without reservation, it would be hard to implement for general $r \times c$ contingency tables. It calls for enriching the reference set by permitting the column margins to vary and then maximising over the unknown marginal probabilities. Such a process is difficult, computationally, for tables of higher dimension than 2×2.

Another way of addressing conservatism is by using 'flexible' significance levels. Conservatism really hinges on approaching data with a fixed significance level (say 5%) in mind. Not all statisticians believe in fixed significance levels for decision making, however. Fisher (1973) stated:

'No scientific worker has a fixed level of significance at which from year to year, and in all circumstances, he rejects hypotheses; he rather gives his mind to each particular case in the light of his evidence and his ideas.'

Barnard (1989) has formalised this principle in terms of the 'flexible Fisher exact test' for the single 2×2 table for comparing two binomials. He proposes that we choose different significance levels for rejecting the null hypothesis depending on the observed sum of successes in the two binomial populations. Flexible Fisher can be shown to be equivalent to the various alternatives that have been proposed over the years to counter the alleged conservatism of Fisher's exact test for 2×2 tables.

A third way of controlling conservatism is by using a continuity correction, such as the mid-P-value, which is obtained by subtracting half the probability of the observed statistic from the exact P-value. This modified P-value has been recommended by many statisticians (see, for example, Barnard, 1989) as a good compromise between reporting a possibly conservative exact P-value and relying on a randomised test to eliminate conservatism completely. However, the mid-p cannot guarantee, theoretically, that the Type 1 error rate will be limited to the desired level. By the same token, researchers have shown empirically that mid-P-values do in fact preserve the Type 1 error rate while reducing the conservatism of exact P-values for a single 2×2 contingency table and in k 2×2 contingency tables. The coverage of the mid-P confidence intervals was not compromised, but they were shorter on average than the corresponding exact intervals.   *CCo/PSe/CM/NP*

Agresti, A. 1992: A survey of exact inference for contingency tables. *Statistical Science* 7, 1, 131–77. **Agresti, A.** 2002: *Categorical data analysis*, 2nd edn. New York: John Wiley & Sons. **Arbuthnot, J.** 1710: An argument for divine providence, taken from the constant regularity observed in the birth of both sexes. *Philosophical Transactions* 27, 186–90. **Barnard, G.A.** 1947: Significance tests for 2×2 tables. *Biometrika* 34, 123–38. **Barnard, G.A.** 1949: Statistical inference. *Journal of the Royal Statistical Society Series B* 11, 115–39. **Barnard, G.A.** 1989: On alleged gains in power from lower P-values. *Statistics in Medicine* 8, 1469–77. **Fisher, R.A.** 1925: *Statistical methods for research workers*. Edinburgh: Oliver and Boyd. **Fisher, R.A.** 1956: *Statistical methods for scientific inference*. Edinburgh: Oliver and Boyd. **Fisher, R.A.** 1973: *Statistical methods and scientific Inference*, 3rd edn. London: Collier Macmillan. **Lehmann, E.L.** 1975: *Nonparametrics: statistical methods based on ranks*. San Francisco: Holden-Day. **Mehta, C.R.** 1994: The exact analysis of contingency tables in medical research. *Statistical Methods in Medical Research* 3, 135–56. **Pearson, K.** 1900: On the criterion that a given system of deviations from the probable in the case of a correlated system of variables is such that it can be reasonably supposed to have arisen from random sampling. *Philosophical Magazine Series 5* 50, 157–75. **Wilcoxon, F.** 1945: Individual comparisons by ranking methods *Biometrics* 1, 80–3. **Yates, F.** 1984: Test of significance for 2×2 contingency tables. *Journal of the Royal Statistical Society Series A* 147, 426–63.

experimental design An experiment is a planned method of collecting data under controlled conditions, carried out so that the influence on the responses of one or more factors (which could for example represent different treatments in a CLINICAL TRIAL) may be assessed. The responses at the various levels of the factors are compared to see whether there are any differences that could indicate that the effect of one level of a factor is different from that of another.

Unlike industrial experimentation, the designs mainly used in medical research tend to be relatively simple in structure. This is partly because experiments involving patients are much more difficult to 'control' than experiments carried out under strict industrial conditions. Patients do not always comply with the medication regime and some may withdraw from treatment because they go on holiday, change GP, move house, change jobs etc. It could even be the case that the benefits of a sophisticated design could be lost in the complexity of the final analysis. Although in the early phases of the development of a new drug, more involved experiments, such as dose-ranging experiments using animals or small numbers of healthy volunteers, might be conducted, it is usually regarded as safer when dealing with patients to employ designs that are simple and not so sensitive to MISSING DATA or incorrectly applied treatments. For this reason, the vast majority of clinical trials are carried out as *comparative randomised controlled* experiments using either a *parallel group* structure (a completely randomised design) or as a simple *cross-over* experiment where each subject is exposed to each treatment using a predetermined specific treatment sequence.

In any design situation, it is important to consider the three basic principles of experimentation (Cox, 1958). These principles underlie all forms of good experimentation and are required if the conclusions are to possess the properties of *validity*, *precision* and *coverage*. To achieve validity, an experiment should be planned so that the conclusions are free from BIAS – either conscious or subconscious. It is not enough that the experimenter feels sure that they have not introduced personal bias or preferences into the experiment, it is a question of using a suitable experimental design and following the procedure laid down in the protocol. The first principle of experimentation is RANDOMISATION, which is used to avoid bias. There should be an allocation of treatment to individual subjects according to some randomisation procedure, which the experimenter cannot influence. Random number tables or a computer-generated randomisation should be used to allocate the treatments to the subjects. In a parallel group experiment, the subjects are randomly allocated to two or more separate arms of the study and receive one specific treatment throughout the treatment period. In a CROSS-OVER TRIAL, patients are randomly allocated to a particular sequence of treatments. The simplest form of cross-over experiment is the two period, two treatment, two sequence cross-over, also known as an AB/BA cross-over. In clinical research, it has become common to use *blinding* as an additional feature to avoid bias. *Single-blinding* is where a treatment has been allocated to the patient at random, without the patient knowing which treatment he has received. *Double-blinding* is where neither the patient nor the investigator (or assessor) is aware of the specific treatment received.

When the object of an experiment is to compare the effects of different treatments, there should be a measure of the *precision* (standard error) of the estimates of the differences between the effects of the treatments. This can only be obtained if there is *replication*, the second principle of experimentation. To achieve this, the same treatment must be applied to different subjects. These repeated applications furnish a measure of the variation in the treatment effects that may be compared with the variation due to random error that would arise even if there were no differences between treatments. One of the main requirements of an experiment, particularly in a medical environment, where it could be unethical to carry out an experiment unless it can be shown that the estimates will have sufficient precision, is that the study must be of a sufficient size. That is, there needs to be enough power in the experiment to detect a clinically important difference, if one exists. A power comparison, determining the sample sizes needed in a planned experiment, is an essential part of a clinical trial protocol (see PROTOCOLS FOR CLINICAL TRIALS).

The precision of an experiment depends not only on the number of replications used in the experiment, but also on the inherent variability of the subjects studied. The variability will be smaller if the subjects are more homogeneous. However, in order to achieve wide *coverage* of the conclusions, the subjects used should be as varied as possible. For example, a trial to compare asthma treatments will tell us very little about the response for elderly patients if it is restricted to a narrow age range of young patients. If the results of the experiment are to apply to all patients, the experiment should include patients from a wide range of age groups. However, the desire to extend the coverage of an experiment may result in systematic errors due to the heterogeneity of the subjects. This would be particularly serious if the randomisation resulted in subjects exposed to one treatment being generally different from (e.g. younger than) those exposed to another treatment. One of the techniques for the control of this non-random systematic error is the technique of *stratifying* the subjects into homogeneous blocks and then randomising the treatments within blocks.

Stratification, the third principle of experimentation, leads to experimental designs in which the effects of different blocks may be taken into account in the analysis. Examples of stratified designs are randomised block designs, Latin square designs and incomplete block designs such as Youden squares, balanced incomplete blocks designs, group divisible designs and cyclic designs (see Cutler, 1998).

Other techniques for allowing for differences in the subjects, and therefore extending the coverage of the conclusions, involve the use of auxiliary information. For example, in a hypertension experiment, patients may be entered into the trial with different initial systolic blood pressures, so a simple comparison of the difference between the average systolic blood pressures for the patient groups after treatment will not give a true comparison of the treatments unless suitable adjustment for their initial (baseline) blood pressures is made. This adjustment can be made using the ANALYSIS OF COVARIANCE.

In addition to the parallel group and cross-over designs already mentioned, FACTORIAL DESIGNS are being used more frequently in medical experimentation. In such experiments, more than one factor is involved, giving rise to treatments formed from different combinations of the factor levels. For example, one factor could be different drug treatments, while a second factor might consist of different levels of patient care. It is important in these designs not only to be able to assess the main effects of the different factors but also any interactions between them. One problem with such designs is that the number of

treatment combinations increases rapidly so that it might be necessary to use fractional replications as well as confounding to reduce the size of the experiment and to accommodate stratification.

Response surface designs (Box and Draper, 1987) are used to model a surface representing the responses at different levels of a set of factors. The object of the experiment might be to determine the best levels at which to set a number of factors that affect the responses. Simple factorial designs may be used to fit first-order response surface models, but more complicated designs such as central composite designs are needed if higher order models are required.

Another type of experimental design, increasingly applied in clinical research, is the sequential design (see SEQUENTIAL ANALYSIS) or sequential group design (Whitehead, 1997), in which parallel groups of patients are studied. Such a trial continues until a clear benefit of one treatment is seen or until it is unlikely that any difference between treatments will emerge. The main advantage of these sequential trials is that they will often be shorter, and therefore involve fewer patients, when there is a large difference in the effectiveness of the two treatments.   *PP*

[See also PHASE I TRIALS, PHASE II TRIALS, PHASE III TRIALS, PHASE IV TRIALS]

Box, G.E.P. and Draper, N.R. 1987: *Empirical model building and response surfaces.* New York: John Wiley & Sons. **Cox, D.R.** 1958: *Planning of experiments.* New York: John Wiley & Sons. **Cutler, D.R.** 1998: Incomplete block designs. In Armitage, P. and Colton, T. (eds) *Encyclopedia of biostatistics.* Chichester: John Wiley & Sons. **Whitehead, J.** 1997: *The design and analysis of sequential clinical trials.* Chichester: John Wiley & Sons.

expert systems Also known as knowledge-based systems, expert systems are computer programs that combine knowledge of some specific application domain with the general capability of drawing inferences from it, so as to be able to assist a decision-making process in specialist domains.

Research in this field originated in the 1960s, flourishing in the 1970s and for some time dominating the mainstream of ARTIFICIAL INTELLIGENCE (AI). Many limitations to this paradigm are now known, along with its advantages.

One of the original motivations for the development of this line of research was the impossibility to build general-purpose problem solvers, mostly due to the surprisingly extensive use of commonsense knowledge that is required in such systems. In a very delimited area of expertise, however, this is much less of a problem. The area of human intellectual endeavour to be captured in an expert system is called the 'task domain' of the expert system.

The primary goal of expert systems research is to make expert knowledge available to decision makers, by incorporating the expertise in an expert system, by means of a process known as 'knowledge extraction'.

Expert systems are often divided into two parts: a task-dependent 'knowledge base' and an 'expert system shell' that is independent of the task domain. In the classic approach the expertise in the knowledge base is represented in a symbolic way (e.g. by means of logic-type rules). The expert system shell, by way of contrast, contains an 'inference engine' that makes use of symbolic manipulations (e.g. logical inference) to reason with the information in the knowledge base. Some expert system shells also contain an explanation system (giving explanations about conclusions drawn and about questions asked) and a knowledge base editor (allowing to make modifications in the knowledge base in an easy way). One last important part of expert system shells is the user interface to allow user-friendly interaction with the expert system.

One of the first and most classical expert systems is PROSPECTOR (Duda, 1980; Duda et al., 1977), which was used to evaluate the mineral potential of a geological site or region.

In medical applications expert systems have first proved their usefulness by the development of MYCIN (Buchanan and Shortliffe, 1984; Shortliffe et al., 1975). This is an interactive program developed at Stanford University that diagnoses certain blood infections, recommends treatment and can explain its reasoning in detail. In a controlled test, its performance equalled that of specialists. Unfortunately, legal and ethical issues related to the use of computers in medicine prevented the system being used in practice. Many other developments resulted from the MYCIN project, however, for example EMYCIN, the first expert shell developed from MYCIN. Another early example of a medical expert system is INTERNIST-I (Miller, Pople and Myers, 1982), which later evolved into Iliad. Today expert systems are used in different applications, including medical diagnosis, design (e.g. of large buildings), planning and scheduling (e.g. in logistics).

Recent research in expert systems focuses on the use of statistical reasoning methods such as belief networks, which in turn fall under the more general header of probabilistic GRAPHICAL MODELS. In modern AI, hence, much of the inferential procedures are based on statistical rather than logical inference. Another, related trend is moving from a knowledge-intensive approach (emphasis on producing a good knowledge base) to a data-intensive approach (letting the system improve by machine learning and data mining). *NC/TDB*

Buchanan, B.G. and Shortliffe, E.H. 1984: Uncertainty and evidential support. In *Rule-based expert systems: the MYCIN experiments of the Stanford heuristic programming project*. Reading, MA: Addison-Wesley. Duda, R.O., Hart, P.E., Nilsson, N.J., Reboh, R., Slocum, J. and Sutherland, G.L. 1977: Development of a computer-based consultant for mineral exploration. Stanford Research Institute Annual Report, Project 5821 and 6415. Duda, R.O. 1980: The PROSPECTOR system for mineral exploration. Menlo Park: Stanford Research Institute Final Report, Project 8172. Miller, R.A., Pople, H.E. and Myers, J.D. 1982: INTERNIST-I, an experimental computer-based diagnostic consultant for general internal medicine. *New England Journal of Medicine*, 19 August. Shortliffe, E.H., Rhame, F.S., Axline, S.G., Cohen, S.N., Buchanan, B.G., Davis, R., Scott, A.C., Chavez-Pardo, R. and van Melle, W.J. 1975: MYCIN: a computer program providing antimicrobial therapy recommendations. *Clinical Medicine* 34.

explanatory variables Variables used as potential explanations of another variable in a statistical model. Thus, when using the simple linear regression model:

$$y = \alpha + \beta x + \varepsilon$$

we seek to explain the variation in the outcome variable, y, according to variation in the explanatory variable, x. Here, α and β are constants which specify how y is related to x; any residual, unexplained, variation is accounted for by the random error term, ε. Due to the widespread use of the symbols in this equation, an explanatory variable is often referred to as an 'x variable'. For example, Woodward and Walker (1994) used sugar consumption per head of population as an explanatory variable in a simple linear regression model to predict the average number of decayed, missing and filled teeth in 90 countries in an ecological study. In the analysis of association between these two variables, sugar consumption was taken as the explanatory variable, because the hypothesis was that consumption of sugar caused dental problems, rather than the other way round.

In general, several explanatory variables may be adopted as potential explanations of the outcome variable. For example, Bolton-Smith et al. (1991) used 15 explanatory variables in a MULTIPLE LINEAR REGRESSION model to predict the level of high-density lipoprotein (HDL) cholesterol in 5236 women. Explanatory variables may be quantitative or categorical; the complete set of explanatory variables may be a mixture. For example, in the HDL-cholesterol study, the 15 variables included continuous measures, such as blood pressure, and categorical classifications, such as marital status.

Sometimes there may be a single explanatory variable that is the subject of the hypothesis of interest and the remaining explanatory variables in the statistical model are confounding, or prognostic, variables. For example, in a SURVIVAL ANALYSIS of the effects of cigarette smoking on lung cancer the explanatory variables in the fitted model might be age and smoking. Here, age is not of interest as a predictive variable in its own right, but is a potential confounder in the relationship between smoking and lung cancer. Including age as an explanatory variable enables adjustment for the effects of age. Sometimes, a model includes certain explanatory variables that represent interactions, for instance an age by smoking interaction might be included in the set of explanatory variables, so as to see whether the effect of smoking differs by age. *MW*

Bolton-Smith, C., Woodward, M., Smith, W.C.S. and Tunstall-Pedoe, H. 1991: Dietary and non-dietary predictors of serum total and HDL-cholesterol in men and women: results from the Scottish Heart Health Study. *International Journal of Epidemiology* 20, 95–104. Woodward, M. and Walker, A.R.P. 1994: Sugar consumption and dental caries: evidence from 90 countries. *British Dental Journal* 176, 297–302.

exploratory factor analysis See FACTOR ANALYSIS

exponential distribution A single-parameter PROBABILITY DISTRIBUTION that often models the length of time to an event. If a random variable, X, takes an exponential distribution with parameter λ then this is sometimes written $X \sim \varepsilon(\lambda)$ for shorthand. The exponential distribution has the density function:

$$f(x) = \lambda e^{-\lambda x} \quad x \geq 0$$

which is monotonically decreasing from the MODE at $x = 0$. The distribution has a MEAN of $1/\lambda$ and VARIANCE of $1/\lambda^2$.

When $\lambda = 0.5$, the distribution is identical to a CHI-SQUARE DISTRIBUTION with two DEGREES OF FREEDOM. Changing λ rescales the density function on both axes, but leaves the shape unchanged. The function always intercepts the y-axis at $y = \lambda$, and the 95th percentile (useful for calculating CONFIDENCE LIMITS) is always approximately $x = 3/\lambda$. (The shape can be seen illustrated in the figure accompanying the entry on chi-square distribution.)

The most interesting property of the exponential distribution is the lack of memory (LOM) property. This means that if the lifetime of a surgical instrument is distributed exponentially with parameter λ, then if after 2 years we note that it is still working, its *remaining* lifetime will be distributed exponentially with parameter λ, i.e. it is as if the process has been reset or the first 2 years have been forgotten.

To illustrate, Ainsworth *et al.* (2000) find that the length of time in days until discharge from high-dependency care for premature babies is exponentially distributed with a median value of 6. The lack of memory property tells us that if a baby has already spent 2 days in such care then its median remaining time in high-dependency care is still 6 days; i.e. the median overall time for babies whose time exceeds 2 days is 8 days.

If one has n random variables that independently have exponential distributions with parameter λ, then their sum will be a GAMMA DISTRIBUTION with parameters λ and n. Coupled with the lack of memory property, this tells us that if the time to an event has an exponential distribution, the time to the second of 2 (or the third of 3 etc.) independent such events will have a gamma distribution. *AGL*

Ainsworth, S.B., Beresford, M.W., Milligan, D.W.A., Shaw, N.J., Matthews, J.N.S., Fenton, A.C. and Ward Platt, M.P. 2000: Pumactant and poractant alfa for treatment of respiratory distress syndrome in neonates born at 25–29 weeks' gestation: a randomised trial. *Lancet* 355, 1387–92. **Leemis, L.M.** 1986: Relationships among common univariate distributions. *The American Statistician* 40, 2, 143–6.

exponential family Distributions, including many of the common ones, whose distribution or density functions can be partitioned in a particular way. These distributions have some attractive features that enable easy computation and manipulation.

A distribution is defined by its distribution function (if a discrete distribution) or its density function (if a continuous distribution). In either case the defining function is a function of the data, x, and some parameters, θ. The distribution is in the exponential family if (1) the function can be written as a function of the parameters (e.g. $a(\theta)$) multiplied by a function of the data (e.g. $b(x)$) multiplied by the exponential of another function of the parameters (e.g. $c(\theta)$) multiplied by another function of the data (e.g. $d(x)$) and (2) the value of the parameters does not alter the range of possible values of the data.

To illustrate condition 1: The EXPONENTIAL DISTRIBUTION is unsurprisingly in the exponential family of distributions. The exponential distribution has the probability density function:

$$f(x) = \lambda e^{-\lambda x} \quad x \geq 0$$

which we need to show can be written in the form:

$$f(x) = a(\lambda)b(x)e^{c(\lambda)d(x)}$$

This can be achieved simply by setting $a(\lambda) = \lambda$, $b(x) = 1$, $c(\lambda) = -\lambda$, $d(x) = x$.

To illustrate condition 2: Consider the continuous uniform distribution between 0 and θ that has the probability density function:

$$f(x) = \frac{1}{\theta} \quad 0 \leq x \leq \theta$$

This can be parameterised in the correct manner, but different values of x become possible given different values of θ (e.g. 7 is possible if $\theta = 8$, but not if $\theta = 6$). Therefore this does not belong to the exponential family of distributions.

Other distributions that are in the exponential family of distributions include the exponential, the NORMAL, the BINOMIAL, the POISSON, the Bernoulli, the UNIFORM (if between fixed points) the BETA and the GAMMA to name only some of the more common members.

In frequentist statistics, the distributions in the exponential family are useful because they possess properties that allow for both straightforward MAXIMUM LIKELIHOOD ESTIMATION and GENERALISED LINEAR MODELS, among others. For BAYESIAN METHODS, one attractive feature is that they are the distributions that have natural conjugate PRIOR DISTRIBUTIONS. *AGL*

Dobson, A.J. 1990: *An introduction to generalized linear models.* London: Chapman and Hall. **Gelman, A., Carlin, J.B., Stern, H.S. and Rubin, D.B.** 1995: *Bayesian data analysis.* Boca Rotan: Chapman and Hall/CRC.

F

factor analysis A generic term for procedures that attempt to uncover whether the associations between a set of observed or manifest variables can be explained by the relationships of these variables to a small number of underlying LATENT VARIABLES (more usually referred to as *common factors* in this context). Factor analysis techniques attempt to discover the number and nature of the latent variables that explain the variation and more specifically covariation in the set of measured variables. The common factors are considered to contain the essential information in the larger set of observed variables.

The factor analysis model postulates that each observed variable can be expressed as a linear function of the common factors plus a residual term, i.e. a MULTIPLE LINEAR REGRESSION model for the observed variables on the common factors. The model implies that the covariances/correlations between the observed variables arise from their mutual relationships to the common factors. The covariance matrix of the observed variables predicted by the factor analysis model is a function of the regression coefficients of the observed variables on the common factors (the factor loadings) and the variances of the residual terms.

Estimation of both factor loadings and residual variances involves making the corresponding elements of the predicted and observed covariance matrices as close as possible in some sense. MAXIMUM LIKELIHOOD ESTIMATION is commonly used and has the advantage of providing a formal test of the number of factors needed to adequately represent the data. In general this test is to be preferred to informal tests such as KAISER'S RULE and the SCREE PLOT (see, for example, Preacher and MacCullum, 2003). After the initial estimation phase an attempt is made to simplify the often difficult task of interpreting the derived factors using a process know as FACTOR ROTATION. In general the aim is to produce a solution having what is known as *simple structure*, i.e. each common factor affects only a small number of specific observed variables. Rotated factors can be allowed to be independent or correlated, with the former often being chosen by default since it appears to provide a simpler solution. In particular circumstances, however, correlated factors might be considered to be a more realistic option.

A medical example of the application of factor analysis is provided in Whittick (1989). Attitudes to caregiving were examined in three groups of carers, mothers caring for a mentally handicapped child, mothers caring for a mentally handicapped adult and daughters caring for a parent with dementia. An attitude questionnaire containing 26 variables was developed and administered by post to 145 carers. The correlation matrix of the observed variables was subjected to factor analysis and a particular form of factor rotation giving independent factors. The three-factor solution could be interpreted as follows:

Factor 1: Negative aspects of caregiving with an emphasis on role conflict, family disruption and resentment about the caring role. Labelled as 'conflict'.

factor analysis *Calculation of factor scores on caregiving data*

Subscale	Mother/ child	Mother/ adult	Daughter/ parent	F
Conflict				
Mean	19.6	21.3	27.8	
SD	6.3	5.8	4.5	19.5
Love				
Mean	24.3	25.0	19.4	
SD	3.9	3.8	4.3	21.3
Institution				
Mean	7.5	8.3	12.9	
SD	3.5	2.9	2.7	34.5

Factor 2: Positive aspects of caregiving with the emphasis on love for the dependant and satisfaction gained from the caregiving role. Labelled as 'love'.

Factor 3: Willingness to accept institutional care with an emphasis on its advantages. Labelled as 'institution'.

These three factors provide a concise and convenient description of a relatively complex dataset and were used as the basis of a further investigation of differences between the three groups of carers. Factor scores were calculated on each of these three factors for all 145 carers in the sample and a one-way ANALYSIS OF VARIANCE applied giving results as shown in the Table.

The analysis of variance showed that there were significant differences between care groups on all three factors.

Factor analysis as described in this section is more accurately called exploratory factor analysis, with the 'exploratory' implying that the investigator uses the analysis with no preconceived ideas about the factor structure to be expected (except, of course, that it will be relatively simple and open to clear interpretation). In some situations, however, the researcher may have a theoretical factor structure in mind to be tested on a dataset. In such a case, CONFIRMATORY FACTOR ANALYSIS may be used. *BSE*

[See also PRINCIPAL COMPONENT ANALYSIS]

Preacher, K.J. and MacCullum, R.C. 2003: Repairing Tom Swift's electric factor analysis machine. *Understanding Statistics* 2, 13–44. **Whittick, J.E.** 1989: Dementia and mental handicap: attitudes, emotional distress and caregiving. *British Journal of Medical Psychology* 62, 181–9.

factor rotation A procedure used in exploratory FACTOR ANALYSIS that aims to allow the factor analysis solution to be described as simply as possible. Such a process is possible because the exploratory factor analysis model does not possess a unique solution. Essentially factor rotation tries to find an easily interpretable solution from among an infinitely large set of alternatives that each account for the variances and covariances of the observed variables equally well. Factor rotation is a way by which a solution is made more interpretable without changing its underlying mathematical properties.

The numerical techniques that are used for factor rotation aim for solutions in which each variable is highly loaded on at most one factor with factor loadings being either large and positive or near zero. In essence they try to alter the initial solution by making large loadings larger and small loadings smaller by optimising some suitable numerical criterion. Some methods of rotation give uncorrelated (orthogonal) factors, while others allow correlated (oblique) factors. As a general rule, if a researcher is primarily concerned with getting results that 'best fit' the data, then the factors should be rotated obliquely. If, however, there is more interest in the generalisability of results, then orthogonal rotation is probably to be preferred. For a full discussion of the pros and cons of the two forms of rotation see Preacher and MacCallum (2003).

We can illustrate factor rotation using the correlation matrix shown in the first Table. The factor loadings in the initial two-factor solution for these correlations are shown in the second Table, as are the rotated factor loadings (an orthogonal rotation was used). The factors in the rotated solution might be labelled as 'verbal' and 'mathematical'.

The lack of uniqueness of the factor loadings from an exploratory factor analysis once caused the technique to be viewed with a certain amount of suspicion (particularly by statisticians!), since, apparently, it allows investigators licence to consider a large number of solutions (each corresponding to a rotation of the factors) and to select the one closest to their *a priori* expectations (prejudices) about the factor structure of the data. But such suspicion is largely misplaced because of the essential 'exploratory' nature of the factor analysis solution that is subjected to rotation. (See Everitt and Dunn, 2001, for further discussion.) *BSE*

Everitt, B.S. and Dunn, G. 2001: *Applied multivariate data analysis*, 2nd edn. London: Arnold. **Preacher, K.J. and MacCallum, R.C.** 2003: Repairing Tom Swift's electric factor analysis machine. *Understanding Statistics* 2, 13–44.

factorial designs

factorial designs A term used in the context of a randomised trial (see CLINICAL TRIALS) to refer to a particular experimental design which allows two or more interventions to be evaluated in a statistically efficient way. In its simplest form, where Treatments A and B are to be compared with their respective placebos (see table), a 2×2 factorial design involves each patient being randomised twice, namely to either active A or Placebo A, and to either active B or Placebo B. This design allows the separate effects of A and B to be assessed in the same sample of patients and, for a given sample size, is more powerful than a trial comparing A versus B versus no treatment.

The analysis of factorial design trials involves a number of steps, which may be illustrated by considering a hypothetical analysis of the trial depicted in the table. The first step is to assess the effects of Treatment A among all patients allocated to A or matching Placebo A. The most powerful means of assessing the effects of A is to compare all those allocated to A (cells AB and A0 in the Table) with all those allocated to Placebo A (0B and 00). Analogously, the effects of B can then be estimated by comparing all those allocated to B (AB and 0B) with all those allocated Placebo B (A0 and 00). This 'marginal analysis' is the most statistically efficient analysis unless an 'interaction' exists such that the effects of A differ among patients allocated to B and among those allocated to Placebo B (or vice versa, namely the effects of B differ among patients allocated to A or Placebo A). It is necessary, therefore, to test for such an interaction in the routine analysis of factorial trials, because in situations where the effects of A are smaller among patients allocated to B than among those allocated to Placebo B, the marginal analysis will underestimate the effects of B (and, similarly the effects of B will be overestimated by the marginal analysis if allocation to B enhances the efficacy of A). In the example given, let us suppose that the primary outcome is binary (for example, mortality), so that a test for interaction would test whether the primary comparison (e.g. relative risk) was statistically significantly different for the comparison of A versus Placebo A among either patients allocated to B (that is, AB versus 0B) or among those allocated to Placebo B (that is, A0 versus 00). In the rare situation where such an interaction is identified, and is clinically significant (that is, its existence is relevant to drug selection), separate analyses of

factor rotation *Correlation coefficients of six school subjects*

Subject	1	2	3	4	5	6
1 French	1.00					
2 English	0.44	1.00				
3 History	0.41	0.35	1.00			
4 Arithmetic	0.29	0.35	0.16	1.00		
5 Algebra	0.33	0.32	0.19	0.59	1.00	
6 Geometry	0.25	0.33	0.18	0.47	0.46	1.00

factor rotation *Unrotated and rotated factor loadings*

Variable	Unrotated loadings 1	Unrotated loadings 2	Rotated loadings 1	Rotated loadings 2
1 French	0.55	0.43	0.20	0.62
2 English	0.57	0.29	0.30	0.52
3 History	0.39	0.45	0.05	0.55
4 Arithmetic	0.74	−0.27	0.75	0.15
5 Algebra	0.72	−0.21	0.65	0.18
6 Geometry	0.59	−0.13	0.50	0.20

factorial designs *Schematic diagram of a 2×2 factorial trial of Treatment A versus Placebo A and of Treatment B versus Placebo B*

	Active A	Placebo A	
Active B	AB	0B	All B
Placebo B	A0	00	All non-B
	All A	All non-A	

[**Commentary on the table**: The marginal analysis for the effectiveness of Treatment A involves comparing the measure of treatment effect among all those allocated Treatment A (the total in the cell labelled 'All A') with the measure of treatment effect among all those not allocated to A (the total in the cell labelled 'All non-A'). The marginal analysis for the effects of B is analogous (All B versus All non-B).

The test for interaction between the effects of A and B involves an appropriate measure of the difference between (i) the effects of A among subjects allocated to B and (ii) the effects of A among patients not allocated B. In the special situation where the outcome is binary (for example, mortality) and treatment effects involve comparisons of proportions, then a ratio can be computed, so that the test in this table would be the ratio of the relative risks (AB/0B) and (A0/00).]

the effects of a treatment should be performed among all those allocated the interacting drug and all those allocated not to receive that drug.

In the past, some authors have expressed concerns about the potential for misleading estimates of effect arising from important interactions in factorial trials (Lubsen and Pocock, 1994). It should be noted, however, that such interactions appear to be quite rare. In a recent systematic review of factorial trials of treatments for myocardial ischaemia, for example, the authors found that only 2 of 31 (6%) comparisons demonstrated a statistically significant interaction between two treatments (McAlister *et al.*, 2003).

The factorial design is an especially versatile experimental design. For example, if there are good *a priori* reasons to suspect that two interventions might act synergistically (i.e. their effects in combination may be greater than strictly multiplicative), then a factorial design is the only design that can establish this reliably. Similarly, if the marginal analysis of a factorial trial suggests that two Treatments A and B are effective, the absence of an interaction between A and B suggests that A will be similarly effective in the presence of B, that is, the combination of A and B is more effective than B alone. The test for interaction between the effects of two treatments has low power and so would only be able to detect large differences in effectiveness when treatments are given alone or in combination. But, provided it can be established reliably that a treatment is effective, the existence of modest variation in the size of that effect (which is, after all, no more than would be expected biologically) may be of less immediate clinical relevance.

While factorial designs might well provide a useful tool for answering clinical questions more efficiently, there may occasionally be circumstances where such a design proves impractical. There are two particular situations to note. First, if two or more interventions are to be assessed in a factorial trial, subjects cannot be randomised if one of the treatments is considered to be definitely indicated (or is contraindicated). This may limit the proportion of a target population that is eligible for a trial. Second, trial participants who believe they have experienced an adverse drug reaction in a factorial trial may simply choose to discontinue both treatments, so if the price of assessing a speculative treatment is a sacrifice in compliance with a more promising treatment, then the price may not be worth paying.   *CB*

Lubsen. J. and Pocock, S.J. 1994: Factorial trials in cardiology: pros and cons. *European Heart Journal* 15, 585–8. **McAlister, F.A., Straus S.E., Sackett, D.L. and Altman, D.G.** 2003: Analysis and reporting of factorial trials: a systematic review. *Journal of the American Medical Association* 289, 2545–53.

false negative rate

A false negative test result in a diagnostic test study occurs when a person who has the disease when measured by a reference standard has a negative test result. The false negative rate is the proportion of individuals with false negative results out of all of those who have the disease. For example, when babies are screened for hearing loss using traditional 'distraction' tests, a number of babies with negative test results will be found later on to have significant hearing loss. These babies have had false negative results and the false negative rate is the number of babies with false negative results divided by the total number of babies with hearing loss. It can also be expressed as 1 – SENSITIVITY.   *CLC*

[See also FALSE POSITIVE RATE]

false positive rate

A false positive test result in a diagnostic test study occurs when a person who does not have the disease when measured by a reference standard has a positive test result. The false positive rate is the proportion of individuals with false positive results out of all of those who are disease free. For example, when newborn babies are screened for congenital hypothyroidism using blood spot tests, a number of babies with initial positive tests will be found to have normal values of thyroid hormone on repeat testing. These babies have had false positive results and the false positive rate is the number of babies with false positive results divided by the total number of babies who do not have congenital hypothyroidism. The false positive rate can also be expressed as 1 – SPECIFICITY.

While it is always desirable to avoid false positive results, this is particularly important in the context of population screening, where apparently healthy individuals are invited to undergo screening. Patients with false positive tests will be harmed, as they are likely to experience anxiety they otherwise would not have felt and, in order to clarify their disease status, will have to undergo further investigations that may carry some risk. Hence evaluations of screening should consider both the benefits to patients correctly identified as being at risk of the adverse consequences of a disease (as measured by the test SENSITIVITY) and the harm to patients with false positive diagnoses (as measured by the false positive rate).   *CLC*

[See also FALSE NEGATIVE RATE]

FDA   See FOOD AND DRUG ADMINISTRATION

F-distribution

The PROBABILITY DISTRIBUTION of the multiple of the ratio of two variables, both of which have a CHI-SQUARE DISTRIBUTION. The F-distribution is defined by two parameters, often denoted m and n, known as the degrees of freedom of the distribution. If A is a random variable with a chi-square distribution with m DEGREES OF FREEDOM and B is a random variable independently distributed as chi-square with n degrees of freedom, then $nA/(mB)$ has an F-distribution with m and n degrees of freedom.

The most common use of the F-distribution is in the ANALYSIS OF VARIANCE, where the ratio of two estimates of the variance, each of which independently has a chi-square distribution, is examined. For example when looking at the effects of historical milk intake on hip bone density, Murphy *et al.* (1994) find that their variance ratio is approximately 3.8. Comparing this to an F-distribution with 2 and 245 degrees of freedom, the probability of such an extreme value is 0.0237.

Fortunately, in the medical literature one seldom has to deal with the density function of the F-distribution. It is useful to know that the mean of the distribution, as defined here, is equal to $n/(n-2)$ as long as n is greater than 2, and that the distribution will be positively skewed but approaches symmetry as m and n become large.

The distribution was named 'F' by Snedecor in honour of R.A. Fisher, and so is occasionally referred to as Snedecor's F-distribution or some similar variant.   *AGL*

Grimmet, G.R. and Stirzaker, D.R. 1992: *Probability and random processes*, 2nd edn. Oxford: Clarendon Press. **Murphy, S., Khaw, K.-T., May, H. and Compston, J.E.** 1994: Milk consumption and bone mineral density in middle aged and elderly women. *British Medical Journal* 308, 939–41.

finite mixture distributions

PROBABILITY DISTRIBUTIONS that result from a weighted sum of a number of component distributions. Such distributions have a long history, apparently first being used by Karl Pearson in the 1890s to model a set of data on ratio of forehead to body length for 1000 crabs. These data were skewed and a possible reason suggested for this skewness was that the sample contained representatives of two types of crab but when the data were collected they had not been labelled as such. This led Pearson to propose that the distribution of the measurements on the crabs might be modelled by a weighted sum of two NORMAL DISTRIBUTIONS, with the two weights being the proportions of the crabs of each type (see Pearson, 1894). In mathematical terms, Pearson's suggested distribution for the measurements on the crabs was of the form:

$$f(x) = pN(x, \mu_1, \sigma_1) + (1 - p)N(x, \mu_2, \sigma_2) \qquad (1)$$

where p is the proportion of a type of crab for which the ratio of forehead to body length has mean μ_1 and standard deviation σ_1, and $(1 - p)$ is the proportion of a type of crab for which the corresponding values are μ_2 and σ_2. In equation (1):

$$N(x, \mu_i, \sigma_i) = \frac{1}{\sqrt{2\pi}\sigma_i}\exp\left[-\frac{1}{2\sigma_i^2}(x - \mu_i)^2\right] \qquad (2)$$

The distribution in (1) will be bimodal if the two component distributions are widely separated or will simply display a degree of skewness when the separation of the components is not so great (see BIMODIAL DISTRIBUTION).

Pearson's original estimation procedure for the five parameters in (1) was based on the method of moments (see Everitt and Hand, 1981), an approach that is now only really of historical interest. Nowadays, the parameters of a simple finite mixture model such as (1) or more complex examples with more than two components or other than univariate normal components would generally be quantified using MAXIMUM LIKELIHOOD ESTIMATION, often involving the EM ALGORITHM. (Details are given in McLachlan and Peel, 2000.)

In some applications of finite mixture distributions the number of component distributions in the mixture is known *a priori* (this was the case for the crab data where two types of crab were known to exist in the region from which the data were collected). But finite mixture distributions can also be used as the basis of a cluster analysis of data (see CLUSTER ANALYSIS IN MEDICINE), with each component of the mixture assumed to describe the distribution of the measurement (or measurements) in a particular cluster, and the maximum value of the estimated posterior probabilities of an observation being in a particular cluster being used to determine cluster membership. In such applications, the number of components of the mixture (i.e. the number of clusters in the data) will be unknown and therefore will also need to be estimated in some way. (This, too, is considered in McLachlan and Peel, 2000.)

As an example of the application of finite mixture distributions we will look at the age of onset of mania to investigate the possibility that there is an early onset group and a late onset group in the data. This subtype model implies that the age of onset distribution for mania will be a mixture with two components. To investigate this model, finite mixture distributions with normal components were fitted to age of onset (determined as age on first admission) of 246 manic patients using maximum likelihood. Histograms of the data showing both the fitted two-component mixture distribution and a single normal fit are shown in the Figure.

The LIKELIHOOD RATIO TEST for number of groups (see McLachlan and Peel, 2000) provides strong evidence that

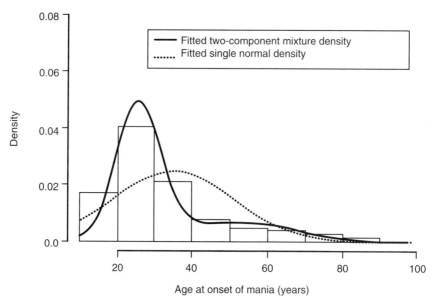

finite mixture distributions *Histograms and fitted mixture distributions for age of onset data*

a two-component mixture provides a better fit than a single normal. *BSE*

Everitt, B.S. and Hand, D.J. 1981: *Finite mixture distributions*. London: Chapman & Hall/CRC. McLachlan, G.J. and Peel, D. 2000: *Finite mixture distributions*. New York: John Wiley & Sons. Pearson, K. 1894: Contributions to the mathematical theory of evolution. *Philosophical Transactions A* 185, 71–110.

Fisher's exact test

A test of the association between the rows and columns of a two-way CONTINGENCY TABLE. The test is 'exact' in the sense that – under the hypothesis of no interaction between the rows and columns – the distribution of the associated test statistic is completely determined. An advantage of such exact methods is that they guarantee preservation of a researcher's pre-specified testing level (in this case, the probability of rejecting the hypothesis of no row and column interaction when the rows and columns are, in fact, not associated). The section EXACT TESTS FOR CATEGORICAL DATA describes exact tests more generally, but one could say that Sir R.A. Fisher – with his method described here – was the father of exact tests. He developed what is popularly known as Fisher's exact test for a single 2×2 contingency table. He motivated his test through a British ritual, the drinking of tea. When drinking tea one afternoon during the 1920s with Sir Fisher and several other university associates, a British woman claimed to be able to distinguish whether milk or tea was added to the cup first. In order to test this claim, she was given 8 cups of tea. In 4 of the cups, tea was added first and in the other 4, milk was added first. The order in which the cups were presented to her was randomised. She was told that there were 3 cups of each type, so that she should make 4 predictions of each order.

This experiment is described by Fisher (1925) and more recently by Salsburg (2001). One possible result of the experiment is shown in the table.

Given this particular performance, could one conclude that she can distinguish whether milk or tea was added to the cup first? The experimental outcome displayed here shows that she guessed correctly more times than not, but, by the same token, the total number of trials is not very large and she might have guessed correctly by chance alone.

A statistically inclined researcher might proceed as follows:

Null hypothesis: The order in which milk or tea is poured in a cup and the taster's guess of the order are independent. Alternative hypothesis: The taster can correctly guess the order in which milk or tea is poured in a cup.

Note that the alternative hypothesis is one-sided. That is, although there are two possibilities, that the woman guesses better than average or she guesses worse than average, we are only interested in detecting the alternative that she guesses better than average.

Suppose that the researcher decides to work at the 0.05 level of significance and decides to use the Pearson CHI-SQUARE TEST of independence. Results are as follows:

Pearson chi-square 2
Degrees of freedom 1
Significance 0.1573

Because the alternative hypothesis is one-sided (that is, we are only interested in evidence in favour of the woman's

Fisher's exact test *Fisher's tea-tasting experiment*

Guess	Pour		Row total
	Milk	Tea	
Milk	3	1	4
Tea	1	3	4
Column total	4	4	4

ability to distinguish between milk first or tea first) one might have the reported significance, thereby obtaining 0.0786 as the observed *P*-VALUE. Because the observed *P*-value is greater than 0.05, the researcher might conclude that there is no evidence that the woman can correctly guess tea-milk order, although the observed level of 0.0786 is only marginally larger than the 0.05 level of significance used for the test.

It is easy to see from inspection of the table that the expected cell count under the null hypothesis of independence is 2 for every cell. Given the popular rules of thumb about expected cell counts (for example, see EXACT METHODS FOR CATEGORICAL DATA), this raises concern about use of the 1 DEGREE OF FREEDOM chi-square distribution as an approximation to the distribution of the Pearson chi-square statistic for the table. Rather than rely on an approximation that has an asymptotic justification, suppose one instead uses an exact approach.

We demonstrate here how this is accomplished. For the 2×2 table, Fisher noted that under the null hypothesis of independence, if one assumes fixed marginal frequencies for both the row and column counts, then a so-called hyper-geometric distribution characterises the distribution of the four cell counts in the 2×2 table. A hyper-geometric distribution can be thought of as the probability model for selecting a particular number of red balls (say x red balls) out of n total selections, without replacement, from a jar that contains r red balls and $m - r$ black balls. This distribution can be derived using basic probability rules, but it provides a useful tool for a variety of applications that include exact inference for contingency tables. (We suppress the details regarding the actual form of the hyper-geometric distribution here, although one may find out more from any book containing a discussion of basic probability.)

In the case of our 2×2 table, if we fix the marginal counts we can see that – under the hypothesis of independence – the selection of milk first or tea first is like choosing red or black balls from a jar. That is, the woman knows that 4 of the 8 cups were prepared with milk first and the other 4 with tea first. If, in fact, she *cannot* tell the difference, then correctly choosing some number of milk-first cups from the 8 cups total is like randomly selecting red balls from a jar containing 4 red balls and 4 black. This fact enables one to calculate an exact *P*-value rather than rely on an asymptotic justification. In fact, the *P*-value for Fisher's exact test of independence in the 2×2 table is the sum of hyper-geometric probabilities for outcomes *at least as favourable to the alternative hypothesis* as the observed outcome.

Let us apply this line of thought to the tea-drinking problem. In this example the experimental design itself fixes both marginal distributions, since the woman was asked to guess which 4 cups had the milk added first and therefore which 4 cups had the tea added first. Note that if we fix the marginal counts we can focus on the cell of the table that corresponds to the number of milk-first cups identified correctly – this value determines the other three cell values. In other words, assuming fixed row and column counts, one could observe the following Table with the indicated probabilities:

Number of milk-first cups correctly identified	Table			Pr(Table)	P-value
0	0	4	4	0.014	1.000
	4	0	4		
	4	4	8		
1	1	3	4	0.229	0.986
	3	1	4		
	4	4	8		
2	2	2	4	0.514	0.757
	2	2	4		
	4	4	8		
3	3	1	4	0.229	0.243
	1	3	4		
	4	4	8		
4	4	0	4	0.014	0.014
	0	4	4		
	4	4	8		

Note that the probability of each possible table in the reference set of 2×2 tables with the observed margins is obtained from the hyper-geometric distribution just described, where the value x in this case represents the number of milk-first cups correctly identified by the woman. That is, she expends four milk-first choices on 8 cups total – 4 of which were *actually* prepared with the milk poured first. The P-values just displayed are the sums of probabilities for all outcomes at least as favourable (in terms of guessing correctly) as the one in question. For example, since the table actually observed has $x = 3$, the exact P-value is the sum of probabilities of all the tables for which x equals or exceeds 3. This works out to 0.229 + 0.014 = 0.243.

Given such a relatively large P-value, one would conclude that the woman's performance does not furnish sufficient evidence that she can correctly guess milk-tea pouring order. Note that the approximate P-value for the Pearson chi-square test of independence was 0.0786, a dramatically different number. The exact test result leads to the same conclusion as the asymptotic test result, but the exact P-value is very different from 0.05 whereas the asymptotic P-value is only marginally bigger than 0.05.

In this example all four margins of the 2×2 table were fixed by design. In many cases, however, the margins are not fixed by design. Nevertheless, the reference set when computing Fisher's exact test is constructed using fixed row and column margins. We stress once again that whether or not the margins of the observed contingency table are naturally fixed is irrelevant to the method used to compute the exact test. In either case, one computes an exact P-value by examining the observed table in relation to all other tables in a reference set of contingency tables whose margins are the same as those of the actually

observed table. We do not imply that other marginal outcomes are impossible under the conditions of the original experiment. However, since the inference is based on hypothetical repetitions of the original experiment, there is no logical problem with imagining that in these repetitions all outcomes whose row and column margins do not match the ones actually observed will be ignored. There are many compelling reasons for this conditioning, including the *ancillarity* principle, the sufficiency principle and the notion of eliminating unknown population characteristics (often called NUISANCE PARAMETERS) from the probability distribution of the test statistic.

Beginning with Fisher, there is a rich body of literature justifying conditional inference along these lines. A more recent treatment of conditioning is provided by Yates (1984). The main advantage of conditioning is that the distribution of the observed table is known, thereby making exact inference possible.

Note further that while Fisher's exact test is traditionally associated with the single 2×2 contingency table, its extension to two-way tables with an arbitrary number of rows or columns was first proposed by Freeman and Halton (1951). Thus it is also known as the Freeman-Halton test. It is hence an alternative to the Pearson chi-square and the likelihood ratio tests for testing independence of row and column classifications in an unordered two-way contingency table.

The idea of conditional inference to eliminate nuisance parameters was first proposed by R.A. Fisher (1925). It is the driving force behind much of exact inference for categorical data. However, Barnard (1945) proposed an exact test which eliminates the nuisance parameter from a single 2×2 contingency table without conditioning on the marginal counts. This has been shown to be less conservative for 2×2 tables than the conditional test. The method is controversial however (see Yates, 1984) and was subsequently disavowed by Barnard himself. Moreover, it does not readily extend to tables of higher dimension than 2×2. For these reasons Fisher's test remains the most widely used exact method for obtaining an exact test of association between two categorical variables. *CCo/PSe/CM/NP*

Barnard, G.A. 1945: A new test for 2×2 tables. *Nature* 156, 177. **Fisher, R.A.** 1925: *Statistical methods for research workers.* Edinburgh: Oliver and Boyd. **Freeman, G.H. and Halton, J.H.** 1951: Note on an exact treatment of contingency, goodness of fit and other problems of significance. *Biometrika* 38, 141–9. **Salsburg, D.** 2001: *The lady tasting tea.* New York: W.H. Freeman. **Yates, F.** 1984: Test of significance for 2×2 contingency tables. *Journal of the Royal Statistical Society Series A* 147, 426–63.

Fisher's linear discriminant function (LDF) DISCRIMINANT FUNCTION ANALYSIS

Fisher's z-transformation See CORRELATION

fishing See POST-HOC ANALYSES

five-number summary See BOX PLOT

fixed effect
One of a set of effects on a response variable corresponding to a finite set of values taken by an EXPLANATORY VARIABLE. Fixed effects are included in a

regression model to acknowledge that response tends to differ between the groups defined by the explanatory variable. By including fixed effects, the investigator can estimate the level of response for each separate group or estimate the effect of another variable of interest while controlling for the differences between groups.

Typical examples of explanatory variables include indicator variables for gender, drug treatment received in a clinical trial, ethnic background, or centre in a multi-centre study. If the variable defines k distinct groups in the dataset, for example k categories of ethnic background, the fixed group effects are incorporated by adding $k-1$ regression parameters to the regression model. Fixed effects are appropriate when the investigator wishes to estimate or control for the effects of the k specific groups defined by the explanatory variable in the dataset of interest. An alternative approach to modelling the differences between groups is to assume RANDOM EFFECTS, by declaring the effects of the grouping variable to be drawn from a distribution of possible effects. This is appropriate when, for example, the 10 hospitals in a study are regarded as a sample drawn from all hospitals and the investigator is interested in the population of hospitals in general rather than the 10 particular hospitals recruited.   *RT*

flexible designs   See DATA-DEPENDENT DESIGNS

Food and Drug Administration (FDA)   The food and drug regulatory body in the USA. Its mission statement is: 'The FDA is responsible for protecting the public health by assuring the safety, efficacy, and security of human and veterinary drugs, biological products, medical devices, our nation's food supply, cosmetics and products that emit radiation. The FDA is also responsible for advancing the public health by helping to speed innovations that make medicines and foods more effective, safer and more affordable; and helping the public to get the accurate science-based information they need to use medicines and food to improve their health.'

For more details see www.fda.gov.   *BSE*

[See also MEDICINES AND HEALTHCARE PRODUCTS REGULATORY AGENCY (MHRA), REGULATORY STATISTICAL MATTERS]

forest plot   A diagram most commonly used in SYSTEMATIC REVIEWS AND META-ANALYSES of CLINICAL TRIAL data, but also used for displaying the results from other types of studies. The plot consists of a diagram that shows both the estimated effect sizes from each study and the corresponding CONFIDENCE INTERVAL. An example from a meta-analysis of 28 CASE-CONTROL STUDIES concerned with the possible association between *Chlamydia trachomatis* and oral contraceptive use is shown in the second Figure (see page 140). Here the effect size is the logarithm of the odds ratio. (Other examples are given in Sutton *et al.*, 2000.)

The point estimates are sometimes marked using square shapes of size proportional to the size of the study represented. This counteracts the viewer's eyes being drawn to the least significant studies, which have the widest confidence intervals and are therefore graphically more imposing. Sometimes, too, the individual lines are ordered by date of study, by some index of quality study or by point estimate of effect size.

The first Figure contains both graphical and tabular elements. Data from each included study are summarised in horizontal rows on the diagram, with estimates of treatment effect marked by a block and associated uncertainty depicted by lines extending between the upper and lower confidence limits. The size of the block varies between studies to reflect the weight given to each in the meta-analysis, more influential studies having larger blocks. The overall estimate of effect is marked at the bottom of the plot as a diamond, the central points indicating the point estimate while the outer points mark the confidence limits. A vertical line is often drawn across the diagram at the meta-analytical point estimate. Forest plots of ratio effect measures (such as odds ratios, risk ratios – see RELATIVE RISK AND ODDS RATIO – and hazard ratios – see SURVIVAL ANALYSIS) are plotted on log scales so that the CONFIDENCE INTERVALS for individual studies and the overall estimate are symmetrical about their point estimates.

In addition to the graphical display, forest plots may numerically report the data for each trial from which the estimate is calculated, the estimate of effect and confidence interval and the percentage weight that the study contributes to the meta-analysis. The overall estimate may

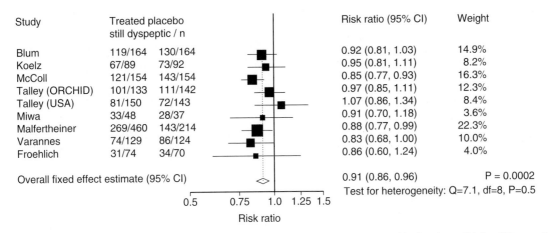

Study	Treated placebo still dyspeptic / n		Risk ratio (95% CI)	Weight
Blum	119/164	130/164	0.92 (0.81, 1.03)	14.9%
Koelz	67/89	73/92	0.95 (0.81, 1.11)	8.2%
McColl	121/154	143/154	0.85 (0.77, 0.93)	16.3%
Talley (ORCHID)	101/133	111/142	0.97 (0.85, 1.11)	12.3%
Talley (USA)	81/150	72/143	1.07 (0.86, 1.34)	8.4%
Miwa	33/48	28/37	0.91 (0.70, 1.18)	3.6%
Malfertheiner	269/460	143/214	0.88 (0.77, 0.99)	22.3%
Varannes	74/129	86/124	0.83 (0.68, 1.00)	10.0%
Froehlich	31/74	34/70	0.86 (0.60, 1.24)	4.0%
Overall fixed effect estimate (95% CI)			0.91 (0.86, 0.96)	P = 0.0002

Test for heterogeneity: Q=7.1, df=8, P=0.5

0.5   0.75   1.0   1.25 1.5
Risk ratio

forest plot   *Forest plot of the nine trials comparing* Helicobacter pylori *eradication therapy with placebo antibiotics (Moayyedi* et al., *2000)*

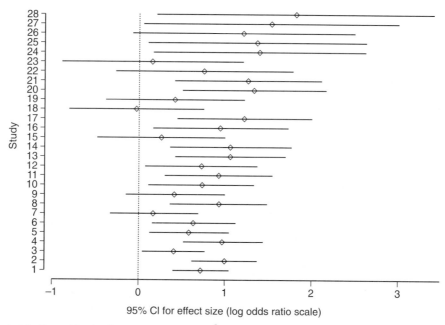

95% CI for effect size (log odds ratio scale)

forest plot *Forest plot of log odd ratios for case-control studies of* Chlamydia trachomatis *and oral contraceptive use*

also be reported numerically stating the point estimate, a confidence interval, a test of statistical significance of the null hypothesis of no treatment effect and a test of homogeneity of no difference in effects between studies. From the plot it is often possible visually to assess the degree of heterogeneity in study results by noting the overlap of confidence intervals of individual studies with the meta-analytical point estimate.

Forest plots may be supplemented in systematic reviews by *L'Abbé plots* (which plot event rates on treatment against event rates on control) and FUNNEL PLOTS. However, none of these diagrams can replace forest plots in their ability to report both the individual study data depicting effect estimates and uncertainty, as well as the meta-analytical summary estimates.

Lewis and Clarke (2001) reviewed the origins of the name 'forest' and identified that both the occasionally encountered spelling as *forrest* and capitalisation are inappropriate. *JD/BSE*

Lewis, S. and Clarke, M. 2001: Forest plot: trying to see the wood and the trees. *British Medical Journal* 322, 1479–80. **Moayyedi, P., Soo, S., Deeks, J., Forman, D., Mason, J., Innes, M. and Delaney, B.** 2000: Systematic review and economic evaluation of Helicobacter pylori eradication treatment for non-ulcer dyspepsia. *British Medical Journal* 321, 659–64. **Sutton, A.J., Abrams, K.R., Jones, D.R., Sheldon, T.A. and Song, F.** 2000: *Methods in meta-analysis.* Chichester: John Wiley & Sons.

forwards regression See LOGISTIC REGRESSION, MULTIPLE LINEAR REGRESSION

frailty A term generally used for unobserved individual heterogeneity, particularly in the analysis of SURVIVAL DATA. Such analysis is usually based on the assumption that the survival times of different individuals are independent and come from the same distribution, i.e. we assume a homogeneous population. In practice, populations are usually heterogeneous. We attempt to explain this heterogeneity by fitting models (such as COX'S REGRESSION MODELS) using explanatory variables. Frequently, even after adjusting for the explanatory variables, substantial heterogeneity remains, either due to lack of knowledge of or inability to measure all explanatory variables.

Frailty models were developed by Vaupel, Manton and Stallard (1979) to take into account this 'extra' variability. Individuals who have the same observed explanatory variable may differ in their underlying unobserved health status or frailty. As time progresses and frail individuals tend to die, the composition of the population with respect to frailty changes. Ignoring this can lead to biased estimation. An unmeasured random variable representing the unknown frailty is generally assumed to act multiplicatively on the baseline hazard function. These types of models are essentially MIXED or RANDOM EFFECT MODELS. The LIKELIHOOD functions for frailty models are quite complex and estimation is generally carried out using the EM ALGORITHM. Much research has been devoted to the choice of distributions for the frailty variable. A common choice is the GAMMA DISTRIBUTION. Klein and Moeschberger (1997) provide SAS macros that estimate the gamma frailty Cox regression model on their website. Other choices are discussed in Hougaard (2000). These frailty models have been widely applied. Hougaard (2000) provides a number of examples, including death due to malignant melanoma and times to catheter removal due to infection, for which the standard Cox regression approach is compared with the use of frailty models.

Frailty models are also used in the analysis of multivariate survival data to model dependence between times (Aalen, 1994). Such data can arise in several different ways. For example, time to recurrent events (such as epileptic seizures) on a subject will generally be dependent. Multivariate data also arises in connection with time to failure of similar organs (right eye, left eye) or lifetimes of related people (related genetically, by a common environment etc.).

For simplicity consider survival data on pairs of twins who are assumed to have a common frailty. This frailty is taken to be a random variable. Given the frailty for a specified pair the individual hazard function is taken to be the multiple of frailty with a baseline hazard. The common frailty (of a pair) creates the dependence between the survival times within pairs. Assuming a distributional form for the frailty and averaging the conditional survival functions over the frailty distribution permits the derivation of a joint survival function. The resulting shared frailty models describe the dependence between the times. Details and more complicated multivariate frailty models are discussed by Hougaard (2000) along with various applications such as twin survival data.   *DF/BR*

Aalen, O.O. 1994: Effects of frailty in survival analysis. *Statistical Methods in Medical Research* 3, 227–43. **Hougaard, P.** 2000: *Analysis of multivariate survival data.* New York: Springer Verlag. **Klein, J.P. and Moeschberger, M.L.** 1997: *Survival analysis.* New York: Springer Verlag. **Vaupel, J.W., Manton, K.G and Stallard, E.** 1979: The impact of heterogeneity in individual frailty on the dynamics of mortality. *Demography* 16, 439–54.

fraud detection in biomedical research

Fraud in biomedical research comes in many guises (Lock and Wells, 1993). The boundary between fraud and simple carelessness is often fuzzy, although fraud is characterised by a *deliberate* attempt to deceive, which may be very hard to prove in the absence of positive external evidence or confession. Data discrepancies such as transcription errors between the source documents and the data collection forms, may potentially be regarded as fraud if they occur in some systematic way or with abnormally high frequency, two circumstances that require a statistical assessment. In the USA, the term 'fraud' implies injury or damage to victims, hence the term 'misconduct' might be preferred. However 'misconduct' also includes practices such as plagiarism, conflicts of interest, misuse of funds and other questionable research practices. In the UK, a Joint Consensus Conference on Misconduct in Biomedical Research held in October 1999 defined research misconduct as 'behaviour by a researcher, *intentional or not*, that falls short of good ethical and scientific standards'. Here the term 'fraud' refers specifically to *data fabrication* (making up data values) and *data falsification* (amending or eliminating data values), a use of the word that is at once more restrictive than is implied in normal conversation and less specific than in legal texts.

Scientific fraud (in the limited sense of data fabrication or falsification) is, in all likelihood, a rare phenomenon in biomedical research, although other misconduct may be more common. Some of the most widely publicised cases of fraud have taken place in randomised CLINICAL TRIALS and have created so much media attention that the uncritical observer may have been misled into thinking that the problem was far worse than it actually is. In all systematic investigations reported by cooperative groups and pharmaceutical companies, the proportion of investigators who were found to have committed fraud was less than 1% (Buyse *et al.*, 1999). In the audits performed by the United States FOOD AND DRUG ADMINISTRATION, the 'for-cause' investigations that followed revealed in most cases

sloppiness or incompetence rather than fraud (Buyse *et al.*, 1999). However, there may be substantial BIAS in estimating the actual prevalence of fraud because of the natural tendency to suppress, conceal or minimise actual cases. In a recent cross-sectional survey of biostatisticians who were members of the International Society for Clinical Biostatistics in 1998, more than half of the respondents stated that they knew of a project in which fraud had occurred in the previous 10 years, while almost one-third of them had been engaged in a project in which fraud took place or was about to take place (Ranstam *et al.*, 2000). All in all, reliable data on the true prevalence of fraud are lacking.

The major difference between fraud and mere error lies in the 'intention to cheat' that defines fraud (Buyse *et al.*, 1999). This difference must, however, be qualified by the nature of the intent. Often investigators fabricate or falsify data to have complete records on all cases, or to eliminate OUTLIERS, not to modify the outcome of the experiment. Such data manipulations, if done independently of treatment assignment (e.g. in a blinded trial) introduce *noise* but no bias in the experiment. More serious cases of fraud involve fabricating complete patients or tampering the data in order to obtain a desirable result. These are cases where there is an expectation of gain in terms of prestige, advancement or money. These cases may also be the easiest to detect statistically, especially in MULTI-CENTRE TRIALS.

Some data items collected in clinical trials seem to be more prone to error and/or fraud than others. *Eligibility criteria* may be 'pushed' a little to make a patient eligible for the trial when in fact that patient does not strictly meet the criteria; many examples of fraud may have occurred because eligibility criteria were excessively restrictive and widening entry standards is often a good solution. *Repeated measurements* are requested repeatedly over time (such as, for instance, a battery of laboratory examinations), in which case data may be 'propagated' from the previous visit if the measurements are missing for a particular visit; such imputation of missing values is questionable at the time of the analysis, but certainly unacceptable when reporting the observations. *Adverse events* are likely to be underreported by some investigators (although such underreporting may reveal lack of interest or differences in interpretation rather than fraud). *Compliance data* are notoriously unreliable if they are based on the number of medications returned ('pill counts'); whenever compliance information is deemed important, it is advisable to use objective measurements based on blood or urine tests. *Patient diaries* in which data fabrication have been detected through the colour and texture of the pen supposedly used on successive days by the patient, the patient's handwriting, etc; the reliability of information collected in patient diaries can often be called into question, although electronic data capture can provide a more reliable alternative.

Some types of fraud are committed in trials conducted in a fastidious way, with lengthy case report forms, excessive requests for data clarification etc. Often randomised clinical trials can be drastically simplified without loss of essential information. For instance: eligibility criteria can be simplified and left to the discretion of the investigator; the amount of data collected in the case report forms can be reduced, e.g. by eliminating much of the medical history and prior medications, concomitant medications, laboratory examinations etc. that are not essential to the interpretation of the trial results; the follow-up of the patients in trials requiring prolonged observation can be as in routine clinical practice.

The traditional approach to fraud detection has involved monitoring visits to the centres or sites participating in the trial (Knatterud *et al.*, 1998). Some such onsite monitoring may be needed and useful, for many types of fraud would remain completely undiscovered were it not for the careful checks carried out during these visits. However, onsite monitoring is labour intensive and expensive and it, too, may fail to pick up fraudulent data. Moreover, the law of diminishing returns suggests that it is not cost effective to demand 100% verification of all source data. Monitoring activities can be limited to some random selection of the data, with the possible exception of data pertaining to the primary ENDPOINT of the trial. The random selection can be done at the level of the centres, the patients or the data items themselves. With such a random sampling scheme, one can estimate the overall data error rate with pre-specified precision and increase the amount of onsite monitoring, if the observed rate exceeds some upper limit. Another approach consists of visiting only the centres in which problems, errors or fraud are suspected.

A more innovative approach to detect fraud relies solely on statistics. The data of randomised clinical trials can be verified using statistical techniques that take advantage of their highly structured nature. Most data-entry and data management software used for clinical trials perform basic checks, such as RANGE and consistency checks, but more extensive data checks typically occur at the end of the study along with other statistical analyses, far too late for corrective action. Batteries of checks using standard statistical techniques could be used early on in the course of a trial without large increases in costs and could save considerable time if problems were detected and corrected early.

The principles involved in uncovering fraud through statistical techniques rest on the difficulty of fabricating plausible data, particularly in high dimensions (Evans, 1998). Univariate observations can always be fabricated to fall close to the mean, although preserving their variance is more of a challenge to the inexperienced. Even the astute cheater who takes care in preserving both the mean and the variance may be tripped up by examination of the KURTOSIS of the distribution. Multivariate observations must in addition be consistent with the correlation structure between their individual components. In general, when data are fabricated to pass certain statistical tests, they are likely to fail on others (Haldane, 1948).

Another observation that can be used to check fabricated data is that humans are poor random number generators. Even informed people seem unable to generate long sequences of numbers that pass simple tests for randomness. Digit preference, especially terminal digit preference, or an excess of round numbers may easily reveal data fabrication. Benford's law may also be used to check the randomness of the first digit of all real numbers reported by a single individual (or a single centre). This law establishes that the probability of the first significant digit being equal to D ($D = 1, ..., 9$) is approximately given by a logarithmic distribution (Hill, 1998):

$$P(D) \approx \log (D + 1) - \log (D)$$

fraud detection in biomedical research *Some statistical techniques that may be used to uncover fraud*

One variable at a time	Descriptive statistics
	Box plot
	Frequency histogram
	Stem-and-leaf plots
	Tests for slippage
Several variables at a time	Cross-tabulation/scatterplot
	Correlation/regression
	Cook's distance
	Mahalanobis' distance
	Cluster analysis
	Discriminant analysis
	Chernoff faces
	Star (needle, spike) plots
	Hotelling's T^2
	Tests for treatment contrasts
Repeated measurements	Autocorrelations
	Profiles
	Polynomial contrasts
	Runs tests
Calendar time	Residual plots
	Cusum
	Control charts

Hence the frequency of 1 as a first digit should be as high as 30%, the frequency of 2 as a first digit should be close to 18%, while that of 9s should be lower than 5%, a result that runs against intuition. More sophisticated techniques are available to check the randomness of digits in a sequence of data values.

Statistical approaches may also take full advantage of the highly structured nature of clinical trials, which are prospective studies, entirely specified in a written protocol and data collection instrument (the 'case report form'), usually involving several centres and, when com-

fraud detection in biomedical research *Some patterns that may reveal fraud in clinical trial data*

One variable at a time	Digit preference
	Round number preference
	Too few or too many outliers
	Too little or too much variance
	Strange peaks
	Data too skewed
Several variables at a time	Multivariate inliers
	Multivariate outliers
	Leverage
	Too weak or too strong correlation
Repeated measurements	Interpolation
	Duplicates
	Invented patterns
Calendar time	Breach of randomisation
	Days of week (Sundays or holidays)
	Implausible accrual
	Time trends

parative, a randomly assigned treatment. Comparing each centre or treatment to the others in terms of the distribution of some variables, either taken in isolation (univariate approach) or jointly (multivariate approach) can detect unusual patterns in the data. Comparisons between centres are particularly informative if there are more than a few observations per centre (in which case fraud in any one centre may have a sizeable impact on the overall result). Such comparisons are useful with different types of fraud; for instance, the presence of outliers or the consistency in the effect of treatment may reveal fraud aimed at exaggerating the effect, while the presence of 'inliers' or under-dispersion in the data may reveal invented cases.

Several univariate statistical techniques may be used to inspect the data (see first Table on page 142).

Statistical checks may reveal unusual data patterns that are often the mark of fraud (see second Table on page 142). Invented or manipulated data tend to have too little VARIANCE, no outliers or an abnormally flat distribution. Their distribution may be too close to a simple but implausible model, such as a NORMAL DISTRIBUTION with round numbers for the MEAN and STANDARD DEVIATION.

Since fraud usually occurs in a single centre (except in the unlikely situation of a coordinated fraud across several centres), statistical checks must be performed within each centre as well as overall. A comparison of the results reported by different centres may reveal too little variability in one or more centres as compared to the overall variability. Perfect compliance with the protocol, for instance, may be the mark of fraud. Such a comparison may also reveal 'slippage' of one or more centres, the null hypothesis being that the means of the variable of interest are equal, but for random fluctuations, to the overall mean (Canner, Huang and Meinert, 1981).

Multivariate statistical techniques offer more checking possibilities, but they are seldom used in clinical trials, if at all. Multivariate statistical methods include correlations between several patient-related variables as well as comparisons between the randomised groups. Simple two-way cross-tabulations or SCATTERPLOTS for various pairs of variables can be compared across centres and any unusual patterns investigated further. Outlying observations, or outlying groups of observations coming from the same centre, can be detected more effectively in multidimensional space than in a single dimension. Moreover, in multidimensional space, inliers can be detected through the use of the Mahalanobis' distance just as well as outliers: inliers have an abnormally low Mahalanobis' distance (they fall too close to the multivariate mean), while outliers have an abnormally high Mahalanobis' distance (they fall too far from the multivariate mean). The detection of inliers may be more useful to detect fraud than the detection of outliers, because fabricated data will tend not to contain outliers that are at higher risk of being detected than are values close to the (multivariate) mean. Robust methods such as using ranks in place of the observations are advisable for the detection of outliers, because these can create severe departures from multivariate normality.

When, as is often the case, some variables are measured repeatedly over the course of the trial on the same patient, these measures lend themselves well to a variety of checks. Here again, an insufficient variability over time may reveal

propagation of previous values rather than genuine observations. Sometimes the fraud involves a mechanism or computer algorithm for making up data.

In any trial with prolonged patient entry and follow-up, one can use calendar time to perform additional checks on the data. Simple checks can be performed on a specific day of the week, for instance, since certain events or examinations are unlikely to have taken place on a Sunday. Time intervals between successive visits and the number of visits per unit time provide further opportunities for checking the plausibility of a sequence of events. A comparison of treatment groups by week or month of RANDOMISATION can reveal suspect periods during which all treatments were not allocated with equal probability. Perfect compliance with the protocol in terms of dates may be a marker of fraud. More advanced checks can be useful, such as the stability of the variance of observations over time.

Randomised clinical trials constitute, by design, the most reliable type of medical experiment and their results are generally robust to occasional cases of data falsification and fabrication at some participating centres. The highly publicised case of fraud in the National Surgical Adjuvant Breast and Bowel Project (NSABP) provides a framework to examine the impact of such fraud on the results of clinical trials. Briefly, one of the investigators in breast cancer trials systematically altered some baseline patient data so that these patients became eligible for entry into the trials. The data subject to falsification were the date of surgery, the date of biopsy and estrogen receptor values. For example, in one study, the delay between the surgery and randomisation had been set to a maximum of 30 days by the trial protocol and dates were falsified for a few patients in whom this limit had been exceeded. The fraud was clearly not aimed at distorting the results of the trials one way or another and, indeed, a careful re-analysis of NSABP trial data with and without the fraudulent centre confirmed that the trial outcomes had not been materially affected by the fraud (Fisher, Anderson, Redmond et al., 1995). In another large published trial in stroke, all data from one centre suspected of fraud were excluded from the analysis, again with negligible impact on the study results (ESPS2 Group, 1997). Yet this centre had contributed to the study of 452 of the 7054 patients involved overall!

Fraud is unlikely to affect the results of a trial if any of the following conditions hold: the fraud is limited to one or a few investigators (perhaps one centre in a multicentre setting) and/or to a few data items, provided that there are many investigators or centres; the fraud bears on secondary variables that have little or no effect on the primary endpoint of the trial; the fraud affects all treatment groups equally, and hence does not bias the results of the trial. Fraud committed without regard to the treatment assignments (e.g. prior to randomisation or in double-blind trials) generates noise but no bias. At least one of these conditions frequently holds and therefore fraud should not be expected to have a major impact on the results of multi-centre clinical trials. One caveat is that where an increase in noise occurs, this can make dissimilar treatments appear similar. With a trend towards using equivalence or non-inferiority trials for licensing purposes this is of concern and could result in ineffective medicines being licensed.   *MB*

Buyse, M., George, S.L., Evans, S., Geller, N., Ranstam, J., Scherrer, B., Lesaffre, E., Murray, G., Edler, L., Hutton, J., Colton, T., Lachenbruch, P. and Verma, B. for the ISCB Subcommittee on Fraud 1999: The role of biostatistics in the prevention, detection and treatment of fraud in clinical trials. *Statistics in Medicine* 18, 3435–52. Canner, P.L., Huang, Y.B. and Meinert, C.L. 1981: On the detection of outlier clinics in medical and surgical trials: I. Practical considerations. *Controlled Clinical Trials* 2, 231–40. Evans, S. 1998: Fraud and misconduct in medical science. In Armitage, P. and Colton, T. (eds), *Encyclopaedia of biostatistics*. Chichester: John Wiley & Sons. ESPS2 Group 1997: European Stroke Prevention Study 2. Efficacy and safety data. *Journal of Neurological Sciences* 151, (Suppl) S1–S77. Fisher, B., Anderson, S. and Redmond, C.K. *et al.* 1995: Reanalysis and results after 12 years of follow-up in a randomised clinical trial comparing total mastectomy with lumpectomy with or without irradiation in the treatment of breast cancer. *New England Journal of Medicine* 333, 1456–61. Haldane, J.B.S. 1948: The faking of genetic results. *Eureka* 6, 21–8. Hill, T.P. 1998: The first-digit phenomenon. *American Scientist* 86, 358–63. Knatterud, G.L., Rockhold, F.W., George, S.L., Barton, F.B., Davis, C.E., Fairweather, W.R., Honohan, T., Mowery, R. and O'Neill, R.T. 1998: Guidelines for quality assurance procedures for multicenter trials: a position paper. *Controlled Clinical Trials* 19, 477–93. Lock, S. and Wells, F. (eds.) 1993: *Fraud and misconduct in medical research*. London: BMJ Publishing Group. Ranstam, J., Buyse, M., George, S.L., Evans, S., Geller, N., Scherrer, B., Lesaffre, E., Murray, G., Edler, L., Hutton, J., Colton, T., Lachenbruch, P. for the ISCB Subcommittee on Fraud 2000: The biostatistician's view of fraud in medical research. *Controlled Clinical Trials* 21, 415–27.

frequency distribution The division of a sample of observations into a number of classes together with a count of the number of observations falling in each class. Acts as a useful tabular summary of the main features of a data set, for example, location, shape and spread.   *BSE*

[See also HISTOGRAM, PROBABILITY DISTRIBUTION]

Friedman test

A non-parametric equivalent to REPEATED MEASURES ANALYSIS OF VARIANCE being an extension of the WILCOXON SIGNED RANK TEST to more than two groups or time points. It examines the ranks within a group and tests if the underlying continuous distribution is the same for each group. The null hypothesis is that there are no differences in medians between the groups. The alternative hypothesis is there is at least one difference in medians. The data should be continuous in nature and should be a randomly selected sample measured at different time points or blocks of matched subjects ran-

domly assigned to a group. Subjects or blocks of subjects should be independent. An extension to the test exists that allows repeated measures on each subject.

The test begins by constructing a two-way table with N (the number of subjects) rows and k (the number of time points) columns. Rank each row from lowest to highest, assigning the average rank to ties in the data. Find the sum of ranks in each of the columns. Calculate:

$$F_r = \frac{12}{Nk(k+1)}\left[\sum_{j=1}^{k} R_j^2\right] - \left[3N(k+1)\right]$$

where:

R_j = the sum of the ranks for column j
N = the number of subjects
k = the number of periods or conditions.

Compare F_r to the critical value in Friedman tables and reject the null hypothesis if F_r is greater than or equal to the critical value. If N and k are sufficiently large then chi-square tables with $k-1$ DEGREES OF FREEDOM can be used instead of Friedman tables.

As an example a study measured FEV_1 at three different times of day to see if there were a difference. Data can be found in the table.

To compute the Friedman test statistic:

$$\begin{aligned} F_r &= \frac{12}{Nk(k+1)}\left[\sum_{j=1}^{k} R_j^2\right] - \left[3N(k+1)\right] \\ &= \frac{12}{7 \times 3 \times (3+1)} \times \left[12^2 + 16.5^2 + 13.5^2\right] \\ &\quad - \left[3 \times 7 \times (3+1)\right] = 1.5 \end{aligned}$$

From the tables ($N = 7$, $k = 3$, $\alpha = 0.05$) the critical value is 7.714, as 1.5 is less than 7.714, there is insufficient evidence to reject the null hypothesis of no difference in medians between the three time points, so the medians can be considered unchanging across the time points.

When the Friedman test gives a significant result it is possible to do POST-HOC TESTING to see where any differences lie. There are two ways of doing this.

Use the Wilcoxon signed rank test pairwise on the groups applying a correction for multiple testing such as a BONFERRONI CORRECTION. Alternatively, the average ranks in each of the groups can be compared. The null hypothesis is rejected if the absolute difference in mean ranks is greater than or equal to the critical value as shown:

$$\left|\bar{R}_i - \bar{R}_j\right| \geq Z_{\alpha/[k(k-1)]} \times \sqrt{\frac{k(k+1)}{6N}}$$

where:

$\bar{R}_i$ = the mean rank in period or condition i
$\bar{R}_j$ = the mean rank in period or condition j
$Z_{\alpha'}$ = the critical Z value for α'
α' = $\alpha/[k(k-1)]$
k = the number of periods or conditions
N = the number of subjects   *SLV*

Conover, W.J. 1999: *Practical nonparametric statistics*, 3rd edn. Chichester: John Wiley & Sons. Pett, M.A. 1997: *Nonparametric statistics for health care research*. Thousand Oaks: Sage.

Friedman test *FEV₁ data from 7 subjects recorded at three times a day*

Morning	Rank	Afternoon	Rank	Evening	Rank
0.25	1	0.4	2.5	0.4	2.5
0.56	1	0.87	2	1.06	3
0.63	2	1.45	3	0.25	1
0.65	2	3.02	3	0.45	1
0.74	2	1.07	3	0.28	1
0.97	1	1.29	2	1.98	3
1.91	3	0.15	1	0.27	2
Rank sum	**12**	—	**16.5**	—	**13.5**

funnel plots   Funnel plots are a graphical device, used to detect publication BIAS in SYSTEMATIC REVIEWS AND META-ANALYSES. For each study in a review the estimated treatment effect is plotted against a measure of trial precision such as the VARIANCE or standard error of the treatment effect or the study sample size (Light and Pillemar, 1984). In a departure from standard graphical practice, the plots conventionally depict precision on the vertical axis and treatment effect on the horizontal axis. The meta-analytical summary may be marked by a vertical line. When all study results are published it is expected that the studies will have a symmetrical distribution around the average effect line, the spread of studies with low precision being larger than that of studies with high precision, yielding a funnel-like shape. Some graphs mark the funnel with lines within which 95% of studies would fall were there no between-study heterogeneity. The choice of the measure of treatment effect (Tang and Liu, 2000) and the measure of precision (Sterne and Egger, 2001) makes a difference to the shape of the plot. Plots of treatment effects against standard errors are usually to be preferred, as the funnel will have straight rather than curvilinear sides.

Studies of the causes of publication bias have indicated non-publication is often linked to studies with non-significant P-VALUES, which tend to be the smaller studies reporting null or small effects (Dickersin, 1997). Suppression of these studies creates a visual hole in the plot. Unless the intervention has no effect, this will bias the meta-analysis and induce asymmetry into the plot. Tests of publication bias, such as the Begg (Begg and Mazumdar, 1994) and Egger tests (Egger *et al.*, 1997), are testing for this asymmetry. The trim-and-fill method of investigating the impact of publication bias (Duval and Tweedie, 2000) imputes missing studies with results designed to remove asymmetry from the plot.

Interpretation of funnel plots is often visually difficult due to there being inadequate numbers of studies. Assessing the causes of funnel plot asymmetry is also difficult as between study heterogeneity, relationships betweens study quality and sample size, as well as publication bias can all cause similar patterns in funnel plots (Egger *et al.*, 1997). An example of a funnel plot is given in the SYSTEMATIC REVIEWS AND META-ANALYSIS entry.   *JD*

[See also FOREST PLOTS]

Begg, C.B. and Mazumdar, M. 1994: Operating characteristics of a rank correlation test for publication bias. *Biometrics* 50, 4, 1088–101. **Dickersin, K.** 1997: How important is publication bias? A synthesis of available data. *AIDS Education and Prevention* 9, (Suppl) 15–21. **Duval, S. and Tweedie, R.L.** 2000: Trim-and-fill: a simple funnel plot based method of testing and adjusting for publication bias in meta-analysis. *Biometrics* 56, 2, 455–63. **Egger, M., Davey Smith, G., Schneider, M. and Minder, C.** 1997: Bias in meta-analysis detected by a simple, graphical test. *British Medical Journal* 315, 7109, 629–34. **Light, R.J. and Pillemar, D.B.** 1984: *Summing up: the science of reviewing research.* Cambridge, MA: Harvard University Press. **Sterne, J.A.C. and Egger, M.** 2001: Funnel plots for detecting bias in meta-analysis: guidelines on choice of axis. *Journal of Clinical Epidemiology* 54, 1046–55. **Tang, J.-L. and Liu, J.L.Y.** 2000: Misleading funnel plots for detection of bias in meta-analysis. *Journal of Clinical Epidemiology* 53, 477–84.

G

gamma distribution A PROBABILITY DISTRIBUTION for non-negative values defined by two parameters, here denoted λ and t (where t must be greater than 1), with the density function:

$$f(x) = \frac{1}{\Gamma(t)} \lambda^t x^{t-1} e^{-\lambda x}$$

Here t defines the shape of the distribution, while λ defines the scale on which the distribution is observed. The $\Gamma(t)$ expression is the gamma function that for integer values of t is equal to $(t-1)!$ (factorial). The MEAN of the distribution is t/λ and the VARIANCE is t/λ^2.

If events take place as part of a Poisson process, i.e. the time between successive events can be modelled as taking the EXPONENTIAL DISTRIBUTION with parameter λ, then the time between any two events will take a gamma distribution. The gamma distribution can then arise as the distribution of the sum of exponentially distributed variables. It is also the case that the exponential distribution is a special case of the gamma distribution. The CHI-SQUARE DISTRIBUTION is also a special case, and given two variables A and B which have gamma distributions, it is possible to create a variable A/(A+B) that has a BETA DISTRIBUTION. Gamma distributions with the same scale parameter will sum to another gamma distribution with that scale parameter.

The gamma distribution is always positively skewed (of little surprise since it is constrained at zero on the left-hand side, but the tail extends to infinity on the right-hand side), but the SKEWNESS diminishes as t tends to infinity where the NORMAL DISTRIBUTION is the limiting distribution. For some illustration of the shapes that the gamma distribution can take see the illustration in the chi-square distribution article.

The gamma is sometimes used to model times to event as has been suggested. For example in Phillips *et al.* (1994) where it is used to model the time to develop AIDS. Often, however, it is merely a convenient distribution for a quantity that cannot be negative. In Bayesian analyses (see BAYESIAN METHODS), it is of use as the conjugate prior for the mean of a POISSON DISTRIBUTION, but most commonly as the conjugate prior for the inverse of the variance of a normal distribution. *AGL*

Gelman, A., Carlin, J.B., Stern, H.S. and Rubin, D.B. 1995: *Bayesian data analysis*. Boca Rotan: Chapman & Hall/CRC. **Grimmet, G.R. and Stirzaker, D.R.** 1992: *Probability and random processes*, 2nd edn. Oxford: Clarendon Press. **Leemis, L. M.** 1986: Relationships among common univariate distributions. *The American Statistician* 40, 2, 143–6. **Phillips, A.N, Sabin, C.A., Elford, J., Bofill, M., Janossy, G. and Lee, C.A.** 1994: Use of CD4 lymphocyte count to predict long-term survival free of AIDS after HIV infection. *British Medical Journal* 309, 309–13.

general fertility rate (GFR) See DEMOGRAPHY

generalised additive models (GAMs) Models that allow possible nonlinear relationships between a response variable and one or more explanatory variables to be accounted for in a flexible manner. Generalised additive models are most useful in situations where the relationship between the variables is expected to be of a complex form, not easily fitted by standard methods or where there is no *a priori* reason for using a particular model. In generalised additive models, the $\beta_j x_i$ term of MULTIPLE LINEAR REGRESSION and LOGISTIC REGRESSION is replaced by a 'smooth' function of the explanatory variable x_i, as suggested by the observed data (Everitt, 2002).

The building blocks of generalised additive models are SCATTERPLOT SMOOTHERS such as locally weighted regression fits and spline functions. Generalised additive models work by replacing the regression coefficients found in other regression models by the fit from one or other of these 'smoothers'. In this way, the strong assumptions about the relationships of the response to each explanatory variable implicit in standard regression models are avoided. Details of how such models are fitted to data are given in Hastie and Tibshirani (1990).

Generalised additive models provide a useful addition to the tools available for exploring the relationship between a response variable and a set of explanatory variables. Such models allow possible nonlinear terms in the latter to be discovered and then perhaps to be modelled in terms of a suitable, more familiar, low-degree polynomial. Generalised additive models can deal with nonlinearity in covariates that are not the main interest in a study and adjust for such effects appropriately. *BSE*

[See also GENERALISED LINEAR MODELS]

Everitt, B.S. 2002: *Modern medical statistics*. London: Arnold. **Hastie, T.J. and Tibshirani, R.J.** 1990: *Generalized additive models*. Boca Raton: CRC Press/Chapman & Hall.

generalised estimating equations GEE is a popular method for analysing clustered data such as REPEATED MEASURES DATA.

Let there be $i = 1, ..., n_j$ observations for each cluster j, $j = 1, ..., N$. In a repeated measures setting, the clusters would typically be subjects. The MEAN or expectation μ_{ij} of the responses y_{ij} given a vector of covariates $\mathbf{x}'_{ij} = (x_{1ij}, ..., x_{pij})$ is modelled using a GENERALISED LINEAR MODEL:

$$g[\mathrm{E}(y_{ij} \mid x_{ij})] \equiv g(\mu_{ij}) = \beta_0 + \beta_1 x_{1ij} + ... + \beta_p x_{pij}$$

where $g(\cdot)$ is a link function and β_0 to β_p are regression parameters. For example, an identity link gives a LINEAR REGRESSION MODEL and a logit link a logistic regression model.

The model is exactly the same as a generalised linear model for independent data. The interpretation of the regression parameters is therefore not affected by the nature of the within-cluster dependence between the responses. This is in contrast to RANDOM EFFECTS MODELS, where the regression parameters represent the *conditional* or *subject-specific* effects of covariates given the random effects. These effects will often differ from the *marginal* or population-averaged *effects* estimated using GEE. This difference is illustrated for a logit link (logistic regression) in the Figure. Here the thin curves represent subject-specific relationships between the probability that the response equals 1 and a covariate x for a random intercept logistic regression model, where the horizontal shifts are due to different values of the random intercept. The thick curve represents the population-averaged relationship, formed by averaging the thin curves for each value of x. The slope of the population-averaged curve is flatter than the slopes of the subject-specific curves. Therefore the population-averaged regression parameters tend to be attenuated (closer to zero) relative to the subject-specific regression parameters. Note that the distinction between subject-specific and population-averaged effects disappears when an identity link is used and, for RANDOM INTERCEPT MODELS, when a log link is used.

As in conventional generalised linear models, the variances of the responses given the covariates are assumed to be $\text{Var}(y_{ij}|x_{ij}) = \phi V(\mu_{ij})$, where the variance function $V(\mu_{ij})$ is determined by the choice of distribution family. For instance, for dichotomous responses, the Bernoulli distribution implies that $V(\mu_{ij}) = \mu_{ij}(1 - \mu_{ij})$, whereas for count data, the POISSON DISTRIBUTION implies that $V(\mu_{ij}) = \mu_{ij}$. Since overdispersion is common in clustered data, the dispersion parameter ϕ is typically estimated even if the distribution requires $\phi = 1$.

The feature of GEE that differs from usual generalised linear models is that different responses y_{ij} and $y_{i'j}$ for a cluster j are allowed to be correlated given the covariates. These correlations are typically assumed to have a simple structure parameterised by a small number of α-parameters. One of the following correlation structures is commonly used.

Independence: The responses are independent given the covariates:

$$\text{Cor}(y_{ij}, y_{i'j}|x_{ij}) = 0$$

Exchangeable: All pairs of responses for the same cluster have the same correlation given the covariates:

$$\text{Cor}(y_{ij}, y_{i'j}|x_{ij}) = \alpha, \; i \neq i'$$

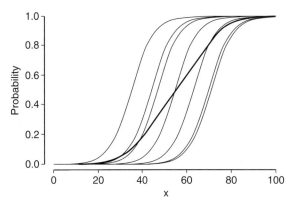

generalised estimating equation *Conditional and marginal logistic relationships*

AR(1): The correlations between pairs of responses for the same cluster (given the covariates) fall off exponentially as the time lag between them increases (for longitudinal data only):

$$\text{Cor}(y_{ij}, y_{i+t,j}|x_{ij}) = \alpha^t, \; |\alpha| < 1 \; t = 0, 1, ..., n_j - i$$

Unstructured: The correlation matrix of the responses given the covariates is estimated freely, without restrictions:

$$\text{Cor}(y_{ij}, y_{i'j}|x_{ij}) = \alpha_{ii'}, \; i \neq i'$$

For given values of the regression parameters β_1 to β_p, the α-parameters of the *working correlation matrix* can be estimated along with the dispersion parameter ϕ (see Zeger and Liang, 1986, for details). These estimates can then be used in so-called *generalised estimating equations* to obtain estimates of the regression parameters. Since estimation of the correlation and dispersion parameters requires knowledge of the regression parameters and vice versa, the GEE algorithm proceeds by iterating between (1) estimation of the regression parameters using the correlation and dispersion parameters from the previous iteration; and (2) estimation of the correlation and dispersion parameters using the regression parameters from the previous iteration. Eventually, the algorithm converges, producing the same estimates in successive iterations.

It has been demonstrated that the estimated *marginal* effects β_1 to β_p are consistent, that is the estimates approach the true values as the number of clusters increases. Importantly, these estimates are 'robust' in the sense that they are consistent for mis-specified correlation structures, assuming that the mean structure is correctly specified. Consistent estimates of the COVARIANCE MATRIX of the estimated marginal effects are next obtained by means of the so-called sandwich estimator.

The Madras Longitudinal Schizophrenia Study followed up 44 female patients monthly after their first hospitalisation for schizophrenia (see RANDOM EFFECT MODELS FOR DISCRETE LONGITUDINAL DATA for the data). We will use GEE to investigate whether the course of illness differs between patients with early and late onset. The three variables considered are: [Month]: number of months since first hospitalisation; [Early]: early onset (1: before age 20, 0: at age 20 or later); [y]: repeated measures of thought disorder (1: present, 0: absent).

Here we consider a subset of the data, namely on whether thought disorder [y] was present or not at 0, 2, 4, 6, 8 and 10 months after hospitalisation. Letting y_{it} be the repeated measurement of thought disorder at occasion i for patient j, we consider a dichotomous logistic regression model:

$$\ln \left(\frac{\text{Pr}(y_{ij} = 1|x_{ij})}{1 - \text{Pr}(y_{ij} = 1|x_{ij})} \right) = \beta_0 + \beta_1 x_{1ij} + ... + \beta_p x_{pij}.$$

We use GEE with independence and exchangeable working correlations to estimate a model with explanatory variables [Month], [Early] and the interaction [Early] × [Month], allowing us to investigate the linear trend of time (for the log odds) as well as differences between times of onset, not just in the overall odds of thought disorder but also in the trend over time (see Table on page 148).

147

generalised estimating equations *Estimated regression parameters from GEE with independence and exchangeable correlation structures*

	GEE independent		GEE exchangeable	
	Est	*('Sandwich' SE)*	*Est*	*('Sandwich' SE)*
β_0 [Cons]	0.69	(0.35)	0.71	(0.35)
β_1 [Month]	−0.27	(0.07)	−0.28	(0.07)
β_2 [Early]	0.04	(0.67)	0.10	(0.69)
β_3 [Early] × [Month]	−0.04	(0.11)	−0.04	(0.11)

The estimates assuming an exchangeable correlation structure suggest that there is a decline over time in the odds of thought disorder in the late-onset patients (odds ratio = exp(–0.28) = 0.76 per month). However, the early-onset patients do not appear to have an appreciably greater odds of thought disorder at baseline (odds ratio = exp(0.10) = 1.11) or a greater decline in the odds over time (odds ratio = exp(–0.04) = 0.96).

A definite merit of GEE is that valid inferences are produced for population-averaged effects as long as the mean structure is correctly specified, even if the dependence structure is mis-specified. However, there are also a number of limitations. The estimates are consistent only under the restrictive assumption that the probability that a response is missing does not depend on other responses for the same cluster. Although GEE is often said to require that responses are missing completely at random (MCAR), missingness may in fact depend on covariates included in the model. Another limitation is that it is in general difficult to assess model adequacy in GEE; likelihood-based diagnostics are for instance not available. The use of GEE should furthermore be reserved to problems where marginal or population-averaged effects are of interest and avoided in analyses of aetiology. This is because causal processes operate at the cluster or individual level, not the population level. Population-averaged effects are therefore merely descriptive and largely determined by the degree of heterogeneity in the population. Finally, the estimated regression parameters are no longer consistent if 'baseline' (initial) responses are included as covariates for longitudinal data (Crouchley and Davies, 1999).

See Diggle *et al.* (2002) for a thorough treatment of GEE and Lindsey and Lambert (1998) for a critical evaluation. *AS/SRH*

Crouchley, R. and Davies, R.B. 1999: A comparison of population average and random effects models for the analysis of longitudinal count data with base-line information. *Journal of the Royal Statistical Society Series A* 162, 331–47. **Diggle, P.J., Heagerty, P., Liang, K.-Y. and Zeger, S.L.** 2002: *Analysis of longitudinal data.* Oxford: Oxford University Press. **Lindsey, J.K. and Lambert, P.** 1998: On the appropriateness of marginal models for repeated measurements in clinical trials. *Statistics in Medicine* 17, 447–69. **Zeger, S.L. and Liang, K.-Y.** 1986: Longitudinal data analysis for discrete and continuous outcomes. *Biometrics* 42, 121–30.

generalised linear model (GLM)

A unified framework for regression models introduced in a landmark paper by Nelder and Wedderburn (1972) over 30 years ago. A wide range of statistical models including ANALYSIS OF VARIANCE, ANALYSIS OF COVARIANCE, MULTIPLE LINEAR REGRESSION and LOGISTIC REGRESSION are included in the GLM framework. A comprehensive technical account of the model is given in McCullagh and Nelder (1989) with a more concise description appearing in Dobson (2001) and Cook (1998).

The term 'regression' was first introduced by Francis Galton in the 19th century to characterise a tendency to mediocrity, that is, towards the average, observed in the offspring of parent seeds and used by Karl Pearson in a study of the heights of fathers and sons. The sons' heights tended, on average, to be less extreme than the fathers' (see REGRESSION TO THE MEAN). In essence, all forms of regression have as their aim the development and assessment of a mathematical model for the relationship between a response variable, y, and a set of q explanatory variables, $x_1, x_2,...,x_q$. Multiple linear regression, for example, involves the following model for y:

$$y = \beta_0 + \beta_1 x_1 +...+ \beta_q x_q + \varepsilon$$

where β_0, β_1, ..., β_q are regression coefficients that have to be estimated from sample data and ε is an error term assumed normally distributed with zero mean and a constant variance σ^2.

An equivalent way of writing the multiple regression model is as:

$$y \sim N(\mu,\sigma^2)$$

where $\mu = \beta_0 + \beta_1 x_1 +...+ \beta_q x_q$. This makes it clear that this model is only suitable for continuous response variables with, conditional on the values of the explanatory variables, a normal distribution with constant variance. Analysis of variance is essentially exactly the same model with x_1, x_2,...,x_q being dummy variables coding factor levels and interactions between factors; analysis of covariance is also the same model with a mixture of continuous and categorical explanatory variables.

The assumption of the conditional normality of a continuous response variable is one that is probably made more often than it is warranted. And there are many situations where such an assumption is clearly not justified. One example is where the response is a binary variable (e.g. improved, not improved), another is where it is a count (e.g. number of correct answers in some testing situation). The question then arises as to how the multiple regression model can be modified to allow such responses to be related to the explanatory variables of interest. In the GLM approach, the generalisation of the multiple regression model consists of allowing the following three assumptions associated with this model to be modified: the response variable is normally distributed with a mean determined by the model; the mean can be modelled as a linear function of (possibly nonlinear transformations) of the explanatory variables, i.e. the effects of the explanatory variable on the mean are additive; the variance of the response variable given the (predicted) mean is constant.

In a GLM, some transformation of the mean is modelled by a linear function of the explanatory variables and the distribution of the response around its mean (often referred to as the *error distribution*) is generalised usually in a way that fits naturally with a particular transformation. The result is a very wide class of regression models. The essential components of a GLM are: a linear predictor, η, formed from the explanatory variables:

$$\eta = \beta_0 + \beta_1 x_1 + \beta_2 x_2 + \ldots + \beta_q x_q$$

A transformation of the mean, μ, of the response variable called the *link function*, $g(\mu)$. In a GLM it is $g(\mu)$ which is modelled by the linear predictor:

$$g(\mu) = \eta$$

In multiple linear regression and analysis of variance, the link function is the identity function. Other link functions include the log, logit, probit, inverse and power TRANSFORMATIONS, although the log and logit are those most commonly met in practice. The logit link, for example, is the basis of logistic regression.

The distribution of the response variable given its mean μ is assumed to be a distribution from the EXPONENTIAL FAMILY. Distributions in the exponential family include the normal distribution, the BINOMIAL DISTRIBUTION, POISSON DISTRIBUTION, GAMMA DISTRIBUTION and EXPONENTIAL DISTRIBUTION.

Particular link function in GLMs are naturally associated with particular error distributions, for example, the identity link with the Gaussian distribution, the logit with the binomial and the log with the Poisson. In these cases, the term *canonical link* is used.

The choice of PROBABILITY DISTRIBUTION determines the relationships between the variance of the response variable (conditional on the explanatory variables) and its mean. This relationship is known as the *variance function*, denoted $\phi V(\mu)$. Both the Poisson and binomial distributions have variance functions that are completely determined by the mean. There is no free parameter for the variance since in applications of the generalised linear model with binomial or Poisson error distributions the dispersion parameter, ϕ, is defined to be one. But in some applications this becomes too restrictive fully to account for the empirical variance in the data; in such cases it is common to describe the phenomenon as overdispersion. For example, if the response variable is the proportion of family members who have been ill in the past year, observed in a large number of families, then the individual binary observations that make up the observed proportions are likely to be correlated rather than independent. This non-independence can lead to a variance that is greater (less) than that on the assumption of binomial variability. And observed counts often exhibit larger variance than would be expected from the Poisson assumption, a fact noted by Greenwood and Yule nearly a century ago (Greenwood and Yule, 1920). Greenwood and Yule's suggested solution to the problem was a model

in which μ was a random variable with a gamma distribution leading to a NEGATIVE BINOMIAL DISTRIBUTION for the count.

Estimation of the parameters in a GLM is usually carried out through MAXIMUM LIKELIHOOD. Details are given in Dobson (2001). Having estimated the parameters the question of the fit of the model for the sample data will need to be addressed. Clearly, a researcher needs to be satisfied that the chosen model describes the data adequately before drawing conclusions and making interpretations about the parameters themselves. In practice, most interest will lie in comparing the fit of competing models, particularly in the context of selecting subsets of explanatory variables so as to achieve a more parsimonious model. In GLMs a measure of fit is provided by a quantity known as the DEVIANCE. This is, essentially a statistic that measures how closely the model-based fitted values of the response approximate the observed values; the deviance quoted in most examples of GLM fitting is actually −2 times the maximised log-likelihood for a model, so that differences in deviances of competing models give a LIKELIHOOD RATIO TEST for comparing the models. A more detailed account of the assessment of fit for GLMs is given in Dobson (2002).

We can illustrate an application of GLM using the data shown in the first Table on page 150, which are given in Haberman (1978) and also in Seeber (1998). They arise from asking randomly chosen household members from a probability sample of a town in the USA which stressful events had occurred within the last 18 months and to report the month of occurrence of these events. A SCATTERPLOT of the data (see first Figure) indicates a decline in the number of events as these lay further in the past, the result perhaps of the fallibility of human memory.

Since the response variable here is a count that can only take zero or positive values it would not be appropriate to use multiple linear regression here to investigate the relationship of recalls to time. Instead, we shall apply a GLM with a log link function so that fitted values are constrained to be positive and as error distribution use the Poisson distribution, which is suitable for count data. These two assumptions lead to what is usually labelled *Poisson regression*. Explicitly, the model to be fitted to the mean number of recalls, μ is:

$$\log(\mu) = \beta_0 + \beta_1 \text{ time}$$

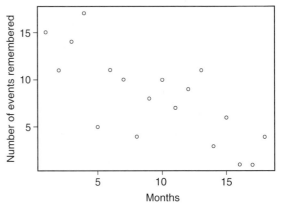

generalised linear model *Plot of recalled memories data*

149

generalised linear model *Distribution by months prior to interview of stressful events reported from subjects; 147 subjects reporting exactly one stressful event in the period from 1 to 18 months prior to interview*

Time	y
1	15
2	11
3	14
4	17
5	5
6	11
7	10
8	4
9	8
10	10
11	7
12	9
13	11
14	3
15	6
16	1
17	1
18	4

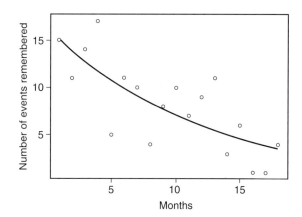

generalised linear model *Recalled memories data showing fitted Poisson regression model*

McCullagh, P. and Nelder, J.A. 1989: *Generalised linear models*, 2nd edn. London: Chapman & Hall. **Nelder, J.A. and Wedderburn, R.W.M.** 1972: Generalised linear models. *Journal of the Royal Statistical Society Series A* 135, 370–84. **Seeber, G.U.H.** 1998: Poisson regression. In Armitage, P. and Colton, T. (eds), *Encyclopedia of biostatistics*. Chichester: John Wiley & Sons.

The results of the fitting procedure are shown in the second Table.

The estimated regression coefficient for time is –0.084 with an estimated standard error of 0.017. Exponentiating this last equation and inserting the estimated parameter values gives the model in terms of the fitted counts rather than their logs, i.e.:

$$\hat{\mu} = 16.5 \times 0.920^{\text{time}}$$

The scatterplot of the original data now also showing the fitted model is given in the second Figure. The difference in deviance of the null model with no explanatory variables and one including time as an explanatory variable is large, which clearly indicates that the regression coefficient for time is not zero.   *BSE*

[See also GENERALISED ESTIMATING EQUATIONS]

Cook, R.J. 1998: Generalised linear models. In Armitage, P. and Colton, T. (eds), *Encyclopedia of biostatistics*. Chichester: John Wiley & Sons. **Dobson, A.J.** 2001: *An introduction to generalized linear models*, 2nd edn. Boca Raton: Chapman & Hall/CRC. **Greenwood, M. and Yule, G.U.** 1920: An inquiry into the nature of frequency distributions of multiple happenings. *Journal of the Royal Statistical Society* 83, 255. **Haberman, S.** 1978: *Analysis of qualitative data*. Vol. I. New York: Academic Press.

generalised linear model *Results of a Poisson regression*

Covariates	Estimated regression coefficient	Standard error	Estimate/SE
(Intercept)	2.803	0.148	18.920
Time	–0.084	0.017	–4.987

Dispersion parameter for Poisson family taken to be 1; null deviance: 50.84 on 17 degrees of freedom; residual deviance: 24.57 on 16 degrees of freedom

genetic epidemiology Study of the genetic aspects of the patterns of disease and other biological traits. Although, conceptually, genetic epidemiology is a branch of epidemiology, it has developed from distinct historical roots and employs different study designs, methods of statistical analysis and terminology.

Genetic epidemiology is usually distinguished from population genetics, which emphasises the genetics of populations over time and its relation to factors such as population structure and selection. The statistical component of these and related areas is referred to as *statistical genetics*.

The central themes in genetic epidemiology are the identification of genes related to disease or other traits and the evaluation of risks associated with different genetic variants. There is a major emphasis in genetic epidemiology on family studies (*pedigree analysis*). Indeed, some authors have considered that familial factors in disease, whether or not genetic, are an essential component of genetic epidemiology. Here we outline some of the main analytical approaches in genetic epidemiology.

A genetic epidemiological analysis often starts with descriptive studies of familial aggregation. *Twin studies* are important in this context, because comparison of MZ and DZ twins allows genetic effects to be separated from shared environmental influences on risk. For binary traits such as diseases, familial aggregation is often described in terms of *familial relative risks*. These are defined as the ratio of the risk of the disease in a relative of affected individual to the risk of the disease in the general population. The size of the familial relative risk and its variation by type of relative can give clues to the genetic model underlying the disease. For quantitative traits, familial aggregation may be described in terms of correlations in trait values between relatives.

Another important statistical approach in genetic epidemiology is SEGREGATION ANALYSIS. The aim of segregation analysis is to fit different genetic models to diseases in pedigrees. These may include models involving a single genetic locus or multiple loci. The models are parameterised in terms of the frequencies of alleles and the risks of disease associated with each genotype. Measured or unmeasured environmental risk factors might also be included in the model. Models are usually fitted by computing likelihoods and using a MAXIMUM LIKELIHOOD APPROACH. Efficient algorithms, called peeling algorithms, are available for likelihood computation in large or complex pedigrees, although alternative approaches, such a MARKOV CHAIN MONTE CARLO algorithm, are sometimes necessary.

An important concept in pedigree analysis is *ascertainment*. Analysis is usually conducted on a series of pedigrees that have been collected because of the presence of some trait. It is important to define the part of the data leading to the ascertainment of the pedigree and make appropriate adjustment for it in the analysis, by constructing the appropriate conditional likelihood.

There are two main approaches to the mapping of disease genes: GENETIC LINKAGE studies and ASSOCIATION studies. Genetic linkage studies are based on the inheritance of traits within families. They rely on the fact that loci that are close together on the same chromosome tend to be co-inherited (linked), whereas loci far apart will be inherited independently, due to process of *recombination* at meiosis. The probability of a recombination between two genetic loci is called the *recombination fraction* (usually represented θ). In a family with multiple cases of a disease, the diseased individuals will tend to share alleles at loci that are close to the disease gene. In this way, the entire genome can be examined for evidence of linkage using a limited number of genetic markers whose position in the genome is known. The statistical analysis of genetic linkage data aims to determine whether the pattern of co-inheritance of disease and marker genotype is different from what one would expect under the null hypothesis of no linkage.

Statistical analysis of genetic linkage studies can be of two types: parametric and non-parametric (or model free). In parametric linkage analysis, a particular disease model is specified and likelihoods are then constructed for different values of the recombination fraction. Linkage evidence is often summarised in terms a *LOD score*, defined as $\log_{10}$ of the ratio of the likelihood of the data for a particular recombination fraction to the likelihood under no linkage.

Model-free linkage analysis is based on the sharing of marker alleles among affected individuals in pedigrees. The aim is to determine whether the number of marker alleles at a given time shared by affected individuals is greater than would be expected by chance. This approach is popular in the study of genetically complex disease where the disease model is unknown. It is often used in the study of affected sibling pairs, which is a common study disease for linkage in complex traits, but the approach has been generalised to more general pedigrees. Linkage analysis is implemented in several programs, including LINKAGE and GENEHUNTER.

Linkage analysis is a good approach for identifying genes that have a large effect on disease risk, but tend to lack power to identify loci that have a moderate effect on risk. Association studies evaluate directly the association between specific genetic variants and the trait of interest. They are the method of choice for identifying genes of weak effect. For diseases these are usually CASE-CONTROL STUDIES with unrelated cases and controls. Such studies can be analysed using standard case-control approaches. It is also possible to conduct association studies using within family controls. This approach can eliminate problems of uncontrolled confounding. One commonly used design is to genotype a series of cases of the disease together with their two parents. The case genotypes are then compared with the alleles in the parents that are not transmitted to the affected case. This approach leads to the transmission distortion test (TDT).

Genetic association may arise due to a causal association with the polymorphism of interest or because of a true association with a neighbouring polymorphism. The latter can arise because genotypes at neighbouring polymorphisms tend to be correlated. Polymorphisms arise by mutation at one point in the history of a population, on a particular chromosome with a particular *haplotype* of marker alleles. A newly arising allele will therefore be in association with the alleles at neighbouring loci and this association will be maintained in the population if the loci are close together. This phenomenon is known as *linkage disequilibrium*. To elucidate fully the association at a particular locus, it may be necessary to extend the analysis to the joint effects of multiple markers.   *DE*

[See also GENOTYPE/PHENOTYPE]

Balding, D.J., Bishop, M. and Cannings, C. (eds) 2001: *Handbook of statistical genetics.* Chichester: John Wiley & Sons. **Khoury, M.J., Beaty, T.H. and Cohen, B.H.** 1993: *Fundamentals of genetic epidemiology.* Oxford: Oxford University Press. **Sham, P.** 1998: *Statistics in human genetics.* London: Arnold. **Terwilliger, J.D. and Ott, J.** 1994: *Analysis of human genetic linkage*, 3rd edn. Baltimore: Johns Hopkins University Press.

genetic linkage The non-independent segregation of the alleles at genetic loci close to one another on the same chromosome. Mendel's law of segregation states that an individual with heterozygous genotype (Aa) has equal probability of transmitting either allele (A or a) to an offspring. The same is true of any other locus with alleles B and b. Under Mendel's second law, that of independent assortment, the probabilities of transmitting the four possible combinations of alleles (AB, Ab, aB, ab) are all equal, namely one-quarter. This law is, however, only true for pairs of loci that are on separate chromosomes. For two loci that are on the same chromosome (known technically as syntenic), the probabilities of the four gametic classes (AB, Ab, aB, ab) are not equal, with an excess of the same allelic combinations as those that were transmitted to the individual from his or her parents. In other words, if the individual received the allelic combination AB from one parent and ab from the other, then he or she will transmit these same combinations with greater probability than the others (i.e. Ab and aB). The former allelic combinations are known as parental types and the latter recombinants. The strength of genetic linkage between two loci is measured by the recombination fraction, defined as the probability that a recombinant of the two loci is transmitted to an offspring. Recombination fraction ranges from 0 (complete linkage) to 0.5 (complete absence of linkage).

Recombinant gametes of two syntenic loci are generated by the crossing over of homologous chromosomes at certain semi-random locations during meiosis. The smaller the distance between two syntenic loci, the less likely that they will be separated by crossing over and therefore the smaller the recombination fraction. A recombination of 0.01 corresponds approximately to a genetic map distance of 1 centiMorgan (cM). The crossing-over rate varies between males and females and for different chromosomal regions, but on average a genetic distance of 1 cM corresponds approximately to a physical distance of one million DNA base pairs. The total genetic length of the human genome is approximately 3500 cM.

For many decades linkage analysis was restricted to Mendelian phenotypes such as the ABO blood groups and HLA antigens. Recent developments in molecular genetics have enabled non-functional polymorphisms to be detected and measured. Standard sets of such genetic markers, evenly spaced throughout the entire genome, have been developed for systematic linkage analysis to localise genetic variants that increase the risk of disease. This is a particularly attractive method of mapping the genes for diseases since no knowledge of the pathophysiology is required. For this reason, the use of linkage analysis to map disease genes is also called *positional cloning*.

Linkage analysis in humans presents interesting statistical challenges. For Mendelian diseases, the challenges are those of variable pedigree structure and size and the common occurrence of MISSING DATA. The standard method of analysis involves calculating the likelihood with respect to the recombination fraction between disease and marker loci or the map position of the disease locus in relation to a set of marker loci, while the disease model is assumed known (e.g. dominant or recessive). Traditionally, the strength of evidence for linkage is summarised as a lod score, defined as the common (i.e. base 10) logarithm of the ratio of the likelihood given a certain recombination fraction to that under no linkage. A lod score of 3 or more is conventionally regarded as significant evidence of linkage. For Mendelian disorders, 98% of reports of linkage that meet this criterion have been subsequently confirmed. Linkage analysis has successfully localised and identified the genes for hundreds of Mendelian disorders.

Locus heterogeneity in linkage analysis refers to the situation where the mode of inheritance, but not the actual disease locus, is the same across different pedigrees. In other words, there are multiple disease loci that are indistinguishable from each other both in terms of manifestations at the individual level and in the pattern of familial transmission. Under these circumstances, the power to detect linkage is much diminished, even with lod scores modified to take account of locus heterogeneity, especially for samples consisting of small pedigrees.

For common diseases that do not show a simple Mendelian pattern of inheritance and are therefore likely to be the result of multiple genetic and environmental factors, linkage analysis is a more difficult task. For such diseases we typically would have an idea of the overall importance of genetic factors (i.e. HERITABILITY) but no detailed knowledge of genetic architecture in terms of the number of vulnerability genes or the magnitude of their effects. There are two major approaches to the linkage analysis of such complex diseases. The first is to adopt a lod score approach, but modified to allow for a number of more or less realistic models for the genotype–phenotype relationship and to adjust the largest lod score over these models for multiple testing. The second approach is 'model free' in the sense that a disease model does not have to be specified for the analysis. Instead, the analysis proceeds by defining some measure of allele sharing between individuals in a pedigree and relating the extent allele sharing to phenotypic similarity. One popular version of model-free linkage analysis is the affected sib-pair method, which is based on the detection of excessive allele sharing at a marker locus for a sample of sibling pairs where both members are affected by the disorder. The usual definition of allele sharing in model-free linkage analysis is 'identity-by-descent, which refers to alleles that are descended from (and are therefore replicates of) a single ancestral allele in a recent common ancestor. Algorithms for estimating the extent of local IBD from marker genotype data have been developed.

Methods of linkage analysis have been developed also for quantitative traits (e.g. blood pressure, body mass index). A particularly simple method is based on a regression of phenotypic similarity on allele sharing. A more sophisticated approach is based on a VARIANCE components model, in which a component of variance is specified to have covariance between relatives that is proportional to the extent of allele sharing between relatives.

Regardless of the statistical method used for the linkage analysis of complex traits, there are two major inherent limitations of the approach. The first is that the sample sizes required to detect a locus with a small effect size are very large, potentially many thousands of families. The second is the low resolving power, in that the region that shows linkage is typically very broad, covering a region with potentially hundreds of genes. For these reasons linkage is usually combined with association strategy in the search for the genetic determinants of multigenic diseases.

PS

[See also ALLELIC ASSOCIATION, GENETIC EPIDEMIOLOGY, HAPLOTYPE ANALYSIS]

Sham, P. 1997: *Statistics in human genetics*. London: Arnold.

genotype Genotype describes the genetic make-up of an individual or organism, usually referring to a particular gene or genetic locus. Different genotypes arise at loci in a genome where there are differences in DNA sequence – such loci are said to be *polymorphic* and the sequence differences are referred to as *alleles*. Alleles that are strongly associated with a particular disease or trait may be referred to as MUTATIONS. The genotype of an individual at a particular locus is then the combination of alleles at that location. In humans and other higher organisms, individuals inherit two copies of each gene, one from each parent (except those on the sex chromosomes in males). A genotype at a single locus therefore refers to a pair of alleles.

For example, the gene encoding the ABO blood group has three commonly recognised alleles, known as A, B and O. There are therefore six possible genotypes: (A,A), (A,B), (B,B), (A,O), (B,O) and (O,O).

One may also consider the genotypes at several loci together. For example, suppose there are two polymorphic loci in a particular gene or region with alleles A1 and A2 at the first locus and B1 and B2 at the second locus.

The multi-locus genotype for an individual may consist of A1-B1 on one chromosome and A2-B2 on the other. The combination of alleles at different loci on a given chromosome (for example, A1-B1) is called a *haplotype*.　　　*DE*

[See also GENETIC EPIDEMIOLOGY]

Balding, D.J., Bishop, M. and Cannings, C. (eds) 2001: *Handbook of statistical genetics*. Chichester: John Wiley & Sons. **Sham, P.** 1998: *Statistics in human genetics*. London: Arnold.

geometric distribution

The PROBABILITY DISTRIBUTION of the number of events required in order to observe a first 'success'. If we have a sequence of events, each of which independently has a probability of success p, then the probability mass function for the number of events required before observing a success is:

$$\Pr(X = x) = p(1 - p)^x$$

and that for the number required to observe the first success is:

$$\Pr(X = x) = p(1 - p)^{x-1}$$

Both are sometimes called the geometric distribution. Here we shall consider the second formula to be the definition. If X has this distribution, the mean of X is $1/p$ and the variance of X is $(1 - p)/p^2$. The geometric distribution is a special case of the NEGATIVE BINOMIAL DISTRIBUTION.

The interpretation of the probability mass function is straightforward. In order to observe the first success on the xth event, the xth event must be a success (with probability p) and the $x - 1$ previous events must be failures (with probabilities $1 - p$). Since the events are independent, the overall probability is obtained by simply multiplying together these individual probabilities (see PROBABILITY).

The event can be almost anything, from a generation of a family (perhaps for the purposes of modelling the number of generations until extinction of a species), to a nucleotide on a chromosome (for the purpose of modelling the length of chromosome before a mutation). Indeed, it is this last definition of event that Hilliker *et al.* (1994) use as they look to model the length of conversion tracts in terms of numbers of nucleotides, the length of a conversion tract being the number of nucleotides required before a termination ('success') of the tract is observed. Indeed the majority of uses of this distribution in the medical sciences appear to be in the field of genetics.

The geometric distribution is a discrete analogue of the EXPONENTIAL DISTRIBUTION and a number of similarities should be apparent, e.g. the function of the distribution in modelling the time to an event. When the probability of a success, p, is small the continuous exponential distribution (with parameter p) can provide a good approximation to the discrete geometric distribution. The construction of the distribution in terms of independent events means that the 'lack of memory' property is also shared. That is, observing two events to be failures does not alter the distribution of how many events need to be observed to have a success (independent events, by definition, cannot influence one another).　　　*AGL*

Grimmet, G.R. and Stirzaker, D.R. 1992: *Probability and random processes*, 2nd edn. Oxford: Clarendon Press. **Hilliker, A.J., Harauz, G., Reaume, A.G., Gray, M., Clark, S.H. and Chovnick, A.** 1994: Meiotic gene conversion tract length distribution within the rosy locus of Drosophila melanogaster. *Genetics* 137, 1019–26.

geometric mean

A MEASURE OF LOCATION used when data exhibit positive SKEWNESS, for example, such that the log-transformed data have an approximate normal distribution. The (arithmetic) MEAN of the logged data is, like the individual values, on the log scale. The geometric mean is calculated by back-transforming (anti-logging) this arithmetic mean.

The histogram in the Figure illustrates the position of the arithmetic mean, geometric mean and MEDIAN of red cell folate measurements made on blood samples from a large random sample of women visiting a clinic. Since the data are skewed the median is a better measure of location than the arithmetic mean. However, the logged red cell folate data are normally distributed; in such circumstances the geometric mean is a good measure of location and is closer to the median than to the arithmetic mean.

Note that the geometric mean can only be used when all data points have values of above zero, since it is impossible without further TRANSFORMATION (e.g. by the addition of an initially large number to all observations) to take the log of zero or a negative number. Logs are typically taken to either base 10 or base e: both are equally valid. If the data are logged to base 10 (denoted *log* on most calculators), then the antilog to calculate the geometric mean must be to base 10 (denoted 10^x). If, however, the data are logged to base e (*ln*), known as the natural logarithm, then the antilog must be to base e (e^x). The red cell folate data were logged to base e and the arithmetic mean of these values was calculated as 5.777. The antilog to base e of 5.777 is $e^{5.777} = 323$.

In a RANDOMISED CONTROLLED TRIAL by Ng *et al.* (2002), the primary outcome was length of hospital stay following computed tomography (CT) scan in patients with acute abdominal pain of uncertain aetiology. Since length of

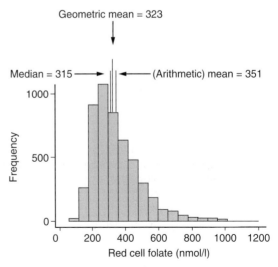

geometric mean *Median, geometric mean and arithmetic mean of red folate measurements on blood samples from 5052 women*

hospital stay was expected to have a skewed distribution, the primary comparison was based on geometric mean length of stay. In their results section, the authors quoted the geometric mean for the two groups involved (5.3 and 6.4 days) but also, since the interpretation of geometric mean is more conducive to relative than absolute differences, this was quoted as a 20% increase in one group's length of stay, with 95% CONFIDENCE INTERVAL from an 8% shorter to a 56% longer stay in hospital.   *SRC*

Ng, C.S., Watson, C.J.E., Palmer, C.R., See, T.C., Beharry, N.A., Howden, B.A., Bradley, J.A. and Dixon, A.K. 2002: Evaluation of early abdominopelvic computed tomography in patients with acute abdominal pain of unknown cause: prospective randomised study. *British Medical Journal* 325, 1387–91.

GLM   See GENERALISED LINEAR MODEL

graphical deception   Graphical displays of data that may mislead the unwary either by design or by error. Consider, for example, the plot of the death rate per million from cancer of the breast, for several periods over the last three decades, shown in the first Figure. The rate appears to undergo a rather alarming increase. However, when the data are re-plotted with the vertical scale starting at zero, as shown in the second Figure, the increase is altogether less startling. The example illustrates that undue exaggeration or compression of the scales is best avoided when constructing graphs if you want to avoid the charge of graphical deception.

A very common form of distortion introduced into the graphics often popular in the media is that where both dimensions of a two-dimensional figure or icon are varied simultaneously in response to changes in a single observed quantity. An example is shown in the third Figure.

Another distortion made popular by graphics packages is the misuse of three-dimensionality, such as in PIE CHARTS, worsened by the ability to rotate the pie and detach slices at will. This can have the effect of inflating or masking a particular sub-category to suit the point being

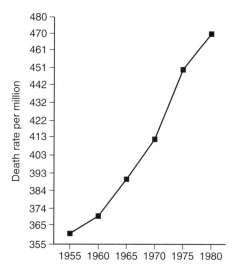

graphical deception *Death rates from cancer of the breast where the y-axis does not include the origin*

The shrinking family doctor
in California

Percentage of doctors devoted solely to family practice

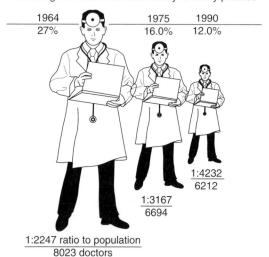

graphical deception *The shrinking family doctor (taken with permission from Tufte, 1983)*

made. Leading journals prohibit the use of such unscientific devices. In the same way, BAR CHARTS and HISTOGRAMS should not have artificial three-dimensionality introduced as it confuses the reader when trying to read off axis values.

Tufte (1983) quantifies the distortion in graphical displays with what he calls the lie factor of the display and defined as follows:

Lie factor = Size of effect in graph/size of effect in data

The lie factor for the shrinking doctors is 2.8.

Some suggested principles for avoiding graphical distor-

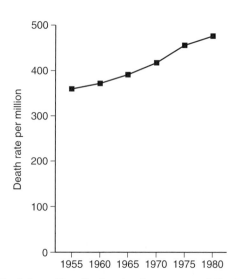

graphical deception *Death rates from cancer of the breast where the y-axis does include the origin*

tion leading to possible graphical deception taken from Tufte (1983) are: representation of numbers, as physically measured on the surface of the graphic itself, should be directly proportional to the numerical quantities represented; clear, detailed and thorough labelling should be used to defeat graphical distortion and ambiguity. Write out explanations of the data on the graphic itself. Label important events in the data; to be truthful and revealing, data graphics must bear on the heart of quantitative thinking, 'compared to what?' Graphics must not quote data out of context; above all else, show the data.   *BSE*

[See also GRAPHICAL DISPLAYS]

Tufte, E.R. 1983: *The visual display of quantitative information*, Cheshire, CT: Graphics Press.

graphical displays Procedures for visually displaying measured quantities by means of the combined use of points, lines, a coordinate system, numbers, symbols, words, shading and colour. It has been estimated that between 900 billion (9×10^{11}) and 2 trillion (2×10^{12}) images of statistical graphics are printed each year. Some of the advantages of graphical methods have been listed by Schmid (1954): in comparison with other types of presentation, well-designed charts are more effective in creating interest and in appealing to the attention of the reader; visual relationships as portrayed by charts and graphs are more easily grasped and more easily remembered; the use of charts and graphs saves time, because the essential meaning of large measures of statistical data can be visualised at a glance; charts and graphs provide a comprehensive picture of a problem that makes for a more complete and better balanced understanding than could be derived from tabular or textual forms of presentation; charts and graphs can bring out hidden facts and relationships and can stimulate as well as aid, analytical thinking and investigation.

The last point in particular implies that perhaps the greatest value of a picture is when it forces us to notice what we never expected to see (although it should not be forgotten that humans are good at discerning subtle patterns that are really there (but equally good at imagining them when they are altogether absent!) – and graphs are sometimes constructed so as to mislead – see GRAPHICAL DECEPTION).

Many graphical displays used in medical research, for example the HISTOGRAM, PIE CHART and SCATTERPLOT, have been around for many years, but during the last two decades a wide variety of new methods have been developed with the aim of making this particular aspect of the examination of data as informative as possible. Graphical techniques have evolved that will provide an overview, hunt for special effects in data, indicate OUTLIERS, identify patterns, diagnose (and criticise) models and generally search for novel and unexpected phenomena. One example of these newer graphical techniques is TRELLIS GRAPHICS.

The current approach to statistical graphics largely arises from the 'visualisation' philosophy expounded by Cleveland (1985, 1993). There are two components to Cleveland's approach to displaying data: (1) *graphing*: visualisation implies a process in which information is encoded in visual displays; and (2) *fitting*: fitting mathematical functions to data is needed as well as just a graphical display. Just graphing raw data, without fitting them and without

graphing the fits and residuals often leaves important aspects of the data undiscovered.

Visualisation is critical to data analysis. It provides a front line of attack, revealing intricate structure in data that cannot be absorbed in any other way and can lead to the discovery of unimagined effects as well as challenging imagined ones.

Good graphics will tell a convincing story about the data. In practice, large numbers of graphs may be needed and computers will generally be needed to draw them for the same reason that they are used for numerical analysis, speed and accuracy.   *BSE*

[See also BOX PLOTS, GROWTH CHARTS, RESIDUAL PLOTS, SCATTERPLOT MATRICES]

Cleveland, W.S. 1985: *The elements of graphing data*. Summit, NJ: Hobart Press. **Cleveland, W.S.** 1993: *Visualizing data*. Summit, NJ: Hobart Press. **Schmid, C.F.** 1954: *Handbook of graphic presentation*. New York: Ronald.

graphical models Also known as *conditional independence graphs*, these models represent interrelationships in multivariate data pictorially. The graphs associated with these models depict the relationships between variables, with nodes representing random variables, and lines between them (*edges*) representing associations between them. The identification of independence between pairs of variables, conditional on the other variables in the model, enables graphs to be simplified by the omission of unnecessary edges. Models for multivariate normal data are called *graphical Gaussian models* or *covariance selection models*. The graphs associated with these models depict partial correlations between variables, conditional on all the other variables. Models for categorical data are based on the multinomial family of distributions and are called *graphical log-linear models*. Here the associations that are depicted are interaction terms in LOG-LINEAR MODELS. *Mixed models* that combine categorical and multivariate normal data (mixed models) can also be fitted.

The first Figure (see page 156) shows some output from MIM, a software package dedicated to this type of analysis (see Edwards, 2002 for further details of the package and of this example, which relates to mathematics exam marks). The first matrix is a correlation matrix for 5 variables (v,w,x,y,z) and it is followed by the partial correlation matrix corresponding to it. The full model with all pairwise partial correlations can be expressed by a model formula as *vwxzy* and the associated graph is shown on the left. A model specified as *vwx,xyz* retains those subsets of variables that are mutually (partially) correlated and sets to zero any insignificant partial correlation. Here, the choice of edges to be omitted (vy,vz,wy,wz) is fairly obvious. However, in a more complex situation the reduced model would typically be found by removing each pair of variables in turn on the basis of their statistical significance. The fitted partial correlation matrix corresponding to this reduced *vwx,xyz* model is shown as the third matrix, with the graph on the right. The position of the variables in the diagram is not important, only the links between them. In the reduced model, one can conclude, for example, that x is needed to predict any of the other variables; also that y and z are not need to predict v, so long as x and w are available.

Graphical models are based not only on statistical dis-

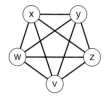 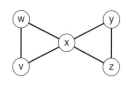

Input correlation matrix

v	1.000				
w	0.553	1.000			
x	0.547	0.610	1.000		
y	0.409	0.485	0.711	1.000	
z	0.389	0.436	0.665	0.607	1.000
	v	w	x	y	z

Partial correlation matrix

v	1.000				
w	0.329	1.000			
x	0.230	0.281	1.000		
y	−0.002	0.078	0.432	1.000	
z	0.025	0.020	0.357	0.253	1.000
	v	w	x	y	z

Partial correlation matrix, 4 elements set to 0

v	1.000				
w	0.332	1.00			
x	0.235	0.327	1.000		
y	0.000	0.000	0.451	1.000	
z	−0.000	−0.000	0.364	0.256	1.000
	v	w	x	y	z

graphical models *A full and a reduced graphical model with associated partial correlation matrices and the initial correlation matrix (mathematics marks data from Mardia et al., 1979, analysed by Edwards, 2002)*

tribution theory, but also on concepts of mathematical graph theory, for example *cliques* and *acyclic graphs*. In this example, the subset of variables *vwx* is a *clique* since (a) all the vertices are joined and (b) no larger subset containing it does not have this property. *Acyclic* means that there are no paths from a node back to itself. Concepts such as these ensure that the illustrative graphs and their associated models do not contain redundant information and can be interpreted unambiguously. *Decomposability* is a criterion sometimes sought. This requires that models can be broken down into series of regressions; it can aid interpretation and allow certain exact significance tests to be applied. Other more familiar criteria may be applied to models. For example, only log-linear models that are *hierarchical* are usually considered, as is the case in standard log-linear analysis.

Graphical chain models, also known as *Bayesian networks*, represent a series of models that have a directional relationship to one another, i.e. one model precedes another in some sense, either through a natural ordering in time or through some assumed causal relationship. The variables for each component model are considered to be in a block and the blocks are ordered to form a chain. Associations within blocks are considered to be non-causal whereas those between blocks are considered potentially causal. From the second block onwards each model is conditional on the other variables in that block and those in all preceding blocks. The edges linking the components are termed *directed* and are denoted by arrows.

The second Figure (see page 157) illustrates a relatively complex graphical chain model concerned with infant mortality in Malaysia (Mohamed, Diamond and Smith, 1998), using categorised data. Note that the convention is to show discrete variables (as they are in this example) as closed circles whereas continuous variables are depicted as open as in the first Figure. The components of chain models are shown as blocks (often enclosed in rectangles). In the second Figure, parts (a) and (c) are simple graphical models showing associations between pairs of variables controlling for the others. The other parts show models that have a temporal or causal relationship with one another. A summary was produced from all the constituent chain models, from which it was concluded that neonatal mortality was directly associated with maternal education, ethnicity, state, year of birth, source of drinking water, birth interval, pre-maturity and sex. However, neonatal mortality was not associated with birth attendant, birthplace and antenatal care.

Estimation of models from data is generally performed by MAXIMUM LIKELIHOOD. Automatic selection of variables can be performed on the basis of the change in likelihood resulting from adding or removing edges in turn. This process typically starts either with the full or saturated model, containing all possible edges, followed by successive elimination of non-significant links, or with the null model followed by successive inclusion of links. In the case of multivariate normal data, summary statistics such as covariance matrices rather than raw data may be sufficient to fit models. However, diagnostic tests based on individual cases and data transformation are then not possible. Such tests include examination of residuals for OUTLIERS and to assess normality if appropriate. *Box-Cox tests* can be used to decide on the appropriate transformation if this is indicated. Graphical Gaussian models assume that there are no interactions (partial correlations depending on the level of a third variable). In the case of continuous variables it may be advisable to dichotomise the data and refit the model as a log-linear or mixed model so that any interactions can be detected.

Many standard statistical techniques can be framed as special cases of graphical models, for example mixtures of multivariate normals (see FINITE MIXTURE DISTRIBUTIONS), or ANALYSIS OF VARIANCE. However, there are two situations in the analysis of medical data for which graphical models may be particularly useful. The first is when little is known about potential ASSOCIATIONS among a group of variables and where an exploratory approach is therefore called for; here a stepwise automatic selection process would probably be used to seek simple models consistent with the data. The other, as in the earlier infant mortality example, is where one has in mind a complex model of associations and causal links, the overall structure of which can be set out even though the details cannot be specified. The ability to depict the associations visually is particularly helpful in these two contexts. The numerical values of effect sizes, for example the partial correlations are of course important, but it may be the qualitative

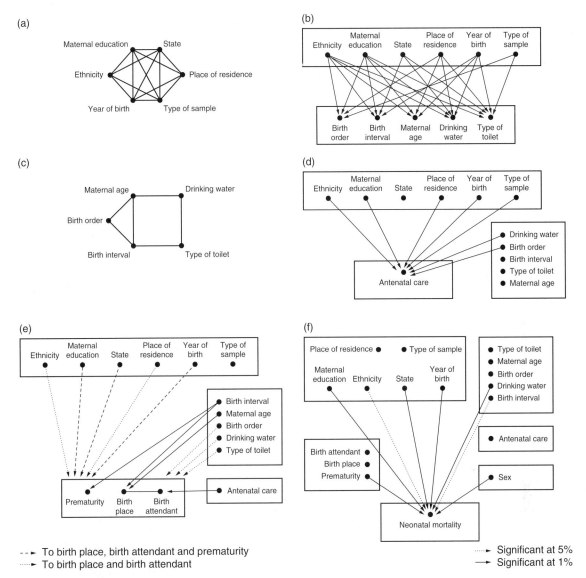

graphical models *Graphical model for each step of an analysis of infant mortality in Malaysia, from Mohamed et al (1998) (a) socio-economic factors – intrablock associations; (b) socio-economic factors and factors before pregnancy – interblock associations; (c) factors before pregnancy – intrablock associations; (d) direct associations between antenatal care and its potential determinants; (e) direct associations between factors at birth and their potential determinants; (f) direct associations between neonatal mortality and its determinants*

information as to which pairs of variables are associated at any level (conditional on the rest) that may be of prime interest. This is most easily represented graphically rather than in tables.

A key paper is by Lauritzen and Wermuth (1989) and Edwards (2002) provides an application-oriented introduction making use of dedicated software MIM. Whittaker (1990) is another general text. Closely related techniques are PATH ANALYSIS and STRUCTURAL EQUATION MODELS. *Bayesian graphical modelling*, in which parameters and latent variables are included in the graph (in addition to the observed quantities), is discussed by Spiegelhalter (1998) and illustrated with an example relating to cancer incidence.   *ML*

Edwards, D. 2002: *Introduction to graphical modelling*, 2nd edn. New York: Springer Verlag. **Lauritzen, S.L. and Wermuth, W.C.** 1989: Graphical models for associations between variables, some of which are qualitative and some quantitative. *Annals of Statistics* 17, 31–57. **Mardia, K.V., Kent, J.T. and Bibby, J.M.** 1979: *Multivariate analysis*. London: Academic Press. **Mohamed, W.N., Diamond, I. and Smith, P.W.F.** 1998: The determinants of infant mortality in Malaysia: a graphical chain modelling approach. *Journal of the Royal Statistical Society Series A* 161, 349–66. **Spiegelhalter, D.J.** 1998: Bayesian graphical modelling: a case-study in monitoring health outcomes. *Applied Statistics* 47, 115–33. **Whittaker, J.** 1990: *Graphical models in applied multivariate statistics*. Chichester: John Wiley & Sons.

gross reproduction rate (GRR)   See DEMOGRAPHY

group sequential methods   See DATA-DEPENDENT DESIGNS, INTERIM ANALYSIS, SEQUENTIAL ANALYSIS

growth charts Graphical displays that present AGE-RELATED REFERENCE RANGES for anthropometry such as height and weight throughout childhood. Growth charts conventionally provide information on 3 or more quantiles of the age-related distribution, including the median and other centiles (percentiles) placed symmetrically about the median. The Figure illustrates a growth chart of infant weight in British boys. There are nine centiles on the chart, equally spaced two-thirds of a unit apart on the standard deviation score scale. There is also the growth curve of an infant followed over a 2-month period, showing marked growth faltering.

The growth chart is used in several distinct ways. First, it is a screening or diagnostic test, corresponding to the way age-related reference ranges are used. Measurements are plotted against age on the chart and children whose measurement lies outside the reference range, i.e. above the top centile or below the bottom centile for the child's age, are considered to be at risk of a growth disorder and are referred for further investigation. The proportion of children screened in depends on the centile used, for

example 2% below the 2nd centile or 9% above the 91st centile. This assumes that the children are representative of the reference population on which the growth chart is based. The population prevalence of a growth disorder is small, so the screening in rate corresponds closely to the FALSE POSITIVE RATE (100% – SPECIFICITY) of the screening test, the vast majority of the selected children being free of the disorder. Note though that the growth chart provides no information of the TRUE POSITIVE RATE (SENSITIVITY) of the screening test, as this needs to be based on a representative sample of growth-disordered children, which is generally not available.

A second use of the growth chart is to quantify the centile position of the individual child, by seeing what centile curve their measurement is close to. For measurements in the body of the distribution the approximate centile can be obtained by interpolating between adjacent centile curves.

The third and most common use of the chart is an extension of this previous use to measurements on two or more occasions, which are plotted on the chart and the

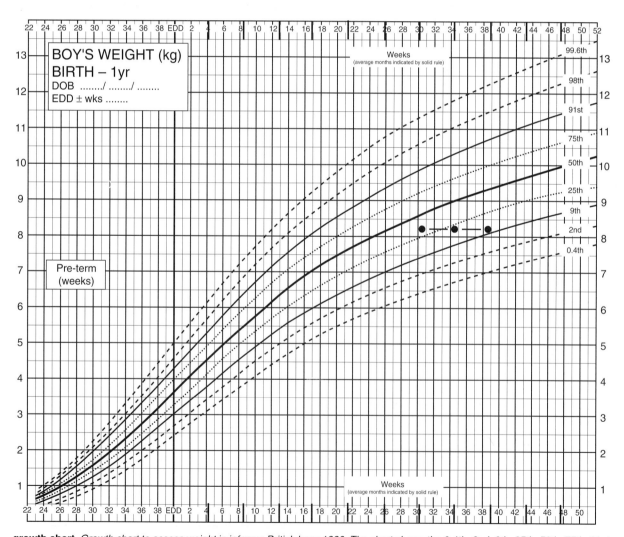

growth chart *Growth chart to assess weight in infancy, British boys 1990. The chart shows the 0.4th, 2nd, 9th, 25th, 50th, 75th, 91st, 98th and 99.6th centiles of the weight distribution by age. Also shown is the growth curve for a child measured at 7, 8 and 9 months (reproduced with permission of the Child Growth Foundation)*

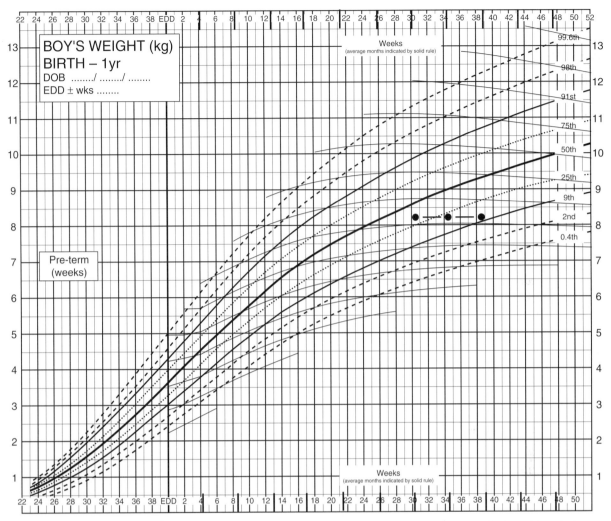

growth chart *Growth chart of the first figure with thrive lines overlaid. The thrive lines quantify the 5th centile for weight velocity over a 4-week period. The infant's growth curve tracks along the thrive lines, corresponding to the 5th weight velocity centile for the first month, and approximately the 1st centile for the whole 2-month period (reproduced with permission of the Child Growth Foundation)*

points joined together to make a growth curve. The child's growth velocity over time is assessed on the assumption of tracking, where the centile is expected to be constant and the growth curve parallel to the centile curves. This constant centile over time corresponds to a growth velocity that is close to the population median, whereas growth-disordered children show 'centile crossing', i.e. they grow more quickly or more slowly than the implied reference median velocity, as seen for example in our first Figure (page 158). It is this use that gives the name to growth charts, quantifying growth in individuals relative to the reference. It should be recognised though that growth charts used in this way lack statistical rigour – the reference data are cross-sectional rather than longitudinal, and contain no information about growth velocity. In addition, the chart does not adjust for regression to the median.

Child centiles followed over time (assumed representative of the reference population) will be subject to regression towards the median, so that for example in a group of children on the 9th centile on one occasion, their mean measurement centile will be closer to the median

when followed up. The size of this centile crossing effect depends solely on the strength of the correlation between measurements on the two occasions. Height, for example, tracks very strongly in mid-childhood before puberty (the year-on-year correlation exceeds 0.97), so most children show very little height centile crossing over time and regression to the median is hard to detect. For more labile measurements such as weight, body mass index or skinfold thickness, and particularly during periods of rapid growth such as early infancy or puberty, the age-on-age correlation may be as low as 0.5 and regression to the median is marked. This emphasises that charts to measure size are not ideal to assess growth and vice versa.

A more useful tool to assess growth velocity is a dedicated velocity chart. Charts to assess growth velocity can be constructed in the same way as charts for size. Here each child from the reference population provides two measurements taken some pre-specified time-interval apart (e.g. 1 year), which are converted to a velocity and then analysed to construct centile charts of velocity for age. The constrained time interval ensures that the contribution of measurement error to the total variability is fixed, as the amount of MEASUREMENT ERROR varies inversely as the time interval. Velocity charts are less satisfactory than size charts for three reasons: (1) the time interval requirement is restrictive as most children are not measured that regularly; (2) the chart does not adjust for regression to the median; and (3) requiring two charts rather than one to assess each child's growth increases resource costs.

An alternative is to assess the child's growth velocity from the size chart. This exploits the principle that velocity is the rate of change of size, so that the slope of the line joining successive measurements is a measure of velocity. Velocity can be assessed in terms of the rate of change of either the measurement or the measurement centile (more correctly the standard deviation score) and the latter corresponds directly to centile crossing. This is the principle behind 'thrive lines', a set of curves analogous to centile curves that are printed on a transparent plastic overlay and placed on the growth (size) chart to detect failure to thrive (i.e. poor growth). Centile curves represent the pattern (or direction) of growth in children who are tracking perfectly, i.e. whose centile remains constant over time. Such children are growing on the median velocity (ignoring regression to the median). In the same way, thrive lines can be drawn to reflect the pattern (or direction) of growth of children growing at some specified velocity centile other than the median. The second Figure (see page 159) shows thrive lines for the 5th velocity centile, superimposed on the infant weight chart of the first figure. The child's growth curve in the second figure tracks along the thrive lines for a period of 4 weeks and this defines his growth rate

as the 5th velocity centile. Only about 1 child in 20 grows more slowly than this. The time period is important and the growth pattern becomes more extreme the longer it tracks the thrive lines. So the child's continuing to track along the thrive lines for a further 4 weeks, i.e. 2 months altogether, means that his velocity over the whole period is near the 1st centile, clearly of much greater concern. Note that the first figure highlights the centile crossing, but gives no clue as to how extreme the velocity centile is.

The main technical concern with growth charts is the representativeness of the underlying reference population. This depends on the nationality, ethnicity and timing of measurement of the child being assessed compared to the reference. For example, the British growth charts (e.g. our first figure) are based on ethnic Caucasian British children measured in 1990. So they are less appropriate for assessing, say, Caucasian Dutch or minority ethnic British children and will become progressively more out of date as time passes, due to the secular trend to increasing height and particularly weight.   *TJC*

[See also AGE-RELATED REFERENCE RANGES]

Cole, T.J. 1998: Presenting information on growth distance and conditional velocity in one chart: practical issues of chart design. *Statistics in Medicine* 17, 2697–707. **Cole, T.J., Freeman, J.V. and Preece, M.A.** 1998: British 1990 growth reference centiles for weight, height, body mass index and head circumference fitted by maximum penalized likelihood. *Statistics in Medicine* 17, 407–29. **Tanner, J.M.** 1978: *Foetus into man: physical growth from conception to maturity*. London: Open Books. **Ulijaszek, S.J., Johnston, F.E. and Preece, M.A.** 1998: *Cambridge encyclopedia of human growth and development*. Cambridge: Cambridge University Press.

Grubbs' test statistic See OUTLIERS

H

haplotype analysis A haplotype refers to a combination of alleles transmitted from a parent to a child through a haploid nucleus in a gametic cell, although the term is often restricted to a combination of alleles that are in tight linkage on the same chromosome. Humans are diploid: an individual's genotype is derived from the union of a haplotype from the father and a haplotype from the mother. Haplotype analysis includes the estimation of population haplotype frequencies from sample genotype data, the inference of an individual's haplotype from genotype data and the investigation of possible associations between haplotypes and disease or other traits.

One important problem in haplotype analysis is that an individual's genotype may be consistent with multiple pairs of haplotypes. Thus, the genotype AaBb is consistent with haplotype pairs AB/ab and Ab/aB. In general, if there are m heterozygous loci in the genotype, then there are 2^{m-1} consistent haplotype pairs. The availability of genotype but not haplotype data can be regarded as a form of incomplete data, so that the estimation of haplotype frequencies from genotype data can be accomplished by an EM ALGORITHM. Other methods to haplotype frequency estimation have also been proposed, including Bayesian approaches that take account of the similarities between the haplotypes.

If the frequency of a haplotype deviates from the product of the frequencies of the constituent alleles, then the alleles are not independent but associated with each other and their loci are said to be in linkage disequilibrium. A number of measures of linkage disequilibrium are available for two diallelic loci, including D (the difference between haplotype frequency and the product of constituent allele frequencies), D′ (D divided by the maximum possible D given the allele frequencies of the two loci) and R (the correlation coefficient between numerically coded values for the alleles of the two loci). The strength of linkage disequilibrium between the markers in a region may reflect the recombination rate in that region (possibly determined by local chromosome structure) and stochastic variation in the recombination and mutation history of the population.

A possible association between haplotype and disease is usually examined by estimating haplotype frequencies in cases and controls and testing whether these can be equated. Often the association between a haplotype and a disease is stronger than the association between any of the constituent alleles and the disease. This happens when the true causal variant had originated in a mutation that occurred on a chromosome containing a particular combination of alleles, or when there is an interaction between the effects of alleles on the same chromosome (called *cis* interactions). Knowledge of haplotype structure is also important for the optimal choice of markers in association studies, leaving out any markers that are predictable by the others because of strong linkage disequilibrium. *PS*

[See also ALLELIC ASSOCIATION, GENETIC EPIDEMIOLOGY, GENETIC LINKAGE]

Sham, P. 1997: *Statistics in human genetics*. London: Arnold.

Hardy-Weinberg law A result concerning the frequency distribution of genotypes at a polymorphic genetic locus in a population under random mating. The Hardy-Weinberg law is an important result in population genetics that was derived independently by the English mathematician, G.H. Hardy, and the German physician, W. Weinberg, in 1908. For a locus with two alternate genetic variants (alleles), the Hardy-Weinberg law states that half the frequency (expressed as a proportion) of the heterozygote genotype is equal to the square root of the product (i.e. the GEOMETRIC MEAN) of the frequencies of the two homozygous genotypes. An alternative way of stating the Hardy-Weinberg law is that the frequency of a homozygous genotype is equal to the square of the frequency of the constituent allele, while the frequency of a heterozygous genotype is equal to twice the product of the frequencies of the two constituent alleles. The Hardy-Weinberg law is therefore the result of the simple rule that the probability of two independent events is equal to the product of the probabilities of the two events.

The Hardy-Weinberg law can be violated in real populations or samples for many reasons. Populations that are made up of non-interbreeding subpopulations with different allele frequencies will tend to have an excess of individuals with homozygous genotypes. The characteristic Hardy-Weinberg ratios can be distorted by selection, where one or more genotypes confer a survival advantage over the others. The overall population ratios can be distorted at a locus that contains disease-predisposing variants, in a sample of patients with the disease. Finally, the apparent distortions of the Hardy-Weinberg ratios can be the result of genotyping errors in the laboratory. *PS*

[See also ALLELIC ASSOCIATION, GENETIC EPIDEMIOLOGY, HERITABILITY]

Sham, P. 1997: *Statistics in human genetics*. London: Arnold.

Hawthorne effect The possible effect that might be produced in an experiment or study simply from subjects' awareness of participation in some form of scientific investigation. That individual behaviours might be altered because they know they are being studied was first said to have been demonstrated in a research project carried out at the Hawthorne Plant of the Western Electric Company in Cicero, Illinois, in the late 1920s. The major finding of the study was that, almost regardless of the experimental manipulation employed, the production of the workers seemed to improve. The implication of the effect is that people who are singled out for a study of any kind may improve their performance or behaviour not because of any specific condition being tested, but simply because of the attention they receive. A medical example suggested by Gail (1998) involves a study of methods to promote smoking cessation, in which it is necessary to contact study participants each year to determine smoking status. The Hawthorne effect could distort study results if this repeated annual contact affected smoking behaviour or the reporting of smoking behaviour.   *BSE*

Gail, M.H. 1998: Hawthorne effect. In Armitage, P. and Colton, T. (eds), *Encyclopedia of biostatistics*. Chichester: John Wiley & Sons.

hazard function   See PROPORTIONAL HAZARDS, SURVIVAL ANALYSIS

health-adjusted life expectancy (HALE)   See DEMOGRAPHY

health services research   Health service research, according to Bowling (2002), 'is concerned with the relationship between the provision, effectiveness and efficient use of health services and the health needs of the population. It is narrower than health research'. It thus entails measuring and evaluating assessing the inputs, processes and outcomes of healthcare provision. While most standard statistical methods are potentially applicable in health services research, some are more useful than others. As shown in some of the examples given in this section, health services research is often relatively complex, involving as it does the analysis of different interventions, outcomes and levels of data simultaneously.

Input and process information that is primarily aimed at assisting healthcare managers and providers, especially when collected on a routine basis, is probably more correctly considered as audit or quality assurance. Generally speaking, such routine data can rarely be used for research purposes, due to difficulties in maintaining standards in data collection. An exception would be a long-term case register containing data on all patients in a given area gathered in a strictly controlled and objective fashion. Outcome studies that investigate a specific research question probably form the most important branch of health services research and these comprise two main types, trials and observational studies. The latter include, for example, CROSS-SECTIONAL SURVEYS, COHORT STUDIES in which groups of patients are followed up over time and CASE-CONTROL STUDIES.

Healthcare trials may be experimental (involving the comparison of randomised groups) or quasi-experimental (involving the comparison of non-randomised groups). Further discussion of the terminology of healthcare trials may be found in Spitzer, Feinstein and Hackett (1975). A contrast between the typical healthcare trial and the typical clinical trial is that the latter is usually focused on the outcome for the individual patient and assesses some particular therapeutic intervention such as a drug, a surgical procedure or a psychological intervention. The remit of a typical healthcare trial, contrariwise, tends to be broader and often involves the evaluation of one or more interventions, the environment in which they take place and the personnel administering them. The outcomes, which may be both clinical and non-clinical, may be measured at the patient level but they may also be measured at other levels, such as the ward, the hospital or the health providing authority, or indeed at several of these levels simultaneously.

In a discussion aimed specifically at psychiatrists, but which is nevertheless generally applicable, Dunn (2001) draws attention to some of the problems inherent in health service trials. One of these is the HAWTHORNE EFFECT, in which there are non-specific or PLACEBO effects that are not directly associated with the specific content of the intervention but are rather due to the mere fact of participation in the study. Dunn points out that, in health service research, providers as well as patients may be subject to such an effect. Avoiding it is often more difficult in healthcare trials compared to clinical trials because blinding of participants may be impractical or unethical.

The definition of outcome is often quite problematic in health services research since interventions may potentially produce multiple and conflicting changes in several dimensions. Important statistical issues in this area are thus dealing with multiple significance testing and combining outcomes into summary statistics. Economic analysis, aimed at balancing the effectiveness of outcomes against the cost of providing interventions, is commonly performed in health services research (see COST-EFFECTIVENESS ANALYSIS). One issue that has to be addressed in this context is whether service use information, such as number of hospital admissions, should be regarded as an outcome in its own right or whether it should be considered purely on the cost side of the equation. The views of clinicians and health economists may differ on this point. Often outcomes are concerned with such concepts as patient satisfaction or quality of life, which may be difficult to define and capture.

Even once they have been defined conceptually, outcomes are not always straightforward to measure and often involve the use of QUESTIONNAIRES. The latter may be prone to test–retest imprecision, due to a subject's inconsistency or, indeed, genuine changes from one time point to the next, or disagreement between raters (in cases where the questionnaires are administered and interpreted by someone other than the subject). Methods for assessing MEASUREMENT ERROR are thus important in health services research. The analysis of the psychometric properties of instruments, such as their reliability and validity (see Streiner and Norman, 1995), may be necessary where instruments have been developed especially for a study. The treatment of MISSING DATA, and data quality in general, is also a relatively common issue arising in health services research. This is because there is generally less control over data collection in the community or a hospital, as opposed to an experimental laboratory or dedicated clinic.

MULTILEVEL MODELS are often required: these allow the investigator to analyse simultaneously data on the various units on which the outcomes may be measured. For example, a survey of patient satisfaction in wards in a number of hospitals might collect data not only from patients, but also on ward environment and overall characteristics of the hospitals. Three nested levels here would be patient, ward and hospital, and these would all need to be taken into account in the analysis. Two other specific types of multilevel data are common: in the first, one is primarily interested in assessing the effect on the lowest level unit but one also has to allow for the associations between these units grouped or 'clustered' at a higher level. For example, clinics may be assigned randomly to one of two interventions, but the outcome is measured on individual patients. The impact of the higher level (clinic) is not of relevance in itself but has to be built into the analysis of the patient data since these are no longer independent. A second specific type of multilevel data is derived from LONGITUDINAL DATA, where the same group of people, or 'panel', is followed in time. Here the lowest level unit is the individual observation (with several observations per patient) and the higher level unit is the patient.

Sometimes the focus in health services research is on aggregate data from high-level units such as hospitals or health authorities. For example, methods for comparing the performance of health providers in league tables may be required. Goldstein and Spiegelhalter (1996) discuss some of the issues arising from the comparison of institutional performance. Methods for analysing spatial statistics are used when the geographical location of the units is also important and such methods may be integrated with a geographical information system (GIS); this is a specialised form of database that holds complex geographical data so as to allow it to be visualised. Such methods may be aimed at identifying outlying disease clusters, examining the impact of area-wide interventions or measuring health inequalities and relating them to other area-wide data such as social deprivation. *ML*

Bowling, A. 2002: *Research methods in health*, 2nd edn. Buckingham: Open University Press. **Dunn, G.** 2001: Statistical methods for measuring outcomes. In Thornicroft, G. and Tansella, M. (eds), *Mental health outcome measures*, 2nd edn. New York: Springer Verlag, 5–18. **Goldstein, H. and Spiegelhalter, D.J.** 1996: League tables and their limitations: statistical issues in comparisons of institutional performance. *Journal of the Royal Statistical Society Series A* 159, 385–443. **Spitzer, W.O., Feinstein, A.R. and Sackett, D.L.** 1975: What is a healthcare trial? *Journal of the American Medical Association* 233, 161–3. **Streiner, D.L. and Norman, G.R.** 1995: *Health measurement scales: a practical guide to their development and use*, 2nd edn. Oxford: Oxford Medical Publications.

heritability In the broad sense, the proportion of the variance of a given trait that is explained by genetic difference. In the narrow sense, genetic differences are restricted to those due to the additive effects of alleles. Heritability is a key concept in population genetics introduced by Sir R.A. Fisher, in close connection with his work on variance partitioning. Non-additive genetic influences, which include interactions between alleles at the same locus (dominance) or at different loci (epistasis), are included in broad but not narrow heritability.

In humans, heritability is usually estimated by twin or adoption studies (see TWIN ANALYSIS). The classical twin design relies on the fact that monozygotic (MZ) twins are developed from the same fertilised egg and are therefore genetically identical, whereas dizygotic (DZ) twins are like ordinary brothers and sisters in being developed from two separate fertilised ova and therefore share on average 50% of their genes. Given this fact, and under some additional assumptions (including the equality of environmental similarity between MZ and DZ twins and the absence of dominance and epistasis), a simple estimate of heritability is given by twice the difference between the MZ and DZ correlations for the trait.

Adoption studies work under the assumption that any correlation between an adoptee and his or her biological family is entirely genetic in origin. Twice the correlation between adoptee and biological parent provides an estimate of heritability.

A high heritability is sometimes misinterpreted as meaning that the trait is unlikely to respond to environmental changes. Heritability reflects on the genetic and environmental differences that exist in a particular population; it cannot be used to predict the consequences of environmental changes outside the normal range for the population. A familiar example is that the mental retardation associated with the genetic condition phenylketonuria can be prevented by the early introduction of a low-phenylalanine diet in early infancy. *PS*

[See also GENETIC EPIDEMIOLOGY, GENETIC LINKAGE, QUANTITATIVE TRAIT LOCI]

Sham, P. 1997: *Statistics in human genetics*. London: Arnold.

hierarchical models See LOG-LINEAR MODELS

histogram A graphical representation of a FREQUENCY DISTRIBUTION in which each class interval is represented by

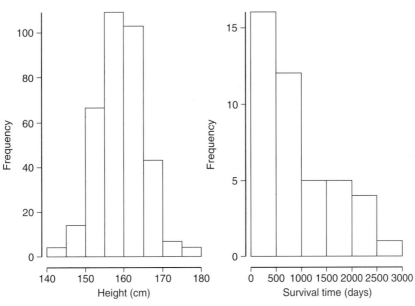

histogram *(a) Heights (cm) of elderly women; (b) survival times (days) of patients with leukaemia*

a vertical bar whose base is the class interval and whose height is the number of observations in the class interval. When the class intervals are unequally spaced the histogram is drawn in such a way that the area of each bar is proportional to the frequency for that class interval. Scott (1979) considers how to choose the optimal number and width of classes in a histogram, for there are matters of choice. Two examples of histograms are shown in the Figure on page 163.

The histogram is generally used for two purposes, counting and displaying the distribution of a variable, although it is relatively ineffective for both, with STEM-AND-LEAF PLOTS being better for counting and BOX PLOTS better for assessing distributional properties. *BSE*

Scott, D.W. 1979: On optimal and data-based histograms. *Biometrika* 66, 605–10.

historical controls   Refers to the use of past data for the purpose of making comparisons with present data in a research context. Unfortunately, despite the appeal of desiring to make efficient use of previously collected resources, with information stored perhaps on a computer database, the use of historical controls is fraught with bias (Pocock, 1983). One cannot make reliable inferences in controlled clinical trials by comparing new data with old. The main reason why bias would be introduced is the lack of comparability at baseline between the two groups. Only concurrent RANDOMISATION of eligible participants can bestow such between-group comparability, since randomising alone can seek to ensure treatment groups are balanced with respect to all the known and (innumerable) unknown risk factors. *CRP*

Pocock, S.J. 1983: *Clinical trials: a practical approach.* Chichester: John Wiley & Sons.

historical demography   See DEMOGRAPHY

history of medical statistics   The first attempts at 'medical statistics' might perhaps be considered the early efforts to keep track of births and deaths through church records of weddings, christenings and burials. But more ambitious statistical procedures than simple counting would have been largely unwelcome to physicians until well into the 17th century simply because they might have raised the unthinkable spectre of questioning the invulnerability most of them still claimed. Medical practices at the time were largely based on uncritical reliance on past experience, *post hoc, ergo propter hoc* reasoning, and veneration of the 'truth' as proclaimed by authoritative figures such as Galen (130–200), a Greek physician whose influence dominated medicine for many centuries. Such attitudes largely stifled any interest in experimentation or proper scientific investigation or explanation of medical phenomena. Even the few clinicians who did strive to increase their knowledge by close observation or simple experiment often interpreted their findings in the light of the currently accepted dogma.

Several authors have pointed out what must qualify as the world's earliest recorded comparative trial. Described in the biblical book of Daniel, hence *circa* 600 BC, Daniel and three colleagues expressed their preference not to be given food that had been prepared contrary to their beliefs. Their study involved a prior hypothesis and pri-

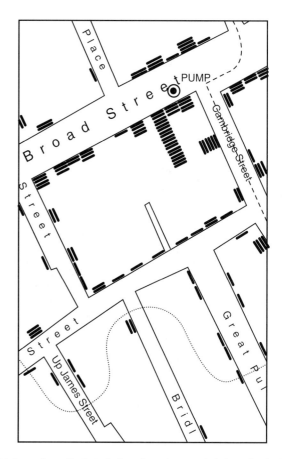

history of medical statistics *Snow's map of cholera deaths in the Broad Street area*

mary ENDPOINT, albeit rather subjective (facial appearance), and the trial duration was limited to just 10 days. The control group, which received the standard fare, was an unknown size, but clearly, the treatment group, which received vegetables and water only, was small, at just 4. The study turned out positively for Daniel. Despite modern-day criticism, notably lack of RANDOMISATION, no one could criticise Daniel for his influential choice of publication. (See Daniel 1: 8–16, Holy Bible.)

But by the late 17th and early 18th centuries, medicine began its slow progress from a sort of mystical certainty, to a scientifically more acceptable uncertainty about many of its procedures. The taking of systematic observations and carrying out of experiments became more widespread. John Graunt (1620–1674), son of a London draper, for example, published his *Natural and Political Observations Made Upon the Bills of Mortality* in 1662 and derived the first ever life table. Graunt was what might today be termed a vital statistician: he examined the risk inherent in the process of birth, marriage and death and used bills of mortality (weekly reports on the numbers and causes of death in an area) to compare one disease with another and one year with another by calculating mortality statistics. Graunt's work and ideas had considerable influence and bills of mortality were also introduced in Paris and other cities in Europe.

Early experimental work in medicine is illustrated by

the example that is often quoted of James Lind's (1716–1794) study undertaken on board the ship the *Salisbury* in 1747. Lind assessed several different possible treatments for scurvy by giving each to a different pair of sailors with the disease. He observed that the two men given oranges and lemons made the most dramatic recovery, although it was to be another 40 years before the Admiralty was convinced enough by Lind's finding to issue lemon juice to members of the British Navy.

The 1700s also saw the first appearance of a procedure that looks remarkably similar to a modern-day significance test, specifically a SIGN TEST. This arose from John Arbuthnot's (1667–1735) endeavours to argue the case for divine providence in the stability of the ratio of number of men to women. Arbuthnot maintained that the guiding hand of a divine being was to be discerned in the nearly constant ratio of male to female christenings recorded annually in London over the years 1629–1710. The data presented by Arbuthnot showed that in each of the 82 years in this period, the annual number of male christenings had been consistently higher than the number of female christenings, but never very much higher. He then essentially tested a null hypothesis of 'chance' determination of sex at birth, against an alternative of divine providence, by calculating, under the assumption that the null hypothesis is true, a probability defined by reference to the observed data. Arbuthnot's representation of chance in this context was the toss of a fair two-sided coin, in which case the distribution of births would be:

$$(1/2+1/2)^{82}$$

so that the observed excess of male christenings on each of 82 occasions had an extremely small probability, thus providing support for the divine providence hypothesis. Arbuthnot offered an explanation for the greater supply of males as a wise economy of nature, as the males are more subject to accidents and diseases, having to seek their food with danger. Therefore, provident nature to repair the loss brings forth more males. The near equality of the sexes is designed so that every male may have a female in the same country and of suitable age.

Other mathematical developments in the 18th century that were of special relevance for medical statistics included Daniel Bernoulli's (1700–1782) development of the normal approximation to the BINOMIAL DISTRIBUTION, which was also used in studies of the stability of the sex ratio at birth.

The power of medical statistics in pursuing reform is illustrated by the work of Florence Nightingale (1820–1907). In her efforts to improve the squalid hospital conditions in Turkey during the Crimean War, and in her subsequent campaigns to improve the health and living conditions of the British Army, the sanitary conditions and administration of hospitals and the nursing profession, Florence Nightingale was not unlike many other Victorian reformers. But in one important respect she was very different, since she marshalled massive amounts of data, carefully arranged, tabulated and graphed and presented this material to ministers, viceroys and others, to convince them of the justice of her case. No other major national cause had previously been championed through the presentation of sound statistical data and those who opposed Florence Nightingale's reforms went down to

defeat because her data were unanswerable; their publication led to an outcry.

Another telling example of how careful arrangement of data was used in the 19th century to save lives is provided by the work of the epidemiologist John Snow (1813–1858). After an outbreak of cholera in central London in September, 1854, Snow used data collected by the General Register Office and plotted the location of deaths on a map of the area and also showed the location of the area's 11 water pumps. The resulting map is shown in the Figure on page 164. Examining the scatter over the surface of the map, Snow observed that nearly all the cholera deaths were among those who lived near the Broad Street pump. But before claiming that he had discovered a possible causal connection, Snow made a more detailed investigation of the deaths that had occurred near some other pump. He visited the families of 10 of the deceased and found that 4 of these, because they preferred its taste, regularly sent for water from the Broad Street pump. Three others were children who attended a school near the Broad Street pump. One other finding that initially confused Snow was that there were no deaths among workers in a brewery close to the Broad Street pump, a confusion that was quickly resolved when it became apparent that the workers drank only beer, never water. Snow's findings were sufficiently compelling to persuade the authorities to remove the handle of the Broad Street pump and, in days, the neighbourhood epidemic that had claimed more than 500 lives had ended.

Later in the 19th century and in the early 20th century, the work of people such as Sir Francis Galton (1822–1911), Wilhelm Lexis (1837–1914) and, in particular, Karl Pearson (1857–1936) began to change the emphasis in statistics from the descriptive to the mathematical. The concept of CORRELATION and its measurement by a correlation coefficient was introduced. Statistical inference began to develop and enter most areas of scientific investigation including medical research. And in 1909 Ronald Aylmer Fisher (later Sir Ronald) (1890–1962) entered Cambridge to study mathematics, the first step to becoming the most influential statistician of the 20th century. Fisher developed MAXIMUM LIKELIHOOD ESTIMATION, worked on evolutionary theory, made massive contributions to genetics and invented the ANALYSIS OF VARIANCE. But Fisher's most important contribution to medical statistics was his introduction of randomisation as a principle in the design of certain experiments. In Fisher's case the experiments were in agriculture and were concerned with which fertilisers led to the greatest crop yields. Fisher divided agricultural areas into plots and randomly assigned the plots to different experimental fertilisers. But the principle was soon adopted in medicine in studies to compare competing therapies for a particular condition, leading, of course, to the randomised CLINICAL TRIAL, described by eminent British statistician Sir David Cox as 'the most important contribution of 20th-century statistics'. The first properly performed randomised clinical trial is now generally acknowledged to be that published in 1948 by another giant of 20th-century medical statistics, Sir Austin Bradford Hill (1897–1991), who investigated the use of streptomycin in the treatment of pulmonary tuberculosis. Nowadays, it is estimated that over 8000 RCTs are undertaken worldwide every year.

At about the time that Bradford Hill was busy with the first randomised clinical trial, another development was taking place that, by revolutionising man's ability to calculate, was to have a dramatic effect on the science of statistics and the work of statisticians. The computer age was about to begin, although it would be some years before statisticians were entirely relieved of the burden of undertaking large amounts of laborious arithmetic on some pre-computer calculator. But, in the 1960s, the first statistical software packages began to appear that made the application of many complex statistical procedures easy and routine.

The influence of increasing, inexpensive computing power on statistics continues to this day and over the last 20 years its almost universal availability has meant that research workers in statistics in general, and medical statistics in particular, no longer have to keep one eye on the computational difficulties when developing new methods of analysis. The result has been the introduction of many exciting and powerful new statistical methods many of which are of great importance in medical statistics. Notable examples to name but a few are BOOTSTRAP, COX'S REGRESSION, GENERALISED ESTIMATING EQUATIONS, LOGISTIC REGRESSION and MULTIPLE IMPUTATION.

In addition, BAYESIAN METHODS, at one time little more than an intellectual curiosity without practical implications because of their associated computational requirements, can now be applied relatively routinely. Many interesting examples are described in Congdon (2001). There seems little doubt that the remarkable success of medical statistics will continue into the 21st century.   *BSE*

[See also DEMOGRAPHY, EPIDEMIOLOGY]

Arbuthnot, J. 1710: An argument for Divine Providence, taken from the constant regularity observ'd in the births of both sexes. *Philosophical Transactions of the Royal Society* 27, 186–90. **Congdon, P.** 2001: *Bayesian statistical modelling.* Chichester: John Wiley & Sons.

hotspot clustering   See DISEASE CLUSTERING

human research ethics board (HREB)   See ETHICAL REVIEW COMMITTEES

hypothesis tests   The testing of hypotheses is fundamental to statistics and arguments about appropriate ways to test hypotheses date back to disputes between the founders of statistical inference, during the first half of the 20th century. R.A. Fisher proposed SIGNIFICANCE TESTS as a means of examining the discrepancy between the data and a *null hypothesis* (for example, the null hypothesis that there is no association between two variables). The *P*-VALUE (*significance level*) is the probability that an ASSOCIATION as large or larger than that observed in the data would occur if the null hypothesis were true. In Fisher's approach the null hypothesis is never proved or established, but is possibly *disproved*. Fisher advocated $P = 0.05$ (5% significance) as a standard level for concluding that there is evidence against the hypothesis tested, although not as an absolute rule:

If *P* is between .1 and .9 there is certainly no reason to suspect the hypothesis tested. If it is below .02 it is strongly indicated that the hypothesis fails to account for the whole of the facts. We shall not

often be astray if we draw a conventional line at .05. (Fisher, 1951)

In fact no scientific worker has a fixed level of significance at which from year to year, and in all circumstances, he rejects hypotheses; he rather gives his mind to each particular case in the light of his evidence and his ideas. (Fisher, 1973)

For Fisher, interpretation of the *P*-value was ultimately for the experimenter: for example a *P*-value of around 0.05 might lead neither to belief nor disbelief in the null hypothesis, but to a decision to perform another experiment. To some extent, use of thresholds for significance resulted from the reduction in the size of statistical tables when only the quantiles of distributions (such as 0.1, 0.05 and 0.01) were tabulated.

Dislike of the subjective interpretation inherent in Fisher's approach led Neyman and Pearson (Neyman and Pearson, 1933) to propose what they called '*hypothesis tests*', which were designed to provide an objective, decision-theoretic approach to the results of experiments. Instead of focusing on evidence against a null hypothesis, Neyman and Pearson considered how to decide between two competing hypotheses; the null hypothesis and a specified *alternative hypothesis*. For example, the null hypothesis might state that the difference between the means of two normally distributed variables is zero, while the alternative hypothesis might state that this difference is 10.

Based on this paradigm, Neyman and Pearson argued that there were two types of error that could be made in interpreting the results of an experiment (see ERRORS IN HYPOTHESIS TESTS). We make a TYPE I ERROR if we reject the null hypothesis when it is, in fact, true, while we make a TYPE II ERROR if we accept the null hypothesis when it is, in fact, false. Neyman and Pearson then showed how to find optimal rules that would, in the long run, minimise the probabilities (the *Type I* and *Type II error rates*) of making these errors over a series of many experiments. The Type I error rate, usually denoted as α, is closely related to the *P*-value since if, for example, the Type I error rate is fixed at 5% then we will reject the null hypothesis when $P < 0.05$. The Type II error rate is usually denoted as β and the POWER of the test (the probability that we do not make a Type II error, if the alternative hypothesis is true) is $1 - \beta$. Based on these ideas, Neyman and Pearson were able to derive tests that were 'best' in the sense that they minimised the Type II error rate, given a particular Type I error rate.

It is important to realise that in this paradigm we do not attempt to infer whether the null hypothesis is true:

No test based upon a theory of probability can by itself provide any valuable evidence of the truth or falsehood of a hypothesis. But we may look at the purpose of tests from another viewpoint. Without hoping to know whether each separate hypothesis is true or false, we may search for rules to govern our behaviour with regard to them, in following which we insure that, in the long run of experience, we shall not often be wrong. (Neyman and Pearson, 1933)

To illustrate the differences between the two approaches, consider the hypothetical controlled trial of a new cholesterol-lowering drug, with results (mean post-treatment cholesterol) summarised in the Table.

Mean cholesterol has been reduced by 15 mg/dl: a reduction of this magnitude might lead to a substantial reduction in the risk of heart disease. An unpaired t-test gives $P = 0.11$. Based on Fisher's approach, the null hypothesis has not been disproved. However a thoughtful investigator might, rather than discarding the drug, proceed to conduct a larger trial.

Application of the Neyman-Pearson approach requires the specification of both Type I and Type II error rates in advance, so we must specify a precise alternative hypothesis, for example, that the mean reduction is 10 mg/dl. An investigator attempting to follow the Neyman-Pearson approach would need to report not only that the test was not significant at the 5% level (Type I error rate 5%), but also the pre-specified Type II error rate. However the power of a study with 15 patients per group to detect a difference of 10 mg/dl is only 19.5%. For a study that is too small, such as this one, there is no choice of Type I and Type II error rates that is satisfactory.

Had we done a POWER calculation on the basis that we wished to detect a difference of 10 mg/dl with 80% power at 5% significance, we would have found that we require a much larger study, with 99 patients in each group. The use of power calculations to ensure that studies are large enough to detect associations of interest is an enduring legacy of Neyman and Pearson's work.

Now that most statistical computer packages report precise P-values, there seems little justification in reporting the results of our drug trial as $P > 0.05$, $P > 0.1$ or 'NS'

hypothesis tests *Results of hypothetical controlled trial of new cholesterol-lowering drug*

Group	Number of participants	Mean cholesterol (mg/dl)	Standard deviation
New drug	15	220	25
Placebo	15	205	25

(non-significant) unless one is following a pre-specified choice of both Type I *and* Type II error rates. This is rarely the case: even in randomised trials we will usually investigate a number of hypotheses beyond the primary one for which the trial was designed. Therefore, in modern medical statistics, it is usual to report the precise P-value, together with the estimated difference and the CONFIDENCE INTERVAL for the difference. For example, for our hypothetical trial we could report that the mean reduction in cholesterol was 15 mg/dl (95% CI −3.7 mg/dl to 33.7 mg/dl, $P = 0.11$). When we examine the confidence interval we see that the results are consistent either with a substantial and clinically important reduction in mean cholesterol or with a modest increase. Examining the confidence interval should help us avoid the common error of equating 'non-significance' with acceptance of the null hypothesis that the drug has no effect, regardless of the power of the study to detect differences of interest.

A number of books and articles discuss in more detail the testing of hypotheses, the arguments between the Fisher and Neyman-Pearson schools of inference and the case for Bayesian reasoning as an alternative (e.g. Cox, 1982; Goodman, 1999a, 1999b; Lehmann, 1993; Oakes, 1986; Sterne and Davey Smith, 2001).   *JS*

Cox, D.R. 1982: Statistical significance tests. *British Journal of Clinical Pharmacology* 14, 325–31. **Fisher, R.A.** 1950: *Statistical methods for research workers*. London: Oliver and Boyd. **Fisher, R.A.** 1973: *Statistical methods and scientific inference*. London: Collins Macmillan. **Goodman, S.N.** 1999a: Toward evidence-based medical statistics. 1: the P-value fallacy. *Annals of International Medicine* 130, 995–1004. **Goodman, S.N.** 1999b: Toward evidence-based medical statistics. 2: the Bayes factor. *Annals of International Medicine* 130, 1005–13. **Lehmann, E.L.** 1993: The Fisher, Neyman-Pearson theories of testing hypotheses: one theory or two? *Journal of the American Statistical Association* 88, 1242–9. **Neyman, J. and Pearson, E.** 1933: On the problem of the most efficient tests of statistical hypotheses. *Philosophical Transactions of the Royal Society Series A* 231, 289–337. **Oakes, M.** 1986: *Statistical inference*. Chichester: John Wiley & Sons. **Sterne, J.A. and Davey Smith, G.** 2001: Sifting the evidence – what's wrong with significance tests? *British Medical Journal* 322, 226–31.

I

ICC Abbreviation for INTRACLUSTER CORRELATION COEFFICIENT.

ICER Abbreviation for incremental cost-effectiveness ratio. See COST-EFFECTIVENESS ANALYSIS

immune proportion The proportion of individuals who may not be subject to death, failure, relapse etc. in a sample of censored survival times. The presence of such individuals may be indicated by a relatively high number of individuals with large censored survival times. FINITE MIXTURE DISTRIBUTIONS can be used to investigate such data. Specifically, the population is assumed to consist of two components. The first, which is present in proportion, p, say, contains those individuals who are susceptible to some event of interest (death, relapse etc.) and have, say, an EXPONENTIAL DISTRIBUTION for the time to the occurrence of the event. These individuals are subject to right censoring. The remaining proportion $1 - p$ of the population is assumed to be immune to, or cured of, the disease and for these individuals the event never happens. Consequently, observations on their survival times are always censored at the limit of follow-up. An important aspect of such analysis is to consider whether or not an immune proportion does in fact exist in the population (see, for example, Maller and Zhou, 1995). *BSE*

[See also CURE MODELS]

Maller, R.A. and Zhou, S. 1995: Testing for the presence of immune or cured individuals in censored survival data. *Biometrics* 51, 181–201.

imputation See MULTIPLE IMPUTATION

incidence The incidence of a disease is the number of new cases of the disease occurring within a specified period of time in a defined population. A time period of 1 year is most commonly used, but any appropriate length of time can be substituted. It is generally presented as a rate. Thus:

$$\text{Incidence rate} = \frac{\text{Number of new cases of the disease in one year}}{\text{Number in the population at risk}}$$

This assumes that the size of the study population remains constant over the time period for which the rate is calculated. Small increases or decreases in population size over a year, for example, can be dealt with by using the mid-year population as the denominator for the incidence rate.

This results in a number between 0 and 1, but for ease of presentation it is often expressed as a rate per 1000, per 100,000 or per 1,000,000 depending on the disease rarity. As an example, the incidence rate of colorectal cancer in males aged 60–64 in Scotland was 200 per 100,000 in the year 2000 compared to 141 per 100,000 in 1990 (Scottish Health Statistics). Thus incidence rates can be used to measure risk and compare risks across time or between different populations.

This definition is rather simplistic because it ignores the fact that when new cases of the disease occur, the subject is no longer at risk and should ideally be removed from the denominator. It is also unsatisfactory for dealing with data from LONGITUDINAL STUDIES in which subjects may be followed up for varying lengths of time. For these studies the incidence rate can be defined as:

$$\text{Incidence rate} = \frac{\text{Number of new cases of the disease in the defined population}}{\text{Total length of time for which subjects have been followed up}}$$

The denominator gives the number of person-years of observation. Incidence rates defined in this way are often expressed as rates per 100 or per 1000 person-years of observation. (A more detailed discussion of incidence and incidence rates is given in Rothman and Greenland, 1998).

Care should be taken to distinguish between incidence and PREVALENCE. Although the definitions appear similar at first sight, they are used for different purposes and it is essential to distinguish between them correctly. *WHG*

Rothman, K.J. and Greenland, S. 1998: *Modern epidemiology*, 2nd edn. Philadelphia: Lippincott Wilkins and Williams. **Scottish Health Statistics:** www.isdscotland.org. **Woodward, M.** 1999: *Epidemiology: study design and data analysis*. Boca Raton: Chapman & Hall.

inclusion and exclusion criteria Criteria that operationalise choice of study group, a choice that lies at the heart of the design of, and inference from, CLINICAL TRIALS. 'Inclusion' criteria define the population of interest; 'exclusion' criteria remove people for whom the study treatment is contraindicated or unlikely to be effective. Collectively, inclusion criteria and exclusion criteria comprise the *entry criteria* or *eligibility criteria*. Biological plausibility, the internal validity of the study, the epidemiological basis for generalisability and statistical POWER all play parts in selecting entry criteria and in making recommendations from the results of the trial. The selection of those to be enrolled in a trial often reflects a deliberate attempt to select a study cohort homogeneous enough to allow a true treatment effect to become manifest, yet heterogeneous enough to permit reliable generalisation to a broader population. Clinical trials necessarily study people with more homogeneous characteristics than the patients to whom clinicians will apply the results.

Strict representativeness is relevant to the *generalisability* of clinical trials but not essential to *inference* from them. In randomised studies, the logical basis for drawing conclusions lies in the act of RANDOMISATION. The process of concluding that the effect seen in a clinical trial will apply to another population is informal and subjective (Cowan and Wittes, 1994).

Homogeneity of the study population differs from homogeneity of treatment effect. The former refers to a study group's sharing similar characteristics; the latter refers to an effect of treatment whose expected magnitude and direction would lead to the same recommendation for use or non-use in identifiable subgroups. If a therapy affects a wide group of people quite similarly, then either a homogeneous or heterogeneous study group will provide similar answers regarding the magnitude of treatment effect.

An ideal study group would consist of a cohort for whom the treatment is effective and corresponding to whom is an identifiable population that will be treated. Defining such a study group before the trial is usually difficult. Available data are rarely sufficiently reliable to provide serious guidance about whom to include.

Early-phase studies typically define narrow entry criteria to establish preliminary safety or to demonstrate proof of concept (see PHASE I TRIALS, PHASE II TRIALS). Such trials often exclude children, pregnant and nursing women, the frail elderly and other vulnerable populations.

Later phase trials with narrow entry criteria specify the type of patient likely to benefit most and then test whether the treatment works for them (see PHASE III TRIALS, PHASE IV TRIALS). A study showing benefit in this narrow group of participants may lead to future trials with wider entry criteria. A treatment with important heterogeneity of effect requires a homogeneous study population.

Trials with wide entry criteria address whether the treatment under study works on average when applied to potential users. Wide entry criteria simplify screening and recruitment. Enrolling a wide range of people is consistent with assuming homogeneity of effect while affording the investigator a tentative glimpse at the likelihood of the truth of that assumption.

Biological plausibility should play a decisive role in selecting the range of people to enrol in a trial. Study entry criteria should aim to achieve heterogeneity when no convincing information at the start of the study suggests that sizeable differential effects are likely. A heterogeneous study group leads to variation in the incidence of endpoints, so increasing heterogeneity generally requires increased sample size.

Defining entry criteria requires an operational definition of the disease in a treatment trial or a specification of who is at risk in a prevention trial. Allowing people with questionable diagnoses to enter a trial tends to attenuate the estimated treatment effect and hence decreases statistical power. Yet often the insistence on unequivocal documentation of diagnosis excludes many people who in fact would receive the treatment if the trial shows benefit (Yusuf, Held and Teo, 1994).

Trials must exclude people known to have contraindications to the treatments under study or those who are particularly vulnerable. Similarly, trials of therapies already known to be effective or ineffective in certain group should exclude those groups of patients. Some randomised trials use an 'uncertainty principle' to guide entry (see MEGA-TRIAL). 'A patient can be entered if, and only if, the responsible clinician is substantially uncertain which of the trial treatments would be most appropriate for that particular patient' (Peto and Baigent, 1998).

Typical PROTOCOLS FOR CLINICAL TRIALS exclude people unlikely to finish a study or to adhere to the protocol.

Many clinical trials have very few participants with some specific characteristics. A trial may exclude racial or ethnic groups not because the entry criteria preclude their participation, but because the clinics involved in the study do not have access to them.

In summary, trial designers should ensure that each entry criterion represents a defensible limitation on the study group; however, the fact of inclusion does not usually provide much information about the effect of treatment in specific groups of people. The argument that only by including, say, women and minorities, can one legitimately apply the results of the trial needs to be tempered with the fact that a trial rarely gives enough information about specific groups to learn much about the effect of treatment for them. When the trial is over, the results should usually be applied quite broadly, both to people whose demographic characteristics are similar and dissimilar to those in the trial; however, the medical community should maintain an intellectual stance open to suggestive data indicating differences.

The situation is more complicated for groups of people defined by such medical or physiologic variable as diagnosis, severity, prognostic features, prior history or concomitant medications, for often apparently biological cogent reasons justify exclusions. Here too a critical questioning of the reasons for exclusion is warranted; in many cases very few data are available to support even strongly held views.

Designers of clinical trials should construct entry criteria bearing in mind the purpose of the current trial, the available knowledge of the study treatments being tested, the likely studies that will follow the trial and how investigators, practising clinicians, patients and regulatory agencies will interpret the results in light of the entry criteria.   *JW*

Cowan, C. and Wittes, J. 1994: Intercept studies, clinical trials, and cluster experiments: to whom can we extrapolate? *Controlled Clinical Trials* 15, 24–9. **Peto, R. and Baigent, C.** 1998: Trials: the next 50 years. *British Medical Journal* 317, 1170–1. **Yusuf, S., Held, P. and Teo, K.K.** 1994: Selection of patients for randomised controlled trials: implications of wide or narrow eligibility criteria. *Statistics in Medicine* 9, 73–86.

incomplete block designs See CROSS-OVER TRIALS

incremental cost-effectiveness ratio (ICER)
See COST-EFFECTIVENESS ANALYSIS

incubation period The time interval between the acquisition of infection and the appearance of symptomatic disease. Examples include the time between exposure to radiation or to a chemical carcinogen and the occurrence of cancer and the time from infection with HIV and the onset of AIDS.

The length of the incubation period depends on the disease, ranging from days, for instance, in the case of malaria to a number of years for HIV. The incubation period typically varies from individual to individual and may depend on the dose of the disease-causing agent received. Given this variability, it makes sense to talk about incubation period distribution. The incubation period distribution $F(t)$ represents the probability that the length of the incubation period is less than or equal to t time units.

Estimation and characterisation of $F(t)$ is important for a number of reasons. For diseases with short incubation periods, such as outbreaks, knowledge of the incubation period is essential to the investigation of the circumstances in which the disease has spread. In the case of diseases with long incubation periods, such as HIV or Creutzfeldt-Jakob disease, information on $F(t)$ is a necessary input to the estimation and projection of the evolution of the epidemic (see BACK-CALCULATION). Finally, it is very important to identify covariates that might affect the length of the incubation period for an effective clinical management of the patient.

The ideal setup to estimate the incubation period distribution is a COHORT STUDY where individuals are uninfected at enrolment and are followed up to observe both the occurrence of infection and the appearance of symptomatic disease. The resulting observations will be right censored as every individual will have either developed the disease or been censored by the end of the follow-up period (see CENSORED OBSERVATIONS). Classical survival analysis can be used to estimate $F(t)$ both non-parametrically, via KAPLAN-MEIER PLOTS, and parametrically, by fitting parametric models to the right-censored data. Usually, especially for diseases with long incubation time, such cohort studies are difficult to set up. Estimation of the incubation period distribution is then carried out either using information on individuals who have already developed symptoms or following up cohorts of individuals who are already infected, but have not yet developed the disease. In either case, biased results can be obtained if estimation does not properly account for the sampling criteria by which individuals are included in the study. *DDA*

Brookmeyer, R. 1998: Incubation period of infectious diseases. In Armitage, P. and Colton, T. (eds), *Encyclopedia of biostatistics* 1, 2011–16. Chichester: John Wiley & Sons. **Brookmeyer, R. and Gail, M.H.** 1994: *AIDS epidemiology: a quantitative approach*. New York: Oxford University Press.

indirect standardisation   See DEMOGRAPHY

individual ethics   See ETHICS AND CLINICAL TRIALS

infant mortality rate   See DEMOGRAPHY

informative censoring/dropout   See CENSORED OBSERVATIONS, DROPOUT, MISSING DATA

informative dropout   Synonym for NON-IGNORABLE DROPOUT.

informed consent   See ETHICS AND CLINICAL TRIALS

instantaneous death rate   Synonym for layered function. See SURVIVAL ANALYSIS

institutional review board (IRB)   See ETHICAL REVIEW COMMITTEES

instrumental variables   A VARIABLE highly correlated with an explanatory variable but has no direct influence on the response variable (i.e. its effect is mediated by the explanatory variable). Consider the so-called endogeneity problem, in which we can assume that a response variable, Y, is linearly related to an explanatory variable, X, as follows:

$$Y = \alpha + \beta X + \varepsilon \tag{1}$$

where ε is a random deviation of a particular value of Y from that expected from its relationship with X. Typically,

we wish to use a sample of (X, Y) pairs of measurements in order to estimate the unknown values of the parameters, α and β. The ordinary least squares (OLS) estimator of β is equivalent to the ratio of the estimated COVARIANCE of X and Y to the estimated variance of X (this ratio is usually calculated by dividing the sum of the cross-products of the Xs and Ys from their respective mean by the sum of squares of the Xs). It is possible to demonstrate that such an estimate is unbiased for β provided certain assumptions hold – the key one being that X and ε are uncorrelated.

Now, if we have an unmeasured confounder, C, such that the true model is, in fact:

$$Y = \alpha + \beta X + \gamma C + \delta \tag{2}$$

where δ is the random deviation of Y from that explained by the model and we still proceed with our naive OLS estimator as for equation (1), we will obtain a biased estimate of β. This is due to the correlation between X and ε no longer being zero. This is an example of what econometricians call endogeneity (see Wooldridge, 2003). In such circumstances, how might we obtain a valid estimate of β? The obvious answer is to measure C and fit equation (2). Another approach (much more common in economics than in medical applications) is to find a variable that is strongly correlated with X, but has no direct effect on the response, Y. Such a variable is called an instrumental variable, or instrument for short.

Now consider a different circumstance. Suppose that the values of X are measured subject to error such that:

$$X = \tau + v \tag{3}$$

where the vs are random measurement errors with zero mean and assumed to be uncorrelated both with each other and with the true values, τ. The relationship we are really interested in is the following:

$$Y = \alpha + \beta \tau + \varepsilon \tag{4}$$

How do we estimate β? Again, using OLS in a regression of Y against X would produce a biased result (see ATTENUATION DUE TO MEASUREMENT ERROR). This is another example of the endogeneity problem. A similar situation holds when we attempt the comparative calibration of two measurement methods, both subject to measurement errors (see METHOD COMPARISON STUDIES). If we were in the fortuitous position of knowing the variance of the measurement errors in X, or the reliability of X, we would be able to make appropriate corrections. Another approach is again to find an instrumental variable. Consider an instrumental variable, Z. The instrumental variable (or IV) estimator of β in (2) or (4) is:

$$\beta_{IV} = \frac{\sum (Z - \bar{Z})(Y - \bar{Y})}{\sum (Z - \bar{Z})(X - \bar{X})} \tag{5}$$

which is equivalent to the ratio of the estimated covariance of Z and Y to the estimated covariance of Z and X. Typically, this estimate is obtained through the use of a two-stage least squares (2SLS or TSLS) algorithm. Wooldridge (2003) gives further details of the method, including the sampling distribution of the IV estimate. This algorithm is available in most large general-purpose software packages. Note that its validity is not dependent on any distributional assumptions concerning either Z or X. Both could be binary (yes/no) indicators, for example.

For linear models, IV estimates can also be obtained using structural equation modelling (see STRUCTURAL EQUATION MODELS).

As an example, an early medical application of instrumental variable methods was provided by Permutt and Hebel (1989). They describe a trial in which pregnant women were randomly allocated to receive encouragement to reduce or stop their cigarette smoking during pregnancy (the treatment group) or not (the control group) – indicated by the binary variable, Z. An intermediate outcome variable (X) was the amount of cigarette smoking recorded during pregnancy. The ultimate outcome (Y) was the birth weight of the newborn child. Readers will be familiar with evaluating the effect of RANDOMISATION on the child's birth weight. But what about the effect of smoking (X) on birth weight? Smoking is likely to have been reduced in the group subject to encouragement, but also in the control group (but, presumably, to a lesser extent). There are also likely to be hidden confounders (e.g. other health promoting behaviours) that are associated with both mother's smoking during pregnancy and the child's birth weight. Smoking (X) is an endogenous treatment variable. The problem is solved by noting that randomisation (Z) is an obvious candidate for the instrumental variable. If the intervention (i.e. encouragement to reduce smoking) works then randomisation should be correlated with smoking during pregnancy. Given the amount of smoking observed it is also a reasonable assumption that the randomisation itself will not have an effect on outcome (the birth weight of the child).

Randomisation (Z) is, in fact, increasingly being used as an instrumental variable in the estimation of the effect of treatment received (X) on outcome (Y) in randomised controlled trials subject to non-adherence or non-compliance with the allocated treatment (see ADJUSTMENT FOR NON-COMPLIANCE IN RANDOMISED CONTROLLED TRIALS). The potential for the use of instrumental variables in epidemiological investigations is illustrated by Greenland (2000). Health economic applications are reviewed by Newhouse and McClellan (1998).

What about MEASUREMENT ERROR problems? Well, first note that for the example provided by Permutt and Hebel (1989) the IV estimate of the effect of mother's smoking on her child's birth weight is not attenuated by the inevitable measurement error in the number of cigarettes smoked by the mother. The IV estimator effectively copes with the simultaneous problems of confounding and measurement error. What about the problem solely due to measurement error? Here an obvious choice for an instrument is a measurement of the characteristic measured as X using a different procedure. Smoking (X) could be measured by self-report (in a diary, for example) and a suitable instrument (Z) might be a measurement of a biomarker of nicotine consumption (cotinine levels in the blood, for example). The key here is to be able to convince oneself of the conditional independence of Z (biomarker measurement) and outcome, Y (health status), given the fallible indicator of exposure, X (self-reported cigarette smoking). Dunn (2004) provides detailed descriptions of the use of instrumental variable methodology in the evaluation of measurement errors, mainly in the context of linear models, but also in latent class modelling of binary diagnostic test results. Non-linear models can be handled too, but are beyond the scope of this section (but see Stefanski and Buzas, 1995). *GD*

Dunn, G. 2004: *Statistical evaluation of measurement errors.* London: Arnold. **Greenland, S.** 2000: An introduction to instrumental variables for epidemiologists. *International Journal of Epidemiology* 29, 722–9 (erratum p. 1102). **Newhouse, J.P. and McClellan, M.** 1998: Econometrics in outcomes research: the use of instrumental variables. *Annual Reviews of Public Health* 19, 17–34. **Permutt, T. and Hebel, J.R.** 1989: Simultaneous-equation estimation in a clinical trial of the effect of smoking and birth weight. *Biometrics* 45, 619–22. **Stefanski, L. and Buzas, J.S.** 1995: Instrumental variable estimation in binary regression measurement error models. *Journal of the American Statistical Association* 90, 541–9. **Wooldridge, J.M.** 2003: *Introductory econometrics: a modern approach*, 2nd edn. Mason, OH: South-Western.

integrated hazard function   See SURVIVAL ANALYSIS

intention-to-treat (ITT)   A principle used in the design, analysis and conduct of randomised CLINICAL TRIALS. It asserts that the effect of an intervention policy can be best assessed by comparing participants according to the intention to treat each participant (i.e. the planned intervention), rather than according to the actual intervention received. When the ITT principle is used, all participants allocated to an intervention group should be followed up, assessed and analysed as members of that group irrespective of their compliance to the planned intervention (ICH E9, 1999). This is the most suitable approach for pragmatic trials (see CLINICAL TRIALS) that aim to measure the *effectiveness* of an intervention policy in routine practice, the overall effect of the policy including protocol deviations and non-compliance. It is less suitable for explanatory trials that aim to measure the *efficacy* of an intervention under equalised conditions, but even here it may be preferable to the alternatives (see later).

The purpose of RANDOMISATION in a controlled trial is to create groups that are similar, apart from chance variation, in all observed and unobserved characteristics that might affect the outcome. If analysis is not performed on the groups produced by the randomisation process, this key feature will be lost, which may lead to a biased comparison. For example, participants may not receive the allocated treatment due to a poor prognosis. In a trial comparing medical and surgical therapy in stable angina pectoris, a particularly high mortality rate was seen in participants allocated to surgery who did not receive it (see first Table). It could be considered unfair to include these deaths in the surgery group, but if we wish to compare the *policy* of surgery with the *policy* of medical treatment then these deaths should be included in the analysis in the surgery group. Participants who died before receiving

intention-to-treat *Coronary artery bypass surgery in stable angina pectoris trial. Mortality at two years after randomisation by allocated and actual intervention (European Coronary Surgery Study Group, 1979)*

Allocated intervention	Medical	Medical	Surgical	Surgical
Actual intervention	Medical	Surgical	Surgical	Medical
Survivors	296	48	353	20
Deaths	27	2	15	6
Mortality	8.4%	4.0%	4.1%	23.1%

surgery were either too sick for surgery or died before surgery could be carried out and exclusion of such participants from one arm only introduces BIAS. The ITT analysis of these data would compare a mortality rate of 7.8% (29/373) in those allocated to medical treatment with a rate of 5.3% (21/394) in those allocated to surgery. If the 6 deaths that occurred in participants allocated to surgical intervention who died before receiving surgery are not attributed to surgical intervention using an intention-to-treat analysis, surgery would appear to have a falsely low mortality rate. Since protocol deviations and non-compliance are likely to occur in routine use of an intervention, ITT analysis can provide an estimate of treatment effect that reasonably reflects what might happen in clinical practice.

Alternatives to ITT include PER PROTOCOL analysis where only participants who comply with the allocated intervention are included, and '*as treated*' analysis where participants are analysed according to the intervention received rather than the randomised allocation. Each of these analyses aims to estimate efficacy, rather than effectiveness as estimated in an ITT analysis. In the trial comparing medical and surgical therapy in stable angina pectoris, intention to treat analysis gives an estimate of 2.5% lower mortality with surgery (95% confidence interval −1.5% to +5.5%). Per protocol and as treated analyses are severely biased by their handling of the 6 deaths in patients randomised to surgery who were too sick or died too soon to receive surgery, giving statistically significant estimated decreases in mortality with surgery of 4.3% and 5.4% respectively (see second Table). (For a discussion of ways to estimate efficacy while avoiding this bias, see ADJUSTMENT FOR NON-COMPLIANCE IN RCTS.)

If some participants lack outcome data, then a full ITT approach will not be possible since all randomised participants cannot then be included in the analysis. Sensitivity analysis should be considered to examine the potential impact of any MISSING DATA (Hollis and Campbell, 1999). Participants with incomplete outcome data can be included by using MULTIPLE IMPUTATION or RANDOM EFFECTS MODELLING.

It is often argued that ITT provides a conservative estimate of treatment effectiveness, that is a smaller effect than the true potential effectiveness of an intervention, since the estimated treatment effect is likely to be reduced by the inclusion of protocol deviations and non-compliance. This may be true for comparisons with PLACEBO, because any switching between groups will tend to dilute

the estimated treatment effect. However, in comparisons between active treatments or when an effective rescue medication is available, an ITT analysis may not be conservative. For example, two equally good treatments will appear different on ITT analysis if clinicians are more likely to supplement one of the treatments with a more powerful agent. Particular care should be taken when using the ITT approach for adverse effects or safety data and for non-inferiority or equivalence trials. In these situations the generally conservative answers provided by ITT may lead to inappropriate conclusions. Other analyses such as PER PROTOCOL analysis should also be carried out in these situations.

Some exclusions from an ITT analysis may be justified, provided that these exclusions are not associated with treatment allocation or outcome (Fergusson *et al.*, 2002). Ineligible participants who are randomised in error could be excluded provided that detection of ineligibility is not more likely in one intervention group or in participants with a particular outcome. It may not always be possible to establish eligibility prior to randomisation. Again, participants found to be ineligible can be excluded provided that the judgement of eligibility is based on information established before randomisation and not influenced by the allocated intervention or outcome. However, if clinical practice requires treatment to be started before eligibility can be determined then the most relevant comparison will usually be between all those randomised to treatment and all those randomised to control. Failure to start the allocated treatment is also sometimes a justified basis for exclusion in a blinded trial, but it could be argued that this does not comply with the basic principle of ITT. If any randomised participants are excluded from an ITT analysis then it should be demonstrated that steps have been taken to avoid bias, such as the use of independent blinded assessment of eligibility. Every effort should be made to minimise post-randomisation exclusions through appropriate design and execution of trials.   *SH/IW*

[See also AVAILABLE CASE ANALYSIS, COMPLETE CASE ANALYSIS]

European Coronary Surgery Study Group 1979: Coronary-artery bypass surgery in stable angina pectoris: survival at two years. *The Lancet* i, 889–93. **Fergusson, D., Aaron, S., Guyatt, G. and Hebert, P.** 2002: Post-randomisation exclusions: the intention to treat principle and excluding patients from analysis. *British Medical Journal* 325, 652–4. **Heritier, S.R., Gebski, V.J. and Keech, A.C.** 2003: Inclusion of patients in clinical trial analysis: the intention-to-treat principle. *Medical Journal of Australia* 179, 438–40. **Hollis, S. and Campbell, F.** 1999: What is meant by 'intention-to-treat' analysis? *British Medical Journal* 319, 670–74. **International Conference on Harmonisation E9 Expert Working Group (ICH E9)** 1999: ICH harmonised tripartite guideline. Statistical principles for clinical trials. *Statistics in Medicine* 18, 15, 1905–42.

interim analysis   Analyses performed at regular intervals for monitoring of data and safety in clinical trials. An interim analysis refers to any analysis performed during the course of a trial and is often intended to compare intervention effects with respect to efficacy and safety prior to the formal completion of a trial. Because the number, methods and consequences of these comparisons affect the interpretation of the trial, all interim analyses should be carefully planned in advance and described in

intention-to-treat   *Different methods of analysis illustrated using mortality at two years after randomisation in the coronary artery bypass surgery in stable angina pectoris trial (European Coronary Surgery Study Group, 1979)*

	Medical % (n/N)	Surgical % (n/N)	Medical vs Surgical difference (95% CI)
Intention-to-treat analysis	7.8% (29/373)	5.3% (21/394)	2.5% (−1.5%, 5.5%)
Per-protocol analysis	8.4% (27/323)	4.1% (15/368)	4.3% (0.7%, 8.2%)
As treated analysis	9.5% (33/349)	4.1% (17/418)	5.4% (1.9%, 9.3%)

the protocol explicitly. When an interim analysis is planned with the intention of deciding whether or not to terminate a trial early, this is usually accomplished by one of three general methods known as group sequential methods, triangular tests and stochastic curtailment procedures.

The goal of such an interim analysis is to stop the trial early if the superiority of an intervention under study is clearly established, if the demonstration of a relevant difference in intervention effects becomes unlikely or if unacceptable adverse effects are apparent. Also as a result of interim analyses, trial interventions may be modified or experimental design such as the enrolment inclusion and exclusion criteria or sample size requirement changed. Ethical obligation to the study participants and even beyond the study demands that results be monitored during the study to protect study participants. If one intervention is substantially superior to the other, if there are unexpected adverse effects on either of the interventions or if the study is unlikely to give definitive answers to the study questions, continuing RANDOMISATION means that participants can be assigned to and subsequently treated with an inferior intervention or put to an unnecessary and unjustifiable experiment. The issues of early stopping due to unexpected adverse effects are less statistical in nature, unless safety is the primary outcome of interest to the investigators.

Suppose the response to intervention is normally distributed with means μ_A and μ_B for intervention arms A and B and known variance σ^2. We want to test the null hypothesis:

$$H_0 : \mu_A = \mu_B$$

against the alternative hypothesis $H_1 : \mu_A \neq \mu_B$ or, equivalently, $H_0 : \delta_\mu = 0$ against $H_1 : \delta\mu \neq 0$ where $\delta_\mu = \mu_A - \mu_B$. Let $\bar{X}_A$ and $\bar{X}_B$ be the sample means respectively for interventions A and B and let n denote the number of participants per intervention per analysis. In a fixed sample study, one may use the test statistic:

$$Z = \frac{\bar{X}_A - \bar{X}_B}{\sqrt{(2\sigma^2/n)}}$$

to test the null hypothesis H_0. For a significance level α, one would reject H_0 if $|Z| \geq z_{1-\alpha/2}$ where $z_{1-\alpha/2}$ is the $1 - \alpha/2$ quantile of the standard normal distribution.

Group sequential methods call for monitoring of the accumulating data periodically after groups of observations. One simple-minded approach is to reject the null hypothesis whenever the P-value is less than 0.05, say. The problem with this approach is that multiple looks at 0.05 level lead to the overall level of significance greater than 0.05. More specifically, the actual TYPE I ERROR probability becomes 0.083 with two looks, 0.142 with five looks and becomes closer and closer to 1 with more and more looks. This phenomenon was aptly described as 'sampling to reach a foregone conclusion' by Anscombe (1954).

Suppose we plan to conduct interim analyses of the accumulating data up to K times after a pre-specified number of participants n on each intervention. The difference in intervention effects is measured at the kth interim analysis by:

$$\bar{X}_{Ak} - \bar{X}_{Bk} \sim N(\delta_\mu, 2\sigma^2/n)$$

where $\bar{X}_{Ak}$ and $\bar{X}_{Bk}$ are the sample means of n observations accumulated between the $(k - 1)$th and the kth interim analyses on interventions A and B, respectively. Or it can be summarised by the standardised difference:

$$Y_k = \frac{\bar{X}_{Ak} - \bar{X}_{Bk}}{\sqrt{(2\sigma^2/n)}} \sim N(\delta^\star, 1)$$

where $\delta^\star = \delta_\mu/\sqrt{(2\sigma^2/n)}$. For the kth interim analysis, we consider the partial sum of independently and identically distributed normal random variables $Y_1, \ldots, Y_k$:

$$S_k = \sum_{j=1}^{k} Y_j \sim N(\delta^\star k, k)$$

or equivalently the standardised test statistic:

$$Z_k = S_k/\sqrt{k} \sim N(\delta^* \sqrt{k}, 1)$$

and decide to reject H_0 or to continue to the next group, up to a maximum of K interim analyses.

The objective of a group sequential design is to derive a group sequential test that has desired operating characteristics, i.e., pre-specified Type I and II error probabilities. Thus a group sequential design for a trial requires choosing group sequential critical values, $c_1, \ldots, c_K$, such that one rejects H_0 after the kth interim analysis if the statistic $|Z_k|$ exceeds c_k for the first time. We do not reject the null hypotheses if $|Z_1| < c_1, \ldots, |Z_K| < c_K$. There are many different designs, that is, many different choices for the group sequential critical values. However, there are a few with known statistical justifications.

The group sequential test by Pocock (1997) uses the same critical value at each interim analysis. Specifically, the Pocock group sequential test rejects H_0 the first time when:

$$|Z_k| \geq c_k \equiv c_P \quad \text{or equivalently} \quad |S_k| \geq b_k = c_P\sqrt{k}$$

Hence one has only to determine c_P as a function of the overall Type I error probability α and the maximum number of interim analyses K.

The group sequential test by O'Brien and Fleming (1979) uses larger critical values at earlier interim analyses so that it is difficult to reject H_0 early in the study and relaxes the criteria until, at the end, the critical value is close to the fixed sample critical value. Specifically, the O'Brien-Fleming group sequential test rejects H_0 the first time when:

$$|Z_k| \geq c_k = c_O\sqrt{(K/k)} \quad \text{or equivalently} \quad |S_k| \geq b_k \equiv c_O\sqrt{K}$$

Again, one has only to determine c_O as a function of α and K.

The standard group sequential method has some limitations because of the requirements in the pre-specified maximum number of interim analyses and the equal increment in statistical information between interim analyses. There are, however, flexible group sequential procedures that make these requirements unnecessary based on the notion of an error spending function as proposed by Lan and DeMets (1983). Especially for trials with censored survival or repeated measures data, it is necessary to be flexible in the group sequential test since typical interim analyses take place after unequal increment in the information fraction. Also recent developments in group sequential methods allow early stopping in order to reject the alternative hypothesis just as the triangular tests do with the required flexibility as proposed by Chang, Hwang and Shih (1998) and Pampallona, Tsiatis and Kim (2001).

Wald's sequential probability ratio test (1947) for $H_0: \theta = \theta_0$ vs. $H_1: \theta = \theta_1$ is optimal in the sense that, among all tests with Type I and II error probabilities α and β, it minimises the expected sample sizes $E(N|\theta_0)$ and $E(N|\theta_1)$ where N is a random variable for the sequential sample size. However, $E(N|\theta)$ can be worse than the corresponding fixed sample size at or near $\theta = (\theta_0 + \theta_1)/2$. Moreover, the sample size is unbounded and, in particular, $\Pr(N \geq n) > 0$ for any given n. Thus the motivation in Anderson (1960) was to find a sequential test that would minimise $E(N|\theta)$ at $\theta = (\theta_0 + \theta_1)/2$, leading to the so-called triangular test. Triangular tests have been further developed in Whitehead (1997) as described below.

In a general problem, efficient score Z for the parameter of interest θ, which typically measures the difference has the following asymptotic distribution according to likelihood theory:

$$Z \overset{a}{\sim} N(\theta V, V)$$

where V denotes Fisher information. For a fixed sample test, the critical value c and Fisher information required for the study are determined to have Type I and II error probabilities α and β, respectively, such that:

$$\Pr(|Z| \geq c; 0) = \alpha \quad \text{and} \quad \Pr(Z \geq c; \theta_1) = 1 - \beta$$

where θ_1 is the hypothesised difference of interest. These two requirements lead to:

$$V = \left(\frac{z_{1-\alpha/2} + z_{1-\beta}}{\theta_1} \right)^2 \quad \text{and} \quad c = \frac{(z_{1-\alpha/2} + z_{1-\beta}) z_{1-\alpha/2}}{\theta_1}.$$

According to Whitehead (1997), a triangular test is defined by the upper and lower boundaries of the form:

$$Z = a + cV \quad \text{and} \quad Z = -a + 3cV$$

respectively, with the apex of the triangle at $Z = 2a$ and $V = a/c$. In the special case where $\alpha/2 = \beta$:

$$a = -2 \log \alpha / \theta_1 \quad \text{and} \quad c = \theta_1/4.$$

A solution is possible for the general case as well when $\alpha/2 \ll \beta$ which is typically the case.

Since interim analyses are performed only a limited number of times, some adjustments need to be made in order to maintain the operating characteristics. This is accomplished by the so-called 'Christmas tree adjustment', which is described later. Suppose that $(Z^\star, V^\star)$ denotes the value of sequential statistics at the time an upper boundary is crossed. The overshoot R is the vertical distance between the final point of the sample path and the continuous boundary defined as:

$$R = Z^\star - (a + cV^\star).$$

In order to account for the discreteness of the interim analyses, the continuous stopping criterion:

$$Z \geq a + cV$$

is replaced by:

$$Z \geq a + cV - A$$

where:

$$A = E(R; \theta).$$

In developing triangular tests, two different power requirements are specified. Traditional accounts of testing the null hypothesis $H_0: \theta = 0$ allow two outcomes in which 'H_0 is accepted' or 'H_0 is rejected'. However, three outcomes are possible in practice. The power function $C(\theta)$ is the probability of rejecting H_0 under the parameter value θ defined as:

$$C(\theta) = C^+(\theta) + C^-(\theta)$$

where $C^+(\theta)$ denotes the probability that H_0 is rejected and it is concluded that the experimental intervention is superior and $C^-(\theta)$ denotes the probability that H_0 is rejected and it is concluded that the experimental intervention is inferior. Obviously, for two-sided tests:

$$C(0) = \alpha \quad \text{with} \quad C^+(0) = C^-(0) = \alpha/2.$$

Two specific power requirements are either $C^+(\theta_1) = 1 - \beta$ or $C^+(\theta_1) = 1 - \beta = C^-(-\theta_1)$. These give rise to asymmetric or symmetric triangular tests for two-sided test of the null hypothesis.

In curtailment sampling, one is interested in assessing the likelihood of a trend reversal. There are two possible ways: deterministic and stochastic. This notion has been found to be useful in consideration of early stopping for futility. In contrast, early acceptance of the null hypothesis is possible based on group sequential methods and triangular tests discussed earlier. An example of deterministic curtailment is curtailed sampling in sampling inspection in which trend reversal is impossible. Let S denote a test statistic which measures difference in intervention effects and let the sample space Ω of S consist of disjoint regions, A and R, such that:

$$\Pr(S \in R | H_0) = \alpha \quad \text{and} \quad \Pr(S \in A | H_1) = \beta.$$

Let t denote the time of an interim analysis and let $D(t)$ denote the accumulated data up to time t. A deterministic curtailment test rejects or accepts the null hypothesis H_0 if:

$$\Pr(S \in R | D(t)) = 1 \quad \text{or} \quad \Pr(S \in A | D(t)) = 1$$

respectively, regardless of whether H_0 or H_1 is true. Note that this procedure does not affect the Type I and II error probabilities.

As an example, consider testing the fairness of a coin, $H_0: \pi = 0.5$ vs $H_1: \pi \neq 0.5$. After tossing a coin 400 times, one will consider the total number of heads S and reject H_0 if $|Z| > 1.96$ at a significance level 0.05 where:

$$Z = \frac{S - 200}{\sqrt{(400 \times 0.5 \times 0.5)}}$$

or equivalently if $|S - 200| \geq 20$. After 350 tosses, we will reject H_0 for sure with 220 heads. With 210 heads, however, it depends on the future outcomes.

Consider a fixed sample test of $H_0: \theta = 0$ at a significance level α with power $1 - \beta$ to detect the difference $\theta = \theta_1$. The conditional probability of rejection of H_0, i.e. conditional power, at θ is defined as:

$$P_C(\theta) = \Pr(S \in R | D(t); \theta).$$

For some $\gamma_0, \gamma_1 > 1/2$, a stochastic curtailment test rejects the null hypothesis if:

$$P_C(\theta_1) \approx 1 \quad \text{and} \quad P_C(0) > \gamma_0$$

or accepts the null hypothesis (rejects the alternative hypothesis) if:

$$P_C(0) \approx 0 \quad \text{and} \quad P_C(\theta_1) < 1 - \gamma_1.$$

According to Lan, Simon and Halperin (1982), the Type I and II error probabilities are inflated but remain bounded from above by:

$$\alpha' = \alpha/\gamma_0 \quad \text{and} \quad \beta' = \beta/\gamma_1.$$

Generally stochastic curtailment is very conservative and if $\gamma_0 = 1 = \gamma_1$, it becomes deterministic curtailment.

A formal significance test is only one factor in the complex decision process of whether to continue, modify or stop a trial. Interim analyses based on group sequential methods, triangular tests or stochastic curtailment procedures provide objective guidelines to the DATA AND SAFETY MONITORING BOARDS.

The choice for the method of interim analyses should depend on the desired operating characteristics of the study in terms of the early stopping property, the maximum sample size requirement and the expected sample size. For example, if the study continues through all K analyses, the group sequential design will accrue more participants than the fixed sample design, which is likely to occur if H_0 is true. However, if the study stops at an earlier interim analysis, the group sequential design will accrue fewer participants on average than the fixed sample design, which is likely to occur if H_1 is true.

A randomised Phase III trial should never be terminated in the early stages of recruitment merely because it is failing to reach the anticipated 'minimal' benefit envisaged at the design stage of the study. This is because early termination of a study in these circumstances will leave the associated CONFIDENCE INTERVAL unacceptably wide, thereby indicating the possibility of a plausible, and maybe worthwhile, advantage to one therapy even when there is no true difference in intervention effects. In such circumstances the level of uncertainty remains unacceptably high. *KK*

[See also DATA AND SAFETY MONITORING BOARDS]

Anderson, T.W. (1960). A modification of the sequential probability ratio test to reduce the sample size. *Annals of Mathematical Statistics* 31, 165–97. **Anscombe, F.J.** 1954: Fixed-sample-size analysis of sequential observations. *Biometrics* 10, 89–100. **Chang, M.N., Hwang, I.K. and Shih, W.J.** 1998: Group sequential designs using both Type I and Type II error probability spending functions. *Communications in Statistics, Part A – Theory and Methods* 27, 1323–39. **Lan, K.K.G. and DeMets, D.L.** 1983: Discrete sequential boundaries for clinical trials. *Biometrika* 70, 659–63. **Lan, K.K.G., Simon, R. and Halperin, M.** 1982: Stochastically curtailed testing in long-term clinical trials. *Sequential Analysis* 1, 207–19. **O'Brien, P.C. and Fleming, T.R.** 1979: A multiple testing procedure for clinical trials. *Biometrics* 35, 549–56. **Pampallona, S., Tsiatis, A.A. and Kim, K.** 2001: Spending functions for Type I and Type II error probabilities of group sequential trials. *Drug Information Journal* 72, 247–60. **Pocock, S.J.** 1977: Group sequential methods in the design and analysis of clinical trials. *Biometrika* 64, 191–9. **Wald, A.** 1947: *Sequential analysis.* New York: John Wiley & Sons. **Whitehead, J.** 1997: *The design and analysis of sequential clinical trials*, 2nd rev. edn. Chichester: John Wiley & Sons.

internal pilot study See PILOT STUDIES, SAMPLE SIZE DETERMINATION IN CLINICAL TRIALS

interquartile range A MEASURE OF SPREAD defined as the interval between the values that are located one-quarter and three-quarters of the way through the sample when the observations are ordered. Thus, it encloses the middle 50% of the data points.

For example, suppose the weights in kilograms of 11 elderly men from a community sample attending a clinic were:

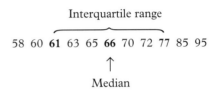

Interquartile range

58 60 **61** 63 65 **66** 70 72 77 85 95

Median

Then, the interquartile range is the interval between the 3rd and 9th values, i.e. 61 kg to 77 kg, a difference of 16 kg.

The interquartile range is most informative if the upper and lower values are both quoted, rather than simply the interval between them. The lower value is known as the lower quartile or 25th percentile and the upper value as the upper quartile or 75th percentile.

If the number of observations + 1 is divisible by 4 then the interquartile range is simple to calculate. If this is not the case then the values for the interquartile range need to be interpolated. In general, the position of the lower quartile is calculated by multiplying the sample size plus one by 0.25, and by 0.75 in the case of the upper quartile. So, if another man attends the clinic with a weight of 100 kg then the lower quartile is now at position $(12 + 1)/4 = 3\frac{1}{4}$.

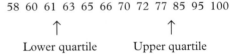

58 60 61 63 65 66 70 72 77 85 95 100

Lower quartile   Upper quartile

Thus the lower quartile lies a quarter of the way between 61 and 63, interpolated as 61.5 kg. Similarly the upper quartile lies three-quarters of the way between 77 and 85, interpolated as 83 kg.

The interquartile range is typically used as a measure of spread around the MEDIAN. Like the median, it is useful when the data are not symmetrically distributed because it is not unduly affected by the presence of SKEWNESS or OUTLIERS. *SRC*

intraclass correlation coefficient See INTRACLUSTER CORRELATION COEFFICIENT

intracluster correlation coefficient (ICC) A measure that quantifies the extent of similarity among individual observations within clusters. For example, when a study collects data on patients from a number of different clinics, the intracluster correlation coefficient (ICC) represents the degree to which patients attending the same clinic are more similar than the patients attending different clinics. Also known as the intraclass correlation coefficient, the ICC takes values between 0 and 1, where the value 0 corresponds to the situation where individuals from the same cluster are no more alike than individuals from different clusters and higher values indicate greater similarity within clusters.

The ICC has been used extensively in several application areas. In health services research, it is used to measure the extent of similarity of patients within administrative units such as hospitals or geographical units such as towns. In family studies, it measures the degree of resemblance among members of the same family. In psychological research, it is used when examining reliability (see MEASUREMENT PRECISION AND RELIABILITY), where the same measurements are taken on subjects by different assessors. When individuals are sampled within clusters such as hospitals or families, the ICC representing within-cluster similarity is defined as the proportion of the variation between individuals that is explained by the variation between clusters.

Formally, this definition assumes a simple random effects model for the ENDPOINT of interest, which includes random cluster effects with variance σ_c^2 and individual residual effects with variance σ^2, and the ICC is defined as $\sigma_c^2/(\sigma_c^2 + \sigma^2)$. The most common approach for estimating the ICC is to obtain estimates for σ_c^2 and σ^2 by fitting the RANDOM EFFECTS MODEL to the data and substitute these into the formula. CONFIDENCE INTERVALS for reporting alongside the ICC estimate are also obtained using the assumptions of the random effects model. In most settings, negative ICC values are regarded as implausible, so negative values obtained for ICC estimates are set to 0 and lower limits of confidence intervals are truncated at 0. When considering the ICC for a binary outcome, for example presence or absence of a disease in family members, an ICC estimate can be obtained as described above, but the methods for constructing confidence intervals are based on different assumptions.

The simple model outlined here is not appropriate for all types of design. When measuring reliability, the definition of the ICC differs according to whether the focus is on 'consistency' or 'absolute agreement' as described by McGraw and Wong (1996). Some study designs require more complex models; for example, when repeated measurements are available on patients within clusters, or when wishing to estimate multiple ICC values simultaneously (Donner, 1986). *RT*

Donner, A. 1986: A review of inference procedures for the intraclass correlation coefficient in the one-way random effects model. *International Statistical Review* 54, 67–82. **Donner, A. and Wells, G.** 1986: A comparison of confidence interval methods for the intraclass correlation coefficient. *Biometrics* 42, 401–12. **McGraw, K.O. and Wong, S.P.** 1996: Forming inferences about some intraclass correlation coefficients. *Psychological Methods* 1, 30–46. **Ridout, M.S., Demetrio, C.G.B. and Firth, D.** 1999: Estimating intraclass correlation for binary data. *Biometrics* 55, 137–48.

ITT Abbreviation for INTENTION-TO-TREAT.

J

Jaccard coefficient   See CLUSTER ANALYSIS IN MEDICINE

jackknife method   The jackknife was originally proposed as a method for estimating biases (Quenouille, 1949); soon afterwards it was applied to estimating standard errors. Subsequently it has been applied more widely. In particular, the 'jackknife after bootstrap', discussed later, is a useful tool for understanding the influence of individual observations on BOOTSTRAP analyses.

Here, we motivate the jackknife using a hypothetical example and illustrate it using a real dataset. We then briefly discuss its relationship to the bootstrap and 'jackknife after bootstrap' analyses.

Suppose we wish to estimate the average adult height in a population, which we denote by θ. To do this, we take a sample of 7 adults from the population and calculate the average height in the sample. Let the first row of the Figure below represent the population, from which 7 adults are sampled. Note that the numbers 1, ..., 7 index the sampled adults, they are not the actual heights. This sample is represented in the box in the second row. The average height of the 7 adults in this sample, denoted by $\hat{\theta}$, is our estimate of θ. Suppose we now wish to calculate an estimate of the variability of $\hat{\theta}$ about θ. Hypothetically, we could do this by drawing a number of further samples, also of size 7, from the population and calculating the average adult heights in each of these.

Of course, this is impractical. However, it suggests an alternative approach. Suppose we draw a number of sub-samples from the data and calculate the average height in each of these sub-samples. The variation of the average height in these sub-samples about the value in the observed data might be a reasonable estimate of the variation of $\hat{\theta}$ about the true adult height, θ.

One method of constructing these sub-samples is the jackknife. The jackknife datasets are constructed by omitting one observation in turn from the observed dataset. Thus if the dataset has 7 observations, there are 7 jackknife datasets. These are shown in the third row in the figure.

Having obtained the jackknife datasets, we simply calculate the average height of the 6 adults in each jackknife dataset. By convention, these are denoted $\hat{\theta}_{(1)}, \ldots, \hat{\theta}_{(7)}$, where the subscript number indicates the *observation that is omitted*. Recall we are interested in estimating the variability of $\hat{\theta}$. Let the average of the jackknife estimates be $\hat{\theta}_{(.)} = (\hat{\theta}_{(1)} + \hat{\theta}_{(2)} + \ldots + \hat{\theta}_{(7)})/7$, and let n equal the sample size (7 in this case). The jackknife estimate of VARIANCE is:

$$\hat{\sigma}_{jack}^2 = \frac{(n-1)}{n} \sum_{i=1}^{n} (\hat{\theta}_{(i)} - \hat{\theta}_{(.)})^2. \qquad (1)$$

(Note, in passing, that by convention, the jackknife estimate of variance differs from the bootstrap estimate by a factor of $(n-1)/n$, but this negligible unless n is small.) Thus the jackknife is motivated by an analogous version of the bootstrap principle (see BOOTSTRAP), in which jackknife datasets replace bootstrap datasets. However, in comparison with bootstrap datasets, jackknife datasets are much less variable. Therefore, extra multiplying factors, like the $(n-1)$ in the numerator of (1) are needed to make the jackknife work.

As an example, consider the data in the first Table on page 178. We will use the jackknife to estimate the variance of the average change in the carbon monoxide transfer factor, which is $(33+2+24+27+4+1-6)/7 = 12.14$.

The 7 jackknife samples, and their corresponding means, are shown in the second table. As the statistic we are using is the mean, it turns out that

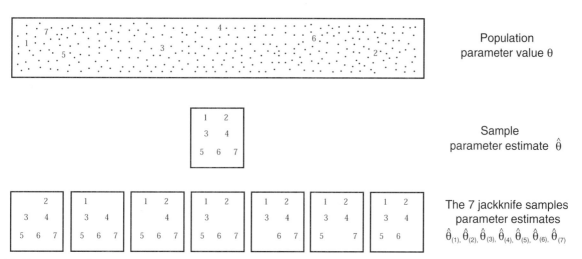

jackknife method   *Schematic illustration of jackknife.*

jackknife method *Data on the carbon monoxide transfer factor for seven smokers with chickenpox, measured on admission to hospital and after a stay of one week (Davison and Hinkley, 1997:67).*

Patient	Entry	Week	Change = (Week–Entry)
1	40	73	33
2	50	52	2
3	56	80	24
4	58	85	27
5	60	64	4
6	62	63	1
7	66	60	–6

$\hat{\theta}_{(.)} = (\hat{\theta}_{(1)} + \hat{\theta}_{(2)} + \cdots + \hat{\theta}_{(7)})/7 = \hat{\theta} = 12.14$. From (1), the jackknife estimate of variance is:

$$\hat{\sigma}^2_{jack} = \frac{6}{7}\left\{(8.67 - 12.14)^2 + (13.83 - 12.14)^2 + \right.$$
$$(10.17 - 12.14)^2 + (9.67 - 12.14)^2 +$$
$$(13.50 - 12.14)^2 + (14.00 - 12.14)^2 +$$
$$\left. (15.17 - 12.14)^2\right\} = 5.81^2.$$

Note that the jackknife estimate of variance agrees exactly with the result obtained using the usual formula for the variance of a mean. This is a feature of the statistic used in this example (the MEAN) and will not occur generally.

Apparent similarities of the jackknife and bootstrap are indicative of a deeper relationship. It turns out that, in situations where the jackknife works, it can be viewed as an approximation to the bootstrap (Efron and Tibshirani, 1993: 146). The attraction of the jackknife is that it is computationally easier (as there are only a finite number of jackknife samples). The disadvantage is that it only works in more restricted situations. In particular, the jackknife only works for statistics whose value changes smoothly as the data changes (Efron and Tibshirani, 1993: 148).

The mean is an example of a smooth statistic. The median is not, however, because as the data values change it does not change smoothly. For example, the median of the change variable in the first Table is 4. Suppose we now increase the second observation from its observed value, 2. While the new value for the second observation is less than 4, the median remains unchanged. As soon as it is greater than 4, the median changes. This lack of smooth-

jackknife method *Jackknife samples for the 'change' data from the first Table.*

								Statistic (mean)
Data from first Table	33	2	24	27	4	1	–6	$\hat{\theta} = 12.14$
1st jackknife sample,	–	2	24	27	4	1	–6	$\hat{\theta}_{(1)} = 8.67$
2nd jackknife sample,	33	–	24	27	4	1	–6	$\hat{\theta}_{(2)} = 13.83$
3rd jackknife sample,	33	2	–	27	4	1	–6	$\hat{\theta}_{(3)} = 10.17$
4th jackknife sample,	33	2	24	–	4	1	–6	$\hat{\theta}_{(4)} = 9.67$
5th jackknife sample,	33	2	24	27	–	1	–6	$\hat{\theta}_{(5)} = 13.50$
6th jackknife sample,	33	2	24	27	4	–	–6	$\hat{\theta}_{(6)} = 14.00$
7th jackknife sample,	33	2	24	27	4	1	–	$\hat{\theta}_{(7)} = 15.17$

ness makes the jackknife fail for the median. By contrast, the bootstrap works for the median.

A useful application of the jackknife is known as the 'jackknife after bootstrap'. Following a bootstrap analysis, the bootstrap datasets are divided into groups: those that do not contain the first observation, those that do not contain the second and so on. In other words, we form jackknife groups from (i.e. after) generating the bootstrap datasets. The analysis of the bootstrap data can then be performed on each of these jackknife groups in turn. Marked differences in the results between the jackknife groups indicate that a particular observation, or group of observations, is strongly affecting the conclusions. For example, if jackknife group 1 (i.e. the group of bootstrap datasets which do not contain the first observation) results in a *P*-VALUE above 0.05, but all the other jackknife groups result in *P*-values below 0.05, this suggests the results critically depend on the first observation and should be interpreted cautiously. In practice, 'jackknife after bootstrap' results are usually displayed graphically (e.g. Carpenter and Bithell, 2000; Davison and Hinkley, 1997: 117).

(For further reading, see Efron and Tibshirani, 1993, or Davison and Hinkley, 1997, both of which discuss the jackknife comprehensively.) *JRC*

[**Acknowledgement:** James R. Carpenter was supported by ESRC Research Methods Programme grant H333 250047, titled 'Missing data in multi-level models'.]

Carpenter, J. and Bithell, J. 2000: Bootstrap confidence intervals: when, which, what? A practical guide for medical statisticians. *Statistics in Medicine* 19, 1141–64. **Davison, A.C. and Hinkley, D.V.** 1997: *Bootstrap methods and their application.* Cambridge: Cambridge University Press. **Efron, B. and Tibshirani, R.** 1993: *An introduction to the bootstrap.* New York: Chapman & Hall. **Quenouille, M.** 1949: Approximate tests of correlation in time series. *Journal of the Royal Statistical Society Series B*, 11, 18–44.

Jonckheere-Terpstra test

A non-parametric test for ordered alternatives with the null hypothesis that there is no difference in group medians and alternative hypothesis that the group medians increase in a specific predetermined sequence. It is used when the assumption that the independent variable is nominal in the KRUSKAL-WALLIS TEST is violated. As it allows the independent variable to have an order it is more powerful than the Kruskal-Wallis test when the groups are ordered.

The method begins by specifying the order of the groups, which need not be equal sized. Then, cast the data into a two-way table with the groups in the pre-specified order, with the group with the lowest median first and the data within the groups ordered from smallest to largest. Find the total number of times each value in the first group precedes a value in the subsequent groups. Add ½ to each precedent count when a tie occurs. Repeat for the remaining groups and sum over the groups to give $\mathcal{J}$, the test statistic. Compare this value to that as found in standard tables, for example, in Siegel and Castellan (1998).

To illustrate, Mcm-2 values were collected in a breast cancer study. The median Mcm-2 value was expected to increase with histological grade (data in the first Table on page 179). This hypothesis was tested using the Jonckheere-Terpstra test, with intermediate calculations shown in the second Table on page 179.

Jonckheere-Terpstra test *Mcm-2 values in a breast cancer study according to increasing histological grade*

| Histological grade | | |
1	2	3
1.99	4.40	6.94
3.01	9.82	8.04
4.17	10.23	9.82
7.13	11.99	15.75
9.82	11.99	18.30
9.91	13.17	25.01
	13.20	26.40
		28.17

Jonckheere-Terpstra test *Derivation of Jonckheere-Terpstra test statistic from data in first Table*

| | Precedent counts | |
Grades 1 and 2	Grades 1 and 3	Grades 2 and 3
7	8	8
7	8	5.5
7	8	5
6	7	5
5.5	5.5	5
5	5	5
		5
Total 37.5	**41.5**	**38.5**

Therefore, $\mathcal{J} = 37.5 + 41.5 + 38.5 = 117.5$. From tables ($n_1 = 6$, $n_2 = 7$, $n_3 = 8$, $\alpha = 0.05$) the critical value is 99. As $117.5 > 99$, there is sufficient evidence to reject the null hypothesis and conclude that there is a significant increase in median Mcm-2 value as histological grade increases.

SLV

Conover, W.J. 1999: *Practical nonparametric statistics*, 3rd edn. Chichester: John Wiley & Sons. **Siegel, S. and Castellan, N.J.** 1998: *Nonparametric statistics for the behavioral sciences*, 2nd edn. Maidenhead: McGraw-Hill.

journals in medical statistics

There are thousands of published articles on medical statistics scattered very widely throughout the statistical and the biomedical literature. They reflect both the diversity and the complexity of this discipline and range from highly theoretical to the most mundane practical applications. This section provides a brief overview of this literature, together with an historical perspective of the rise of journals in medical statistics.

Papers on aspects of medical statistics have been published in the biomedical literature since the late 1920s. Their purpose is to explain and illustrate specific techniques, to point out incorrect applications and to make the readership generally aware of how, and why, statistics can lead to poor experimental designs, incorrect analysis and unjustified conclusions. Publication within the biomedical (instead of statistical) literature enables direct contact with researchers and greater impact through explanation within a specific medical context. These papers can be grouped broadly into 7 areas (see Johnson and Altman, 1998, for more details): isolated papers on a particular statistical issue, (for example, the CHI-SQUARE TEST and INTENTION-TO-TREAT analysis); series of thematic papers dedicated to a narrow statistical area (for example, systematic reviews and CONFIDENCE INTERVALS); series of papers covering broad areas of medical statistics (such as that by Bradford Hill published in *The Lancet* in 1937); guidelines (a recent example is CONSORT for reporting clinical trials); surveys of published papers reporting the frequency of usage of statistical techniques (and the statistical knowledge required to understand the research literature); reviews of published papers examining critically aspects of design, analysis, conduct, presentation and summary (all general medical journals, and many of the specialist ones, have been the subject of these); and SYSTEMATIC REVIEWS AND META-ANALYSIS incorporating assessment of methodological quality.

Papers on the general theory of techniques employed within medical statistics, as well as specific applications, have been published for over a century in statistical journals such as *Journal of the American Statistical Association* and those produced by the Royal Statistical Society, London. However, the origins of medical statistics lie in the older disciplines of biometry, psychometry, epidemiology, public health medicine, demography and actuarial science, and it is the journals in these specialties that published many of the early papers in medical statistics; some of them continue to do so today (see Table on page 180 for some examples).

Biometrika (from the Biometrika Trust) publishes papers 'containing original theoretical contributions of direct or potential value in applications', while *Biometrics* (journal of the International Biometrics Society) 'promotes and extends the use of mathematical and statistical methods in pure and applied biological sciences'. The *Biometrical Journal*, also published over many years, aims for papers 'on the development of statistical and related methodology and its applications to problems arising in all areas of the life sciences, in particular medicine'. The three psychology journals, *Psychological Bulletin* (from American Psychological Association), *Psychometrika* (from Psychological Society) and *British Journal of Mathematical and Statistical Psychology* (from British Psychological Society), all publish articles on the development of quantitative methods in psychology.

The principal applications of medical statistics are within epidemiology and clinical trials and it was the journals within these specific areas that next took up publication of papers on the broadest aspects of medical statistics, as it applied within each of them. The Table on page 180 provides a list of the principal (English-language) journals in these areas together with some details of the size of the volumes published in 2003. All the epidemiological and clinical trials journals publish papers describing methodological developments. Such papers are also found in the more specialised journals devoted to specific disease areas, for example, *British Journal of Cancer* and *International Journal of Cancer*.

It was not until the 1980s that the discipline of medical statistics was finally recognised by publication of its own journals. *Statistics in Medicine*, which 'presents practical applications of statistics and other quantitative methods to medicine and its applied sciences, together with all aspects of the collection, analysis, presentation, and interpretation of medical data, and aims to enhance communication between statisticians, clinicians and medical researchers', started in 1981 and was soon followed by the review jour-

journals in medical statistics *Journals publishing papers in medical statistics*

Title	1st vol.	2003			
		Publisher	Volume (issues)	Pages	Papers
Biometrika	1901	Biometrika Trust	90 (4)	994	81
Psychological Bulletin	1904	APA	129 (6)	972	41
American Journal of Epidemiology [1]	1921	OUP	157/158 (24)	1230	284
Psychometrika	1936	Psychometric Society	68 (4)	636	31
Biometrics [2]	1945	IBS	59 (4)	1198	128
Journal of Epidemiology and Community Health [3]	1947	BMJ	57 (12)	996	204
British Journal of Mathematical and Statistical Psychology [4]	1947	BPS	56 (2)	388	21
Journal of Clinical Epidemiology [5]	1955	Elsevier	56 (12)	1260	166
Biometrical Journal	1959	Wiley-VCH	45 (8)	1042	72
Clinical Pharmacology & Therapeutics	1960	Elsevier (Mosby)	73/74 (12)	1206	121
Clinical Trials and Meta-Analysis [6]	1964	Elsevier	–	–	–
Drug Information Journal [7]	1966	DIA	37 (4)	450	46
International Journal of Clinical Pharmacology and Therapeutics [8]	1967	Dustri-Verlag	41 (12)	626	86
International Journal of Epidemiology	1972	OUP	32 (6)	1134	140
Epidemiologic Reviews	1979	OUP	25 (1)	98	9
Controlled Clinical Trials: Design, Methods, and Analysis	1980	Elsevier	24 (8)	904	66
Statistics in Medicine	1982	Wiley	22 (24)	3932	247
Annals of Epidemiology	1990	Elsevier	13 (11)	742	100
International Journal of Methods in Psychiatric Research	1991	Whurr (online)	12 (4)	–	20
Journal of Biopharmaceutical Statistics	1991	Dekker	13 (4)	816	54
Statistical Methods in Medical Research	1992	Arnold	12 (6)	554	30
Lifetime Data Analysis	1995	Kluwer	9 (4)	412	22
Journal of Epidemiology and Biostatistics [9]	1996	–	–	–	–
Biostatistics	2000	OUP	4 (4)	650	44
BioMed Central (BMC) Medical Research Methodology	2001	[Online]	3	–	27
Statistical Modelling	2001	Arnold	3 (4)	324	17
Pharmaceutical Statistics	2002	Wiley	2 (4)	308	25
Understanding Statistics	2002	Lawrence Erlbaum	2 (4)	280	16
Clinical Trials: Journal of the Society for Clinical Trials	2004	Arnold	–	–	–

Paper counts for some journals are approximate as some Editorials and Commentaries have been excluded.
[1] Previously *American Journal of Hygiene*; *Journal of Hygiene*; [2] previously *Biometrics Bulletin*; [3] previously *British Journal of Social Medicine*; *British Journal of Preventive and Social Medicine*; *Journal of Epidemiology and Community Medicine*; *Epidemiology and Community Health*; [4] previously *British Journal of Psychology: Statistical Section*; *British Journal of Statistical Psychology*; [5] previously *Journal of Chronic Diseases*; [6] previously *Clinical Trials Journal* and from 1995 incorporated within *Controlled Clinical Trials*; [7] previously *Drug Information Bulletin*; [8] previously *International Journal of Clinical Pharmacology and Biopharmacy*; *International Journal of Clinical Pharmacology and Therapeutics*; *International Journal of Clinical Pharmacology, Therapy and Toxicology*; [9] later *Journal of Cancer Epidemiology and Prevention*.

nal, *Statistical Methods in Medical Research*. The launch of these journals coincided with a period of huge increase in both the demand for medical statisticians and in the development of sophisticated modelling techniques, enabled particularly by increased computing power and fuelled by the need to forecast the requirements for future healthcare and the extent of the AIDS epidemic. By the turn of the century, the capacity of the current journals could not forestall further specialisation, represented by *Pharmaceutical Statistics*, 'concerned with the application and use of statistics in all stages of drug development', and *Statistical Modelling*, or the need for another journal of biostatistics and another for clinical trials.

Medical statistics interacts with all quantitative areas of biomedicine and many qualitative areas as well. It is no surprise that in addition to the publications mentioned already, many papers are also found in established journals, such as *Medical Decision Making*, *Journal of Theoretical Biology* and *Multivariate Behavioural Research*, as well as those that lie at the interfaces with computing (*Computers in Biology and Medicine*, *Journal of Biomedical Computing* and *Statistics and Computing*); artificial intelligence; quality of life; and health economics, as well as the comparatively recent areas represented by *Evidence-Based Medicine* and *Journal of Bioinformatics*. More journals will appear in the future some as paper, others electronic, the latter supplementing the online journals that exist already, for example, at BioMed Central (BMC).   *TJ*

Johnson, T. and Altman, D.G. 1998: Statistical articles in medical journals. In Armitage, P. and Colton, T. (eds), *Encyclopedia of biostatistics*. Chichester: John Wiley & Sons.

K

Kaiser's rule A rule for selecting number of common factors in FACTOR ANALYSIS and the number of components in PRINCIPAL COMPONENTS ANALYSIS. The rule is to retain as many factors or components derived from the sample correlation matrix that have variances greater than one. The rationale for this rule is that factors (components) with variances greater than one account for at least as much variability as can be explained by a single observed variable. Those factors (components) with variances less than one account for less variability than does a single observed variable and so will usually be of little interest to the investigator. Further discussion of the rule is given in Floyd and Widaman (1995) and Preacher and MacCallum (2003). *BSE*

Floyd, F.J. and Widaman, K.F. 1995: Factor analysis in the development and refinement of clinical assessment instruments. *Psychological Assessment* 7, 286–99. **Preacher, K.J. and MacCullum, R.C.** 2003: Repairing Tom Swift's electric factor analysis machine. *Understanding Statistics* 2, 13–44.

Kaplan-Meier estimator Also known as the product limit estimator, it is one of the most commonly reported methods for describing (estimating) the survival distribution or survivor function (see SURVIVAL ANALYSIS), $S(t)$, of a homogeneous population in time-to-event (survival) studies, with right-CENSORED OBSERVATIONS. Kaplan and Meier introduced it in 1958 as a non-parametric method for using the exact survival (or event) times of those subjects uncensored in the calculation of the survival (or event-free) probabilities. The method takes appropriate account of the information contained in censored observations through the definition of the number at risk. It requires, however, that the assumption of independent censoring hold to be validly applied.

The Kaplan-Meier estimator is based on the partitioning of the time during which subjects are observed into a sequence of non-overlapping time bands (or time intervals), where each time band contains only one distinct (unique) uncensored event time and this event time is taken to occur at the start of the interval. If censored and uncensored times are tied, the convention is to consider the uncensored times to have occurred just before the censored times. The Kaplan-Meier estimate for the probability of surviving up to time t, $S(t)$, is then given by the product of CONDITIONAL PROBABILITIES for surviving each of these time intervals (given survival through the preceding time intervals) before or including t.

More precisely, suppose that there are n subjects drawn randomly from the population of interest, with observed survival times (both uncensored and censored) $t_1, \ldots, t_n$. Assume that there were d events occurring and that the r unique event times corresponding to these events can be arranged in ascending order as $t_{(1)} < t_{(2)} < \ldots < t_{(r)}$. Let the kth time band, I_k, start from $t_{(k)}$ and end at a time just before $t_{(k+1)}$, written $I_k = [t_{(k)}, t_{(k+1)}]$. Also let n_k and d_k be the number of subjects at risk just before $t_{(k)}$ (i.e. at the beginning of the kth time band) and the number who experience the event of interest at $t_{(k)}$ (i.e. the number of events occurring in the kth time band) respectively. Then, the probability of surviving up to time t is estimated as:

$$S(t) = \prod_{j=1}^{k} \left(\frac{n_j - d_j}{n_j} \right),$$

for t lying within the kth time band, I_k. $S(t)$ is defined to be equal to 1 for any time less than the smallest uncensored time, $t_{(1)}$. If the largest observed survival time is an uncensored observation, then for all t greater than or

Kaplan-Meier estimator *Survival times (days) of 10 small-cell lung cancer patients*

Survival times (days)	9	35	40	63	110	151	212	284	305	365
Status (1 = dead; 0 = censored)	1	0	0	1	1	1	1	0	1	0

Kaplan-Meier estimator *Kaplan-Meier estimate of the survivor function for the data given in the first Table*

Interval	Time interval	Number at risk	Deaths	Censored	Conditional probability of surviving	Cumulative probability	Standard error
k	I_k	n_k	d_k	c_k	$(n_k - d_k)/n_k$	$S(t)$	
1	0 –	10	0	0	1	1	—
2	9 –	10	1	2	0.900	0.900	0.0949
3	63 –	7	1	0	0.857	0.771	0.1442
4	110 –	6	1	0	0.833	0.643	0.1679
5	151 –	5	1	0	0.800	0.514	0.1769
6	212 –	4	1	1	0.750	0.386	0.1732
7	305 –	2	1	1	0.500	0.193	0.1615

equal to $t_{(r)}$, $S(t) = 0$. However, if the largest observed time is a censored observation, then the Kaplan-Meier estimate is not defined past this censored time. Note also that the probability of 'surviving' remains constant throughout any given interval. Finally, note that standard errors based on a formula due to Greenwood can be attached to the Kaplan-Meier estimates of the survival probabilities so as to reflect the uncertainty inherent in them.

The information obtained from the Kaplan-Meier estimator can be displayed in tabular format or graphically as a KAPLAN-MEIER PLOT. The second Table on page 181 illustrates the use of the Kaplan-Meier estimator for the data in the first table describing a hypothetical study of 10 patients followed up for 365 days from diagnosis of small-cell lung cancer to death, if it has occurred. The notation c_k denotes the number of censored observations in the kth time band. Observe in the second table that the estimate $S(t)$ in the kth interval is obtained by multiplying the estimate of the conditional probability obtained in the kth interval to the estimate of $S(t)$ in the $(k-1)$th interval. *BT*

Collett, D. 2003: *Modelling survival data in medical research*, 2nd edn. Boca Raton: Chapman & Hall/CRC. **Kaplan, E.L. and Meier, P.** 1958: Nonparametric estimation from incomplete observation. *Journal of the American Statistical Association* 53, 457–81.

Kaplan-Meier plot

A popular way of displaying 'survival' information obtained from the KAPLAN-MEIER ESTIMATOR, the Kaplan-Meier plot or curve is a graph in which the horizontal axis represents the survival (or event) times and the vertical axis represents the survival (or event-free) probabilities. The plot starts from 1 (100% of subjects event free) at time 0 and declines towards 0 (all subjects have experienced the event of interest) with increasing time.

It is plotted as a step function, since the survival probability remains constant between successive (uncensored) event times and only drops instantaneously any time an event occurs. The graph only reaches 0 if the subject with the longest observed survival time experiences an event, otherwise the survival curve is undefined after this time. Note that CENSORED OBSERVATIONS occurring in the interval between two successive event times have no effect on the survival probability calculated for this interval, but will have an impact on the calculation of the survival probability at the start of the next interval, through the number at risk. The Figure shows an example of a Kaplan-Meier curve.

The Kaplan-Meier curve is the best description of the survival experience of a homogeneous group of subjects in a study. The reading of the curve is straightforward. For example, if the estimated median survival time (see SURVIVAL ANALYSIS) is to be reported (i.e. the time beyond which 50% of the subjects in the study are expected to survive or be event free), then this can be found by extending a horizontal line from the survival probability of 0.5 on the vertical axis, to the point where the curve and this line intersect and then dropping a vertical line to the time axis. The estimated median time is the point at which the vertical line cuts the time axis. This is illustrated in the Figure. If, however, the survival curve is horizontal at the probability 0.5, then no unique value can be identified for the median survival time. In this situation, a reasonable estimate of the median time is the midpoint of the time interval over which the survival curve has a probability of 0.5.

Note that the survival curve shows the *pattern of mortality* (if death is the outcome of interest) *over time* and not the details. Thus any conclusions made based on the finer details of the curve are likely to be inaccurate. In particular, if the 'tail' of the survival curve is 'flat', then this does not mean that the risk to subjects still alive is non-existent (i.e. evidence of a 'cured fraction' of patients). In fact, this may occur because the number of subjects under observation along the tail is small and therefore reliable estimates of the survival probabilities along it are not obtained. Also, drastic drops and large flat sections in other parts of the curve may be due to a large proportion of censored observations and may indicate inappropriate censoring.

Hence the survival curve is unreliable if based on small numbers at risk. Also, there is a natural tendency for the

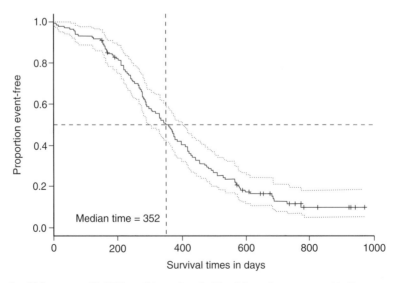

Kaplan-Meier plot *Kaplan-Meier curve with 95% confidence bands. The tick marks correspond to the occurrence of censoring*

eye to be drawn to the right-hand end of the curve where it is least reliable. Therefore it is wise not to place too much confidence in the finer details of the curve, unless there is a valid reason (based possibly on prior knowledge) to do so. The overall picture is more reliable. Pocock, Clayton and Altman (2002) advocate placing confidence bands (or standard error bars) at a few regularly spaced time points on the curve in order to highlight the uncertainty in the estimated survival probabilities. In addition, they recommend that the number at risk at select time points should also be displayed. They further discuss whether 'survival curves' should go up or down (for it is sensible when events are rare to consider plotting the event rate instead of the event-free rate) and how far in time to extend the plot.

Finally, note that presenting more than one survival curve on a single diagram (e.g. curves for treated and untreated) is a useful way of informally comparing the survival experiences of different groups of homogeneous subjects and can be very informative. However, this diagram alone will not allow us to say with any confidence whether or not there are any real differences between these groups. The observed differences may be true differences, but equally could be due merely to chance variation. Assessing whether or not there are any real differences between groups can only be done, with any degree of confidence, by utilising formal statistical tests, such as the log rank test (Armitage, Berry and Matthews, 2002). *BT*

Armitage, P., Berry, G. and Matthews, J.N.S. 2002: *Statistical methods in medical research*, 4th edn. Oxford: Blackwell Science. **Collett, D.** 2003: *Modelling survival data in medical research*, 2nd edn. London: Chapman and Hall/CRC. **Matthews, D.E. and Farewell, V.T.** 1996: *Using and understanding medical statistics*, 3rd edn. New York: Karger. **Pocock, S.J., Clayton, T.C. and Altman, D.G.** 2002: Survival plots of time-to-event outcomes in clinical trials: good practice and pitfalls. *The Lancet* 359, 1686–9.

kappa and weighted kappa

Rating scales are commonly used for assessment of subjective variables, such as well-being, pain and satisfaction. Experts use scales in diagnostic judgements, for example, concerning the severity of disease and in classification of physical, mental and social status. How reliable are judgements on scales? *Reliability* expresses the extent to which repeated assessments yield similar results. The Cohen's coefficient kappa (κ) is an agreement measure that takes into account that two assessments could agree by chance. Kappa is defined as the ratio between the percentage agreement (p_o) after excluding chance expected (p_e) agreement and the chance-corrected maximum possible agreement

$$\kappa = (p_o - p_e)/(1 - p_e).$$

Possible values range between −1 and 1, where the agreement that could occur by chance is zero kappa and a higher agreement than the chance is zero kappa and a positive value.

Kappa was developed for *categorical classifications*, where a disagreement to any other category is equally likely, but is commonly used for *ordered categorical (ordinal)* classifications, where disagreeing classifications concern adjacent rather than extreme categories. In the weighted kappa (κ_w) all observations are weighted and included in the calculation. Cicchetti (1976) proposed linear agreement weights; maximum weight (= 1) for observations of total agreement and minimum (= 0) for the most extreme disagreeing observations. For example, observations representing a disagreement of one, two and three categories between two four-point scale assessments are weighted 2/3, 1/3 and 0, respectively. A set of disagreement weights will have the opposite order. The κ_w with quadratic disagreement weights equals *the intraclass correlation coefficient*, provided equal marginal distributions (unbiased raters).

There are limitations with kappa. The maximum kappa, $\kappa = 1$, is obtainable only when unbiased raters agree completely. Kappa depends on the marginal distributions and on the number of categories; kappa increases when the number of categories decreases. Therefore, kappa values from different studies are not comparable and using rules for interpretation saying that kappa larger than 0.6 represents good agreement is not meaningful. The κ_w depends on the choice of weights. Two disagreement patterns inspired by data from a reliability study in neuro-radiology illustrate the limitations of a summary measure of reliability.

Two experts, X and Y, independently judged 59 objects on a four-point scale, here labelled A, B, C and D. Two hypothetical frequency distributions of the pairs of judgements are given in the Figures ((a) and (b)). The disagreement patterns differ, but the percentage agreements are similar, 75% (44 of 59) in (a), 76% (45 of 59) in (b). The chance-expected agreement is determined by the marginal distributions and the number of chance-expected agreeing observations in (a) is ($4 \times 7 + 9 \times 12 + 12 \times 12 + 34 \times 28)/59 = 20.88$ and $\kappa = 0.61$. The kappa value of (b) is 0.60. Hence, the agreement measures are

	Expert X						Expert X				
(a)	A	B	C	D	Total	(b)	A	B	C	D	Total
D				28	28			1	3	30	34
C			6	6	12		1	1	7	3	12
B		6	6		12		1	6	1	1	9
A	4	3			7		2	1	1		4
Total	4	9	12	34	59		4	9	12	34	59

(Expert Y labels the rows)

kappa and weighted kappa *Two examples of paired distributions of assessments made by experts X and Y when classifying 59 subjects in the ordered-scale categories A, B, C and D*

almost the same, but the observations are more dispersed in (b) than in (a). In (a) the experts agree completely in 44 and disagree just one category in 15 judgements, so, using Cicchetti weights, the weighted agreement is (44 + (15 × 2/3)) = 54 and $\kappa_w = 0.84$, correspondingly $\kappa_w = 0.68$ in (b).

Besides the measures of kappa, the two patterns have different explanations. The marginal distributions in (a) differ, which indicates a systematic inter-rater disagreement concerning the use of the scale; X tends to use a higher categorical level than Y. Equal marginal distributions in (b) means lack of such bias so the disagreement between the experts can be regarded as occasional. For a detailed evaluation of inter-rater reliability the approach by Svensson *et al.* (1996) that identifies and measures the level of systematic disagreement separately from occasional disagreements could be considered.   *ES*

[See also MATCHED PAIRS ANALYSIS, ORDINAL DATA, RELIABILITY, RATING SCALES]

Altman, D.G. 2000: *Practical statistics for medical research.* Boca Raton: Chapman & Hall/CRC. **Cicchetti, D.V.** 1976: Assessing inter-rater reliability for rating scales: resolving some basic issues. *British Journal of Psychiatry* 129, 452–6. **Cohen, J.** 1960: A coefficient of agreement for nominal scales. *Educational and Psychological Measurement* 20, 37–46. **Maclure, M. and Willett, W.C.** 1987: Misinterpretation and misuse of the kappa statistic. *American Journal of Epidemiology* 126, 161–9. **Svensson, E., Starmark, J.-E., Ekholm, S., von Essen, C. and Johansson, A.** 1996: Analysis of inter-observer disagreement in the assessment of subarachnoid blood and acute hydrocephalus on CT scans. *Neurological Research* 18, 487–94.

Kendall's tau   See CORRELATION

kernel density estimation   See DENSITY ESTIMATION

k-nearest neighbour rule (kNN)   See DISCRIMINANT FUNCTION ANALYSIS

knowledge discovery in databases (KDD)
Synonym for data mining.

[See also DATA MINING IN MEDICINE]

knowledge-based systems   Synonym for expert systems. See EXPERT SYSTEMS

Kolmogorov-Smirnov test   A non-parametric, goodness-of-fit test that takes two different forms, the one-sample and the two-sample form. The one-sample test compares the observed cumulative distribution function with a theoretical cumulative distribution function, for example the NORMAL DISTRIBUTION. The two-sample test compares two observed cumulative distribution functions with each other. The Kolmogorov-Smirnov test assumes that the theoretical distribution is completely specified, i.e. for each observed value, the value of the theoretical distribution can be calculated.

The parameters (e.g. the mean) of the theoretical distribution should be specified in advance and not derived from the data. For the one-sample case the null hypothesis is that there is no difference between the observed and the theoretical distribution. For the two-sample case, the null hypothesis is that there is no difference between the two distributions. The alternative hypothesis can be directional or non-directional.

For the one-sample case, the method begins by ordering the observations from smallest to largest. Then calculate the empirical distribution function $S(x)$, which is the proportion of observations less than or equal to x.

Kolmogorov-Smirnov test *Raw data, expected cumulative distribution function, F(x), here normal with mean 3.5, standard deviation 1.75, empirical distribution function, S(X), their difference and absolute difference*

Mcm-2, x	F(x)	S(x)	[F(x) − S(x)]	[S(x) − F(x)]	|S(x) − F(x)|
0.54	0.045	0.05	0.045	0.005	0.005
0.97	0.074	0.1	0.024	0.026	0.026
1.27	0.101	0.15	0.001	0.049	0.049
1.99	0.194	0.2	0.044	0.006	0.006
2.02	0.199	0.25	−0.001	0.051	0.051
2.42	0.269	0.3	0.019	0.031	0.031
2.89	0.364	0.35	0.064	−0.014	0.014
3.01	0.39	0.4	0.04	0.01	0.01
3.13	0.416	0.45	0.016	0.034	0.034
3.26	0.445	0.5	−0.005	0.055	0.055
3.59	0.521	0.55	0.021	0.029	0.029
4.15	0.645	0.6	0.095	−0.045	0.045
4.17	0.649	0.65	0.049	0.001	0.001
4.27	0.67	0.7	0.02	0.03	0.03
4.3	0.676	0.75	−0.024	0.074	0.074
4.4	0.696	0.8	−0.054	0.104	0.104
4.68	0.75	0.85	−0.05	0.1	0.1
5.63	0.888	0.9	0.038	0.012	0.012
6.73	0.968	0.95	0.068	−0.018	0.018
6.94	0.975	1	0.025	0.025	0.025
Max	–	–	0.095	0.104	0.104

Kolmogorov-Smirnov test *Frequency distributions and empirical distribution functions, their differences and absolute difference*

Category	n_1	n_2	$S_1(x)$	$S_2(x)$	$[S_1(x) - S_2(x)]$	$[S_2(x) - S_1(x)]$	$\|S_1(x) - S_2(x)\|$
1	14	35	0.060	0.310	0.250	−0.250	0.250
2	43	45	0.245	0.708	0.463	−0.463	0.463
3	61	5	0.506	0.752	0.246	−0.246	0.246
4	29	10	0.631	0.841	0.210	−0.210	0.210
5	16	14	0.700	0.965	0.265	−0.265	0.265
6	70	4	1.000	1.000	0.000	0.000	0.000
Max	–	–	–	–	0.463	0.000	0.463

Calculate the value of the theoretical cumulative distribution function, $F(x)$. Calculate the test statistic

$$T = \max |F(x) - S(x)|$$

and compare this value to standard tables. This is a two-sided test with alternative hypothesis

$$F(x) \neq S(x).$$

There are two alternative one-sided tests and the hypotheses for these are $F(x) \leq S(x)$ and $S(x) \leq F(x)$, with test statistics

$$T_1 = \max [S(x) - F(x)] \text{ and } T_2 = \max [F(x) - S(x)],$$

respectively.

For the two-sample case, calculate $S(x)$ for each group and the test statistic is $T = \max |S_1(x) - S_2(x)|$, this can be compared to the tables and is a two-sided test. For a one-sided test, the test statistics are

$$T_1 = \max [S_1(x) - S_2(x)] \text{ and } T_2 = \max [S_2(x) - S_1(x)],$$

depending on which distribution is expected to be greater.

As an example, Mcm-2 values are collected in a study. It is thought that they come from a normal distribution with mean 3.5 and standard deviation 1.75. The Kolmogorov-Smirnov one-sample test will be used to test this hypothesis. Therefore, $F(x)$ is calculated from a normal distribution with mean 3.5 and standard deviation 1.75 (see Table on page 184).

The test statistic is shown in the final row of the first Table as the maximal value of the final column for the two-sided case. $T = \max |F(x) - S(x)| = 0.104$. Comparing $T = 0.104$ to standard tables ($n = 20$, $\alpha = 0.05$) gives the value 0.294. As $0.104 < 0.294$, there is insufficient evidence to reject the null hypothesis. Therefore it can be concluded that it is plausible for these data to have come from a normal distribution with mean 3.5 and standard deviation 1.75.

Data for a two-sample example classified into six categories are shown in the second Table.

$$T = \max |S_1(x) - S_2(x)| = 0.463.$$

As the sample size is too large for the tables use the formula for $\alpha = 0.05$, of

$$1.36\sqrt{\frac{N_1 + N_2}{N_1 N_2}} = 1.36\sqrt{\frac{233 + 113}{233 \times 113}} = 0.156.$$

As $0.463 > 0.156$ there is sufficient evidence to reject the null hypothesis that the distributions are the same, therefore it is concluded that the distributions are different.

Further information, including standard tables, is available in textbooks such as Conover (1999), Pett (1997) and Siegel and Castellan (1998) or in the software manual for StatXact (Mehta and Patel, 1998).   *SLV*

Conover, W.J. 1999: *Practical nonparametric statistics*, 3rd edn. Chichester: John Wiley & Sons. **Mehta, C. and Patel, N.** 1998: *Stat-Xact 4 for Windows user manual.* Cytel Software Corporation. **Pett, M.A.** 1997: *Nonparametric statistics for healthcare research.* Thousand Oaks: Sage. **Siegel, S. and Castellan, N.J.** 1998: *Nonparametric statistics for the behavioural sciences*, 2nd edn. Maidenhead: McGraw-Hill.

Kruskal-Wallis test A non-parametric method that is the extension of the MANN-WHITNEY RANK SUM TEST to more than two groups. It is more sensitive than the median test as it uses the magnitude of the differences rather than the direction. It is less sensitive than the JONCKHEERE-TERPSTRA TEST if the groups have an inherent order, as Kruskal-Wallis looks for a difference between groups and the Jonckheere-Terpstra test looks for an increase over the groups. Kruskal-Wallis is derived from one-way ANALYSIS OF VARIANCE but uses ranks rather than the actual observations. It tests if k groups are drawn from populations with the same median and assumes that the data are a randomly selected set of observations, that the data are continuous in nature and in more than two groups. It also assumes an independence of the groups and observations within a group and that the groups have similarly shaped distributions.

To use the test, rank the whole sample from smallest to largest. Calculate the sum of the ranks in each group, the average rank in each group, $\bar{R}_i$ and the average rank for the whole sample, $\bar{R}$. Calculate the test statistic H:

$$H = \frac{12 \sum_{i=1}^{k} n_i (\bar{R}_i - \bar{R})^2}{N(N + 1)}$$

where n_i = the number of observations in group i, and N = the total sample size. Compare H to the critical value of the CHI-SQUARE DISTRIBUTION with $k-1$ DEGREES OF FREEDOM. Reject the null hypothesis if H is bigger than the critical value.

To illustrate, suppose that, within a study, age is an important predictor and so whether there is a difference in age between three groups needs to be decided. The ages are shown in the Table on page 186, as are the ranks for each observation and the sum of the ranks and the average rank in each group.

From standard tables, the critical value of the chi-

Kruskal-Wallis test *Ages and their overall ranks within three groups*

Group 1	Rank	Group 2	Rank	Group 3	Rank
55	18	59	25.5	53	15.5
51	13	40	3.5	62	29
60	27.5	48	11	55	18
34	1.5	56	20	58	23
45	7.5	44	6	58	23
55	18	42	5	57	21
51	13	58	23	46	9.5
60	27.5	67	30	51	13
34	1.5	59	25.5	53	15.5
45	7.5	40	3.5	46	9.5
Rank sum	135		153		177
(average)	(13.5)		(15.3)		(17.7)

$$\bar{R} = \frac{N+1}{2} = \frac{30+1}{2} = 15.5$$

$$H = \frac{12 \sum n_i (\bar{R}_i - \bar{R})^2}{N(N+1)}$$

$$= \frac{12 \times (10 \times (13.5 - 15.5)^2 + 10 \times (15.3 - 15.5)^2 + 10 \times (17.7 - 15.5)^2)}{30 \times (30+1)}$$

$$= 1.15$$

square distribution with 2 degrees of freedom is 5.99, 1.15 < 5.99, therefore there is not sufficient evidence to reject the null hypothesis that the median age is the same in the three groups.

For further details, refer to texts by Conover (1999), Pett (1997) or Siegel and Castellan (1998). *SLV*

Conover, W.J. 1999: *Practical nonparametric statistics*, 3rd edn. Chichester: John Wiley & Sons. **Pett, M.A.** 1997: *Non-parametrics for healthcare research*. Thousand Oaks: Sage. **Siegel, S. and Castellan, N.J.** 1998: *Nonparametric statistics for the behavioural sciences*, 2nd edn. Maidenhead: McGraw-Hill.

kurtosis

A term that describes 'peakedness' of a FREQUENCY DISTRIBUTION or a PROBABILITY DISTRIBUTION. Data that have high kurtosis have a sharp peak and decline rapidly at either side to leave long tails ((a) in the Figure). Data with low kurtosis are flatter ((b) in the Figure).

Mathematical measures of kurtosis can be used to describe distributions. The kurtosis of a normal distribution is 3 and of a uniform distribution is 1.8. However, some formulae for kurtosis subtract 3, so that the kurtosis of a normal distribution is 0 and that of a uniform distribution is −1.2. *SRC*

[See also DESCRIPTIVE STATISTICS]

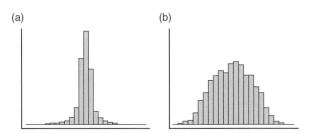

kurtosis *Histogram of distributions having (a) high and (b) low kurtosis*

L

L'Abbé plots See FOREST PLOT

large simple trial (LST) See MEGA-TRIAL

latent variables Variables that cannot be measured directly but that are assumed to be related to a number of observable or manifest variables. Consider, for example, a concept such as 'racial prejudice'. Clearly, direct measurement of this concept is not possible; however, one could, for example, observe whether a person approves or disapproves of a particular piece of government legislation designed to achieve a greater degree of racial equality, whether he or she numbers members of some ethnic minority among his or her friends and acquaintances etc. and assume that these are, in some sense, indicators of the more fundamental variable, racial prejudice.

Although latent variables are the basis of FACTOR ANALYSIS and STRUCTURAL EQUATION MODELS, scepticism about methods based on such variables (particularly factor analysis) has not been uncommon among statisticians over the years. Latent variable modelling has often been viewed as a dubious exercise fraught with unverifiable assumptions and naive inferences regarding causality. For such critics the only thing in favour of latent variable models is that they occupy a rather obscure area of statistics, primarily confined to psychometrics. There are, however, a number of reasons that such criticisms are mistaken: ignoring latent variables often implies stronger assumptions than including them, latent variable modelling then being viewed as a sensitivity analysis of a simpler analysis excluding latent variables; many of the assumptions in latent variable modelling *can* be empirically assessed and some can be relaxed; latent variable modelling pervades modern mainstream statistics and are widely used in different disciplines – not only medicine but also economics, engineering, psychology, geography, marketing and biology (see Skrondal and Rabe-Hesketh, 2004).

This 'omnipresence' of latent variables is commonly not recognised, perhaps because latent variables are given different names in different areas of application, for example, RANDOM EFFECTS, common factors and latent classes. In fact, latent variables can be used to represent a variety of phenomena, for example: true variables measured with error; hypothetical constructs; unobserved heterogeneity; latent responses underlying categorical variables; and MISSING DATA, to name but a few. *BSE*

Skrondal, A. and Rabe-Hesketh, S. 2004: *Generalized latent variable modeling*. Boca Raton: Chapman & Hall/CRC.

lead time bias See BIAS, SCREENING STUDIES

learn-as-you-go designs See DATA-DEPENDENT DESIGNS

least squares estimation A general method for estimating regression parameters in a model for expected outcomes (e.g. a linear regression model). Parameter values are chosen to minimise the sum of squared differences between the observed and expected outcomes. Least squares estimation is, for instance, the standard method of estimation in MULTIPLE LINEAR REGRESSION where observations y_i are approximated by a linear function of explanatory variables x_i, e.g. $\beta_1 x_{i1} + \ldots + \beta_k x_{ik}$ with $\beta_1, \ldots, \beta_k$ unknown. When the model is linear and outcomes are independent and normally distributed with constant variance around their expectation, the method coincides with MAXIMUM LIKELIHOOD ESTIMATION and is efficient in large samples, i.e. yields precise estimators.

More generally, least squares estimators (LSE) can be studied for any type of outcome distribution around the regression curve. They are also useful outside the context of statistical models. Least squares lines are for instance typically drawn as the best fitting line through a cloud of points. This is illustrated in the Figure on page 188, where we depict the LSE of a linear regression curve of body weight (in kg) in function of body height (in cm) based on a random sample of 250 American men (Penrose, Nelson and Fisher, 1985). The curve is obtained by minimising the sum of squared distances e^2 over all observations. It contains the point where the sample averaged body weight is predicted for men of average body height. Within the context of a regression model, predictions on the estimated regression curve are most precise at the centre of the data, but may be imprecise towards the tails. Extrapolations beyond the range of the data often cannot be trusted.

Least squares estimators are attractive due to their strong intuitive appeal, the stability and efficiency of the algorithm and their sound statistical properties in large samples. Under mild regularity conditions, large samples yield an LSE that is subject to normal variation around the true parameter. A 95% CONFIDENCE INTERVAL then becomes the LSE plus or minus 1.96 times the standard error.

When outcome variation is known to differ between observations, a more precise estimator is obtained by a weighted least squares estimator (WLSE), which minimises a sum of *weighted* squared differences between observed and expected outcomes. When the model is linear and the outcomes are independent, weights chosen as the inverse of the individual variances yield the most efficient estimator. When furthermore the outcomes are normally distributed, this WLSE then also coincides with the maximum likelihood estimate (MLE). In other instances, e.g. with logistic regression and many other generalised linear models, the optimal weights depend on the target parameter. Because the latter is unknown, a method of iteratively re-weighted least squares is usually applied, whereby weights in each iteration depend on previous estimates for the unknown parameter.

Even though the LSE may be less precise than the MLE under certain models, least squares estimation is popular because it does not require a complete description of the sampling distribution of the observed data. For example, it is not necessary to assume that outcomes are normally distributed to derive least squares estimates of the

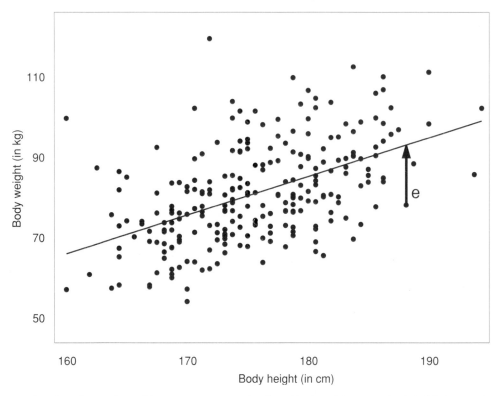

least squares estimation *Scatterplot and least squares regression line of body weight versus body height in a random sample of 250 American men*

unknown regression coefficients in the MULTIPLE LINEAR REGRESSION model. The model of interest for the means is all that is needed. The LSE is therefore immune to mis-specification of the sampling distribution, unlike the MLE.

Further modifications of least squares estimation have been devised to achieve additional goals. For instance, to enhance ROBUSTNESS to outlying observations, L_1-regression is based on minimising the average absolute deviation between the observations and the regression function. *SV/EG*

Bland, M. 2000: *An introduction to medical statistics*, 3rd edn. Oxford: Oxford University Press. **Penrose, K.W., Nelson, A.G. and Fisher, A.G.** 1985: Generalized body composition prediction for men using simple measurement techniques. *Medicine and Science in Sports and Medicine* 17, 189. **Woolson, R.F. and Clarke, W.R.** 2002: *Statistical methods for the analysis of biomedical data*, 2nd edn. New York: John Wiley & Sons.

leave-one-out cross-validation See DISCRIMINANT FUNCTION ANALYSIS

length-biased sampling A form of sampling that arises when items are sampled in proportion to their values on some variable of interest. For example, a sampling scheme based on number of patient visits. A BIAS may be introduced because some individuals are more likely to be selected than others simply because they make more frequent visits. The problem arises in SCREENING STUDIES where the sample of cases detected is likely to contain an excess of slow-growing cancers compared to the sample diagnosed positive because of their symptoms. If length-

biased sampling is ignored, the estimate of the true population mean can be greatly inflated. *BSE*

[See also BIAS, BIAS IN OBSERVATIONAL STUDIES, SAMPLING METHODS – AN OVERVIEW]

Levene's test Used to test whether two or more groups have equal variance. The null hypothesis states that the variance of all groups is equal; the alternative hypothesis states that the variances are unequal for at least one pair. Equal variance of two or more groups is a frequent assumption for parametric tests, ANALYSIS OF VARIANCE for example, and so Levene's test can be used to verify this assumption. Levene's test is relatively simple and robust to departures from normality.

To perform Levene's test we begin by finding, for each group, the absolute differences between the observed values and the median, mean or trimmed mean. The groups need not be of equal size. Whether to use the median, mean or trimmed mean depends on the underlying distribution of the data. If the data are symmetric and moderate tailed the mean provides the best power, using the trimmed mean performs best if the data are heavy tailed and the median performs best if the data are skewed. However, using the median provides good ROBUSTNESS for many types of non-normal data while retaining good power. We complete Levene's test by performing an analysis of variance on these absolute differences (see Table on page 189).

For example, for treatment 1 a score of 23 differs by 4.5 points from the median, while a score of 14 also differs by 4.5 points from the median. The idea is that the larger the

Levene's test *Data resulting from applying Levene's test on three different treatment groups*

Group 1	Absolute differences	Group 2	Absolute differences	Group 3	Absolute differences
24	5.5	22	0.5	8	5
23	4.5	21	0.5	12	1
19	0.5	18	3.5	14	1
18	0.5	25	3.5	15	2
14	4.5	18	3.5	12	1
6	12.5	22	0.5	13	0
5	13.5	16	5.5	7	6
21	2.5	17	4.5	14	1
23	4.5	26	4.5	13	0
10	8.5	23	1.5	15	2
Median **18.5**		**21.5**		**13**	

differences in some groups compared to others, the more the spread and, hence, the more likely it will be that the variance in the populations, from which they arose, is not the same. So a *one-way analysis of variance* on these differences will test this.

This results in an *F*-statistic of 4.21 with an associated *P*-value of 0.026 so we reject the null hypothesis that the variance of the groups is equal. *MMB*

Brown, M. and Forsythe, A. 1974: Robust tests for the equality of variances. *Journal of the American Statistical Association* 69, 346, 364–7. **Wilcox, R.** 1998: Trimming and Winsorisation. In Armitage, P. and Colton, T. (eds), *Encyclopedia of Biostatistics*. Chichester: John Wiley & Sons.

Lexis diagram

A descriptive tool used in epidemiology and demography, being a plot of individuals in a study on two timescales simultaneously. These timescales are most commonly calendar time and age.

Each individual is then represented by a diagonal line at 45° to each axis, which begins at the calendar time and age at enrolment and ends at the calendar time and age at the event of interest (e.g. death) or censoring.

As an example, the Table shows the year of birth, age at enrolment and age at death/censoring of 4 individuals enrolled in a study that began in 1975 and ended follow-up in 2004. The corresponding Lexis diagram is shown in the Figure. A death is shown by a filled circle and a censoring event by an empty circle.

One use of the Lexis diagram relates to estimating, or adjusting for, the effects of age and calendar time on mortality (or morbidity) rate. In this application, age is divided into (for example, 5-year) bands and calendar time is divided into (for example, 5-year) periods.

It is assumed that the mortality rate (or baseline mortality rate) is piecewise constant, i.e. is constant on each

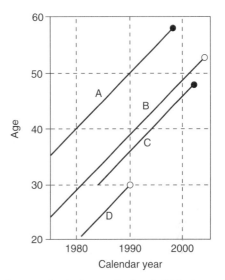

Lexis diagram *Lexis diagram for four individuals*

combination of age band and calendar period. To estimate the mortality rate in each of these band-period combinations, it is necessary to calculate the number of deaths and total time at risk in each band period.

For example, if age bands and calendar periods of 10 years' duration are adopted, individual C joins the cohort in 1984 aged 30. He changes calendar period after 6 years, in 1990. Then he changes age band 4 years later, in 1994. Finally, he changes calendar period 6 years later, in 2000, and dies 2 years later, in 2002.

The Lexis diagram representation makes it easy to see when he changes from one band-period to another: this happens whenever his diagonal line crosses a horizontal or vertical line. Individual C contributes 6, 4, 6 and 2 years at risk, respectively, to 4 band-periods and a death event to the last of these.

Variations on this simple Lexis diagram may be obtained by changing the timescales represented by the axes, by marking other symbols on the diagonal lines to represent other events of interest or by introducing colour to differentiate periods spent by an individual in different states. *SRS*

Lexis diagram *Study data for 4 individuals*

Individual	Birth year	Age at enrolment	Status	Age at death or censoring
A	1940	35	Died	58
B	1951	24	Censored	53
C	1954	30	Died	48
D	1960	21	Censored	30

Clayton, D. and Hills, M. 1993: *Statistical models in epidemiology.* Oxford: Blackwell Science Publications. **Goldman, A.I.** 1992: Events charts: visualizing survival and other timed-events data. *The American Statistician* 46, 13–18. **Keiding, N.** 1990: Statistical inference in the Lexis diagram. *Philosophical Transactions of the Royal Society of London Series A* 332, 487–509.

life tables

Life tables are models that conveniently summarise the level of mortality in a population of interest. Their best known function, life expectancy, has a ready intuitive meaning. Life table functions are independent of the age structure of the population whose mortality level they are used to summarise.

Period life tables are used to summarise the mortality experience during a given period, e.g. a calendar year. Cohort life tables summarise the experience of a defined cohort as it ages through calendar time. For the necessary mortality observations to be available to construct them, the relevant cohort has to be at least towards the end of its life span.

Full life tables have one row for each year of life, usually to age 110 (see Figure on page 191). Abridged life tables typically have one row for each 5 years of life except that there are usually separate rows for ages 0 to 1 and 1 to 5.

Constructing life tables. There are two main steps to building a life table.

First, the 'preliminary computation', in which the observed age and sex-specific death rates during the period of interest are converted into corresponding risks of death between 2 exact ages. Suppose, for example, that the observed central death rate in the population of interest for persons aged 40 to 44 last birthday is 0.003404. (This is $_5M_{40}$, in lifetable notation, when referring to observations made in the population of interest, and is conventionally taken to be an unbiased estimator of the corresponding lifetable function $_5m_{40}$.) The risk of death between exact age 40 and exact age 45 is given by

$$_nq_x = \frac{n._nm_x}{1+(1-_na_x)n._nm_x} = \frac{5._5m_{40}}{1+(1-_5a_{40})5._5m_{40}}$$

$$= \frac{5\times0.003404}{1+(1-0.59)5\times0.003404} = 0.01690$$

where $_5a_{40}$ is the fraction of the age interval lived, on average, by those who die during it. The risk of death across the age interval is close, but not equal to, the central death rate. (In this case, the central death rate times 5 – to take account of the age interval width – equals 0.01702, slightly greater than the risk.)

Second, the computation of the life table proper (see Figure on page 191). In constructing the life table an initial hypothetical cohort of 100,000 (l_0, known as the radix) is subjected across each successive age interval to the calculated risks of death. So, starting at birth ($x = 0$), 100,000 are exposed to the risk of death before exact age 1, i.e. $_1q_0$, which in this example equals 0.02006. This results in 2006 deaths in the interval ($_1d_0$). The person time lived in the interval ($_1L_0$) is 1 year for all who survived it ($l_1 = 97994$) plus the time lived by those who died in the interval – which equals $_1d_0 \times _1a_0$ (the fraction of the interval lived by those who died within it) or 2006×0.129 which equals 98252, as shown, when added to l_1). (For economy $_na_x$ is not shown in the table: it is 0.129 for the

first year of life and approximately 0.5 thereafter.) The $_nL_x$ column is calculated in this way, row at a time, to the end of the lifespan. A special rule is then needed for closing the last open-ended interval – representing, on the table shown, the person time lived beyond 109 – $_\infty L_{109}$. This is estimated by $l_{109}/_\infty M_{109}$. (The justification for this is that the remaining survival time is taken to be distributed exponentially with a mean of $1/_\infty M_{109}$.)

T_x is then summed back from the end of the lifespan, beginning, in this example, with T_{109} which equals L_{109}. Moving up one row, T_{108} then equals $T_{109} + _1L_{108}$ and so on back to T_0. T_0 represents all the person-time lived by the 100000 who set out, so the average person-time lived, or life expectancy e_0, is T_0/l_0 and more generally for any age x, $e_x = T_x/l_x$.

Life table populations can be interpreted in two ways: 1) as fully hypothetical constructs or models in which 100,000 individuals are imagined, as it were, to be born in the same instant and then instantaneously subjected to the relevant risks of death throughout their hypothetical lifespans; or 2) as representing stationary populations experiencing constant, and equal, birth and death rates. In this latter interpretation, $_nL_x$ gives the expected number of individuals aged x to $x+n$ and T_0 gives the total population size. In such stationary populations there are l_0 births each year, so the birth rate = l_0/T_0 – the inverse of the life expectancy. Thus the

Crude birth rate = crude death rate = $1/e_0$

Uses of the life table. The l_x and q_x columns have many uses in summarising mortality risks in populations of interest. Thus infant mortality, conceptually defined as the risk of death before the first birthday is $_1q_0$. The under 5 mortality 'rate' (actually the risk of death before age 5) is $1-l_5/l_0$. The adult mortality 'rate' ($_{45}q_{15}$, or the probability of death between 15 and 60) is $1-l_{60}/l_{15}$. Similarly, the probability of survival between any 2 ages i and j is given by l_j/l_i.

Life tables have long been used to provide comparable summaries of mortality risks in populations. They are also serving as the basis of newer 'summary measures of average population health' which combine information on both the risks of premature death and of non-fatal illness and injury. Such summary measures may be either 'health expectancies' (such as 'health adjusted life expectancy') or 'health gaps' (such as DALYs (disability adjusted life years) lost).

The d_x and l_x functions when plotted for a given population at successive time intervals show how the distribution of age at death changes as life expectancy has risen. One interpretation of recent trends in low mortality countries is that the rise in e_0 has been disproportionately due to a reduction of the more premature adult deaths. As this process continues, a larger and larger proportion of each generation survives until closer to the maximum lifespan. The distribution of deaths by age at death becomes concentrated at a high age – manifest as a reduced dispersion in the distribution of deaths by age (d_x) in the life table. The corresponding shift in pattern for the survivorship (l_x) function is for it to remain high till closer to the maximum lifespan and then fall sharply – a process described as the 'rectangularisation of the survival curve'. This 'optimistic' interpretation of recent trends is taken to imply that there has been no extension of the average duration of ill-health in the period immediately before death. *JP*

Lifetable functions and notation

x is exact age x, i.e. the xth birthday.

n refers to the width of the age interval being considered. In a full life table where $n = 1$ it may be omitted.

e_x is life expectancy at exact age x.

$_nm_x$ is the central death rate for persons aged between x and $x + n$ in the hypothetical lifetable population. It is estimated by $_nM_x$ (below).

$_nM_x$ is the observed central death rate in the population of interest.

l_x is the number of persons still alive at exact age x.

$_nq_x$ is the risk (probability) of death between exact ages x and $x + n$.

$_np_x$ is the risk of surviving from exact age x to $x + n$ (equals $1 - {_nq_x}$).

$_na_x$ is the average fraction of the interval lived by those who die between x and $x + n$.

$_nL_x$ is the number of person years lived between exact ages x and $x + n$.

T_x is the number of person years lived between exact age x and the extinction of the hypothetical cohort.

life tables *Extract of first 6 and last 10 rows of a full life table for US white males in 1970*

| Age interval, period of life between 2 ages, x and x+n | Width of age interval in years | Proportion of persons alive at the beginning of age interval dying during interval* | Of 100000 born alive | | In stationary (life table) population with 100000 born into it each year | | Average number of years of life remaining at beginning of age interval (life expectancy) |
| | | | Number living at beginning of age interval | Number dying during age interval | Number of person years of life lived in age interval | Number of person years of life lived in this and all subsequent intervals | |
x	n	$_nq_x$	l_x	$_nd_x$	$_nL_x$	T_x	e_x
0	1	.02006	100000	2006	98252	6793828	67.94
1	1	.00116	97994	114	97037	6695576	68.33
2	1	.00083	97880	81	97840	6597639	67.41
3	1	.00072	97799	71	97763	6499799	66.46
4	1	.00059	97728	57	97700	6402036	65.51
5	1	.00054	97671	52	97645	6304336	64.55
⋮	⋮	⋮	⋮	⋮	⋮	⋮	⋮
100	1	.35479	189	67	155	415	2.20
101	1	.36553	122	45	100	260	2.13
102	1	.37550	77	29	62	160	2.08
103	1	.38471	48	18	39	98	2.02
104	1	.39320	30	12	24	59	1.98
105	1	.40101	18	7	15	35	1.94
106	1	.40818	11	5	8	20	1.90
107	1	.41475	6	2	5	12	1.86
108	1	.42075	4	2	3	7	1.82
109	∞	1.00000	2	2	4	4	1.79

* a_x is 0.129 for the first year of life and approximately 0.5 for all subsequent years

Preston, S.H., Heuveline, P., and Guillot, M. 2001: *Demography: measuring and modeling population processes,* Oxford: Blackwell. **Elandt-Johnson, R.C. and Johnson, N.L.** 1980: *Survival models and data analysis,* New York: Wiley. **Peeters, A., Barendregt, J.J., Willekens, F., Mackenbach, J.P., Al Mamun, A. and Bonneux, L.** 2003: Obesity in adulthood and its consequences for life expectancy: a life-table analysis, *Ann. Intern. Med,* 138, 24–32. **Lopez, A.D., Ahmad, O.B., Guillot, M., Ferguson, B.D., Salomon, J.A., Murray, C.J.L. and Hill, K.H.** 2003: Life Tables for 191 Countries for 2000: Data, Methods, Results, in *Health systems performance assessment: debates, methods and empiricism.* Murray, C.J.L. and Evans, D.B. (eds.), Geneva: World Health Organization, pp. 335–53.

likelihood The likelihood function plays two roles in statistics. First, in its own right it provides a means for estimating unknown parameters by finding the value of the unknown parameter(s) that maximises it (maximum likelihood) as well as for comparing hypotheses (likelihood ratio). Second, it has a role in Bayesian statistics (see BAYESIAN METHODS).

Suppose interest lies in learning about the response of patients suffering from influenza symptoms to a new treatment. Data are collected from 10 patients, of whom 6 respond positively. What can be said about the unknown probability of positive response π? By definition, the probability of a positive response is π and, of a negative response, $1 - \pi$. Suppose that we have observed 6 positive response and 4 negative responses in that order. The likelihood of this happening is $\pi^6 (1 - \pi)^4$. In practice, the order of observation of the responses is arbitrary and we could account for this multiplying the likelihood we have calculated by the number of ways 6 positive responses and 4 negative responses could occur. If this is done the likelihood becomes:

$$\frac{6!}{4!2!}\pi^6(1 - \pi)^4 = 15\pi^6(1 - \pi)^4$$

which corresponds to a probability from a BINOMIAL DISTRIBUTION. For different values of π we can determine the likelihood and on this basis find the most likely value.

For example, if π has the value 0.1 the likelihood is $15 \times 0.2^6 \times 0.8^4 = 0.0000098$ and for the values of $\pi = 0.3, 0.5, 0.7$ and 0.9 the corresponding likelihood values are $0.00263, 0.0146, 0.0143, 0.00080$ respectively. So, of these four values, 0.5 is the most likely. In fact, we can plot the likelihood values for all potential values of π and choose that value that gives the maximum, as in the first Figure. From the Figure, we can conclude that the most likely value for π is 0.6, as it gives the largest likelihood value. This value is the maximum likelihood estimator.

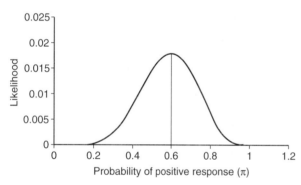

likelihood *Likelihood function based on 6 positive responses out of 10*

The same approach can be used for other types of data. For example, Altman gives the following data on daily energy intake (kJ) of 11 healthy women: 5260, 5470, 5640, 6180, 6390, 6515, 6805, 7515, 7515, 8230, 8770.

Assuming that these data arise from a NORMAL DISTRIBUTION with a common MEAN denoted μ and known STANDARD DEVIATION 1100 we can determine the likelihood as a function of the unknown μ and plot it as before. The second Figure illustrates this in which the maximum likelihood occurs at the value 6754.

In Bayesian statistics, the likelihood works to modify the PRIOR DISTRIBUTION to yield the POSTERIOR DISTRIBUTION and represents the information contained in the experiment about the parameter of interest. In a formal way, Bayesian analysis proceeds by calculating:

$$p(\theta \mid \text{Data}) \propto p(\text{Data} \mid \theta)p(\theta)$$

in which p(θ) is the prior distribution expressing initial beliefs in the parameter of interest, θ, p(θ | Data) is the corresponding posterior distribution of beliefs and $p(\text{Data} \mid \theta)$ is the likelihood. If there is great prior uncer-

tainty about the parameter of interest so that the prior distribution is essentially flat relative to the region in which the likelihood is peaked then it has little impact on modifying prior beliefs. In such circumstances, the posterior distribution is essentially proportional to the likelihood so that posterior beliefs about the parameter are dictated by the location and shape of the likelihood. In particular, the posterior mode, the value believed to be the most likely after collecting data, is essentially equivalent to the value that maximises the likelihood, that is, the maximum likelihood estimate. *AG*

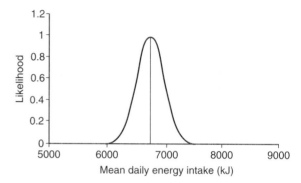

likelihood *Likelihood function for the mean daily energy intake based on a sample of 11 values*

likelihood ratio The likelihood ratio provides a method for comparing competing hypotheses based on the LIKELIHOOD calculated from experimental data. It also plays a role in Bayesian hypothesis testing (see BAYESIAN METHODS).

Suppose interest lies in learning about the response of patients suffering from influenza symptoms to a new treatment. Data are collected from 10 patients of whom 6 respond positively. What can be said about the competing hypotheses H_1: $\pi = 0.3$ and H_2: $\pi = 0.7$? The likelihood of obtaining 6 positive results and 4 negative results is:

$$\frac{6!}{4!2!}\pi^6(1 - \pi)^4 = 15\pi^6(1 - \pi)^4$$

and this can be determined for the competing values of π under the pair of hypotheses. For hypothesis H_1 the value is 0.00263, while that for H_2 is 0.0143. The ratio of these values is 5.44, the likelihood ratio of H_2 against H_1 indicating, in this instance, that hypothesis H_2 is almost 5½ as likely as H_1, which is strong evidence in favour of H_2 rather than H_1.

The Bayesian equivalent to this form of hypothesis testing is based on determining the ratio of the posterior probabilities of the hypotheses. Formally, we calculate:

$$p(H_i \mid \text{Data}) \propto p(\text{Data} \mid H_i)p(H_i), \, i = 1,2$$

in which $p(H_i)$ is the prior probability of hypothesis H_i, expressing initial beliefs in its veracity, $p(H_i \mid \text{Data})$ is the corresponding posterior probabilities and $p(\text{Data} \mid H_i)$ is the likelihood of the hypothesis giving rise to the data. By taking the ratio of the two expressions just given, the ratio of the posterior probabilities of the two hypotheses can be expressed as:

$$\frac{p(H_2 \mid \text{Data})}{p(H_1 \mid \text{Data})} = \frac{p(\text{Data} \mid H_2)}{p(\text{Data} \mid H_1)} \times \frac{p(H_2)}{p(H_1)}$$

The left-hand side of this expression is the posterior odds ratio, the first term on the right-side is the likelihood ratio and the second term the prior odds ratio.

This form of Bayesian analysis is familiar in diagnostic testing. In that context the likelihood ratio is expressed as:

$$\text{Likelihood ratio} = \frac{\text{Probability(positive test result} \mid \text{disease)}}{\text{Probability(positive test result} \mid \text{no disease)}}$$

$$= \frac{\text{sensitivity}}{1 - \text{specificity}}$$

AG

Altman, D.G. 1991: *Practical statistics for medical research.* London: Chapman and Hall.

Likert scales

Scales that are used to measure the extent to which an individual agrees with a statement. A Likert scale typically has five levels, ranging from 'strongly disagree' to 'strongly agree'. One common alternative is to use an even number of options in order to avoid having a 'neutral' option. A typical Likert scale questionnaire item with five levels is the following:

In a proposed study of mild asthma, it is ethically acceptable to give some participants a placebo treatment.

- strongly disagree
- disagree
- neither agree nor disagree
- agree
- strongly agree

The data from a Likert scale are often coded as a number (e.g. 1 to 5) and it is typical for responses from multiple items to be summed or averaged to provide an overall score related to an underlying issue or LATENT VARIABLE.

When there are multiple items, it is recommended that the order of responses be reversed for some items, to help prevent subjects falling into a simple pattern of responses (e.g. always select 'strongly agree').

The data from one or more Likert scale items are often analysed as interval data. For this to be a justifiable approach, it is important to trial and develop the items properly, perhaps using a pilot study and test for validation and reliability (see MEASUREMENT PRECISION AND RELIABILITY). *PM*

[See also FACTOR ANALYSIS]

DeVellis, R.F. 1991: *Scale development: theory and applications.* London: Sage. **Streiner, D.L. and Norman, G.R.** 1995: *Health measurement scales: a practical guide to their development and use,* 2nd edn. Oxford: Oxford University Press.

limits of agreement

An approach developed by Bland and Altman (1986) to assess agreement in method comparison studies. This approach, based on both graphical techniques and straightforward statistical calculations, is simple to apply and interpret. It quantifies agreement between two methods through the mean difference (i.e. the estimate of the systematic bias of one method relative to the other), and the standard deviation of the differences between measurements taken by the methods on the same subjects (i.e. an indication of the variability of these differences across subjects).

The information provided by these summary statistics is commonly presented visually in a *Bland–Altman plot*, where the difference between measurements are plotted against

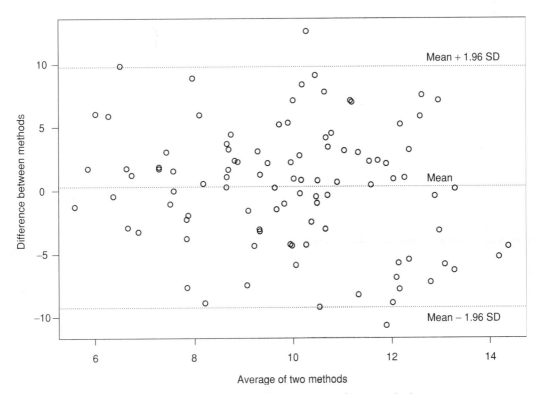

limits of agreement *Bland and Altman plot of the difference against the average for two methods*

the average of the measurements taken by the methods on the same subjects (see Figure). This summary information is displayed on the plot by three horizontal lines indicating the mean difference, and the mean difference ± 1.96 standard deviation of the differences. The latter two lines represent the 95% limits of agreement. That is, a range within which one would expect 95% of the differences to lie, under the assumptions of Normally distributed differences and the uniformity of systematic bias and standard deviation across the whole range of measurements (as indicated by no evidence in the Bland and Altman plot of a relationship between the difference and the average in measurements taken by the two methods on each subject).

The assumption of Normality of the differences is generally reasonable, as a lot of the between subject variation is removed by the differencing of the measurements between methods, and therefore what remains is the measurement error. However even if this assumption is violated, there may not be any serious consequences resulting from the constructing of the limits of agreement as already described. 5% of the differences will still be expected to lie outside the range created by these limits, although most of these differences may be in the same direction.

If there is found to be a relationship between the difference and average, for example, the plot shows a 'fanning out' effect of the differences as the average increases (i.e. the variability of the differences is increasing with the size of the measurement), then application of the limits of agreement method, as described above, would produce limits that would be wider apart than needed for lower values of the average, and narrower than expected at higher values. Thus it is better to try to either accommodate this relationship or remove it by suitably transforming the data (e.g. using a logarithmic transformation).

Bland and Altman provide comprehensive expositions about the limits of agreement approach, the issues that result when the assumptions of Normality and uniformity of the bias and standard deviation are violated, and the ways to overcome these obstacles in their approach. They also discuss repeatability and replication, and further extensions to their approach. The reader is referred to their articles for more information. (See references below.)

Before concluding this article, further mention must be made of the purpose behind the limits of agreement approach. In medicine interest often lies in comparing two (or more) different methods or techniques for measuring some clinically important quantity, such as carotid stenosis or blood pressure. One of the methods may be already routinely established in clinical practice (e.g. Intra-arterial Digital Subtraction Angiography (DSA)), while the other may be a new technique (e.g. Contrast-Enhanced Magnetic Resonance Angiography (CEMRA)) that needs to be evaluated. Both however measure the true quantity of interest with error. Thus neither is a true gold standard, and therefore the question of interest is not whether the new method, say CEMRA, accurately measures stenosis of the carotid artery, as assessed by the established method, DSA. But it is instead 'Do the different methods of measurement agree sufficiently closely to allow either the new method to replace the old or both to be used interchangeably, with little or no differences arrived at in clinical conclusions or decisions?' For example, if CEMRA is shown to give sufficiently close measurements to DSA, then, as the latter is an invasive and expensive technique

that carries with its use a small, but significant risk of stroke or death, justification for using CEMRA, which is a non-invasive technique, over DSA is obtained. Note finally that the setting of the level of acceptable agreement depends on the clinical context of the study, and should be made based on clinical judgement, not on statistical grounds. Further this decision should be made, in general, *a priori* of the commencement of the study. *BT*

Altman, D.G. 1991: *Practical statistics for medical research*, London: Chapman & Hall. **Altman, D.G. and Bland, J.M.** 1983: Measurement in medicine: the analysis of method comparison studies. *The Statistician* 32, 307–17. **Bland, J.M. and Altman, D.G.** 1986: Statistical methods for assessing agreement between two methods of clinical measurement. *Lancet* i, 307–10. **Bland, J.M. and Altman, D.G.** 1999: Measuring agreement in method comparison studies. *Statistical Methods in Medical Research* 8, 135–60.

linear mixed-effects models

Regression models that include both FIXED EFFECTS and RANDOM EFFECTS, which are also known as MULTILEVEL MODELS or hierarchical models. Mixed-effects models are fitted to data that have a hierarchical or clustered structure, in which individual observations are correlated within clusters. Examples of application areas include longitudinal data, where the measurements taken repeatedly on patients over time are correlated within patients, and multicentre studies, where the measurements taken on patients within centres are correlated. Mixed-effects models include random effects to allow for the correlation of observations within clusters. To illustrate the basic structure, we consider a simple example of a linear mixed-effects model. In a clinical trial comparing the effects of active treatment and control over time, suppose that y_{ij} is the response measured on subject j ($j = 1, ..., J$) at time t_{ij} ($i = 1, ..., I_j$), and let the treatment group allocated to each subject be indicated by $x_{ij} = 0/1$. A simple mixed-effects model for the data y_{ij} includes random effects for patients to acknowledge that response tends to differ between patients and that repeated measurements taken on the same patient are therefore alike. This model is written as

$$y_{ij} = (\alpha + u_j) + \beta t_{ij} + \gamma x_{ij} + e_{ij}$$

where the u_j are random patient effects and the e_{ij} are random residual effects which represent the variability between measurements within patients. The parameters α, β and γ are fixed effects that represent, respectively, the overall mean response in the control group (where $x_{ij} = 0$), the trend in response over time and the treatment effect, which is constant over time. The two sets of random effects u_j and e_{ij} are independent and it is usual to assume these to be normally distributed, $u_j \sim N(0, \sigma_u^2)$ and $e_{ij} \sim N(0, \sigma_e^2)$. This basic mixed-effects model for the data can be extended in a number of interesting ways. For example, we could allow the trend in response over time to vary from one patient to another, we could include additional explanatory variables, or we could allow the effect of treatment to vary over time. For a range of extended mixed-effects models and guidance on their interpretation, readers are referred to the full entry on this subject area titled multilevel models (see also Everitt and Pickles, 2000; Pinheiro and Bates, 2000). This entry provides details of methods and software for estimation of mixed-effects models and also covers topics such as handling of missing data and complex applications. *RT*

[See also GENERALISED ESTIMATING EQUATIONS, MULTI-LEVEL MODELS]

Everitt, B.S. and Pickles, A. 2000: *Statistical aspects of the design and analysis of clinical trials*. London: Imperial College Press. Pinheiro, J.C. and Bates, D.M. 2000: *Mixed effects models in S and S-PLUS*. New York: Springer Verlag.

linear regression See MULTIPLE LINEAR REGRESSION

linkage disequilibrium See ALLELIC ASSOCIATION

LISREL See STRUCTURAL EQUATION MODELLING SOFTWARE

local research ethics committee (LREC) See ETHICAL REVIEW COMMITTEES

locally weighted regression See SCATTERPLOT SMOOTHERS

loess See SCATTERPLOT SMOOTHERS

logistic discrimination See DISCRIMINANT FUNCTION ANALYSIS

logistic regression A form of regression analysis to be used when the response is a binary variable. Medical outcomes often have only two possibilities. Whether a patient is dead or alive is the most obvious, but presence or absence of particular diagnoses, symptoms or signs are also examples of binary or dichotomous variables. Hypertension, obesity and airways obstruction are diagnoses that result from observing that a particular measurement is above or below a particular value, thus creating a binary outcome from a continuous measurement.

Methods for the analysis of binary data differ from those for continuous variables. First, the summary statistic to describe the results is a proportion or percentage of individuals who are dead (or alive), have the symptom or in general have the designated outcome. Data from a continuous variable are summarised by the MEAN and STANDARD DEVIATION or MEDIAN and INTERQUARTILE RANGE, as how variable the values are is required as well as a typical value, while for binary data the proportion or percentage tells us everything. Second, when we analyse a binary outcome in relation to EXPLANATORY VARIABLES we cannot use STUDENT t-TESTS, ANALYSIS OF VARIANCE or MULTIPLE LINEAR REGRESSION, as the data are not normally distributed, do not have the same variance for groups with different outcome proportions and predictions of proportions must not fall outside the range zero to one, which can happen if multiple linear regression of a proportion is used.

Binary data can be analysed in relation to a single categorical explanatory variable using the CHI-SQUARE TEST, but very frequently it is necessary to analyse a binary outcome in relation to several explanatory variables, some or all of which may be continuous. For example, in a study that investigated whether reported wheeze is related to the use of gas for cooking it would be desirable to take age and gender into account, also conditions in the home, such as an extractor fan, that might affect the concentration of the combustion product thought to be responsible for any increase in symptoms. Alternatively, we might want to analyse wheeze in relation to use of gas for cooking and passive smoking simultaneously. To analyse binary data and adjust the relation to the factor of primary interest for confounding variables or to determine to which of several potential explanatory variables the outcome is related, an analogue of analysis of variance and multiple regression is required. Logistic regression meets these requirements.

An explanation of the method is easiest in relation to an example. Logistic regression has been used to describe the distribution of age at menarche in girls and the factors associated with early or delayed menarche. Roberts, Rozner and Swan (1971) carried out a cross-sectional survey of girls in South Shields, County Durham, in 1967. Data are shown in the first Table.

logistic regression *Number of girls, and number recorded as menstruating, by age group*

Age group	No. of girls	No. menstruating	% menstruating
11 – <12	82	4	4.9
12 – <13	304	76	25.0
13 – <14	366	178	48.6
14 – <15	351	285	81.2
15 – <16	216	209	96.8

The percentage of girls who had reached menarche, of course, increased with age, being very low in the youngest age group and very high in the oldest. Had younger age groups been included the percentage menstruating would have been less than 4.9% and 0% if sufficiently low. Similarly, the percentage would have been close to 100% in older age groups. The relation of proportion or percentage menstruating to age can be described by an S-shaped (or 'sigmoid') curve. The data from the first table are plotted together with a fitted smooth sigmoid curve in the Figure.

The curve shown is a cumulative logistic curve, selected from the family of such curves so that it best describes the data. Its formula is:

$$\pi = \frac{1}{1 + e^{-(\alpha + \beta x)}}$$

where π is the proportion menstruating by age x and α and β are the parameters that describe the best fitting curve. These parameters were estimated to be -18.40 and 1.37,

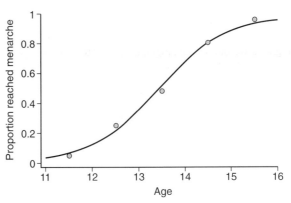

logistic regression *Cumulative logistic curve*

respectively, to fit the curve shown. Median age at menarche is estimated at $\pi = 0.5$, i.e. where $-(\alpha + \beta x) = 0$, or $x = -\alpha/\beta$, so was 13.4 years from these data. As the logistic distribution is symmetric this is an estimate of mean age at menarche.

The equation defining π can be rewritten:

$$\log_e \frac{\pi}{1 - \pi} = \alpha + \beta x$$

The left-hand side of this equation is known as the *logistic transformation* of the proportion π. Its effect is to stretch the scale, so that the transformed variable can take values from minus infinity $(-\infty)$, corresponding to $\pi = 0$, to plus infinity $(+\infty)$, corresponding to $\pi = 1$, and also to linearise the relation with age. Fitting the logistic curve can therefore be achieved by least squares regression of the logistic transform of π on age (see LEAST SQUARES ESTIMATION), except that the transformation does not achieve homogeneity of variance and so iteratively weighted least squares regression is required. However, most modern computer programs use MAXIMUM LIKELIHOOD ESTIMATION, which also requires iteration, and individual rather than grouped data are usually analysed. Full specification of the binary outcome y for individuals requires that y is distributed as a binomial distribution with parameter 1 (here also known as a Bernoulli distribution) and success probability π.

The logistic curve is not the only curve that could be fitted to describe the data. A fitted cumulative NORMAL DISTRIBUTION would be almost indistinguishable from the logistic curve. Fitting a normal distribution before the days of electronic computing was known as *probit analysis* (see PROBIT MODELS), a probit being a normal equivalent deviate with 5 added to avoid negative numbers and was developed for use in pharmacology (Finney, 1971). The distribution of the dose of a toxic substance required to kill a given strain of animal is known as the *tolerance distribution*. It cannot usually be observed directly, but if groups of animals are given different doses of the drug and the proportions dying are recorded, then a sigmoid curve of proportion with dose is observed that describes the cumulative tolerance distribution.

Finney (1964) ascribed the logistic transformation to Berkson and showed the close agreement of the normal and logistic distributions, but favoured the normal distribution to describe the tolerance distribution of drug toxicity. Hence, in general, the normal or probit transformation was used when there was an underlying tolerance distribution. An exception was age at menarche; it became accepted that the logistic transformation should be used (Finney, 1971) as one study apparently found a better fit of the logistic than of the normal distribution.

Just as linear regression can be extended to multiple regression and also incorporate categorical explanatory variables, so can logistic regression. A multiple logistic regression equation can be written:

$$\log_e \frac{\pi}{1 - \pi} = \alpha + \beta_1 x_1 + \beta_2 x_2 + \beta_3 x_3 \ldots.$$

where the x_i can be continuous or DUMMY VARIABLES to indicate categories of groups. For example Roberts, Danskin and Chinn (1975) analysed age at menarche in relation to family size, in categories of one, two, three, four and at least five children. In the model shown graphically in the paper, x_1 was age, and four dummy variables x_2 to x_5 were used to describe the differences in median age at menarche between the five family size groups, corresponding to fitting parallel sigmoid curves. The estimates b_i of the β_i are known as LOGISTIC REGRESSION coefficients.

To return to our first example: if presence or absence of wheeze is the outcome and presence or absence of a gas cooker the independent or explanatory variable, with no other factors considered for the moment, then if the dummy (indicator) variable x is 0 for absence and 1 for presence of a gas cooker, then we have:

$$\log_e \frac{\pi_{nogas}}{1 - \pi_{nogas}} = \alpha$$

$$\log_e \frac{\pi_{gas}}{1 - \pi_{gas}} = \alpha + \beta$$

Hence:

$$\log_e \left[\frac{\pi_{gas}}{1 - \pi_{gas}} \right] - \log_e \left[\frac{\pi_{nogas}}{1 - \pi_{nogas}} \right] = \beta$$

Each of the terms within brackets is an odds and a difference in log odds, when anti-logged, is an odds ratio. Anti-logging both sides of the equation gives:

$$\frac{\pi_{gas}(1 - \pi_{nogas})}{\pi_{nogas}(1 - \pi_{gas})} = e^{\beta}$$

The odds ratio on the left-hand side of this equation is the odds of having wheeze in the presence of a gas cooker divided by the odds of having wheeze if no gas cooker is present. It will approximate the relative risk, or risk ratio, of wheeze in the presence of a gas cooker compared to no gas cooker provided that the prevalence of wheeze is low. This relative risk is estimated by e^{β}. The differences of this example from the age at menarche example are that π for wheeze is unlikely to be greater than, say 0.2, and no 'tolerance distribution' analogous to that of age at menarche is directly specified, although one can envisage this being the distribution of whatever product of combustion of gas is responsible for increased wheeze in people in homes with gas cookers. Even with such a distribution specified, it is unlikely that exposure would ever be high enough to cause 100% wheeze, so, in practice, only the lower portion of the sigmoid curve is relevant.

As with applications in general, it was the availability of software that led to an expansion in the use of logistic regression, in particular GLIM (Generalised Linear Interactive Modelling) in the early 1970s. Although now largely superseded, notably but not exclusively by STATA, GLIM enabled unbalanced analysis of variance, multiple linear regression and multiple logistic regression models to be fitted within the same framework. The application of logistic regression in epidemiology and public health journals showed a steep rise from around 1980 (Chinn 2001; Hosmer, Taber and Lemshow, 1991). Odds ratios were used in epidemiology and, in particular, for the results of a CASE-CONTROL STUDY, before the widespread availability of computers and statistical software, enabled easy fitting of multiple logistic regression models, and therefore logistic regression was readily adopted by epidemiologists. It was also established as the appropriate method for the analysis of case-control studies with adjustment for confounding. When cases and controls are individually matched the method of analysis is conditional logistic regression. Most statistical software for logistic regression requires the binary outcome to be coded 0 and 1, with 1 for the 'positive' outcome.

Like all estimates from a sample, an odds ratio has an associated CONFIDENCE INTERVAL. The null hypothesis of no relation to an explanatory variable is an odds ratio of one or equivalently zero for the corresponding logistic regression coefficient. Older papers gave logistic regression coefficients with standard errors or 95% confidence intervals, but more recent papers give odds ratios with 95% confidence intervals. For example, Somerville, Rona and Chinn (1988) gave logistic regression coefficients in a study of passive smoking by children in survey of 5- to 11-year-old children in England and Scotland. One result is shown in the first line of the second table. The logistic regression coefficient of the symptom, reported by a parent in a self-administered questionnaire, 'chest ever sounds wheezy or whistling', on passive smoking as measured by the total number of cigarettes per day reported to be smoked by the parents, was 0.011 with a standard error of 0.005. By calculating the coefficient $\pm 1.96 \times$ standard error, a 95% confidence for the logistic regression coefficient can be obtained. Anti-logging (base e) the coefficient and each limit of its confidence interval gives the odds ratio and its 95% confidence interval in the second line. However, the odds ratio associated with exposure to just one cigarette a day is not very useful; 20 cigarettes a day represents a more common exposure of children who are exposed to passive smoking. To obtain the odds ratio associated with exposure to 20 cigarettes a day, multiply both the logistic regression coefficient and its standard error by 20 and repeat the confidence interval calculation and anti-logging to obtain the third line of the table.

Although the evidence against the null hypothesis was not strong ($P \sim 0.028$) and the 95% confidence interval correspondingly wide, the results in the third line show that the size of the likely effect is not negligible, which could not be easily appreciated from either of the first two rows. Note that the confidence interval for the logistic regression coefficient is symmetric around the estimate, but that that for an odds ratio is not.

It is tempting to interpret the third line of the second table as meaning that exposure to 20 cigarettes smoked a day in the home results in an increased risk of wheeze of between 2.4% and 51.6%. This is interpreting an odds ratio as if it were a relative risk, which is only justified if the prevalence of wheeze is low, say less than 10% (Zhang and Yu, 1998). In this case it was 10.9%, so perhaps not too misleading, but it is easy to find examples of incorrect interpretation of odds ratios in the medical literature (Chinn, 2001). Although the fact that the odds ratio is biased away from the null value of 1 as an estimate of relative risk is well known to statisticians and epidemiologists, it is often conveniently ignored in the medical literature, especially in the reporting of results of CROSS-SECTIONAL STUDIES. In fact, it is possible to estimate relative risk directly, by binomial regression, but at the expense of the iterative model fitting sometimes failing to converge (Chinn, 2001).

Logistic regression is essential for the analysis of unmatched case-control studies and is likely to continue to be the most used method for the analysis of binary outcomes in cross-sectional studies. Statistically it cannot be faulted; it is in the reporting, and the fact that an odds ratio does not estimate relative risk directly, that the problem lies. Binary outcomes in COHORT STUDIES should be analysed by SURVIVAL ANALYSIS, unless the follow-up time is constant, which is rarely the case.

The P-VALUE associated with the odds ratio, to test a difference from 1, can be obtained by dividing the logistic regression coefficient by its standard error and comparing the result with the normal distribution, as the null hypothesis value for the logistic regression coefficient is zero. Note that the normal distribution is used rather than the t-distribution, as no residual standard deviation is estimated. This is because a binomial distribution is assumed for the observations, which is specified only by the expected proportion, and does not involve a standard deviation. Alternatively, if the model were fitted by MAXIMUM LIKELIHOOD, the LIKELIHOOD RATIO test can be used and will usually give approximately the same answer for a single parameter. If model 1 is the model with the factor of interest included, with likelihood l_1, and model 2 that with it omitted with likelihood l_2, then $-2\log(l_2/l_1)$ has a chi-squared distribution with DEGREES OF FREEDOM equal to the difference in the number of fitted parameters. This can be used to test equivalence of several parameters, for example equal median age at menarche for girls from different size of family (Roberts, Danskin and Chinn, 1975).

Related to testing for association of outcome with risk factors is that of goodness of fit of the model. This is more difficult to assess than with a linear regression model, as individual values are each 0 or 1, so a plot of observed against fitted values, or of residuals, is uninformative. For associated reasons the overall likelihood ratio statistic cannot be used. Hosmer, Taber and Lemeshow (1991) give a number of plots that can be used and the necessary calculations are implemented in Stata.

Logistic regression as described here for a binary outcome is a special case of the more general multinomial, or polytomous, logistic regression for a categorical outcome with three or more possible values (see LOGIT MODELS FOR ORDINAL RESPONSES). It is also closely related to the LOG-

logistic regression *Alternative presentations of result of logistic regression analysis, illustrated by 'chest EVER sounds wheezy or whistling' in relation to passive smoking for children in the National Study of Health and Growth (Somerville, Rona and Chinn, 1988)*

Quantity presented	Result
Logistic regression coefficient $\pm$ standard error on total number of cigarettes smoked at home by father and mother	0.011 ± 0.005
Odds ratio per cigarette smoked (95% confidence interval)	1.011 (1.001 to 1.021)
Odds ratio per 20 cigarettes smoked (95% confidence interval)	1.246 (1.024 to 1.516)

LINEAR MODEL, which assumes a POISSON DISTRIBUTION for the count in each cell of a contingency table. Each is an example of a GENERALISED LINEAR MODEL.

Medical journals now frequently report results from multiple logistic regression, showing odds ratios, P-values and confidence intervals. These need to be read carefully, as seemingly similar tables may be used in different situations. The lines of the table may be for different binary outcomes or independent analyses of the same outcome with different explanatory variables. The odds ratios will often be adjusted, for a list of stated variables such as age and sex, although unadjusted odds ratios may also be shown. An example is shown in Table 2 of Lawlor, Patel and Ebrahim (2003), in which odds ratios of falls in women aged 60 to 79 with drug use are given. Each row of the table gives results for one class of drug, while there are columns for 'crude', i.e. unadjusted, and fully adjusted odds ratios for each of three outcomes: any falls, two or more falls and falls where medical attention was given. The variables used to adjust the fully adjusted odds ratios are listed as a footnote to the table.

Other papers give odds ratios that are mutually adjusted for other factors shown in the same table of results, i.e. all the results come from a single multiple logistic regression and full information is given, while Lawlor, Patel and Ebrahim (2003) (described earlier) appear to have carried out 21 adjusted analyses (three outcomes by seven drug classes). (For an example of mutually adjusted odds ratios see Slap et al. (2003), Table 1 in the abridged printed version, Table 2 in the full electronic version.)

Particularly where all results shown are 'statistically significant' (SS), the reader needs to ascertain whether all factors in the model are shown and whether the final model was selected from a set of possible models. This is appropriate if either the question is 'What factors are associated with the outcome?' or a parsimonious model is required for prediction purposes and selected either by forwards or backwards stepwise elimination. However, as with a similar procedure with multiple regression, it must be understood that prediction on a further dataset will not be as good as on the one from which the prediction was derived and exclusion or inclusion of factors with P-values close to the chosen critical value may not be reproducible.

By the same token, however, when there is a stated hypothesis, the odds ratio of interest should ideally be adjusted for all factors determined *a priori* to be of potential importance. Some of these may not be associated with outcome in the data at the conventional level of statistical significant, but adjustment can still affect the odds ratio of interest. It is useful when there may be controversy over the number of potentially confounding variables to be included to give both unadjusted, fully adjusted and, perhaps also, partially adjusted odds ratios. *SC*

Chinn, S. 2001: The rise and fall of logistic regression. *Australasian Epidemiologist* 4, 7–10. **Finney, D.J.** 1964: *Statistical method in biological assay*, 2nd edn. London: Griffin. **Finney, D.J.** 1971: *Probit analysis*, 3rd edn. Cambridge: Cambridge University Press. **Hosmer, D.W., Taber, S. and Lemeshow, S.** 1991: The importance of assessing the fit of logistic regression models: a case study. *American Journal of Public Health* 81, 1630–5. **Lawlor, D.A., Patel, R. and Ebrahim, S.** 2003: Association between falls in elderly women and chronic diseases and drug use: cross-sectional study. *British Medical Journal* 327, 712–15. **Roberts, D.F., Rozner, L.M. and Swan, A.V.** 1971: Age at menarche, physique and environment in industrial north-east England. *Acta Paediatrica Scandinavica* 60, 158–64. **Roberts, D.F., Danskin, M.J. and Chinn, S.** 1975: Menarcheal age in Northumberland. *Acta Paediatrica Scandinavica* 64, 845–52. **Slap, G.B., Lot, L., Huang, B., Daniyam, C.A., Zink, T.M. and Succop, P.A.** 2003: Sexual behaviour of adolescents in Nigeria: cross-sectional survey of secondary school students. *British Medical Journal* 326, 15–18. **Somerville, S., Rona, R.J. and Chinn, S.** 1988: Passive smoking and respiratory conditions in primary school children. *Journal of Epidemiology and Community Health* 42, 105–10. **Zhang, J. and Yu, K.F.** 1998: What's the relative risk? *Journal of the American Medical Association* 280, 1690–1.

logit models for ordinal responses

A regression model is a statistical model for describing the relationship between one or more explanatory variables and the response (dependent) variable. The purpose of statistical modelling is to fit the best model from a medical and epidemiological point of view that describes this relationship. The statistical modelling of how the relationship between the explanatory variables and the response variable could be described depends on how the response variable is recorded. The *linear regression model* assumes continuous quantitative response values. When the response variable has only two possible values or is measured on a rating scale, a *logit transformation* of the response values will meet the assumption of continuity.

A simple *linear regression model* describes how much a continuous quantitative response variable (y) depends on the explanatory (x) variable by the expression $y = a + bx$, where a is a constant, the *intercept*, and b is the *regression coefficient*, which contains the important information about the dependence of y on x. According to the model y will change b units when x increases 1 unit. In a *multiple regression model* a linear combination of several explanatory variables are included. The purpose could be to investigate how the response variable depends on all explanatory variables together. Some of the variables could also be included in the model as *confounding* factors, which means that they would disturb the relationship of interest if not being adjusted for.

In case of only two responses; success/failure or diseased/non-diseased, the range of possible response values is between zero and one; for example when the probability of success is $p = 0.8$, then the probability of failure is $(1 - p) = 0.2$. As the modelling assumes unlimited possible continuous values, the explanatory variable will be linked to the response variable by a *logit transformation*. Then the *odds* of success is the ratio between the probability of success and the probability of failure; odds $= p/(1 - p)$. The logit of the proportion p is defined as the *log odds* $=$ logit(p) $= ln \dfrac{p}{1 - p}$, where ln denotes the logarithm to the base e. The regression model is called a (linear) LOGISTIC REGRESSION MODEL, logit $(p) = a + bx$, and the multiple logistic regression model is logit$(p) = a + b_1x_1 + b_2x_2 + \ldots + b_kx_k$, when k explanatory variables are included. The interpretation of the relationship between an explanatory variable x and the probability p of success is that when x increases 1 unit, then the odds will change e^b. For example logit$(p) = 3.2 + 1.3\ x$, means that the logit(p), or the *log odds*, is predicted to change 1.3 for each unit of increase in x and hence the *odds* of success will change $e^{1.3} = 3.7$.

Logistic regression is commonly used to compare the odds of success between two groups of subjects with and without some prognostic property, such as smoking habits. For illustration, consider a model for having a specific disease, $\text{logit}(p) = 3.2 + 1.3$ age + 0.4 smoking, where the prognostic variables are age (years) and smoking habits coded as (smokers = 1, non-smokers = 0). Assuming the same age in the two groups, the logit for smokers is $\text{logit}(p_s) = 3.2 + 1.3$ age + 0.4, and for non-smokers $\text{logit}(p_{non-s}) = 3.2 + 1.3$ age + 0. The difference between these logits is $\text{logit}(p_s) - \text{logit}(p_{non-s}) = 0.4$, which is a difference between the log odds of disease in smokers and non-smokers.

This difference between logarithms is the same as a ratio, in this case the log odds ratio, lnOR. Thus, lnOR = 0.4, which was the regression coefficient associated with the variable smoking, then OR = $e^{0.4}$ = 1.5. According to this example, we can predict that the odds of having the disease are related to smoking habits and are predicted to be 1.5 times larger in smokers than in non-smokers, after adjustment for age.

The logit transformation makes it possible to model how a dichotomous response variable depends on the explanatory variables. The logit transformation is also suitable for *ordered categorical (ordinal) responses*, provided dichotomisation of the response categories. Consider a four-point scale with the categories 'none', 'slight', 'moderate' and 'severe'. Assume that the numbers of observations in the categories are n_1, n_2, n_3 and n_4 respectively and the total number of observations is n. The *cumulative, continuation-ratio* and the *adjacent-categories logits* are three approaches to creating dichotomous datasets considering the ordered structure of the ordinal responses.

In the *cumulative logit*, also called *the proportional odds model*, the probability of being in the lower categories is compared with the probability of being in the higher. Empirically, the number of observations in categories representing lower levels is compared with the number of observations in the higher levels of the scale. There are $(m - 1)$ possible cut-off points between categories in a scale with m categories when creating cumulative logits. In the four-point scale there are three possible cumulative logits; when the cut-off point is the first category, 'none', the cumulative logit is $\ln \dfrac{n_1}{n_2 + n_3 + n_4}$; by moving the cut-off point one category at a time the cumulative logits will be $\ln \dfrac{n_1 + n_2}{n_3 + n_4}$ and $\ln \dfrac{n_1 + n_2 + n_3}{n_4}$. In cumulative logits, all data are used in each logit.

The first cumulative logit could be interpreted as the log odds of the response 'none', as compared with 'slight', 'moderate' and 'severe'. If the variable is pain this cut-off point seems reasonable. Absence of pain is compared with presence of pain, but the other cumulative logits could also be of interest in a logistic model.

In the *continuation-ratio approach*, the number of observations in one category is compared with the number of observations in all categories representing lower levels. In the four-point scale the continuation-ratio logits are $\ln \dfrac{n_2}{n_1}$, $\ln \dfrac{n_3}{n_1 + n_2}$ and $\ln \dfrac{n_4}{n_1 + n_2 + n_3}$.

In the *adjacent-categories logit*, adjacent categories are compared; in the four-point scale the logits are $\ln \dfrac{n_2}{n_1}$, $\ln \dfrac{n_3}{n_2}$ and $\ln \dfrac{n_4}{n_3}$ and this approach is also applicable to categorical/nominal data.

After dichotomisation the logits for ordinal data can be used in the logistic regression model for dichotomous data and with corresponding interpretation of odds ratios, when evaluating possible relationship between dichotomised ordinal responses and some prognostic variable, when controlling for other prognostic or disturbing background variables. *ES*

[See also LINEAR REGRESSION, LOG-LINEAR MODELS, MULTIPLE REGRESSION MODELS]

Agresti, A. 1984: *Analysis of ordinal categorical data*. New York: John Wiley & Sons. Altman, D.G. 2000: *Practical statistics for medical research*. Boca Raton: Chapman & Hall/CRC. Campbell, M.J. 2001: *Statistics at square two*. Bristol: BMJ Books.

log-linear models Models that serve to describe the relationships between frequencies (counts) and one or more variables that affect their size. In practice, log-linear models are most often used in connection with CONTINGENCY TABLES to describe the nature of associations between multiple nominal categorical variables. The analysis of contingency tables formed from three or more categorical variables will be the primary concern of this section, since two-way contingency tables are dealt with in the entry mentioned earlier.

When a sample from some population is classified with respect to more than two qualitative variables, the resulting data can be displayed as a multi-way contingency table. As an example, we consider the three-way contingency table resulting from classifying 1330 patients according to blood pressure, serum cholesterol and coronary heart disease (see first Table). In three-way tables 'layering' is used to accommodate the levels of the third categorical variable (heart disease).

log-linear models *Cross-classification of patients with respect to three clinical variables discussed in Ku and Kullback (1974)*

Coronary heart disease	Blood pressure	Serum cholesterol				Total
		< 200 mg/100cc	200–219	220–259	> 260	
Yes	<127 mm Hg	2	3	3	4	12
	127–146	3	2	1	3	9
	147–166	8	11	6	6	31
	>167	7	12	11	11	41
Total		20	28	21	24	93
No	<127 mm Hg	117	121	47	22	307
	127–146	85	98	43	20	246
	147–166	119	209	68	43	439
	>167	67	99	46	33	245
Total		388	527	204	118	1237
Overall total		408	555	225	142	1330

199

Several independence hypotheses might be of interest in the three-way contingency table. These correspond to different combinations of *first-order relationships* between pairs of categorical variables:

(1) *mutual independence* of the three variables, i.e. none of the pairs of variables is associated;

(2) *partial independence*, i.e. an association exists between two of the variables, both of which are independent of the third;

(3) *conditional independence*, i.e. two of the variables are independent in each level of the third, but each may be associated with the third variable;

(4) *mutual association*, i.e. each pair of variables is associated within each level of the third variable.

In addition, the three variables in a three-way contingency table may display a more complex form of association, namely, what is known as a *second-order relationship*. This means that the type and/or degree of association between two categorical variables is different in some or all levels of the remaining variable. In theory, in a k-dimensional table relationships up to $(k-1)$th order can be investigated but the interpretation of higher order relationships becomes increasingly more difficult.

For some of the hypotheses of interest in multi-way tables, the corresponding expected values under the null hypothesis can be calculated directly from appropriate marginal totals, but for other some form of iterative fitting algorithm is needed (see Everitt, 1992, for details).

The basic idea of log-linear modelling is to translate the different hypotheses of interest in a multi-way table into a sequence of statistical models so as to provide a systematic approach to the analysis of complex multidimensional tables and, in addition, to provide estimates of the magnitudes of effects of interest.

The analysis of three-dimensional tables poses entirely new conceptual problems as compared with those in two dimensions. However, the extension from tables of three dimensions to four or more while becoming more complex in analysis and interpretation poses no further new problems and here description of the analysis of higher order contingency tables will be in terms of those arising from three categorical variables.

The nomenclature used for dealing with the $r \times c$ table is easily extended to deal with a three-dimensional $r \times c \times l$ contingency table having r rows, c columns and l layers. The observed frequency in the ijkth cell is now represented by n_{ijk} for $i = 1,2,\ldots,r$, $j = 1,2,\ldots,c$, $k = 1,2,\ldots,l$. The general model is:

$$\ln(F_{ijk}) = \text{linear function of parameters}$$

where F_{ijk} are theoretical expected frequencies in a three-way table under a particular hypothesis. A *saturated model* for the F_{ijk}, that is a model that explains all the variation in the data, is given by:

$$\ln(F_{ijk}) = u + u_{1(i)} + u_{2(j)} + u_{3(k)} + u_{12(ij)} + u_{13(ik)} + u_{23(jk)} + u_{123(ijk)}$$

where u is an unknown parameter referred to as an 'overall mean effect' since all the other model terms are restricted to be deviation terms; $u_{1(i)}$ with $\sum_i u_{1(i)} = 0$ is an unknown deviation term that varies with the level of variable 1 and is called the 'main effect of variable 1'; $u_{2(j)}$ with $\sum_j u_{2(j)} = 0$ is an unknown deviation term that varies with the level of variable 2, the so-called 'main effect of variable 2'; $u_{3(k)}$ with $\sum_k u_{3(k)} = 0$ is an unknown deviation term that varies with the level of variable 3, the so-called 'main effect of variable 3'; $u_{12(ij)}$ with $\sum_i u_{12(ij)} = 0$ for all $j \in \{1,\ldots,c\}$ and $\sum_j u_{12(ij)} = 0$ for all $i \in \{1,\ldots,r\}$ is a further unknown deviation term for the ith category of variable 1 and the jth category of variable 2, the so-called 'interaction between variables 1 and 2'; $u_{13(ik)}$ with $\sum_i u_{13(ik)} = 0$ for all $k \in \{1,\ldots,l\}$ and $\sum_k u_{13(ik)} = 0$ for all $i \in \{1,\ldots,r\}$ is a further unknown deviation term for the ith category of variable 1 and the kth category of variable 3, the so-called 'interaction between variables 1 and 3'; $u_{23(jk)}$ with $\sum_j u_{23(jk)} = 0$ for all $k \in \{1,\ldots,l\}$ and $\sum_k u_{23(jk)} = 0$ for all $j \in \{1,\ldots,c\}$ is a further unknown deviation term for the jth category of variable 2 and the kth category of variable

log-linear models *Identification of an adequate log-linear model for the data in the first table*

	Model comparison			LR test		
	Model change	Simpler model	More complex model	DF	Deviance change	P-value
Step 1	Add interaction between blood pressure and cholesterol	Minimal model (4): mutual independence	Model (5): partial independence of heart disease	9	24.45	0.0036
Step 2	Add interaction between blood pressure and heart disease	Model (5): partial independence of heart disease	Model (6): conditional independence of heart disease and cholesterol	3	30.45	< 0.0001
Step 3	Add interaction between cholesterol and heart disease	Model (6): conditional independence of heart disease and cholesterol	Model (7): mutual association between blood pressure, cholesterol and heart disease	3	19.28	0.0002
Step 4	Add three-way interaction	Model (7): mutual association between blood pressure, cholesterol and heart disease	Saturated model (8): all first-order and second-order relationships	9	4.77	0.85

3, the so-called 'interaction between variables 2 and 3'; $u_{123(ijk)}$ with $\sum_i u_{123(ijk)} = 0$ for all j and k, $\sum_j u_{123(ijk)} = 0$ for all i and k and $\sum_k u_{123(ijk)} = 0$ for all i and j is yet another unknown deviation term for the ith category of variable 1 within the jth category of variable 2 and the kth category of variable 3, the so-called 'three-way interaction'.

The main effect terms in the second to fourth of these terms serve to model the single variable marginal distributions. The two-way interaction terms in the fifth to seventh model the first-order relationships. Different combinations of absence/presence of the three two-way interactions correspond to the mutual, partial, conditional independence or mutual association hypotheses. The three-way interaction term in the eighth models the two-way relationship. For example, for the data in our first Table we might compare the following sequence of models:

(1) all cell frequencies are the same:

$$\ln(F_{ijk}) = u;$$

(2) marginal totals for variable 2 (say cholesterol) and 3 (say heart disease) are equal:

$$\ln(F_{ijk}) = u + u_{1(i)};$$

(3) only marginal totals for variable 3 (heart disease) are equal:

$$\ln(F_{ijk}) = u + u_{1(i)} + u_{2(j)};$$

(4) the variables blood pressure, cholesterol and heart disease, are mutually independent:

$$\ln(F_{ijk}) = u + u_{1(i)} + u_{2(j)} + u_{3(k)};$$

(5) variables 1 (blood pressure) and 2 (cholesterol) are associated and both are independent of variable 3 (heart disease):

$$\ln(F_{ijk}) = u + u_{1(i)} + u_{2(j)} + u_{3(k)} + u_{12(ij)};$$

(6) variables 2 (cholesterol) and 3 (heart disease) are conditionally independent given the level of variable 1 (blood pressure):

$$\ln(F_{ijk}) = u + u_{1(i)} + u_{2(j)} + u_{3(k)} + u_{12(ij)} + u_{13(ik)};$$

(7) all pairs of variables are associated:

$$\ln(F_{ijk}) = u + u_{1(i)} + u_{2(j)} + u_{3(k)} + u_{12(ij)} + u_{13(ik)} + u_{23(jk)};$$

(8) saturated model for the three-way table, including the second-order relationship:

$$\ln(F_{ijk}) = u + u_{1(i)} + u_{2(j)} + u_{3(k)} + u_{12(ij)} + u_{13(ik)} + u_{23(jk)} + u_{123(ijk)}.$$

The model is analogous to a two-way ANALYSIS OF VARIANCE (ANOVA) – hence the use of the ANOVA terminology – but differs in a number of important respects: first, the data consist of counts rather than a score for each subject on some dependent variable; second, the model does not distinguish between independent and dependent variables. All categorical variables are treated alike as 'response' variables whose mutual associations are to be explored; third, whereas a linear combination of parameters is used in an ANOVA or regression model, in multi-way tables the natural model is multiplicative and hence the counts are log-transformed to obtain a model in which parameters are combined additively; lastly, whereas the errors in an ANOVA or regression model are assumed to follow a normal distribution, appropriate distributions to model cell counts are the MULTINOMIAL DISTRIBUTION (for fixed sample size) or POISSON DISTRIBUTION (for random sample size).

The purpose of modelling a three-way table is to find the unsaturated model with fewest parameters that adequately predicts the observed cell frequencies. The LIKELIHOOD RATIO test principle can be employed formally to assess the improvement in model fit of a more complex model against a simpler model. The DEVIANCE of a model is defined as minus twice the log-likelihood ratio between the model fitted and a saturated model and represents a measure of model fit. For cell counts from a contingency table the deviance or log-likelihood ratio statistic for a particular model is calculated as:

$$X^2_{LR} = 2 \sum_{i=1}^{r} \sum_{j=1}^{c} n_{ij} \times \ln(n_{ij}/E_{ij})$$

where the E_{ij} denote maximum likelihood estimates of the expected cell counts under the model. The likelihood ratio (LR) principle then states that an asymptotic test for a null hypothesis, that amounts to zero difference between two competing nested models, can be derived by comparing the difference in deviances with a CHI-SQUARE DISTRIBUTION with DEGREES OF FREEDOM equal to the number of extra parameters in the more complex model.

We carry out a series of LR tests to compare the sequence of models shown in the second Table, on page 200. Model (4), which allows the marginal totals of all three variables to vary, is a good starting point since we are interested in the relationships between the variables rather than their marginal distributions. This model is usually referred to as the *minimal model* for a table. Adding the two-way interaction terms improves the model fit significantly compared to the simpler model in the previous step. Model (7), which includes all first-order relationships but no second-order relationship, provides an adequate fit for the data since the comparison with the saturated model does not indicate any lack of fit ($p = 0.85$).

It is important to note that attention must be restricted to HIERARCHICAL MODELS. These are such that, whenever a higher order effect is included in a model, the lower order effects composed from variables in the higher effects are also included. However, in practice, this restriction is of little consequence, since most tables can be described by a series of hierarchical models.

Identified associations are best understood by constructing tables of estimated cell counts under the final model. The final model for the data in the first table states that the association between blood pressure and cholesterol is the same for patients with or without heart disease, the association between blood pressure and heart disease the same for each level of cholesterol and the association between cholesterol and heart disease the same for each level of blood pressure. We can therefore assess three two-way tables of estimated cell counts (third Table, on page 202). For each of these two-way tables the levels of the third variable have been 'averaged out' (on the log scale) to provide a picture of the two-way interaction. To understand the nature of the interactions, odds of the categories of one variable can be calculated (e.g. of coronary heart disease) and compared between the categories of the second variable.

In essence the results indicate that there is a positive association between high blood pressure and the occurrence of coronary heart disease and, similarly, a positive

log-linear models *Cell counts estimated by best log-linear model 'averaged' over level of third variable: (a) association between blood pressure and cholesterol; (b) association between heart disease and cholesterol; (c) association between heart disease and blood pressure*

(a)	Serum cholesterol			
Blood pressure	< 200 mg/100cc	200– 219	220– 259	> 260
< 127 mm Hg	20.12	20.59	11.08	7.51
127–146	14.25	15.90	9.36	6.4
147–166	27.83	47.37	20.90	17.53
> 167	22.6	33.38	21.55	19.74
Odds				
127–146 vs > 167	0.63	0.48	0.43	0.32

(b)	Serum cholesterol			
Heart disease	< 200 mg/100cc	200– 219	220– 259	> 260
Yes	4.5	5.75	4.31	4.53
No	94.29	125.13	50.15	28.46
Odds	0.048	0.046	0.086	0.159

(c)	Blood pressure			
Heart disease	< 127 mm Hg	127– 146	147– 166	> 167
Yes	2.95	2.24	7.57	10.1
No	62.82	52.09	91.77	56.09
Odds	0.047	0.043	0.082	0.18

association between high serum cholesterol level and coronary heart disease. The odds of coronary heart disease are estimated to more than triple when comparing the highest cholesterol (blood pressure) category with the lowest. The nature of the detected association between blood pressure and cholesterol is less clear. However, looking at the estimated odds of the second lowest blood pressure category to the largest it would appear that the odds of high blood pressure increase with increasing cholesterol level. When it has been decided how best to describe an interaction the relevant odds ratios and preferably confidence intervals should be reported. Associations between categorical variables can also be displayed graphically using CORRESPONDENCE ANALYSIS.

Log-linear modelling of cell counts is appropriate when a sample is classified with respect to several categorical variables and associations between their levels are of interest. In other words, all categorical variables are treated as dependent variables and none of the marginal totals is fixed by design. When one variable is viewed as the single dependent variable and the others as explanatory variables, either as a result of a study design that fixed some of the marginal totals (for example, a COHORT STUDY) or simply because a directional relationship is of interest, models such as LOGISTIC REGRESSION for binary dependent variables and *multinomial logistic regression* for dependent variables with more than two categories are warranted. (For more details, see Agresti, 1996, and LOGIT MODELS FOR ORDINAL RESPONSES.)

While log-linear modelling of cell counts is most often used to analyse associations between categorical variables

the concept extends to any count data and also allows for effects of continuous variables. The total incidence is usually not fixed by design in such applications and the modelling is more generally referred to as POISSON REGRESSION. Even more general all the modelling approaches for counts mentioned so far can be considered special cases of GENERALISED LINEAR MODELS where a *link function* (e.g. the logarithm) is used to avoid predictions outside the possible range and the data modelled by a distribution from a class of distributions (e.g. Poisson or binomial). (For more details, see McCullagh and Nelder, 1989.) *SL*

Agresti, A. 1996: *An introduction to categorical data analysis.* New York: John Wiley & Sons. **Everitt, B.S.** 1992: *The analysis of contingency tables*, 2nd edn. Boca Raton: Chapman & Hall. **Ku, H.H. and Kullback, S.** 1974: Log-linear models in contingency table analysis. *American Statistician* 28, 115–22. **McCullagh, P. and Nelder, J.** 1989: *Generalized linear models*, 2nd edn. London: Chapman & Hall.

lognormal distribution A PROBABILITY DISTRIBUTION such that the natural logarithms of observations from the distribution are normally distributed. As a result the distribution is always positively skewed (see SKEWNESS) and only produces positive observations. The distribution is usually defined by the standard parameters of the associated NORMAL DISTRIBUTION, so X is lognormally distributed with parameters μ and σ^2 if log(X) is normally distributed with parameters μ and σ^2. The density function of X is then:

$$f(x) = \frac{1}{x\sigma\sqrt{2\pi}}\exp\left(-\frac{(\log(x)-\mu)^2}{2\sigma^2}\right)$$

Although the need for an extra x in the leading denominator (compared to the density function of a normal distribution) may not be obvious, it becomes apparent that it is required when one considers the effective change of parameterisation that has taken place and its effect on the integral that defines the cumulative density function of the normal distribution. The distribution has mean $\exp(\mu + \sigma^2/2)$ and variance $\exp(2\mu + 2\sigma^2) - \exp(2\mu + \sigma^2)$.

If Y (= log(X)) has a normal distribution, this is often because Y is the result of summing many independent but similarly distributed variables. The lognormal distribution then can arise from the multiplication of many independent but similarly distributed variables. Object sizes may often be lognormally distributed if they are the result of repeated (multiplicative) erosion processes or coagulation processes. Many sources of positively skewed data, e.g. survival times (see SURVIVAL ANALYSIS), may be adequately approximated by a lognormal distribution, although this is not a sufficient criterion for assuming the lognormal distribution can model any positively skewed data. Marubini (1994), in fact, finds that breast cancer survival times can be modelled as coming from the lognormal distribution.

One particularly common use of the lognormal distribution is for modelling ratios. In particular, the CONFIDENCE INTERVALS for odds ratios and relative risks are often calculated by assuming that the ratio has come from a lognormal distribution.

It should be noted that lognormal data are often subjected to a log TRANSFORMATION and then treated as normal rather than explicitly trying to use the density function given earlier. *AGL*

Bland, M.J. and Altman, D.G. 1996: Statistics notes: transforming data. *British Medical Journal* 312, 770. **Marubini, E.** 1994: When patients with breast cancer can be considered to be cured. *British Medical Journal* 309, 554–5.

LogXact LogXact is a companion product to STATXACT featuring exact inference for binary data in the presence of covariates. An underlying LOGISTIC REGRESSION model is assumed. Both exact and asymptotic solutions are provided. LogXact additionally allows modeling of polychotomous responses (that is, outcomes with more than two categories).

LogXact handles matched case-control data under general M:N matching using conditional LIKELIHOOD inference. Asymptotic inference is based on maximising the unconditional likelihood function for unstratified data and on maximising the conditional likelihood function for stratified data. Exact inference is based on generating the conditional distributions of the sufficient statistics for the regression coefficients of interest, NUISANCE PARAMETERS being eliminated by fixing their respective sufficient statistics at the observed values.

For a detailed discussion of the theory underlying exact logistic regression, references to numerical algorithms that perform the computations and several examples involving the analysis of biomedical data by LogXact, refer to Mehta and Patel (1995). LogXact also provides exact and asymptotic inference for Poisson regression. Reviews of LogXact are given by Lemeshow (1994) and Oster (2002).

The current version, LogXact 6, uses powerful Monte Carlo procedures that enable fast exact inference for a much larger class of datasets than those for which exact inference was previously thought feasible. For example, LogXact actually provides two variations of the Monte Carlo procedure. Neither dominates the other in terms of efficiency – for a given data analysis, the choice of model and the available computing memory will determine which computational method yields a solution the fastest. Moreover, LogXact gives the user flexibility in switching from one computational method to another without having to begin the analysis from the beginning. As exact conditional logistic regression can be time consuming, the incorporation of these refinements can allow an investigator to achieve significant time savings.

LogXact runs on Microsoft Windows NT/2000/XP as a stand alone product. In addition, a special version, PROC-LogXact for SAS Users, is available as an external

procedure that can be used with SAS for Microsoft Windows. *CCo/PSe/CM/NP*

Lemeshow, S. 1994: LogXact-Turbo: logistic regression software featuring exact methods. *Epidemiology* 5, 2, 259–60. **Mehta, C.R. and Patel, N.R.** 1995: Exact logistic regression: theory and applications. *Statistics in Medicine* 14, 2143–60. **Oster, R.A.** 2002: An examination of statistical software packages for categorical data analysis using exact methods. *The American Statistician* 56, 3, 235–46.

longitudinal data Data having the distinguishing feature that the response variable of interest and a set of explanatory variables (factors and/or covariates) are measured repeatedly over time. Such data arise frequently in medical studies, particularly, for example, from CLINICAL TRIALS. The main objective in collecting such data is to characterise change in the response variable over time and to determine the covariates most associated with any change. In many clinical trials, for example, primary interest will centre on the effect of treatment group on changes in the response.

Because observations of the response variable are made on the same individual at different times, it is likely that these measurements will be correlated with each other rather than independent. This correlation must be accounted for adequately in order to draw valid and efficient inferences about how the covariates affect the response. Consequently models for longitudinal data (LINEAR MIXED-EFFECTS MODELS, GENERALISED ESTIMATING EQUATIONS) generally have two components: the first is essentially a regression model linking the average response to the covariates; the second is a model for the assumed covariance structure of the repeated measurements of the response. The estimated regression coefficients in the first part will be the parameters of most interest, with the parameters modelling the covariances being of less concern (they are essentially NUISANCE PARAMETERS). But selecting an unsuitable model for the covariance structure of the repeated response values, i.e. one that does not match the observed structure, can adversely affect inferences on those parameters in which the investigator is most interested.

Several examples of the analysis of longitudinal data from clinical trials are given in Everitt and Pickles (2000). *BSE*

[See also DROPOUTS]

Everitt, B.S. and Pickles, A. 2000: *Statistical aspects of the design and analysis of clinical trials.* London: ICP.

M

machine learning Branch of ARTIFICIAL INTELLI-GENCE (AI) concerned with developing algorithms that can learn and generalise from examples. By 'learning' one means the acquisition of domain-specific knowledge resulting in increased predictive power.

The use of learning algorithms for data analysis can generally be divided in two stages. First, a training set of data is provided to the algorithm, and used for selecting a 'hypothesis' (the learning phase). Then the selected hypothesis is validated on a set of known data to measure its predictive power (the validation phase) or used to make predictions on unseen data (the test phase).

A major problem in this setting is the risk that the selected hypothesis reflects specific features of the particular training set that are present due to chance instead of due to the underlying source generating it. This is called 'overfitting' or 'overtraining' and leads to reduced predictive power or generalisation. This risk is naturally higher with smaller training samples.

Motivated by the need to understand overfitting and generalisation, the last few years have seen significant advances in the mathematical theory of learning algorithms that have brought this field very close to certain parts of statistics, and modern machine learning methods tend to be more motivated by theoretical considerations (as is the case for SUPPORT VECTOR MACHINES and GRAPHICAL MODELS) and less by heuristics or analogies with biology (as was the case – at least originally – for NEURAL NETWORKS or genetic algorithms).

Modern machine learning is a very theoretical discipline, whose connections with AI are sometimes less obvious than its connections with multivariate statistics. Limited to the setting when the examples are all given together at the start, it is a valuable tool for data analysis (see also DATA MINING IN MEDICINE).   *NC/TDB*

Mitchell, T. 1995: *Machine learning.* Maidenhead: McGraw-Hill. **Shawe-Taylor, J. and Cristianini, N.** 2004: *Kernel methods for pattern analysis.* Cambridge: Cambridge University Press (www.kernel-methods.net). **Witten, I.H. and Frank, E.** 1999: *Data mining: practical machine learning tools and techniques with Java implementations.* San Francisco: Morgan Kaufmann.

Mallows' C_p

A criterion used for the automated selection of variables in MULTIPLE LINEAR REGRESSION (Gorman and Toman, 1966; Mallows, 1973). Subsets of differing numbers of variables p are considered, from $p = 1$ to $p = k$, where k is the maximum number of variables. At each stage the criterion determines the optimal subset and a stopping rule is then used to decide on the value of p.

Mallows' C_p criterion identifies the best subset of size p, i.e. the one that minimizes the following quantity:

$$C_p = \frac{SS_{res(p)}}{s^2} + 2\,(p-1) - n,$$

where $SS_{res(p)}$ is the residual sum of squares based on a p-variable regression, s^2 is an estimate of σ^2 (the residual variance based on the full model with all k variables) and

n is the sample size. The term $2(p-1) - n$ has the effect of penalising more complex models, the aim being to produce the simplest model that fits the data adequately. A plot of C_p versus p allows the various competitor subsets to be judged for different values of p and a formal stopping rule for p may be applied.

The rule suggested by Mallows is to stop when C_p is 'small' or close to $p - 1$. Gilmour (1996) discusses stopping rules and argues that the subset corresponding to the lowest C_p will tend to include at least one unimportant predictor variable; he proposes a modification of C_p to take account of this.

An example of the use of the criterion is given by Sutcliffe *et al.* (2001), who used multiple regression to determine cost predictors for patients with systemic lupus erythematosus. Mallows' C_p was used to determine how many variables were required in the model and the best fitting model with this number of predictors. The next four best fitting models with that number of predictors and the four best fitting models with one more than this number were also found. This provided a set of candidate models for further analysis.

There are many alternative methods for subset selection. Hocking (1976) describes the advantages and disadvantages of several of them, including 'best subsets', which is computationally very intensive but globally optimal, and the more usual forward selection or backward elimination (or combination) stepwise methods based on F-tests for individual variables (see AUTOMATIC SELECTION METHODS). The latter are very widely used because of their inclusion in software packages but they have been criticised by Hocking and many other statisticians as being potentially misleading. The Mallows' C_p criterion, while not globally optimal, is stepwise optimal and may be preferable to such methods.   *ML*

[See also ALL SUBSETS REGRESSION]

Gilmour, S.G. 1996: The interpretation of Mallows' C_p statistic. *The Statistician* 45, 49–56. **Gorman, J.W. and Toman, R.J.** 1966: Selection of variables for fitting equations to data. *Technometrics* 8, 27–51. **Hocking, R.R.** 1976: The analysis and selection of variables in linear regression. *Biometrics* 32, 1–49. **Mallows, C.L.** 1973: Some comments on C_p. *Technometrics* 15, 661–75. **Sutcliffe, N., Clarke, A.E., Taylor, R., Frost, C. and Isenberg, D.A.** 2001: Total costs and predictors of costs in patients with systemic lupus erythematosus. *Rheumatology* 40, 37–47.

Mann-Whitney rank sum test

The non-parametric version of the independent samples t-test, also known as the Wilcoxon rank sum test and the Mann-Whitney U test. Mann and Whitney, and Wilcoxon independently, derived the test, so the test statistic takes two different forms. The U statistic of Mann and Whitney is usually preferred as it has a useful interpretation. The Mann-Whitney test is applied to two independent samples, testing for a difference in shape and spread of the data between the two groups. With the addition of the assumption that the data from the two groups are similarly distributed, it also tests for a difference in medians or means between the two groups. The other assumptions are that the data are randomly selected observations and that the data must be either continuous or ordinal in nature.

To carry out the test, first rank all the data from the smallest to the largest. Assign the average rank to any ties in the data. Calculate the sum of the ranks in each of the groups. Calculate U_1 and U_2:

$$U_1 = n_1 n_2 + \frac{n_1(n_1 + 1)}{2} - R_1$$

$$U_2 = n_1 n_2 + \frac{n_2(n_2 + 1)}{2} - R_2$$

where n_1 = the number of observations in group 1; n_2 = the number of observations in group 2; R_1 = the sum of the ranks assigned to group 1; and R_2 = the sum of the ranks assigned to group 2.

Calculate $U = min\,(U_1, U_2)$. Compare U with the critical value of the Mann-Whitney U tables. The null hypothesis is rejected if the value of U is less than or equal to the critical value in the tables. The value of $U/n_1 n_2$ can be interpreted as the probability that a new observation from group 1 is less than a new observation from group 2.

As an example, data in the table show Mcm2 levels in two groups of people, 7 with and 8 without fibrosis of the liver. The groups do not have similar distributions. Note the assigned rank for the lowest Mcm2 value observed, due to the tie, is midway between 1 and 2, exemplifying the convention mentioned earlier.

Mann-Whitney rank sum test *Mcm2 levels in 2 groups of people, one with and one without fibrosis of the liver*

	With fibrosis (Group 1)	Without fibrosis (Group 2)
Mcm2 value	3 11 9 14 7 11 11	32 27 25 33 14 4 24 3
Rank	1.5 7 5 9.5 4 7 7	14 13 12 15 9.5 3 11 1.5
Sum of ranks	41	79

$$U_1 = 7 \times 8 + \frac{7 \times (7 + 1)}{2} - 41 = 44$$

$$U_2 = 7 \times 8 + \frac{8 \times (8 + 1)}{2} - 79 = 13$$

Hence, $U = min(44, 13) = 13$. From tables ($n_1 = 7$, $n_2 = 8$, $\alpha = 0.05$), the critical value is 10. As $13 > 10$, there is not sufficient evidence to reject the null hypothesis. Therefore, there is no evidence of a difference in spread or location between the two groups. There is a probability of 0.23 (= 13/56) that a new observation from group 1 will be less than a new observation from group 2.   *SLV*

Hart, A. 2001: Mann-Whitney test is not just a test of medians: differences in spread can be important. *British Medical Journal* 323, 391–3. **Pett, M.A.** 1997: *Nonparametric statistics for health-care research.* Thousand Oaks: Sage. **Swinscow, T.D.V. and Campbell, M.J.** 2002: *Statistics at square one*, 10th edn. London: BMJ Books.

Mann-Whitney *U* test Synonym for MANN-WHITNEY RANK SUM TEST.

MANOVA See ANALYSIS OF VARIANCE

Mantel-Haenszel methods A collection of statistical methods for stratified, categorical data. When analysing data from an epidemiological study, one should be aware of the danger of confounding.

For example, in a CASE-CONTROL STUDY of the association between an industrial chemical and a particular cancer, 100 cases and 100 controls are recruited. When the data are analysed, the odds ratio associated with the chemical is 0.91, suggesting no association or a possible protective effect. However, it is noticed that when the data are stratified by sex, the odds ratio in men is 1.29 and in women is 1.38, suggesting a possible harmful effect (data are shown in the table). The reason for this reversal in the odds ratio is that sex is a confounder in the association between exposure and disease. The disease is more common in women, but women are less likely to be exposed, and so exposure appears protective if one does not adjust for sex.

Mantel-Haenszel methods *Summary data from case-control study, stratified by sex*

	Men		Women		Total	
	Case	Control	Case	Control	Case	Control
Exposed	7	11	4	1	11	12
Unexposed	34	69	55	19	89	88

One method for overcoming confounding is to stratify the data, as in this case where stratification was by sex. The statistic of interest (e.g. the odds ratio) is calculated for each stratum separately. It is then often desirable to combine these stratum-specific statistics into a single overall measure, to calculate a standard error for this and also to test a null hypothesis (e.g. that the odds ratio is one). If the number of subjects in each stratum is large, this may be done using MAXIMUM LIKELIHOOD METHODS (e.g. LOGISTIC REGRESSION), by introducing an additional parameter into the model for each stratum. However, when data are sparser, i.e. when the number of subjects in a stratum may be small, maximum likelihood may give biased estimates. In this situation, it is necessary to use either conditional maximum likelihood methods or Mantel-Haenszel methods. The latter have the advantage of being very straightforward to calculate and, for this reason, are popular. Mantel-Haenszel methods do not require that the numbers of individuals in each stratum be large, only that the total number of subjects be large enough. However, if even the total number of subjects is small, it is necessary to use 'exact' methods (see EXACT METHODS FOR CATEGORICAL DATA).

Mantel-Haenszel methods are available for estimating odds ratios from case-control data, rate ratios or rate differences from cohort data and odds ratios or risk ratios from case-cohort data. They may also be useful when analysing repeated-measures designs. When the exposure and the outcome (disease) are both binary, the analysis of a case-control study with stratification is an example of the analysis of multiple 2×2 tables: one table for each stratum and, in each table, two rows for exposure and two columns for outcome. Mantel-Haenszel methods also exist for the more general situation of multiple $I \times \mathcal{J}$ tables, e.g. a case-control study with more than two possible exposure (or treatment) levels ($I > 2$) and/or more than two possible outcomes ($\mathcal{J} > 2$). Both the exposure and outcome variables can be treated as either nominal or ordinal categorical variables.

Finally, when combining several stratum-specific estimates to form a single overall estimate, it is important to consider whether this is sensible. If the odds ratio (or other measure) appears to vary greatly from one stratum to another, possibly even being much greater than one in some strata and much less than one in other strata and this variation is more than would be expected by chance, a single summary measure may not be very meaningful. In this situation it is better to report the odds ratio estimate for each stratum separately. Thus, before calculating the overall odds ratio (or other measure), it is worth testing the null hypothesis of homogeneity, i.e. that the odds ratio does not vary from one stratum to another. The Breslow-Day test is one such test. *SRS*

Clayton, D. and Hills, M. 1993: *Statistical models in epidemiology.* Oxford: Blackwell Science Publications. **Kuritz, S.J., Landis, J.R. and Koch, G.G.** 1988: A general overview of Mantel-Haenszel methods: applications and recent developments. *Annual Review of Public Health* 9, 123–60. **Rothman, K.J. and Greenland, S.** 1998: *Modern epidemiology*, 2nd edn. Philadelphia: Lippincott-Raven Publishers.

Markov chain Monte Carlo (MCMC)

BAYES' THEOREM (1) provides a means for combining data, y, in the form of the LIKELIHOOD, $p(y|\theta)$, with external evidence in the form of a prior distribution for θ, $p(\theta)$, to produce a posterior distribution, $p(\theta|y)$ (see BAYESIAN METHODS). However, in order to make inferences about either the posterior distribution itself or to obtain the posterior expectation of a function of the model parameters, θ, using (2), we have to evaluate often high-dimension integrals, which are only rarely analytically tractable. Consequently, much of Bayesian statistics over the last 30 years has been concerned with either parameterising models such that the integrals simplify or with the use of approximation methods (Bernardo and Smith, 1994). Such approximate methods fall into three broad categories: asymptotic approximations, for example Laplace approximations; numerical integration techniques, for example Gaussian quadrature; or simulation methods, for example Monte Carlo simulation (Bernardo and Smith, 1994).

$$p(\theta|y) = \frac{p(\theta)p(y|\theta)}{\int p(\theta)p(y|\theta)d\theta} \qquad (1)$$

$$E[f(\theta)|y] = \int f(\theta)p(\theta|y)d\theta \qquad (2)$$

Given a sample of values for θ from the joint posterior distribution, $p(\theta|y)$, $\{\theta^{(m)}, m=1,...,M\}$, then the posterior expectation of $f(\theta)$ can be approximated by:

$$E[f(\theta)|y] \approx \frac{1}{M}\sum_{m=1}^{M}f(\theta^{(m)}) \qquad (3)$$

While the use of (3) appears appealing, in practice, generation of samples from often high-dimensional joint posterior distributions can be difficult. However, for (3) to hold, the samples generated need not be independent, but

rather be from a Markov chain whose stationary distribution is, in fact, the posterior distribution. A Markov chain is a sequence of random variables $\{\theta^{(1)}, \theta^{(2)},...\}$ such that $\theta^{(i)}$ only depends on $\theta^{(i-1)}$ and not the rest of the random variables. Constructing such a chain then gives rise to Markov chain Monte Carlo simulation (Brooks, 1998; Casella and George, 1992).

The construction of a Markov chain with a stationary distribution that is the posterior distribution is relatively straightforward and was initially proposed by Metropolis *et al.* (1953) and later generalised by Hastings (1970) and is now referred to as the *Metropolis-Hastings algorithm*. At the ith of m iterations generate a candidate value for θ, $\theta^{\star}$, from a *proposal* distribution, $g(\theta|\theta^{(i-1)})$, and then with probability $\alpha(\theta^{(i-1)}, \theta^{\star})$ accept $\theta^{\star}$, i.e. $\theta^{(i)} = \theta^{\star}$ or reject it, i.e. $\theta^{(i)} = \theta^{(i-1)}$, where $\alpha(\theta^{(i-1)}, \theta^{\star})$ is given by (4). In practice, this is achieved by generating a value u from a uniform [0,1] distribution and if $u \leq \alpha(\theta^{(i-1)}, \theta^{\star})$ accept $\theta^{\star}$:

$$\alpha(\theta^{(i-1)}, \theta^{\star}) = \min\left[1, \frac{p(\theta^{\star}|y)g(\theta^{(i-1)}|\theta^{\star})}{p(\theta^{(i-1)}|y)g(\theta^{\star}|\theta^{(i-1)})}\right] \qquad (4)$$

Clearly if $g(.)$ is still a multivariate distribution, the generation of samples may still be difficult. In practice, most applications of the Metropolis-Hastings algorithm use a single component proposal distribution (Gilks, Richardson and Spiegelhalter, 1996).

If the Metropolis-Hastings algorithm is *irreducible* then regardless of where it starts it will sample from the entire domain of $p(\theta|y)$ within a finite number of iterations and produce samples from the stationary distribution, i.e. $p(\theta|y)$. Thus, it should not be dependent on the starting values. Clearly, one way in which to verify irreducibility is to use the algorithm a number of times with different starting values and inspect the samples obtained. Even if the algorithm is irreducible it has to be run long enough so that it will 'forget' its starting values and, in practice, this is achieved by running the algorithm for a 'burn-in' period and discarding the first n samples and basing inferences on only the last m–n samples. Of crucial importance, therefore, is the question of how large m and n should be. In practice, a combination of formal methods that have been advocated, together with knowledge of the statistical model and inspection of the samples obtained via sensitivity analyses to choices of m, n and the starting values, is the most pragmatic approach (Cowles and Carlin, 1996; Gilks, Richardson and Spiegelhalter, 1996).

Examination of the auto-correlation between the samples at various numbers of iterations apart can reveal algorithms which are *mixing* slowly, i.e. covering the whole of $p(\theta|y)$ and thus need to be run for considerable numbers of iterations. An alternative, often preferred, option is to consider the re-parameterisation of the statistical model in order to increase the rate of mixing. In linear regression models, centring of covariates, and in the case of hierarchical models, *hierarchical centring*, have been shown to have dramatic effects of the rate of mixing (Gelfand, Sahu and Carlin, 1995; Gilks, Richardson and Spiegelhalter, 1996).

A special case of the single component Metropolis-Hastings algorithm is the Gibbs sampler in which the proposal distributions are the set of full conditionals and the acceptance probability (4) is always equal to 1 (Gelfand and Smith, 1990; Geman and Geman, 1984). Thus, given a set of initial or starting values for the p parameters in a statistical model, $\{\theta_1^{(0)}, \ldots, \theta_P^{(0)}\}$, the Gibbs sampler at each iteration draws sample from each of the conditional distributions in turn. Thus:

$$\theta_1^{(1)} \leftarrow p(\theta_1 \mid \theta_2^{(0)}, \theta_3^{(0)}, \ldots, \theta_P^{(0)}, y)$$
$$\theta_2^{(1)} \leftarrow p(\theta_2 \mid \theta_1^{(1)}, \theta_3^{(0)}, \ldots, \theta_P^{(0)}, y) \qquad (5)$$
$$\vdots$$
$$\theta_P^{(1)} \leftarrow p(\theta_P \mid \theta_1^{(1)}, \theta_2^{(1)}, \ldots, \theta_{P-1}^{(1)}, y)$$

Thus, the realisations $\{\theta_1^{(1)}, \ldots, \theta_1^{(m)}\}, \ldots, \{\theta_P^{(1)}, \ldots, \theta_P^{(m)}\}$ after m iterations provide samples from the marginal posterior distributions and on which inferences can be based. Sampling from the conditional distributions in (5) can be difficult unless they are univariate, although for many hierarchical models they are, or log-concave, in which case *adaptive rejection sampling* may be used (Gilks, Richardson and Spiegelhalter, 1996). One particular appeal of the Gibbs sampler is that, in essence, it is simple to implement and while it can be programmed in a variety of computer languages and software packages, the development of user-friendly software such as BUGS AND WINBUGS has promoted its widespread use in numerous applied settings in biomedical research (Gelman and Rubin, 1996). *KRA*

Bernardo, J.M. and Smith, A.F.M. 1994: *Bayesian theory.* Chichester: John Wiley & Sons. **Brooks, S.P.** 1998: Markov chain Monte Carlo method and its applications. *Journal of the Royal Statistical Society Series D* 47, 69–100. **Casella, G. and George, E.** 1992: Explaining the Gibbs sampler. *American Statistician* 46, 167–74. **Cowles, M.K. and Carlin, B.P.** 1996: Markov Chain Monte Carlo convergence diagnostics: a comparative review. *Journal of the American Statistical Association* 91, 883–904. **Gelfand, A.E. and Smith, A.F.M.** 1990: Sampling-based approaches to calculating marginal densities. *Journal of the American Statistical Association* 85, 398–409. **Gelfand, A.E., Sahu, S.K. and Carlin, B.P.** 1995: Efficient parameterisations for normal linear mixed models. *Biometrika* 82, 479–88. **Gelman, A. and Rubin, D.B.** 1996: Markov chain Monte Carlo methods in biostatistics. *Statistical Methods in Medical Research* 5, 339–55. **Geman, S. and Geman, D.** 1984: Stochastic relaxation, Gibbs distributions and the Bayesian restoration of images. *IEEE Transactions on Pattern Analysis and Machine Intelligence* 6, 721–41. **Gilks, W.R., Richardson, S. and Spiegelhalter, D.J.** 1996: *Markov chain Monte Carlo methods in practice.* New York: Chapman & Hall. **Hastings, W.K.** 1970: Monte Carlo sampling methods using Markov chains and their applications. *Biometrika* 57, 97–109. **Metropolis, N.,** **Rosenbluth, A.W., Teller, M.N. and Tellet, A.H.** 1953: Equations of state calculations by fast computing machine. *Journal of Chemical Physics* 21, 1087–91.

matched pairs analysis

Different types of designs may lead to matched pairs analysis. Individually matched subjects in prospective studies, individually matched controls to cases in retrospective studies and pairs of data obtained when the same individual is measured twice are examples of matched pairs (see MATCHED SAMPLES). A sample of matched pairs consists of statistically dependent data and in statistical analysis the pair, not single subjects, should be the unit. Matched pairs analysis may concern concepts like change, difference, odds, but also agreement and ASSOCIATION.

Questions of change could include: Is there a difference in outcome due to different treatments between individually matched subjects? Is there a change in outcome within subjects before and after a treatment? Do patients prefer one treatment better than another? Statistical methods for matched pairs analysis of quantitative, ordered categorical and dichotomous data, respectively, will be presented.

The cholesterol level was measured in 20 students before and after a period of having a diet that was supposed to have cholesterol-lowering effect. As each student was measured twice, the difference between the two values was the outcome variable. The changes in cholesterol ranged from −1.0mmol/L (increase) to 0.8mmol/L (decrease). The Table shows three different statistical approaches to matched pairs analysis of quantitative data:

The mean approach. Provided that the dataset of differences is a sample from a NORMAL DISTRIBUTION, the paired STUDENT'S t-TEST of the null hypothesis of zero mean change can be used. The observed mean change was 0.23mmol/L and according to the test (see table) one can conclude that the diet significantly will decrease the mean cholesterol level in a representative population of about (0.04 to 0.42) mmol/L, which is the 95% CONFIDENCE INTERVAL (CI).

The median approach. The WILCOXON SIGNED RANK TEST requires no assumptions about distribution of the differences in quantitative data. The median change was 0.2mmol/L and according to the test the null hypothesis of no median change can be rejected ($P = 0.01$).

The dichotomisation approach. The cholesterol level

matched pairs analysis *Three different approaches to matched pairs analysis of change in S-cholesterol in a sample of 20 students*

Mean approach	Median approach	Dichotomisation approach
Mean change 0.23mmol/L	Median change 0.2mmol/L	Negative changes, 3 Positive changes, 16
Standard deviation 0.41mmol/L	Quartiles (Q_1;Q_3) (0.1; 0.5)mmol/L	
Student's paired t: 2.527 significance level $P = 0.02$	Wilcoxon signed rank/ matched pairs/test $P = 0.01$	The exact sign test, $P = 0.004$ The approximate sign test: $z_c = 2.75$, $P = 0.006$
The 95% CI of mean change: (0.04 to 0.42)mmol/L	The 95% CI of median change: (0.1 to 0.5)mmol/L	The 95% CI for the proportion students with decreased value: 62% to 94%.

decreased in 16, increased in three and was unchanged in one student. If the null hypothesis of unchanged values were true one would expect about the same numbers of positive as negative differences and this comparison is performed by a *sign test*. Unchanged values provide no information about the direction of change and will be excluded. The BINOMIAL DISTRIBUTION is used for exact calculation of the probability of getting the observed or even more extreme unbalance in negative and positive differences when the null hypothesis is true. The table shows that the probability of the observed or more extreme unbalance was 0.004, which is strong evidence that the diet will change the cholesterol level. The large sample approximation of the *one-sample sign test* can be written $z_c = \dfrac{|r - np| - \frac{1}{2}}{\sqrt{np(1 - p)}}$, where r is the number of differences of one sign among n non-zero differences, p is the probability under the null hypothesis of having the actual sign ($p = \frac{1}{2}$). In the example, $r = 16$, $n = 19$ and $z_c = 2.75$. The proportion of students with a decrease in cholesterol was 84% and the 95% CI (see Newcombe and Altman, 2000) deviates from that of the null hypothesis (50%) (see the table).

Matched pairs analysis of ordered categorical data is applied to a dataset from a study in diagnostic radiology (Svensson *et al.*, 2002). The patient's perceived difficulty during each of two radiological examinations, here denoted CT and CO, was rated on a scale with the categories 'not at all', 'slightly', 'fairly' and 'very' difficult. Each of the 108 patients underwent both examinations, which means paired data (see the figure).

Data from scale assessments have an ordered structure only, which means that change is not defined by the difference. Therefore, the same statistical methods as for paired dichotomous data will be used. A common expression for *the sign test* is $z_c = \dfrac{|b - c| - 1}{\sqrt{b + c}}$, where b and c denote the number of pairs with different categories. A MCNEMAR'S TEST is an equivalent test. One approach to dichotomise the data is to compare the numbers of pairs below and above the diagonal of unchanged categories. For the data in the Figure, the 17 patients, which rated the CT a higher level of difficulty than the CO are compared

with the 45 pairs above the diagonal. According to the sign test ($z_c = 3.43$, $P = 0.0006$), this observed unbalance in changes gives evidence enough to conclude that the CT is perceived as significantly less difficult than the CO examination.

An alternative way of dichotomising is by grouping the data in two categories; 'not at all difficult' (+), and 'difficult' (−), which contains three categories of difficulty. The table is simplified in two concordant and two discordant combinations of categories. The discordant pairs of 32 CT(+), CO(−) and 13 CT(−), CO(+) contain information about the difference in perceived difficulty between the examinations. The sign test ($z_c = 2.68$, $P = 0.007$) confirms that more patients will find the CT examination as 'not at all difficult' when compared with their rating of the CO examination.

As is evident from the figure, a larger proportion of the patients (17%) judged the CT as being 'not at all difficult', as 48 patients (44%) rated the CT and 29 (27%) rated the CO 'not at all difficult'. The 95% CI for the difference in the paired proportions, Δp, was from 5% to 29% according to the expression $\Delta p \pm 1.96 \times \mathrm{SE}(\Delta p)$. The standard error is $SE(\Delta p) = \dfrac{1}{n}\sqrt{b + c - \dfrac{(b - c)^2}{n}}$, n is the total number of patients ($n = 108$), b and c are the numbers of discordant pairs.

In order to use a pair-matched CASE-CONTROL STUDY method we are interested in the exposure to the risk factor. Using retrospective case-control studies, individuals having a specific disease (e.g. lung cancer) are compared with individuals without the disease. Both the outcome variable (diseased, non-diseased) and the exposure to the risk factor (exposed, not exposed) are dichotomous. Within each pair, there are four possible combinations of disease status and exposure. Two sets of pairs are concordant, but information about the relationship between exposure and disease is given by the pairs with different exposure. Denote the number of pairs with only the case exposed n_{+-} and the number of pairs with the case unexposed n_{-+}. Providing non-zero numbers of discordant pairs, the odds ratio in matched pairs is calculated by $OR = \dfrac{n_{+-}}{n_{-+}}$. An OR larger than unity indicates a relationship between exposure and disease, that is a higher odds of developing disease when exposed. *ES*

[See also CORRELATION, KAPPA AND WEIGHTED KAPPA MATCHING, MATCHED SAMPLES]

Altman, D.G. 2000: *Practical statistics for medical research.* Boca Raton: Chapman & Hall/CRC. **Bland, M.** 1996: *An introduction to medical statistics*, 2nd edn. Oxford: Oxford Medical Press. **McNeil, D.** 1999: *Epidemiological research methods.* New York: John Wiley & Sons. **Newcombe, R.G. and Altman, D.G.** 2000: Proportions and their differences. In Altman, D.G., Machin, D., Bryant, T.N. and Gardner, M.J., *Statistics with confidence*, 2nd edn. Bristol: BMJ Books, 45–57. **Svensson, M.H., Svensson, E., Lasson, A. and Hellström, M.** 2002: Patient acceptance of CT colonography and conventional colonoscopy: prospective comparative study in patients with or suspected of having colorectal disease. *Radiology* 222, 337–45.

matched samples A set of observations in which each observation in one sample is individually matched with one in every other sample. Paired samples consist of individually pair-matched observations. The individually

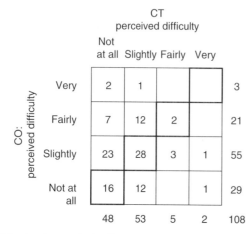

CT
perceived difficulty

	Not at all	Slightly	Fairly	Very	
Very	2	1			3
Fairly	7	12	2		21
Slightly	23	28	3	1	55
Not at all	16	12		1	29
	48	53	5	2	108

CO: perceived difficulty

matched pairs analysis *Frequency distribution of paired data from evaluation concerning perceived difficulty concerning two radiological examinations (CT, CO)* matched observations are *statistically dependent* and should be regarded as one unit in statistical analysis, which means that the matched samples might be regarded as one group of dependent data. Hence, matched samples have an equal number of observations.

Different types of study, such as CROSS-SECTIONAL, CASE-CONTROL and *reliability* STUDIES, can be designed as matched samples. Self-pairing studies lead to matched samples, for example CROSS-OVER TRIALS, *test-retest*, intra-observer studies and studies on paired organs. The purpose of matching is to create homogeneous pairs of observations with regard to important background properties, so the remaining difference between the observations within a pair could be ascribed the source of interest (effect of treatment, exposure, time etc). The choice and the number of matching variables should be carefully considered, as the matching variables cannot be used in the statistical evaluation of possible relationship or explanation regarding the main variable.

Cross-over design is ideal in randomised CLINICAL TRIALS for evaluation of the difference in effect between two treatments; one of the treatments could be a placebo treatment. The variability between individuals in the sample is eliminated as each individual is its own control (*self-pairing*). Cross-over studies are also called *change-over, within-subject* and *AB/BA cross-over studies*. Each individual will get the two treatments, A and B, in random order with a wash-out period in between in order to prevent the effect of the first treatment to interact with the second (carry-over effect) (see the Figure). The important assumption is that the patients will be in the same state when they receive each treatment. Therefore, this design is suitable for chronic states only. An alternative way of creating homogeneous pairs is by using individually matched pairs.

The aim of using matched pairs in cross-sectional studies is to evaluate the difference in effect between two or more treatments. Matching pairs is a preferable alternative method when the self-pairing cross-over design is not appropriate to perform. The matched paired sample consists of individually matched pairs of subjects regarding some prognostic variables where each member of a pair is randomly given one of the treatments (see Figure). The

comparison of the effects between the two treatments is made within each pair and could be defined as the difference in effect between the two treatments (additive effect) or as the ratio of the two treatment effects (multiplicative effect). Hence, each pair is treated as one unit in the statistical analysis.

Matched case-control studies. One aim of epidemiological studies is statistically to evaluate associations between risk factors and disease outcomes among individuals. Patients with a disease (cases) are compared with subjects without the disease (control) and the question of interest is their past experience of exposure to possible risk factors. Matched case-control studies consist of an individually matched control to each case. In the case of rare events, each case may be individually matched with more than one control. The first table shows the four different combinations of outcome and exposure in a matched pair case-control study, when the total number of pairs is n.

The distribution of data from unmatched case-control studies is also commonly presented in a 2×2 table. However, unmatched case-control data should be treated as two independent groups of data (one group of cases and one group of controls), which means that the number of observations equals the total numbers of cases and controls. The second Table shows the frequency distribution of exposed and unexposed cases and controls respectively, when the matched pairs data of the first table are treated as unmatched.

Matched samples of ordered categorical data. Studies that involve *rating scales*, questionnaires and other types of categorical classifications often produce matched or paired

matched samples *Four different combinations of outcome and exposure in a matched case-control study*

| | | Case | |
		Exposed	Unexposed
Control	*Exposed*	n_{++}	n_{-+}
	Unexposed	n_{+-}	n_{--}

n

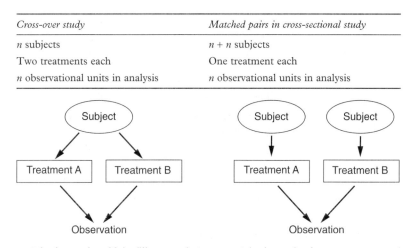

Cross-over study	Matched pairs in cross-sectional study
n subjects	$n + n$ subjects
Two treatments each	One treatment each
n observational units in analysis	n observational units in analysis

matched samples *Main differences between matched samples from cross-over and matched pairs design*

matched samples *2 × 2 frequency table of an unmatched case-control study, showing frequency distribution of the matched case-control data of the first table when treated as unmatched*

	Case	Control
Exposed	$n_{++} + n_{+-}$	$n_{++} + n_{-+}$
Unexposed	$n_{-+} + n_{--}$	$n_{+-} + n_{--}$
Total	n	n

samples of observations. *Quality* assessments of rating scales concern matched samples of ordered categorical data. In inter-observer *reliability studies* the agreement between observers in their classifications of the same subjects is evaluated. The pairs of classifications of each subject are dependent. Agreement studies could also concern an inter-scale comparison, which is comparison between different scales for the same variable. Comparisons between self-rated ability and an expert-rated ability of the patient or between a child's opinion and the parents' judgement of it are also examples of the large variations of paired samples involving ordered categorical data. Matched samples are a natural consequence when multi-item instruments for qualitative variables, such as pain and quality of life are used.

To sum up: a large number of different types of study create matched samples. The important feature they all have in common is that matched/paired samples of observations are dependent, a fact that should be taken into account in the statistical analysis. *ES*

[See also KAPPA AND WEIGHTED KAPPA, MATCHED PAIRS ANALYSIS, MATCHING]

Altman, D.G. 2000: *Practical statistics for medical research.* Boca Raton: Chapman & Hall/CRC. **McNeil, D.** 1999: *Epidemiological research methods.* New York: John Wiley & Sons. **Senn, S.** 2000: *Cross-over trials in clinical research.* Chichester: John Wiley & Sons. **Svensson, E.** 2001: Construction of a single global scale for multi-item assessments of the same variable. *Statistics in Medicine* 20, 3831–46.

matching A study design technique of creating pairs of subjects that are homogeneous with respect to important background variables, which are not interesting for the actual study but could interfere with the variable of interest. Matching normally means that each subject is individually paired with another. In prospective clinical studies where the effects of two treatments are to be compared and the two treatments cannot be given to the same individual, matching means that two subjects with the same background properties (e.g. age, gender and some prognostic variables) are paired, one of whom is randomly given the treatment of interest and the other the placebo or standard treatment. The main aim of the matching is to make the two treatment groups comparable by reducing the variability and possible systematic differences that could occur due to disturbing background variables (*confounding bias*). This means that the remaining difference of interest between the two members of a pair would be due to the different treatments.

In *retrospective* CASE-CONTROL STUDIES, matching means that each case is individually paired with a control subject with respect to the background variables and their exposure to the risk factor of interest is compared. Matching

twins or siblings provides genetically similar individuals, which can be important in both clinical and epidemiological studies. Individually matched pairs can be regarded as 'artificial twins'.

A continuous matching variable, such as age, can be transformed into categories before pairing individuals, but the matching criterion for one subject to be matched with another can also be expressed in terms of a specified tolerance interval (*caliper matching*).

The two individuals in a matched pair should be regarded as one unit and the data should be treated as dependent (paired) in the statistical analysis. *ES*

[See also MATCHED PAIRS ANALYSIS, MATCHED SAMPLES]

Altman, D.G. 2000: *Practical statistics for medical research.* Boca Raton: Chapman & Hall/CRC. **McNeil, D.** 1999: *Epidemiological research methods.* New York: John Wiley & Sons.

maximum likelihood estimation This refers to a general method of estimation for unknown parameters in a probabilistic/statistical model for observed data, for instance a linear regression model. A well-chosen parameterisation of a discrete probability or continuous density ensures that different parameter values determine different chances (densities) of observing a given dataset. The parameter value that maximises this chance (density) for an observed dataset is deemed most likely and known as the maximum likelihood estimate (MLE).

The MLE is often derived in closed form by maximising the logarithm of the likelihood of the data in function of the unknown model parameters. The first Figure depicts this log likelihood function for mean body weight based on a random sample of 250 American men (Penrose, Nelson and Fisher, 1985) with weights that are normally distributed with known standard deviation equal to 12.3 kg. The solid vertical line indicates the MLE at 81.2 kg. With two parameters, the graph of the loglikelihood becomes a surface. In the second Figure (see page 211), we show contour lines of this surface for the intercept and slope in a linear model for the regression of body weight (in kg) on height (in cm). We assume that weights corresponding to fixed height measurements are normally distributed with known standard deviation equal to 10.5 kg. The fitted regression curve is displayed in the entry on LEAST SQUARES ESTIMATION (and seen in the Figure there).

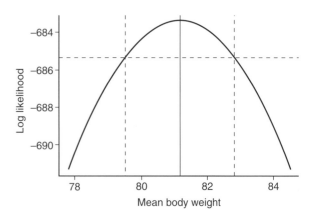

maximum likelihood estimation *Log likelihood function for mean body weight estimation based on a random sample of 250 American men*

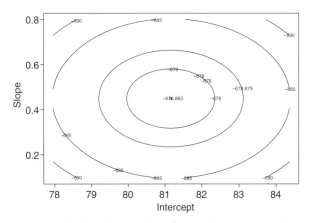

maximum likelihood estimation *Contour lines of the surface for the intercept and slope estimation in a linear model for the regression of body weight (in kg) on height (in cm)*

To maximise the loglikelihood in practice, one can set its derivative with respect to the target parameter, i.e. the score function, equal to zero and solve this for the unknown parameter. Alternatively, computational algorithms can search numerically for the maximum of the loglikelihood function or for a zero of the score function.

Maximum likelihood estimation plays a central role in statistics. It is the standard method of estimation, for instance, in linear, log-linear and LOGISTIC REGRESSION. This is due to its strong intuitive appeal and nice statistical properties in large samples. Under quite general conditions, the MLE becomes normally distributed around the true parameter value as the sample size increases. Hence, 95% CONFIDENCE INTERVALS are obtained as the MLE plus or minus 1.96 times its STANDARD ERROR. For a p-dimensional parameter estimate beta with covariance V, the Wald confidence region is the ellipsoid consisting of $beta_0$-values whose distance from the estimator beta, i.e. $(beta-beta_0)^T V^{-1}$ $(beta-beta_0)$, stays within the 95% percentile of the CHI-SQUARE DISTRIBUTION with p DEGREES OF FREEDOM.

More accurate p-dimensional 95% confidence regions are usually obtained as the set of values that are so likely that twice the loglikelihood is no further removed from the maximum achievable than the 95% percentile of the chi-square distribution with p degrees of freedom. In the first Figure we depict this maximum deviation by the dashed horizontal line. The dashed vertical lines mark the 95% confidence interval (79.5–82.8) kg for mean body weight in American men. In the second Figure, such 95% confidence region for the intercept and slope contains all values enclosed by the contour at −679.879.

A flat loglikelihood in the neighbourhood of the MLE makes it hard to pinpoint the MLE and reveals limited information. Hence, a useful summary of the information about the target parameter is the curvature at the estimated value: minus the second derivative of the loglikelihood function with respect to the unknown parameter, evaluated at the MLE. This is called the 'observed information'. Its expected value under the assumed model is known as the Fisher information. Its inverse approximates the variance of the MLE. The inverse of the observed information is often thought to yield the better variance estimate as it sits closer to the data.

The MLE is efficient when the assumed model holds and

the sample size is large. This means that among all estimators expected to equal the true parameter value in large samples, no estimator will have smaller variance. The bad news is that the MLE relies on the correct specification of the probability model and may be biased otherwise. The MLE is usually also sensitive to outlying observations. To address these problems, alternative estimation techniques have been devised, such as least squares estimation, L1-regression or the generalised method of moments. These avoid specifying the entire sampling distribution of the observed data and trade robustness against outlying observations for efficiency. *SV/EG*

Clayton, D. and Hills, M. 1993: *Statistical models in epidemiology*. Oxford: Oxford University Press. **Cox, D.R. and Hinkley, D.V.** 1979: *Theoretical statistics*. Boca Raton: CRC Press. **Jewell, N.P.** 2004: *Statistics for epidemiology*. Boca Raton: CRC Press. **Penrose, K.W., Nelson, A.G. and Fisher, A.G.** 1985: Generalized body composition prediction for men using simple measurement techniques. *Medicine and science in sports and medicine* 17, 189.

McNemar's test An approximation to the exact binomial test (see BINOMIAL DISTRIBUTION) used in situations where there are two paired outcomes of a binary nature (e.g. yes/no, dead/alive, infected/not infected). The test looks to see if the proportions of the response levels are the same in the two groups being considered.

This might occur when we have measurements taken on the same individuals at two different time points (i.e. the status of a recurrent condition), when two treatments are being tested on the same individuals (e.g. in CROSS-OVER TRIALS), when paired individuals are entering a trial, when two tests are being performed on individuals (e.g. whether the individual has high blood pressure or is overweight) or when comparing the SENSITIVITY/SPECIFICITY of two classification methods. It should be clear that this is not an exclusive list.

Assuming that we have a set of paired yes/no outcomes, McNemar's test looks to answer the question as to whether the proportion of 'no's is different across the two groups/treatments/times. It does so by considering the discordant pairs, i.e. those pairs that return a yes and a no (as opposed to two 'no's or two 'yes's). If the proportion of 'no's is the same between two treatments, then for every 'yes–no', we would expect to see a 'no–yes'. Otherwise, there would be an imbalance in the number of 'no's between the two treatments and thus evidence that the proportions are not the same.

If we were to have 12 discordant pairs, 6 'yes–no's and 6 'no–yes's would be expected if the proportions were the same between the two groups. Deviation from this even split would be evidence of a difference in proportions and McNemar's test uses a normal approximation to evaluate the statistical significance of that evidence.

For example, Nicholson *et al.* (1998) perform a cross-over trial to see if a vaccine for influenza can trigger asthma exacerbations. Individuals receive both the vaccine and a placebo (in random order) and are observed to see in each case whether an exacerbation occurs. Of 256 people in the trial, 242 had the same reaction after both treatments and so provide no direct information about the difference between the treatments. Eleven have an exacerbation after the vaccine but not after the placebo and 3 after the placebo but not after the vaccine.

Under an assumption that there is no difference in proportions, we would expect these 14 discordant pairs to have a 7–7 split rather than the 11–3 split observed. However, the McNemar test is non-significant with a reported P-VALUE of 0.06.

The data for McNemar's test are typically displayed in a CONTINGENCY TABLE, as below. There are various forms of the test statistic. Essentially, one is looking to compare $(b - c)/\sqrt{(b + c)}$ to the normal standard distribution (mean zero and variance one) or, equivalently, $(b - c)^2/(b + c)$ to the CHI-SQUARE DISTRIBUTION with one DEGREE OF FREEDOM (d.f.). These statistics are usually modified to incorporate a continuity correction, the most commonly used of which is to subtract one from the absolute value of the numerator or the positive square root of the numerator, respectively.

McNemar's test *Tabulated paired binary outcome data*

| | | Response from treatment 1 | |
		No	Yes
Response from	No	242 (a)	11 (b)
treatment 2	Yes	3 (c)	0 (d)

For the example of Nicholson *et al.* (1998), the statistic is $(|11 - 3| - 1)^2/(11 + 3) = 3.5$, which when compared to the chi-squared statistic with d.f. 1, gives a P-value of 0.06 as previously stated. (Note that in order to have attained statistical significance at the usual 0.05 level, the statistic would have to exceed the value 3.84.)

As is common when data are well paired, it is the case here that the number of discordant pairs is small. This means that the normal approximation may not perform well. If one's only resource is a table of the normal distribution, then McNemar's test is clearly convenient, but today it is unlikely that researchers will not have the capability to perform the exact binomial test. Much literature is devoted to the problem of powering such trials and it is true that it is a simpler task to power for McNemar's test, but again, with modern computing resources, powering the exact binomial test is practicable. It is, therefore, difficult to advocate the use of this test.

McNemar's test is used for the study of paired dichotomous outcomes. For other types of paired data, other methods are available (see STUDENT'S t-TEST or WILCOXON RANK SUM TEST, for example). If the data are matched triples rather than pairs, or in even greater numbers, then the COCHRAN Q-TEST is applicable. *AGL*

McNemar, Q. 1947: Note on the sampling error of the differences between correlated proportions or percentages. *Psychometrika* 12, 153–7. **Nicholson, K.G., Nguyen-Van-Tam, J.S., Ahmed, A.H., Wiselka, M.J., Leese, J., Ayres, J., Campbell, J.H., Ebden, P., Eiser, N.M., Hutchcroft, B.J., Pearson, J.C.G., Willey, R.F., Wolstenholme, R.J. and Woodhead, M.A.** 1998: Randomised placebo-controlled crossover trial on effect of inactivated influenza vaccine on pulmonary function in asthma. *The Lancet* 351, 326–31. **Zar, J.H.** 1999: *Biostatistical analysis*, 4th edn. Englewood Cliffs, NJ: Prentice Hall.

mean A MEASURE OF LOCATION giving a typical value of a set of observations and what is usually meant when the 'average' is referred to, although other DESCRIPTIVE STATISTICS can also be used as averages.

Technically, the term 'mean' is shorthand for the 'arithmetic mean', to differentiate it from the GEOMETRIC MEAN. It is calculated by dividing the sum of all observations by the *number* of observations. For example, the ages in years of 7 students in an undergraduate seminar are recorded as 18, 19, 19, 19, 20, 20 and 21. The mean age of the students is:

$$\frac{18 + 19 + 19 + 19 + 20 + 20 + 21}{7} = 19.4 \text{ years}$$

The mean is a suitable measure of location to use when the variable being summarised has an approximately symmetrical distribution. However, if SKEWNESS or OUTLIERS are present then the use of the mean is inappropriate, since it is unduly affected by a small number of values. For example, if a mature student aged 51 joins the undergraduate seminar just described then the mean age of the students becomes:

$$\frac{18 + 19 + 19 + 19 + 20 + 20 + 21 + 51}{8} = 23.4 \text{ years}$$

Here, a mean of 23.4 is not a suitable summary of the typical age of the students since it is strongly influenced by the age of the mature student. In such cases, measures of location such as the MEDIAN or geometric mean may be more appropriate. Again, the median may be preferred when summarising discrete data, such as family size, for no one has, say, 2.4 children!

The mean is usually denoted $\bar{x}$ or μ, although the latter technically refers to the mean of a population, rather than a sample (see SAMPLING DISTRIBUTION).

Altman (1991) suggests that a mean should not normally be quoted to more than one decimal place more than the raw data. The STANDARD DEVIATION is typically used as a MEASURE OF SPREAD around the mean.   *SRC*

Altman, D.G. 1991: *Practical statistics for medical research*. London: Chapman & Hall.

measurement error A collective term for many different phenomena that arise when a measurement of a particular variable is made, but the measured value fails to match the true value for the subject. When someone's blood pressure is measured, for instance, the equipment for measuring it might be less than perfect or the observer may not be using it correctly. A sufficient indication of measurement error occurs when a repeat reading returns a different value from that obtained on the first occasion, even when the subject's *true* blood pressure has not changed.

The effect of measurement error is wide ranging and is relevant both for research studies and for clinical practice on individual patients. Measurement error might be systematic or random. Systematic error is where the measurement has a consistent tendency to overestimate (or consistently underestimate) the true value. A clock that is always five minutes fast would be an example of systematic overestimation of time of day. Systematic error may be identified by comparing measured values with known true values. In principle, it could then be removed by recalibrating the measuring instrument. This approach may be feasible if true values could be obtained from an alternative measuring instrument ('gold standard'). In practice, however, gold standards do not often exist and studying the agreement between two measuring instruments is the most realistic approach to quantifying systematic measurement error. The mean difference is a measure of systematic variation between the measuring instruments.

Random error is by its nature less predictable. In this scenario, the measured value neither consistently overestimates nor underestimates the true value, but may depart from the true value in an unpredictable manner. When two or more readings are taken on each of a number of individuals, random measurement error may be quantified in terms of a within subject STANDARD DEVIATION (SD). This SD has the advantage of being expressed in the same units as the variable of interest, making it readily interpretable for clinicians with an intuitive grasp of the clinical meaning of the units; it is an absolute measure of measurement error. Its practical usefulness may be less, however, for a score derived from a subject's response to a questionnaire, since the score may not be used in routine clinical care. Few clinicians would hold an intuitive grasp of the meaning of values for such a score. One alternative approach, then, is to measure the amount of measurement error relative to the variability of subjects' true values, for example by use of the intraclass correlation coefficient (see INTRACLUSTER CORRELATION COEFFICIENT). This equals the ratio of between-subject variance to the sum of between- and within-subject variances.

Measurement error, of course, also occurs with categorical variables; the relative lack of agreement is popularly quantified using the kappa statistic (see KAPPA AND WEIGHTED KAPPA). Absolute measures of agreement for categorical variables are less well established. If quantifying systematic error in measurement of a categorical variable representing presence or absence of a condition, SENSITIVITY and SPECIFICITY are required. Again, they depend on a gold standard measure for presence or absence of the condition.

In clinical medicine, knowledge of the likely size of measurement error for a particular variable will help interpretation of a single reading. An observer may know with 95% confidence that the observed value for the subject is within two standard deviations of that subject's true value. Apparent changes in readings from one occasion to another may occur; if they are larger than twice the standard deviation of differences, they are likely to be true changes. Smaller apparent changes could be attributable to measurement error alone. It may, therefore, be more useful to carry out studies that assess intra-observer variation (within the observer) and inter-observer variation (between observers) for this reason.

Many studies of measurement error will encounter both systematic and random error. Comparing two methods of measurement of the same variable may demonstrate a consistent tendency for method A to measure higher values than method B. If d represents the value given by method A minus that given by method B for a given subject, then $\bar{d}$ (the mean of d for all the subjects studied) can be calculated. If $\bar{d}$ is non-zero, systematic differences between methods A and B are suggested. However, the SD of d is also unlikely to equal zero; in other words, method A will not return exactly the same number of units higher than method B on every subject. This suggests that random differences, as well as systematic differences, exist between methods A and B. Bland and Altman (1986) have, therefore, recommended the calculation of approximate 95% limits of agreement, which are to be represented by $\bar{d} \pm 2\times$ SD (d).

Knowledge of size of measurement error is also required for interpretation of relationships between two or more variables, within research studies. Much of epidemiological research involves understanding the relationship between an 'exposure variable' and an outcome. Inappropriate use of a single measure of exposure may lead to REGRESSION DILUTION BIAS if the exposure is not measured precisely. In other words, the estimate of the effect of exposure will be too conservative. However, if the size of the measurement error can be quantified, the true magnitude of relationship between the exposure and outcome can be properly estimated.

If the outcome variable in epidemiological or clinical studies is measured imprecisely, the estimate of the effect of exposure would not necessarily be biased, but the standard errors of estimates of exposure effects would be inflated. Thus CONFIDENCE INTERVALS would be too wide and P-VALUES too conservative.

Still further issues arise in epidemiological studies where a potential confounding variable is measured with error and included in an analysis of the relationship between an exposure and an outcome of interest. It is possible that the measurement error in the confounding variable fails to adjust for its effect properly, a phenomenon known as 'residual confounding'. *RM/JE*

[See also ATTENUATION TO MEASUREMENT ERROR, MEASUREMENT PRECISION AND RELIABILITY]

Bland, J.M. and Altman, D.G. 1986: Statistical methods for assessing agreement between two methods of clinical measurement. *The Lancet* 1, 8476, 307–10. **Clarke, R., Shipley, M., Lewington, S., Youngman, L., Collins, R., Marmot, M. et al.** 1999: Underestimation of risk associations due to regression dilution in long-term follow-up of prospective studies. *American Journal of Epidemiology* 150, 4, 341–53. **Phillips, A.N. and Smith, G.D.** 1991: How independent are 'independent' effects? Relative risk estimation when correlated exposures are measured imprecisely. *Journal of Clinical Epidemiology* 44, 11, 1223–31.

measurement precision and reliability If we repeatedly measure the concentration of glucose in a given blood sample, for example, or measure a patient's blood pressure on each of several successive days, then we are likely to obtain a set of measurements that are similar but not identical. The greater the similarity of the series of measurements then the more precise is the measurement procedure or method producing them. If we measure the variability of the replicated measurements by their variance (or STANDARD DEVIATION) then we can define the method's precision as the reciprocal of that variance (or standard deviation).

In the context of laboratory assays, say, if we hold the measurement conditions (laboratory, batch of reagents, equipment, equipment operator, temperature etc.) as constant as possible then the measurements are being made under what are usually known as *repeatability conditions* (International Standards Institute, 1994a, 1994b). The precision of the measurements is then assessed from an estimate of the repeatability variance or repeatability standard deviation. The latter is often known for short as the *repeatability of the process*. The repeatability standard deviation is analogous to the psychometricians' standard error of measurement (Dunn, 2004). If the repeated measurements are taken in different laboratories, at different times, with different equipment, reagents and equipment operators then the resulting variability of the measurements provides an assessment of reproducibility or generalisability of the measurement process (International Standards Institute, 1994a, 1994b). This is provided by an estimate of the reproducibility variance or reproducibility standard deviation (reproducibility, for short).

One key characteristic of a measuring instrument's or method's precision (the reciprocal of the repeatability variance or reproducibility variance, for example) is that it is scale dependent. If we measure weight in kilograms we will get a precision that is 1000 times as great as the precision if it were measured in grams (the standard deviation for measures using the former scale being one-thousandth of that for those using the latter). It is essential, therefore, that if we are interested in the relative precision of alternative methods of measurement then the scale of measurement is taken into account. Often the scale of measurement of one method relative to another is not defined *a priori* but needs to be established by experiment (see METHOD COMPARISON STUDIES).

Quite often investigators are interested in the precision of their instrument or method compared to the variability of the characteristic in the population under clinical or scientific investigation. We postulate the following simple model for the observed measurement (X_i) on the ith individual within a population:

$$X_i = \tau_i + \varepsilon_i \qquad (1)$$

Here τ_i is the ith individual's true value for the characteristic and ε_i is a random measurement error. We might be interested in a measure of precision relative to the variability of τ_i, i.e. the ratio $\sigma_\tau^2/\sigma_\varepsilon^2$ where the numerator is the variance of the true values and denominator the variance of the measurement errors. A more familiar index of relative precision is given by the reliability ratio or reliability coefficient defined by:

$$\kappa_X = \sigma_\tau^2 / (\sigma_\tau^2 + \sigma_\varepsilon^2) \qquad (2)$$

If the measurement errors are uncorrelated with each other and with the true values then:

$$\sigma_X^2 = \sigma_\tau^2 + \sigma_\varepsilon^2 \qquad (3)$$

The reliability ratio (or reliability, for short) is the proportion of the variation in the observed measurements that is explained by the variability in the underlying true values. It provides a measure of the attenuation that might be expected in the calculation of correlation between error-prone measurements or the attenuation in a regression coefficient when the independent variable is subject to measurement error (see ATTENUATION DUE TO MEASUREMENT ERROR). Note that reliability is not a fixed characteristic of a method or process (even if σ_ε^2 is assumed to be constant). The reliability ratio is a measure of how well the measurements distinguish between members of the relevant population and as the heterogeneity of the population goes up (i.e. as σ_τ^2 increases) so does κ_X. As the homogeneity of the population increases (as σ_τ^2 decreases towards 0) the reliability tends towards zero. With a fixed σ_ε^2 it is quite straightforward to calculate the change in reliability as one arbitrarily changes the value of σ_τ^2. (A readable introduction to reliability theory can be found in Carmines and Zeller, 1979.)

Supposing that the variance of the measurement errors (σ_ε^2) is not independent of the characteristic (i.e. τ) being measured? It is, in fact, quite common to observe that the variance of the errors increases with the value of τ (i.e. the precision goes down with increasing τ). In this situation, we need to be able to design a relatively sophisticated precision study (often an inter-laboratory precision study) to provide data that can be used to model the relationship between the two. (This is beyond the scope of this entry, but see Dunn, 2004, for a detailed examination of the topic.)

Reliability ratios are usually estimated from data involving repeated measurements on each of an appropriate sample of subjects. The analysis usually involves the estimation of the relevant variance components (either using the traditional one-way analysis of variance or RANDOM EFFECTS MODEL) and then using these to calculate the required reliability. The reliability as defined by (2) is equivalent to the correlation between repeated measurements and this can be estimated by calculating an intraclass correlation coefficient (usually via a one-way analysis of variance). Generalisations of reliability (and various versions of intraclass correlation (see INTRACLUSTER CORRELATION COEFFICIENT)) can be found in Dunn (2004). In the case of binary measurements the intraclass correlation (intraclass kappa) is equivalent to one of the chance-corrected agreement coefficients – Scott's π-statistic (Kraemer, 1979). *GD*

Carmines, E.G. and Zeller, R.A. 1979: *Reliability and validity assessment.* Thousand Oaks: Sage. **Dunn, G.** 2004: *Statistical evaluation of measurement errors.* London: Arnold. **International Standards Institute** 1994a: *International standard ISO 5725-1. Accuracy (trueness and precision) of measurement methods and results. Part 1: General principles and definitions.* **International Standards Institute** 1994b: *International standard ISO 5725-2. Accuracy (trueness and precision) of measurement methods and results. Part 2: Basic method for the determination of the repeatability and reproducibility of a standard measurement method.* **Kraemer, H.C.** 1979: Ramifications of a population model for κ as a coefficient of reliability. *Psychometrika* 44, 461–71.

measures of central tendency   See MEASURES OF LOCATION

measures of dispersion   See MEASURES OF SPREAD

measures of fertility   See DEMOGRAPHY

measures of location   Also known collectively as 'averages', these are single-figure summaries intended to describe the typical or representative level of a set of observations. There are four measures of location commonly encountered.

As part of a study of childhood development, the IQ of 210 mothers was measured. The average IQ of the population is 100, but the average IQ in the sample of mothers was 106. This information indicates that on the whole these women had slightly higher IQs than would be expected from a truly representative sample.

The MEAN is what is usually being referred to when talking about the 'average'; the average mothers' IQ quoted above was technically the mean mothers' IQ. The other averages commonly used are the MEDIAN, GEOMETRIC MEAN and MODE.

The mean is calculating by dividing the sum of all the

observations by the number of observations. However, the mean is not an appropriate summary statistic when SKEWNESS or OUTLIERS are present.

The median is an alternative measure of location in situations when the mean is not suitable. The median is the value that comes halfway when the observations are ordered. It is based on the ranks of the data and is therefore not dependent on the distribution of observations.

In the special case where the data are positively skewed such that the log-transformed data have a NORMAL DISTRIBUTION, the geometric mean is an alternative measure of location. The geometric mean is calculated by back-transforming (anti-logging) the (arithmetic) mean of the logged values.

The fourth measure of location commonly used in statistics is the mode. This is simply the value that occurs most often and it is therefore useful in summarising categorical rather than continuous data. Its usefulness can, however, be limited. For instance, we could not say much in a study of smoking if the modal number of cigarettes smoked in a sample happened to be zero.

A MEASURE OF SPREAD is often quoted alongside a measure of location to give information about the variability of observations around the average. *SRC*

measures of mortality See DEMOGRAPHY

measures of spread
Once the average of a set of observations has been defined using a MEASURE OF LOCATION, it is helpful to know how widely the data are scattered around this typical value. Measures of spread are used to summarise this information numerically.

The most straightforward measure of spread is the RANGE: the interval between the minimum and maximum values in a set of observations. Although the range has the advantage of simplicity, it is only influenced by the most extreme observations in a dataset and is therefore not generally considered a good way of quantifying variability.

Instead, in the case where the data are approximately symmetrically distributed, the STANDARD DEVIATION is often quoted. This measure has the useful property that, especially when the data follow a NORMAL DISTRIBUTION, approximately 95% of the observations lie within two standard deviations of the mean.

The INTERQUARTILE RANGE is an alternative measure of spread used in situations when the standard deviation is not suitable, due to SKEWNESS or the presence of OUTLIERS. It is the interval between the values that are located a quarter and three-quarters of the way through the sample when the observations are ordered. Since it is based on the ranks of the data it is not dependent on the distribution of observations.

The VARIANCE is the square of the standard deviation. Although this quantity is frequently used in statistical analysis, it is not as useful as the standard deviation in describing the spread of observations because it is not in the same units as the original data. Whereas one can have an intuitive feel for, say, cm^2, it is less obvious how to cope with units such as years^2 or mmHg^2. *SRC*

median
The median is a MEASURE OF LOCATION, being the central or 'halfway' value when the observations are ordered. Thus it is the middle value – in other words, half the data lie below it and half above. The median is also known as the *50th percentile*.

For example, in the following dataset, the heights of 11 women are recorded in centimetres:

154 157 157 158 159 **160** 161 162 162 163 169
↑
Median

The median is the 6th value when they are ordered, i.e. 160 cm.

If there is an even number of observations then the median is, by convention, the arithmetic mean of the *two* central values. Without such a convention, any value of an infinite number, lying between the two central observations would be a median, but it is preferable to have a definition enforcing a unique value.

The MEAN is generally used as a measure of location when the data have a symmetrical distribution. If this is not the case then the median is often quoted because it is not unduly affected by the presence of SKEWNESS or OUTLIERS. For instance, a woman who is 185 cm tall is added to the heights dataset in our previous example:

154 157 157 158 159 **160 161** 162 162 163 169 185
Median = 160.5

This changes the median to 160.5 cm, a value that still gives a good indication of the average height of the women.

The INTERQUARTILE RANGE is typically used as a MEASURE OF SPREAD around the median. *SRC*

median survival time See SURVIVAL ANALYSIS

medical statistics – an overview
Statistics may be defined as the science of collecting, analysing and interpreting numerical data. Medical statistics is the application of this science to medicine.

Statistics began as information concerning the state and this aspect is still a central part of medical statistics, as we collect and analyse information on national rates of birth, death and notifiable diseases. The term expanded to include many types of numerical data, collected for the purposes of administration (bed occupancy), research (clinical trials) and pleasure (batting averages) or any combination of the three. I was unable to think of a medical example for pleasure, so I will leave that as an exercise for the reader. To the statistician, statistics is all pleasure anyway.

Statistics is a skill as well as a science and a good statistician can take what seems to its owner a bewildering mass of data and find structure and meaning within it. What the data owner has to provide is the question that needs to be answered. The statistician can seldom provide that. Indeed, when the statistician starts to wonder more about the substantive medical question than how to answer it, he or she ceases to be a statistician and becomes an epidemiologist, trialist or health service researcher. The true statistician is much more interested in the process of answering the question than the answer itself, in the journey rather than the destination.

Statistics is unusual among academic subjects in that its entire purpose is to solve problems in other disciplines. Medical statistics is a collaboration between statisticians and those whose main object is to increase understanding of disease, health and healthcare. In the history of statistics, many important innovations were made by those wishing to answer a question arising in their own discipline. Most of us cannot aspire to be such polymaths, however, and must content ourselves with providing one aspect of the collaboration. Most people from health fields who wish to use statistics really need to acquire two things: the ability to apply a few day-to-day statistical procedures correctly and a vocabulary with which to communicate with their statistician.

We can include in collecting data the design of studies: the decisions as to what data to collect and from where or whom and how they should be collected. A frequent complaint of consulting statisticians is that their clients do not come to them early enough (see CONSULTING A STATISTICIAN). The researcher arriving with the referee's comments on a rejected paper may be too late. If the design were fundamentally flawed, there is probably very little that can be done to rectify matters.

There is no substitute for sound design (see EXPERIMENTAL DESIGN) and statistics has a lot to offer. One of the greatest of all contributions to medicine is surely the invention and development of the randomised CLINICAL TRIAL, which, for the first time, enabled medical researchers to obtain reliable evidence on the relative efficacy of clinical treatments.

The basic principles of study design are fairly straightforward and easily understood, unlike other aspects of medical statistics. In experimental biological studies, whether clinical trials on human subjects or laboratory experiments on animals, tissue samples or cell cultures, randomisation with blind allocation is the key. We neglect it at our peril. Most medical experiments use very simple designs, such as fully randomised two group comparisons or two period cross-overs (see CROSS-OVER TRIALS). At most, we might have a simple factorial design, where two treatments are given in combinations of none, one or both. Much more complex designs are used in other areas of application, such as agriculture or the chemical industry.

RANDOMISATION quickly gets complicated, however, as we often want improve the comparability of groups by stratification or are forced by the nature of the treatment to have patients allocated in clusters rather than individually. We may want, within small blocks of patients, to allocate equal numbers to each of the treatments, to ensure that numbers in treatment groups are always similar. In a small trial on a variable subject group we may decide to improve comparability by minimisation, ensuring that certain key variables will be balanced between the groups. These modifications are in turn require changes to the planned analysis and hence to the sample size estimation. They must not be ignored.

In medical observational studies the usual statistical approach of random sampling is seldom possible, but this does not mean we should ignore sampling issues, rather that we should consider very carefully the representativeness of our sample. As in experimental design, the principles of epidemiological designs such as CASE-CONTROL, COHORT, CROSS-SECTIONAL and ecological studies are easy to understand, but the details of their implementation using cluster or STRATIFIED SAMPLES, matched one to one or one to many, often require statistical insight and input. Clinical designs are often similar to those in epidemiology,

but used for a different purpose: case series may be used to describe clinical experience, cohort studies may be used to describe the natural history of a disease, case-control designs arise in the evaluation of diagnostic tests, cross-sectional studies are used to investigate the properties of measurement methods.

Data collection is very important and here the principle is to ensure that what we collect is accurate, with a minimum of bias and error. BIAS can be reduced by blind assessment, where the observer is unaware of the subject's status, and by blinding the subject to things that may influence response. In an experiment we may achieve this by concealing treatment allocations, for example with a placebo, leading to the ideal of the double-blind randomised trial. In an observational study this is more difficult, but we may, for example, include the questions on our key outcome variable among many others to reduce the apparent emphasis. Statistics offers techniques to ensure that we cannot be certain what individual respondents have told us while still obtaining data for the sample as a whole, such as secret ballots and randomised response, but they are seldom used in healthcare studies. Perhaps the most important thing we must do is to convince our respondents that their answers are absolutely confidential.

Training of observers is also very important in maintaining data quality and we may wish to estimate the degree of observer variation and the effects of using different observers. To reduce measurement error we may need to consider the frequency of measurement and we can weigh the relative advantages of increasing the number of subjects and increasing the number of measurements made on each.

Sample size is one aspect of study design on which statisticians are asked to advise, but often far too late for them to have any real input. A question about the sample size the day before the deadline for a grant application is typical, when all that can be done is to provide some kind of justification for the sample size already chosen on feasibility grounds. To change it at that stage is usually quite impractical. To decide on sample size we need to think about the purpose of the study, what outcome variable we intend to use and the analysis that we propose to carry out. This is, in any case, an excellent discipline for any investigation. Too often people collect data without any idea of how they are to be analysed. It can be a shock when they discover that they have collected data for which the possible analysis is very complex, difficult to interpret, time consuming and expensive and cannot answer their most important questions.

Statistical analysis begins with simple graphical methods, such as HISTOGRAMS and scatter diagrams (see SCATTERPLOT), and tabulations, which begin to reveal the structure of data. To make this more manageable, we then use summary statistics such as MEANS, STANDARD DEVIATIONS, centiles and proportions. An analytical method of peculiarly medical application is the Kaplan Meier survival method (see KAPLAN-MEIER ESTIMATOR), which enables us to estimate the cumulative survival of a group of subjects, some of whom are still surviving and who have been observed for varying lengths of time. Kaplan and Meier (1958) has been reported to be the most highly cited statistical paper ever (Ryan and Woodall, 2005). Comparison of these summary statistics between different groups of subjects leads to the use of differences and ratios between groups. Investigating the strength of relationships between variables observed in tabulations can be done using RELATIVE RISKS AND ODDS RATIOS, investigating those observed in scatter diagrams by regression and correlation.

A frequent problem in medical data is that the variable of interest may be influenced by another, not of any interest in itself. National mortality data provide a good example, where the age structure of the population has a profound effect. Special age-standardisation methods have been developed for this, producing age-standardised mortality rates and standardised mortality ratios. Much more generally applicable to deal with such problems are MULTIPLE LINEAR REGRESSION (see LOGIT MODELS FOR ORDINAL RESPONSES) and its many offspring: logistic, ordered logistic, multinomial, Poisson (see GENERALISED LINEAR MODEL), COX'S REGRESSION MODEL, LOGISTIC REGRESSION, etc. Such techniques also allow us to analyse situations where we are interested in several predicting variables and want to look at their relative importance as predictors.

A key question in analysis of data is the correct unit of analysis. In a trial, for example, if we randomise individual patients to treatment, the patient will be the unit of analysis. But if we allocate a group of patients together, forming a cluster, we must take this into account in the analysis. For example, we might allocate all the asthma patients in a primary care centre to receive an educational intervention or all to act as controls; the primary care centre becomes the unit of analysis. We might calculate the average of our outcome measurement for the cluster of patients in the practice and then compare two groups of clusters. If we want to include information collected at the level of the individual patient in such a study, we may have to use more complex, multilevel techniques. The same problem arises when we have multiple observations on a few patients or several tissue samples taken from each of a few organs. Ignoring the correct unit of analysis may be seriously misleading (see MULTILEVEL MODELS).

Another area when statistical analysis becomes essential is when we have several outcome variables and no clear primary one. This might happen if we have a battery of psychological tests or a questionnaire with many items. We may want to investigate the structure of these, summarise them into a single scale or analyse them all as a group. Methods developed in psychology, such as FACTOR ANALYSIS, enable us to do this.

In medical statistics, we usually have a sample of observations from some larger population, about which we want to draw some conclusion. For example, in a clinical trial the subjects are a sample of all the patients to whom we might wish to give the trial treatments, now and in the future. We use the trial to tell us about what would happen in this larger population. Even when we have data on the whole population, as in the case of national mortality rates, we often think of them as a sample of a hypothetical larger population so that we can investigate the reliability of differences and relationships found. This process of drawing conclusions about the larger population from the sample is called statistical inference. Users of statistics often find the concepts involved in inference quite difficult to master.

Most inference in the medical literature takes the form of CONFIDENCE INTERVALS and significance tests. These are methods from the frequentist formulation of statistics, one of two conceptual frameworks in which statistical inference is carried out. In this approach, we regard our sample as one of many we could have taken and then make deductions from the sample we do have about the many samples we do *not* have and hence about the population from which they would all be drawn. The alternative is the Bayesian conceptual framework (see BAYESIAN METHODS). In this, we try to describe what we already know about the answer to our question in probability terms, then see how these probabilities are modified by the data we have collected. Both approaches provide ways to take data from a sample and decide what they can tell us about the population. Both involve difficult concepts which can take years to master. Fortunately, it is possible to analyse data adequately even with a quite poor understanding of the underlying philosophy.

In the past, statisticians were divided into two warring camps, the Bayesians claiming that their methods had a securer philosophical foundation and frequentists claiming that Bayesian methods were impractical for real problems. In recent years the development of powerful computer-intensive Bayesian methods and computers fast enough to carry them out has led many more statisticians to make use of the Bayesian approach and the barriers are coming down.

Much statistical methodology consists of techniques to apply these fundamental concepts to inference for different types of design and data. The first methods developed were for large samples, estimating and comparing means, rates and proportions. These were followed by t-distribution-based methods for means of small samples, where the distribution of the observations themselves was important. This led to the use of transformations to persuade data into a form where we knew how to analyse them. It led also to the development of alternative methods, such as those based on rank order, which did not require such strong assumptions about the data. Small samples for proportions led to the development of exact probability methods such as FISHER'S EXACT TEST, methods that the advent of powerful and convenient computers has made feasible for large datasets, too. The list of statistical methods is long and growing. Almost all the analysis methods have inference attached to them, so that it is often not explicit which aspect of statistics we are doing.

When we have decided what our data can tell us about the wider world, we usually want to understand why the relationships that we have discovered have arisen. This brings us back in a circle to the design.

If we have a randomised, double-blind experiment we can usually conclude that that evidence supports the difference in treatment causing the difference in outcome. We do not, of course, conclude unequivocally that there is cause and effect; statistics is a discipline that instils caution and it is always possible, however unlikely, that we have an extreme sample producing a result atypical of its population. Statistics enables us to assess how cautious we need to be. If we have a study that is not blinded or randomised, we must consider very carefully the possible biases that may have been introduced.

If we have an observational study, we must always be very cautious in the interpretation. We must ask how good our sampling is and how comparable our groups are. We must remember that just because there is an ASSOCIATION between two variables we should not conclude that one causes the other. We must consider other factors that may be responsible for the relationship we have observed. If we are studying the aetiology of disease, in particular, we must beware of a rush to judgement. Guidelines for assessing the evidence for causality are available (such as BRADFORD HILL CRITERIA), but it takes data from several different sources before we can apply them.

In the era of evidence-based healthcare, all healthcare professionals, whether doctors, nurses or therapists, must be able to understand and interpret the research evidence on which their practice should be based. Much of this evidence is quantitative and statistics is the key skill needed. Not only has the number of statistical analyses published and the number of statistical methods employed increased greatly, but also these analyses have achieved much greater prominence. They are no longer confined to the methods and results sections of papers, but now fill the abstracts, too. Familiarity with basic statistical ideas is inescapable for the healthcare professions.

Healthcare research, whether medical, nursing or therapy, is unusual in that it is mainly initiated and carried out by healthcare professionals. Medical research is done by doctors, nursing research by nurses. This does not happen in other fields. Educational research is not done by teachers, social research by social workers or agricultural research by farmers, but rather by professional researchers in academia and industry. It is quite an attractive idea that it is part of the role of doctors to add to medical knowledge, but it puts a great responsibility on them to do this to a high standard. Unfortunately, this is often not the case. Statistical analysis requires quite different habits of mind to those required for diagnosis and the training of doctors, nurses and others is aimed at developing ways of thinking different to those learned by the mathematicians who specialise in statistics. Healthcare research requires many different skills and aptitudes and is much better done by collaboration between people from the disciplines possessing these. Rather than attempt to train a clinician in statistics to the level required for high-quality medical research, we should employ a statistician. Not only is this more effective, it is, regrettably, cheaper – they are not paid as much (or enough).

To work together, clinicians require familiarity with statistical ideas and vocabulary and close collaboration with statisticians should enhance this. Statisticians need to be familiar with the problems of carrying out research on particularly vulnerable human beings, whose needs must always be paramount, and the many special techniques that have been developed to do this. Close collaboration with clinical researchers should further the education of the statisticians too. Working together benefits clinicians, statisticians and the research itself and hence is to the good of all of us. *JMB*

Kaplan, E.L. and Meier, P. 1958: Nonparametric estimation from incomplete observations. *Journal of the American Statistical Association* 53, 457–81. Ryan, T.P. and Woodall, W.H. 2005: The most-cited statistical papers. *Journal of Applied Statistics*. (In press.)

Medicines and Healthcare products Regulatory Agency (MHRA)

The Agency was formed on 1 April 2003 as the amalgamation of the former Medicines Control and Medical Devices Agencies, which were, respectively, the UK government agencies responsible for the assessment and licensing of pharmaceutical and biological human medicines and (human) medical devices. The Agency has a variety of responsibilities including assessment of new medicines/products, assessment of changes to existing medicines, post-marketing surveillance (see PHARMACOVIGILANCE), inspection of CLINICAL TRIAL conduct and manufacturing facilities, enforcement of regulations and so on.

The legal framework for the Agency's work is set out in the Medicines Act 1968: for medicines, an applicant is required to demonstrate adequate evidence of safety, quality and efficacy. To this end, the Agency employs a large number of quality, pre-clinical and clinical assessors. Most of the statistical work is done in conjunction with the clinical assessors, although statistical considerations often come into other areas such as assessment of pre-clinical safety studies, determination of product shelf-life and assessment of marketing/advertising claims. Companies apply for a 'marketing authorisation' (formerly called simply a 'licence'). Agency staff assess data and prepare assessment reports, which are considered by the Committee on Safety of Medicines (CSM) and some of its expert sub-committees. The CSM is a panel of independent experts (including practising doctors, pharmacologists, statisticians and lay members) that meets every two weeks and advises on the granting, or otherwise, of a marketing authorisation. The final decision on granting is made by the government minister responsible for health. In certain circumstances, companies may appeal against unfavourable decisions and either make presentation before the CSM or appeal to the Medicines Commission.

MHRA works in close collaboration with other European national agencies and the European Medicines Agency (EMEA), which is based in London. There are a variety of routes by which companies can apply for a marketing authorisation within Europe – including national licences in as many (or as few) EU member states as they wish or a centralised licence covering all member states. In the latter case, two member states will be allocated to complete a comprehensive assessment of the application but all other member states are given the opportunity to raise concerns. The European counterpart to the CSM is the Committee for Human Medicinal Products (CHMP), which meets monthly. MHRA and EMEA also work with other agencies across the world and, in particular, contribute to and follow guidelines jointly prepared by the International Conference on Harmonization (a collaborative effort between the major geographical regions of Europe, Japan and the USA).

The assessment of safety and efficacy from clinical trials is similar to that for refereeing a paper for a medical journal but explores much more detail (see REGULATORY STATISTICAL MATTERS). The law requires companies to submit details of all trials that have been conducted. Each of these trials will have detailed study reports running to hundreds of pages and further extensive appendices including: a copy of the protocol and any amendments; individual case reports for serious adverse events/reactions; line listings of individual patient data; possibly efficacy results presented separately for each participating centre; copies of investigators' curriculum vitae; documentation of quality and purity of product used in the trials; and so on. These appendices may run to hundreds of volumes and, hence, the need for a variety of disciplines within the assessment teams.

More information about the Agency, its work and regulations pertaining to medicinal products and medical devices is available at the MHRA website: www.mhra.gov.uk. *SD*

Medicines Control Agency (MCA) See MEDICINES AND HEALTHCARE PRODUCTS REGULATORY AGENCY

mega-trial A large-scale randomised trial (generally involving several thousand subjects) that is designed to detect the effects of one or more treatments on major ENDPOINTS, such as death or disability. The need for mega-trials arises because the vast majority of treatments have only moderate effects on such endpoints, typically producing relative reductions of, at most, a quarter. Any study aiming to detect such a moderate effect needs to be able to guarantee that any biases and random errors inherent in its design are substantially smaller than the expected treatment effect (Collins and MacMahon, 2001). This will ensure that the results of the study either confirm the presence of a moderate effect convincingly or, if the treatment is ineffective, provide clear evidence that this is so.

For a study to avoid moderate biases requires RANDOMISATION using a method which precludes knowledge of each successive allocation. Randomisation in CLINICAL TRIALS is intended to maximise the likelihood that each type of patient will have been allocated in similar proportions to the different treatment strategies being investigated (Armitage, 1994). Randomisation requires that trial procedures are organised in a way that ensures that the decision to enter a patient is made irreversibly and without knowledge of which trial treatment a patient will be allocated. Even when studies are randomised, however, moderate biases can still be introduced by inappropriate analysis or interpretation.

The requirements for reliable assessment of moderate treatment effects are as follows: *negligible biases*, i.e. guaranteed avoidance of moderate biases involves proper randomisation (non-randomised methods cannot guarantee the avoidance of moderate biases); analysis by allocated treatments (i.e. an INTENTION-TO-TREAT analysis); chief emphasis on overall results (with no unduly data-derived subgroup analysis); and systematic meta-analysis of all the relevant randomised trials (with no unduly data dependent emphasis on the results from particular studies). For *small random errors*, i.e. guaranteed avoidance of moderate random errors involves: use of large numbers (with minimal data collection since detailed statistical analyses of masses of data on prognostic features generally add little to the effective size of a trial); and systematic meta-analysis of all the relevant randomised trials.

One well-recognised circumstance is when patients are excluded after randomisation, particularly when the prognosis of the excluded patients in one treatment group differs from that in the other (such as might occur, for example, if non-compliers were excluded after randomisation).

While avoidance of moderate biases requires careful attention both to the randomisation process and to the analysis and interpretation of the available trial evidence, a study can only avoid moderate random errors if it accumulates a sufficiently large number of events. When major endpoints such as death affect only a small proportion of those randomised, very large numbers of patients need to be studied before estimates of treatment effect can be guaranteed to be statistically (and hence medically) convincing. In these circumstances, when a treatment has the potential to be used widely and hence confer large benefit (or harm), a mega-trial is the only type of study that is sufficiently reliable. For example, for an event that is expected to occur among 10% of subjects without active treatment, over 20,000 subjects are required to demonstrate a 20% relative risk reduction (that is, from 10% to 8%) reliably (that is, with 90% POWER at a TYPE I ERROR rate of 1%).

For a mega-trial to randomise large numbers of trial subjects, the main barriers to rapid recruitment need to be removed. To facilitate this, the information recorded at entry should be brief and should concentrate on those few clinical details that are of paramount importance (including at most only a few major prognostic factors and only a few variables that are thought likely to influence substantially the benefits or hazards of treatment). Similarly, the information recorded at follow-up should be limited to serious outcomes, adverse events and to approximate measures of compliance. (Other outcomes, such as surrogate endpoints, that are of interest but do not need to be studied on such a large scale may best be assessed in separate smaller studies or in subsets of these large studies when this is practicable.) Keeping a trial as simple as possible increases the likelihood that it will be able to recruit large numbers of patients. For this reason, mega-trials are also known as 'large simple trials'.

For ethical reasons, randomisation is appropriate only if both the doctor and the patient feel substantially uncertain as to which trial treatment is best. The 'uncertainty principle' maximises the potential for recruitment within this ethical constraint. This says that a patient can be entered if, and only if, the responsible physician is substantially uncertain as to which of the trial treatments would be most appropriate for that particular patient. A patient should not be entered if the responsible physician or the patient are for any medical or non-medical reasons reasonably certain that one of the treatments that might be allocated would be inappropriate for this particular individual (either in comparison with no treatment or in comparison with some other treatment that could be offered to the patient in or outside the trial).

If many hospitals are collaborating in a trial then wholehearted use of the uncertainty principle encourages heterogeneity in the resulting trial population and this, in mega-trials, may add substantially to the practical value of the results. Among the early trials of fibrinolytic therapy, for example, most of the studies had restrictive trial entry criteria that precluded the randomisation of elderly patients, so these trials contributed nothing of direct relevance to the important clinical question of whether treatment was useful among older patients. Other trials that did not impose an upper age limit, however, did include some elderly patients and were therefore able to show that age alone is not a contraindication to fibrinolytic therapy (Fibrinolytic Therapy Trialists' Collaborative Group, 1994). Mega-trials adopting the uncertainty principle to determine eligibility maximise heterogeneity of the study sample, which in turn ensures that their results are relevant to a very diverse range of future patients. *CB*

[See also ETHICS AND CLINICAL TRIALS]

Armitage, P. 1982: The role of randomisation in clinical trials. *Statistics in Medicine* 1, 345–52. **Collins, R. and MacMahon, S.** 2001: Reliable assessment of the effects of treatment on mortality and major morbidity, I: clinical trials. *The Lancet* 357, 373–80. **Fibrinolytic Therapy Trialists' Collaborative Group** 1994: Indications for fibrinolytic therapy in suspected acute myocardial infarction: collaborative overview of early mortality and major morbidity results from all randomised trials of more than 1000 patients. *The Lancet* 343, 311–22.

meta-analysis See SYSTEMATIC REVIEWS AND META-ANALYSIS.

meta-regression Analysis of the relationship between study characteristics and study results in the context of a META-ANALYSIS.

Independent studies of the same problem, for example multiple CLINICAL TRIALS of a particular drug or multiple CASE-CONTROL STUDIES of the same exposure-disease association, will inevitably differ in many ways. Some of the variation may cause the effects being evaluated to be different in different studies, a situation commonly known as heterogeneity. Meta-regression analyses are similar to traditional linear regression analyses, a conceptual difference being that entire studies, rather than individuals, are the units of analysis. Characteristics of studies are used as explanatory (independent) variables and estimates of effect are used as outcome (dependent) variables. Regression coefficients describe how the effects across the studies increase per unit increase in the characteristic. Study characteristics might include numerical summaries of types of participants, variation in the implementation of an intervention or different methodological features. Estimates of effect may be, for example, odds ratios, hazard ratios or differences in mean responses, depending on the type of study and the nature of the outcome data. Ratio measures of effect are usually analysed on the (natural, or base e) log scale. Studies are weighted in the analysis to reflect imprecision in their results, the weights typically involving the inverse variances of the effect estimates.

A meta-regression may be a primary reason for assembling multiple studies, although meta-regressions are perhaps most commonly used as secondary analyses to investigate heterogeneity when a traditional meta-analysis was the primary objective of a review of studies. The study characteristics may be categorical or quantitative and several may be included in the same analysis. For categorical characteristics, meta-regression may be viewed as a generalisation of subgroup analyses, where the sub-grouping is by studies rather than by participants. Meta-regression should ideally be conducted only as part of a thorough systematic review to ensure that the studies involved are reliably identified and appraised.

Notable examples of meta-regression analyses include an investigation of the dose-response relationship between aspirin and secondary prevention of stroke. Among clinical trials administering aspirin at different doses, no relationship was apparent between aspirin dose and the relative risk of recurrence (Johnson *et al.*, 1999). A second example is provided by Zeegers, Jellema and Ostrer (2003), who present a meta-analysis of observational studies comparing prostate cancer risk between people with and without family history of prostate cancer. They used meta-regression to perform several subgroup analyses to assess the ROBUSTNESS of their finding that a family history of the disease is associated with roughly a doubling of risk. Studies were broken down by study design, year of publication and ethnic group, among other characteristics. A third example that has inspired development of meta-regression methodology is an analysis describing a relationship between the geographical latitude of studies of the BCG vaccine and the relative risk of tuberculosis in those vaccinated versus those not (Berkey *et al.*, 1995).

A convenient illustration of a meta-regression analysis for a single characteristic is a simple SCATTERPLOT as in the Figure, which shows the result of the BCG vaccine meta-regression. The circles represent studies, with the size of each circle proportional to the precision of the relative risk estimate from that study. The meta-regression line illustrates that the vaccine was observed to be more effective further away from the equator.

Meta-regression analyses involve observational comparisons across studies, and may suffer from BIAS due to confounding, since studies similar in one characteristic may be similar in others. Causal relationships between characteristics and results can seldom be drawn with confidence. A particular problem is that in most situations the number of studies in a meta-regression is small while the number of potentially important characteristics is large. Thus any meta-regression analyses performed should be driven by a strong scientific rationale and ideally pre-specified and limited in number. It may be necessary to control for the possibility of false-positive findings since the risk of a TYPE I ERROR increases substantially when multiple meta-regression analyses are undertaken.

It is possible to summarise participant-level characteristics at the level of a study for use in a meta-regression. Thus the mean age of participants, the proportion of females or the average length of follow-up might be used as study-level characteristics. Such analyses should be interpreted carefully, as they may not adequately reflect true associations. For example, suppose the effect of an intervention truly depends on a patient's age. If several clinical trials each include a wide range of ages, but if the mean age is similar across trials, then a meta-regression relating mean age to size of effect will fail to detect the

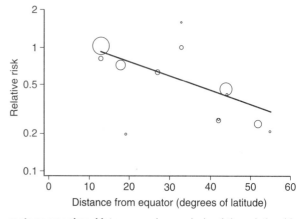

meta-regression *Meta-regression analysis of the relationship between effectiveness of BCG vaccine and latitude of study (data from Berkey et al., 1995)*

relationship that would be evident from within-trial analyses. When interest focuses on participant-level characteristics, a meta-analysis of individual participant level data is the most reliable method of separating within-study from among-study relationships. Potential limitations of meta-regression, including those already mentioned, are discussed by Thompson and Higgins (2002).

In common with meta-analysis, meta-regression may be conducted assuming either a FIXED EFFECT model or a RANDOM EFFECTS MODEL. A fixed effect meta-regression assumes the study characteristic(s) explain all of the inter-study variation in effects. It may be performed using weighted linear regression of the effect estimates on the study characteristics, weighting by the inverse variances of the effect estimates. However, the standard errors of the regression coefficients need to be corrected to account for the fact that the variances are known, by dividing them by the mean square error from the weighted regression.

A random effects meta-regression allows for variation in study effects that is not explained by the study characteristics. Such 'residual heterogeneity' of effect is commonly assumed to follow a normal distribution analogous to a random effects meta-analysis. Random effects meta-regression requires more specialised software, although a convenient implementation is available for STATA (Sterne, Bradburn and Egger, 2001). Since it is unlikely that heterogeneity can be fully explained by a finite selection of study characteristics, random effects meta-regression has been recommended as the default choice (Thompson and Higgins, 2002).

Meta-regression may be performed using alternative methods specific to the nature of the individual level outcome data when these are available. For example, when the outcome data from individuals in the studies are binary, then meta-regression may be undertaken using logistic regression.

Implementations of meta-regression that require special consideration include the relationship between effect estimates and underlying risk (due to correlation between effect estimates and risks), investigations of publication bias (again due to possible correlation between effect estimates and measures of precision) and non-independent outcomes (for example, entering subgroups from the same study). *JPTH*

Berkey, C.S., Hoaglin, D.C., Mosteller, F. and Colditz, G.A. 1995: A random effects regression model for meta-analysis. *Statistics in Medicine* 14, 395–411. **Johnson, E.S., Lanes, S.F., Wentworth III, C.E., Satterfield, M.H., Abebe, B.L. and Dicker, L.W.** 1999: A metaregression analysis of the dose-response effect of aspirin on stroke. *Archives of Internal Medicine* 159, 1248–53. **Sterne, J.A.C., Bradburn, M.J. and Egger, M.** 2001: Meta-analysis in Stata™. In Egger, M., Davey Smith, G. and Altman, D.G. (eds), *Systematic reviews in health care: meta-analysis in context*, 2nd edn. London: BMJ Publication Group. **Thompson, S.G. and Higgins, J.P.T.** 2002: How should meta-regression analyses be undertaken and interpreted? *Statistics in Medicine* 21, 1559–73. **Zeegers, M.P.A., Jellema, A.M. and Ostrer, H.** 2003: Empiric risk of prostate carcinoma for relatives of patients with prostate carcinoma: a meta-analysis. *Cancer* 97, 1894–903.

method comparison studies

At its simplest, a method comparison study involves the measurement of a given characteristic on a sample of subjects or specimens by two different methods. To take a simple and familiar example, we could imagine a study in which the body temperature of each of, say, n patients was assessed once using an old mercury thermometer, calibrated in degrees Fahrenheit (F), and again using a modern thermometer, calibrated in degrees Celsius (C). If the true temperature of the ith individual (in degrees Celsius) is τ_i then the resulting set of measurements might be represented by the following two equations:

$$C_i = \tau_i + \delta_i$$
$$F_i = 32 + 1.8\tau_i + \varepsilon_i \qquad (1)$$

The numbers 32 and 1.8 follow from the temperatures of freezing and boiling water (i.e. $0°$ Celsius $\equiv 32°$ Fahrenheit; $100°$ Celsius $\equiv 212°$ Fahrenheit). The key characteristic of the design is that the resulting data are a series of paired measurements (C_i, F_i). The δs and εs in these two equations correspond to random measurement errors that are assumed to be uncorrelated both with each other and with the patient's true temperature. They are both assumed to have an average value of zero. They cannot be determined individually but statistical methods can be used to assess their variability (their variances, σ^2_δ and σ^2_ε, respectively).

But now we complicate matters by choosing to measure a characteristic, such as tissue enzyme, using two different assay methods with indeterminate scales. Arbitrarily choosing one, say X, to be the standard (or, indeed, it may be already recognised as the standard against which a new assay is being compared) and another, say Y, to be the comparator, a realistic statistical model might have the form:

$$X_i = \tau_i + \delta_i$$
$$Y_i = \alpha + \beta\tau_i + \varepsilon_i \qquad (2)$$

Here the values 32 and 1.8 have been replaced by unknown constants α and β, respectively. Our task is now to take the n pairs of measurements (X_i, Y_i) and use statistical methods to estimate α and β, together with the variances, σ^2_δ and σ^2_ε. These are the parameters of the MEASUREMENT ERROR model (possibly with the addition of the variance of the true scores, σ^2_τ, depending on how the patients or specimens have been selected). Before describing how we might attempt to carry out this estimation, however, it will be useful to discuss briefly what we might wish to learn or decide from the results of a method comparison study.

We might wish to estimate the parameters of a relative calibration or measurement error model such as that described by the pair of equations in (2). It would obviously be of interest to know the values of α and β so that we might know how to convert the scale of X to that of Y, or vice versa. In particular, we might wish to establish whether $\alpha = 0$ or $\beta = 1$ or both (in other words, are the scales the same?). If the scales of measurement *are* the same, then the two measurement methods are mean or average equivalent. In this case, we might also wish to know whether the two methods are equally precise (or whether one is more precise than the other) by comparing the estimates of the variances of the measurement errors (i.e. comparing estimates of σ^2_δ and σ^2_ε). If two methods are mean equivalent, and their precisions are the same, then they are fully individually equivalent. In the theory of psychometric tests (applicable to the measurement of

221

depression or anxiety, for example), tests with mean equivalent or individual equivalent are referred to as being τ-equivalent or parallel, respectively. Measurements using alternative methods that are individually equivalent or parallel are fully interchangeable without any loss of information.

Suppose, however, we wish to evaluate and compare the precisions of two methods that are known not to be mean equivalent? How, for example, do we compare the performance (precision) of an old thermometer calibrated in degrees Fahrenheit with a new one in degrees Celsius? We would need first to convert the Fahrenheit measurements to degrees Celsius (or vice versa) and only then compare the variances of the measurement errors. For methods X and Y, the relevant ratio (i.e. relative precision) for this comparison is $\sigma^2_\varepsilon/\beta^2\sigma^2_\delta$. Here a direct comparison of σ^2_δ and σ^2_ε would provide the answer to the wrong question.

A less stringent question might involve asking whether the two measurements on a given patient are close enough. We do not ask whether two methods are exactly equivalent but whether, for all practical purposes, they are interchangeable. In this situation, we may abandon the measurement model in (2) entirely and concentrate on the paired differences $(X_i - Y_i)$ as indicators of agreement between the two methods (Bland and Altman, 1986; 1999). If the agreement is good enough then we can, for all practical purposes, replace a measurement made using one of the methods by a corresponding measurement using the other one.

This is the rationale for the construction of LIMITS OF AGREEMENT (Bland and Altman, 1986; 1999). A very useful graphical summary to accompany these calculations is what is usually known as the Bland-Altman plot – a plot of the difference between the two measurements, $X_i - Y_i$, against their mean, $(X_i + Y_i)/2$ (Bland and Altman, 1986; 1999). In addition, one might wish to produce a simple Y versus X SCATTERPLOT, together with an estimate of their product-moment correlation and concordance correlation (Lin, 1989).

Many investigators, however, will wish to go beyond testing for equivalence. They will wish to know, for example, whether Y is better than X. Is the new method an improvement on the old one? Or, contrariwise, is it worse? If this is the aim then we have no option but to collect the relevant data (the design might need to be more informative than those discussed so far), postulate realistic statistical models for the measurements and proceed to test whether the models are appropriate and, if so, what do the estimates of the model's parameters tell us about the performance of the methods.

Returning to the statistical model described in (2), how do we estimate the parameters, and test hypotheses concerning them, given a set of paired measurements (X_i, Y_i)? The simple answer is that we cannot. There is insufficient information provided by the data to enable us to estimate these parameters. The technical phrase for this is 'the problem of model under-identification'. The only way to proceed is by making various assumptions concerning some of the parameters to produce a model that is identified and then to estimate the remaining parameters. Examples of these assumptions include (a) knowing the variance of the measurement errors of the standard (or its reliability), (b) assuming a common scale of measurement

(i.e. that $\beta = 1$) or (c) knowing the relative sizes of the two measurement error variances (i.e. the ratio $\sigma^2_\varepsilon/\sigma^2_\delta$).

The trouble with each of these assumptions is that we are assuming something about the measurement methods that we would ideally have wished to study as part of the method comparison study. The other problem is that if the chosen assumption is not actually valid we are likely to finish up with the wrong conclusions. Consider, for example, the assumption that we know the ratio of the error variances. This leads to the use of a method known as orthogonal or *Deming's regression* (very popular in clinical chemistry). Typically, the measurement error variances are estimated for each of the methods by repeatedly measuring the relevant characteristic on the same individual(s) or specimen(s). This enables us to estimate repeatability variances. These are only valid estimates of the measurement error variances (σ^2_ε and σ^2_δ) if the repeated measurements do not have correlated measurement errors. Correlated measurement errors are almost universal and one should be very wary of the use of Deming's regression when they are known to be a possibility (Carroll and Ruppert, 1996).

Better is to use a more informative design involving one or more of the following features: replication using each of the methods, the use of INSTRUMENTAL VARIABLES, and the use of more than three different methods of measurement within the study. The other key feature of these studies should be an adequate sample size. Most method comparison studies are too small. Statistical analyses for the data arising from more of the informative designs, with more realistic measurement models, are beyond the scope of this section. The methods typically involve software developed for covariance structure modelling (see STATISTICAL PACKAGES). These methods, and those relevant for the comparison of binary measurements (diagnostic tests), are described in Dunn (2004). *GD*

Bland, J.M. and Altman, D.G. 1986: Statistical methods for assessing agreement between two methods of clinical measurement. *The Lancet* i, 307–10. **Bland, J.M. and Altman, D.G.** 1999: Measuring agreement in method comparison studies. *Statistical Methods in Medical Research* 8, 135–60. **Carroll, R.J. and Ruppert, D.** 1996: The use and misuse of orthogonal regression in linear errors-in-variables models. *The American Statistician* 50, 1–6. **Dunn, G.** 2004: *Statistical evaluation of measurement errors*. London: Arnold. **Lin, L.I.-K.** 1989: A concordance correlation coefficient to evaluate reproducibility. *Biometrics* 45, 255–68 (see Corrections in *Biometrics* 56, 324–5).

MHRA See MEDICINES AND HEALTHCARE PRODUCTS REGULATORY AGENCY

microarray experiments Studies in microbiology that are designed to measure the expression levels of genes in a particular organism, generally in response to some stimuli or conditions believed to stimulate the organism's genes. Presently, two technologies have been developed to measure these expression levels; both are based on the biological concept of hybridisation between matching nucleotides.

The biological basis for these experiments is the same for both *cDNA slides* and *oligonucleotide arrays*. Genes are organised strings of nucleotides (A = adenine, C = cysteine, G = guanine, T = thymine), arranged in triplets that code for the 20 amino acids that form strings of peptides in proteins. The genes are arranged in a helical structure, with complementary base pairs on either side of the double helix (deoxyribonucleic acid, or DNA) in the nucleus of a cell. The cDNA slides and oligonucleotide arrays contain multiple copies of single-stranded genes or gene fragments, called probes. In response to a stimulus requiring the need for proteins, the coding genes in the DNA of a sample of cells are transcribed and transmitted outside the nucleus as messenger RNA (mRNA). When this cellular mRNA is denatured (i.e. split into its separate strands and reverse-transcribed into its more stable form, complementary DNA, or cDNA), the complementary strand is placed onto the slide or chip containing the gene probes and the nucleotides in the sample cDNA bind (hybridise) to their matching partners. Spots on the slide or chip where hybridisation has occurred indicate genes that were expressed in the mRNA in response to the stimulus. With either technology, the reported intensity level at a particular location on the slide or chip is a summary of fluorescence measurements detected in a series of pixels.

The two technologies for measuring gene expression differ in the material that is used to make the probes on the slide or chip. In cDNA slides, the process for obtaining the probes requires subjecting the cellular DNA to restriction enzymes that splice the DNA at specific locations corresponding to specific genes. Once isolated, the DNA fragments undergo a series of complex processes that amplify and multiply their numbers, resulting in a gene 'library' for a given laboratory, which is then used for thousands of slides. In oligonucleotide arrays, the gene fragments consist of 'known' strings of manufactured nucleotides that are placed on the chip using photolithography. For both the chip and the slide, as many as 20,000 and more gene probes are placed in an array of rows and columns, hence the term 'microarray'.

The technologies also differ in the experimental protocol that yields the data on gene expression levels. In cDNA experiments, a target sample contains a mixture of two types of cell, control and experimental, whose messenger RNA (mRNA) is reverse-transcribed into the more stable cDNA and then labelled with two different fluorophores: the control cells are often labelled with Cyanine 3, or Cy3 (green dye), and the experimental cells (e.g., cells that have been subjected to some sort of treatment, such as stress, heat, radiation or chemicals) are often labelled with Cyanine 5, or Cy5 (red dye). When mRNA concentration is high in the genes of these cells, their cDNA will bind to their corresponding probes on the spotted cDNA slide; an optical detector in a laser scanner will measure the fluorescence at wavelengths corresponding to the green and red dyes (532nm and 635nm, respectively). Good EXPERIMENTAL DESIGN will interchange the dyes in a separate experiment to account for imbalances in the signal intensities from the two types of fluorophores and the expected degradation in the cDNA samples between the first scan at 532nm (green) and second scan at 635nm (red). The ratio of the relative abundance of red and green dyes at these two wavelengths on a certain spot indicates relative mRNA concentration between the experimental and control genes. Thus, the gene expression levels in the target cells can be compared directly with those from the control cells.

Oligonucleotide arrays circumvent the possible inaccuracies that can arise in the preparation of a gene 'library' and the control and experimental samples for spotted array slides, by using 16–20 predefined and pre-fabricated sequences of (usually 25) nucleotides for each gene. Rather than circular-shaped spots, these probes are deposited onto the chip in square-shaped cells. The probe cells measure 24×24 or 50×50 micrometers square and are divided in 8×8 pixels; cells from the target sample, labelled again with a fluorophore, will hybridise to those squares on the chip that correspond to the complementary strands of the target sample's single-stranded cDNA. For these experiments, the target sample contains only one type of cell (e.g. treatment, or control); the assessment of expression is in comparison to the expression level on an adjacent probe, which is exactly the same as the gene probe except for the middle (13th) nucleotide. This 'mismatch' (MM) for the 'perfect match' (PM) sequence is only rough, since a target sample with elevated mRNA concentration for a certain gene may hybridise sufficiently to both the PM and MM probes. However, the results are believed to be less variable, since the probes on the chips are manufactured in more carefully controlled concentrations. Gene expression levels are measured again by a laser scanner that detects the optical energy in the pixels at the various probes (PM and MM) on the chip.

The analysis of the data (fluorescence levels at the various locations on the slide or chip) depends on the technology. For cDNA experiments, the analysis usually involves the logarithm of the ratio of the expression levels between the target and control samples. For oligonucleotide experiments, the analysis involves a weighted linear combination of the logarithm of the PM expression level and the logarithm of the MM expression level (with some authors choosing zero for the weights of the MM values). Several authors have discussed analysis of gene expression data from various standpoints, e.g. image analysis of pixel data on cDNA slides (Yang et al., 2002a), experimental design of multiple cDNA slides (Kerr and Churchill 2001a; 2001b; Yang and Speed, 2002), data transformations (Kafadar and Phang, 2003; Yang et al., 2002b), statistical methods for data from cDNA microarrays (Amaratunga and Cabrera, 2001; Dudoit et al., 2002) and from oligonucleotide microchips (Efron et al., 2001; Irizarry et al., 2002), LINEAR MIXED-EFFECTS MODELS (Wolfinger et al., 2001), adjustments for MULTIPLE COMPARISONS (Reiner, Yekutieli and Benjamini, 2002; Storey, 2003) and finite mixture models. The 'low-level' analysis consists of the necessary 'pre-processing' steps, including data transformation (usually the logarithm) to address partially the non-normality of the expression levels and normalisation and background correction methods to adjust for different signal intensities across different microarray experiments and sources of variation arising from the chip manufacturing process and background intensity levels. The 'high-level' analysis usually involves clustering (see CLUSTER ANALYSIS IN MEDICINE) the gene expression levels into groups of genes that are believed to respond similarly (www.linus.nci.nih.gov/-brb/TechReport.htm; Nguyen and Rocke, 2002). Due to the enormous number of normalisation, clustering and dimension-reduction algorithms for multivariate data, no real consensus has been reached on the best methods for gene expression data and statistical research continues on the development of tools for analysing data from microarray experiments. *KKa*

223

Amaratunga, D. and Cabrera, J. 2001: Analysis of data from viral DNA microchips. *Journal of the American Statistical Association* 96, 456, 1161–70. **Dudoit, S., Yang, Y.H., Callow, M.J. and Speed, T.P.** 2002: Statistical methods for identifying differentially expressed genes in replicated cDNA microarray experiments. *Statistica Sinica* 12, 111–39. **Efron, B., Tibshirani, R., Storey, J.D. and Tusher, V.** 2001: Empirical Bayes' analysis of a microarray experiment. *Journal of the American Statistical Association* 96, 1151–60. **Irizarry, R.A., Hobbs, B., Collin, F., Beazer-Barclay, Y.C., Antonellis, K.J., Scherf, U. and Speed, T.P.** 2002: Exploration, normalization, and summaries of high density oligonucleotide microarray probe level data. *Biostatistics* 19, 185–93. **Kafadar, K. and Phang, T.** 2003: Transformations, background estimation, and process effects in the statistical analysis of microarrays. *Computational Statistics and Data Analysis* 44, 313–38. **Kerr, M.K. and Churchill, G.** 2001a: Experimental design for gene expression arrays. *Biostatistics* 2, 183–201. **Kerr, M.K. and Churchill, G.** 2001b: Statistical design and the analysis of gene expression microarray data. *Genetics Research* 77, 123–8. **Nguyen, D.V. and Rocke, D.M.** 2002: Tumor classification by partial least squares using microarray gene expression data. *Bioinformatics* 18, 39–50. **Reiner, A., Yekutieli, D. and Benjamini, Y.** 2002: Identifying differentially expressed genes using false discovery rate controlling procedures. *Bioinformatics* 19, 3, 368–75. **Storey, J.D.** 2003: The positive false discover rate: a Bayesian interpretation and the q-value. *Annals of Statistics* 31, 2013–35. **Wolfinger, R.D., Gibson G., Wolfinger, E.D., Bennett, L., Hamadeh, H., Bushel, P., Afshari, C. and Paules, R.S.** 2001: Assessing gene significance from cDNA microarray expression data via mixed models. *Journal of Computational Biology* 8, 625–38. **Yang, Y.H. and Speed, T.P.** 2002: Design issues for cDNA microarray experiments. *Nature Reviews* 3, 579–88. **Yang, Y.H., Buckley, M.J., Dudoit, S. and Speed, T.P.** 2002a: Comparison of methods for image analysis on cDNA microarray data. *Journal of Computational and Graphical Statistics* 11, 108–36. **Yang, Y.H., Dudoit, S., Luu, P. and Speed, T.P.** 2002b: Normalization for cDNA microarray data: a robust composite method addressing single and multiple slide systematic variation. *Nucleic Acids Research* 30, E15.

mid-*P*-value See EXACT METHODS FOR CATEGORICAL DATA

MIM See GRAPHICAL MODELS

minimisation A method sometimes used to balance RANDOMISATION in a CLINICAL TRIAL when there are several factors on which it is considered necessary to try to force balance across the treatment groups. Simple randomisation will, in theory (or in 'the long run'), ensure that treatment groups are equally represented with respect to all known and unknown prognostic factors but, for any particular trial, this balance may not be as good as we would hope. When there are only a few factors for which balance is necessary (such as gender or stage of disease) then simple stratified randomisation may be sufficient. However, if there are more than two or three factors on which to try to balance, then the number of strata becomes excessive and the logistics of the trial become overwhelming. Minimisation was a method proposed by Taves (1974) and, more extensively, by Pocock and Simon (1975) as a way of balancing simultaneously for several factors (see also Pocock, 1983: 84–6).

It is important to realise that in most trials, patients arrive sequentially, rather than all being available as a 'pool' of patients at the beginning. Hence, when a patient of a certain demographic and/or disease state enrols, we do not know when (or even if) a similar patient will enrol subsequently. However, if two similar patients were to be available for a trial, it would be desirable to allocate one to each of the treatment groups (a method easily extendable to more than two treatment groups). If there were only one factor on which to balance the randomisation then for patients within each stratum we would (optimally) allocate them alternately between the treatments. If there is more than one factor (e.g. gender [male/female] and disease stage [early/progressive/advance] we have to 'trade off' the benefits of allocating to one treatment in order to ensure an equal balance of males/females across the treatment groups – and simultaneously to ensure an equal balance of early/progressive/advanced patients across the treatment groups. Often to balance gender, we might be better off allocating the patient to one treatment but to balance for disease stage we might be better off allocating the patient to the other. Hence the term 'minimisation': to try to minimise the degree of imbalance across all the identified factors.

The following example is described by Day (1999) and concerns a trial randomising general practitioners to an intervention group or to control (see also Steptoe *et al.*, 1999). Three factors were identified on which to balance the groups: the Jarman score (a level of social status), the ratio of number of patients to hourly nurse practice hours ('low' or 'high') and the fundholding status of the practice (in three categories). Assume we are partway through the trial and the first 18 practices have been allocated as in the table. Balance looks reasonably good. Now assume that the next (the 19th) practice is of type: low Jarman score, high patient–practice nurse hours and is a non-fundholder. We calculate 'scores' for these types of practice, which are $4 + 5 + 3 = 12$ for the intervention group and $3 + 4 + 3 = 10$ for the control group. Imbalance is 'in favour' of intervention, so by allocating this practice to control, we minimise the imbalance.

When Taves and then, the following year, Pocock and Simon published their early papers on this topic, they explained how simple the method is to use and, in particular, how, for a single institution, it is quite possible to 'minimise' on several factors with a simple card index system. In a MULTICENTRE TRIAL this would effectively be

minimisation *Allocation of first 18 general practices and profile of 19th practice indicated*

	Prognostic factor	Intervention group	Control group	
	Jarman score			
→	Low	4	3	←
	Middle	3	5	
	High	2	1	
	Patient–practice hours per week			
	Low	4	5	
→	High	5	4	←
	Fundholding status			
→	Non-fundholder	3	3	←
	1st wave entry	4	3	
	2nd wave entry	2	3	

'minimisation, stratified by centre'. With modern telephone and computer systems used for central randomisation it becomes even easier to use minimisation across centres (possibly using 'centre' as one of the minimisation factors).

It was mentioned earlier how an 'optimal' allocation could easily be determined in the case of a single factor but that would only be optimal in the sense of minimising the imbalance. Maintaining blinding is also important and most minimisation algorithms – particularly those run on computers – incorporate an element of randomisation within them so that, even with complete knowledge of all the patients in the study so far, it is not possible to guarantee correctly guessing the next patient assignment. Minimisation is not without controversy. Including such a random component satisfies most critics but some (such as Rosenberger and Lachin, 2002) still consider that all the theoretical aspects of how the analysis should be done have not been fully worked out.   *SD*

Day, S. 1999: Treatment allocation by the method of minimisation. *British Medical Journal* 319, 947–8. **Pocock, S.J.** 1983: *Clinical trials: a practical approach.* Chichester: John Wiley and Sons. **Pocock, S.J. and Simon, R.** 1975: Sequential treatment assignment with balancing for prognostic factors in the controlled clinical trial. *Biometrics* 31, 103–15. **Rosenberger, W.F. and Lachin, J.M.** 2002: *Randomization in clinical trials.* New York: John Wiley and Sons. **Steptoe, A., Doherty, S., Rink, E., Kerry, S., Kendrick, T. and Hilton, S.** 1999: Behavioural counselling in general practice for the promotion of healthy behaviour among adults at increased risk of coronary heart disease: randomised trial. *British Medical Journal* 319, 943–7. **Taves, D.R.** 1974: Minimization: a new method of assigning patients to treatment and control groups. *Clinical Pharmacology and Therapeutics* 15, 443–53.

missing at random (MAR)   See DROPOUTS, MISSING DATA

missing completely at random (MCAR)   See DROPOUTS, MISSING DATA

missing data   Well-designed statistical studies draw a representative sample from the study population by following a sampling plan and a detailed protocol. Often, however, some of the planned data are unavailable or otherwise absent from the database, hence the term 'missing data'. The data that would be observed if all intended measurements were obtained will be called 'potential data'. The potential data that are not missing, combined with a response indicator of availability of each planned response form the 'observed data'. The name 'missing data' may suggest that the data analyst can simply forget these data, but nothing could be further from the truth.

Missing data form one of the hardest challenges for data analysts. This is because missing data can be intrinsically different from observed data in ways that are hard to predict and thus leave a biased sample. For instance, when studying the evolution of CD4 counts over time, AIDS patients may fail to return for planned clinic visits not only when they are sick as a result of low CD4 counts, but also when they feel good and no longer in need of treatment. In view of this, three types of missing data are typically distinguished (Little and Rubin, 2002): (i) The simplest situation occurs when the risk of missing a certain part of the data is the same for all subjects,

regardless of their potential data values. This process is known as 'missing completely at random' (MCAR). It happens, for instance, in a study where very expensive outcome measures are, by design, only gathered in a random subsample. In that case, missing observations can simply be deleted from the dataset and ignored in further analyses. (ii) A more realistic situation occurs when the risk of missing a certain part of the data does not depend on the missing potential data, given the ones that were observed. This condition is easily interpreted when dealing with baseline covariates that are always observed and a single outcome that can be missing. It becomes complex with non-monotone missingness patterns. In either case, the data are then called 'missing at random' (MAR). This happens for instance in two-stage sampling designs where a subgroup of patients is invited to the second study cycle, depending on their first outcome. A naive data analysis, which ignores missing data, may then be misleading, unless it conditions on the correct subset of observed data. (iii) When neither of these two constraints holds, missingness is fundamentally informative or non-ignorable (NI). In a health survey, for instance, one may lose the uninterested or very busy respondents who have their own disease profile.

Under each of these three scenarios, the popular MAXIMUM LIKELIHOOD ESTIMATION method can be used for unbiased estimation of parameters in the study population. The challenge is then to propose a (parsimonious) model relating the distribution of observed and potential data. Typically, one chooses either a so-called 'selection model' or a 'pattern-mixture' model (Little and Rubin, 2002). The former adds to the usual model for the distribution of the potential data, a model for the conditional distribution of being observed, given the potential data. The latter models the conditional distribution of the potential data for each level of the response indicator and adds to it a model for the distribution of the response indicator. In both cases, one averages over all possible values of the missing data to find the observed data distribution that enters the maximum likelihood procedure. One useful property of MAR is that maximum likelihood estimation can avoid the need to model the probability of being observed and still allow for inference on the potential data, a feature making maximum likelihood estimation very popular in this setting.

Nonetheless, observed data likelihoods under MAR may have complex forms not covered by standard statistical packages. To help avoid lengthy computations in routine practice, the EM ALGORITHM and imputation techniques have been devised (see MULTIPLE IMPUTATION). EM is an iterative algorithm that replaces the usual loglikelihood of the potential data by its conditional expectation, given the observed data. Maximum likelihood estimates are then obtained by maximising it in the usual way and the expected loglikelihood is updated. Imputation methods 'fill in' the missing data by simulating from their distribution conditional on the available data. The resulting 'completed' dataset is then analysed using standard software as if no data were missing. The loss of information due to the missing data must, however, be recognised when standard errors are derived. Corrected standard errors have therefore been proposed based on the variation in estimates over different random imputations (Little and Rubin, 2002).

One drawback of the maximum likelihood approach is that estimates can be biased when the potential data model is mis-specified. One may therefore choose to specify fewer features of the model and follow the Horvitz-Thompson principle, which helps achieve robustness against model mis-specification (Preisser, Lohman and Rathouz, 2002). Here, the completely observed data are upweighted by the inverse conditional probability of being observed, given the potential data, to compensate for similar counterparts that are missing. This line of research has seen extensive developments in recent years and is entering statistical practice as software becomes more readily available.

Regardless of the adopted approach, observed data alone seldom contain information that distinguishes MAR from NI. One is, statistically speaking, blind and must rely on guidance from other sources to make progress. This is made abundantly clear by the pattern mixture approach. Indeed, the pattern with unobserved response completely lacks information on the data distribution and unbiased inference needs unverifiable assumptions regarding the dependence of missingness on the potential data. Reassurance that 'missed' data are comparable to observed ones is found when data are 'missing by design', but is hard to obtain otherwise. It is hence very important to plan to gather such information that helps determine the distribution of the missed data at the design stage. In experimental studies, one seeks to gather data over time that can help predict. Furthermore, a sensitivity analysis can be conducted by examining how estimates vary as different choices are postulated for the unknown outcome distribution in non-responders. This practice of describing how conclusions vary over plausible but untestable assumptions is recommended (Kenward, Goetghebeur and Molenberghs, 2001; Scharfstein and Daniels, 2003).

While enormous progress has been made in statistical methodology for dealing with missing data, many problems remain both in practice and in theory. The term 'missing data' is often misunderstood or the methods are abused. When answers to certain questions are intrinsically meaningless or undefined in certain categories of people (e.g. blood pressure of dead patients), it is hard to justify missing data constructions that give non-responders the outcome distribution of responders and base conclusions on outcomes averaged over both groups. Furthermore, the MAR assumption is frequently adopted for mathematical convenience but may be difficult to interpret or justify. The goal and relevance of any analysis, along with justified assumptions, must come first. In causal inference, for instance, missing data constructs can be exploited (Vansteelandt and Goetghebeur, 2004). At other times, one ignores valuable and simple MAR methods to fall for simplistic analyses that can be very misleading. Due caution is always necessary, additional thought is required in model selection and, with regard to missing data in general, the familiar adage holds: prevention is better than cure. *EG/SV*

[See also DROPOUTS]

Kenward, M.G., Goetghebeur, E. and Molenberghs, G. 2001: Sensitivity analysis for incomplete categorical data. *Statistical Modeling* 1, 31–48. Little, R.J.A. and Rubin, D.B. 2002: *Statistical analysis with missing data.* New York: John Wiley & Sons. Preisser, J.S., Lohman, K.K. and Rathouz, P.J. 2002: Performance of weighted estimating equations for longitudinal binary data with drop-outs missing at random. *Statistics in Medicine* 21, 3035–54. Scharfstein, D.O., Daniels, M.J. and Robins, J.M. 2003: Incorporating prior beliefs about selection bias into the analysis of randomized trials with missing outcomes. *Biostatistics* 4, 495–512. Vansteelandt, S. and Goetghebeur, E. 2004: Sense and sensitivity when correcting for observed exposures in randomized clinical trials. *Statistics in Medicine*, electronic pre-publication by Wiley, 28 October 2004, www3.interscience.wiley.com/cgibin/jissue/96515927

mixed effects models See LINEAR MIXED EFFECTS MODELS

MLWin See MULTILEVEL MODELS

mode The mode is a MEASURE OF LOCATION. It is simply the value that occurs most often. For example, the hair colour of 573 babies born at a UK maternity hospital is shown in the table. In this example, the mode is 'medium brown'.

Hair colour	Frequency
Blond	41
Pale brown/blond	147
Medium brown	244
Dark brown	121
Black	14
Red	6

The mode, however, is of limited value in summarising continuous data. In contrast to the MEAN, the mode is not sensitive to outliers but need not be a unique value, as a distribution of data may be bimodal or multimodal (having two or more modes, respectively). *SRC*

MPLUS See STRUCTURAL EQUATION MODELLING

multi-centre research ethics committee (MREC)
See ETHICAL REVIEW COMMITTEES

multicentre trials Studies that are carried out in several distinct centres, sites or units (hospitals, clinical departments etc.). The first trials of new therapies in man (Phase I) require few subjects who must be monitored very tightly, therefore they are almost always carried out in a single centre. These trials are typically followed by medium sized multicentre efficacy trials (Phase II). If the results of these early trials are promising, then larger multicentre trials are carried out to confirm the efficacy and safety of the new therapies (Phase III).

Multicentre trials are often performed in several countries or even several continents. The conduct of multicentre trials can be overseen by a steering committee, headed by the study chair and consisting of persons designated to represent study centres, disciplines or activities.

Multicentre trials are needed primarily to accrue the number of subjects or patients required for the study over a reasonably short time period. For common diseases, multicentre trials may have several centres with large numbers of subjects per centre or, in the case of rare diseases, they may have a large number of centres with very few subjects per centre. Patients treated at different centres (let alone different countries or continents) may be expected to differ substantially in terms of their ethnicity, exposure to aetiologic or risk factors, living conditions and access to health resources etc.

Such heterogeneity may be a drawback for two main reasons: first, the variance of the outcome of interest is increased because of the heterogeneity and, second, a treatment benefit in some patient subpopulation might be missed in a trial that accrued other patient subpopulations as well. On closer inspection, neither of these two reasons argues against multicentre trials. The increase in sample size that results from heterogeneity is usually negligible compared to the potential number of patients available at multiple centres. In many situations, no centre would be able to accrue the required number of patients, hence a single centre trial would be infeasible. In addition, the results of a multicentre trial are more readily generalisable than those of a single centre trial, because they are obtained in a patient sample more likely to reflect the population of interest. If a treatment is thought *a priori* to exert its benefit selectively in a patient subpopulation, a multicentre trial is still indicated with prior exclusion of patients unlikely to benefit.

An added advantage of multicentre trials is their ROBUSTNESS to fraud, delinquencies and other quality problems that may arise at a few centres. This was illustrated by a series of large multicentre trials in early breast cancer, in which exclusion of a fraudulent centre did not have any sizeable impact on the trial results (Peto *et al.*, 1997). In contrast, another highly publicised case of fraud in a trial of high-dose chemotherapy for advanced breast cancer had disastrous consequences, because its results were completely dominated by fraudulent data. Very few centres had taken part in this trial and fraud from a single investigator was sufficient to cause dramatic bias in the reported results (Weiss *et al.*, 2000). Published results of well-conducted multicentre trials often have a direct impact on clinical practice, while single-centre trials generally require to be reproduced on a larger scale before their results are accepted as valid.

The clinical trial protocol should encourage the participating centres to put the same procedures in place as regards patient management, measurement of treatment effects and other aspects of the study that may have a bearing on the therapeutic results. Some heterogeneity is unavoidable in multicentre trials, but such heterogeneity is unimportant so long as it does not directly affect the outcome of interest. In a randomised trial, in particular, differences between centres are ignorable if they do not impact the treatment effects of interest. Thus if one centre tended to recruit patients of poor prognosis and another centre tended to recruit patients of good prognosis, this difference would not compromise the trial results if the treatment effects were independent of prognosis. Such independence is generally unknown but postulated before the trial and it can, in fact, be studied within the trial itself. In the example just given, differences in prognostic mix between centres might be confounded by other centre-specific factors (such as concomitant medications, supportive care etc.), hence the need to standardise trial procedures across all participating centres to the extent possible.

The logistics of a multicentre trial can be fairly complex and provisions must be made for drug shipment and storage, trial material distribution, ethical approval and compliance to local regulations, training of investigators and local staff to avoid variation in patient management, evaluation criteria, follow-up schemes etc. All these issues can be discussed at investigator meetings and monitoring visits during the trial.

Statistical quality control checks can also be performed to identify discrepancies between centres that may call for more thorough investigations, especially in centres that are found to be clear OUTLIERS. Such checks are best performed while the trial is ongoing, so that remedial action can be taken early and this can be facilitated by electronic data capture that feeds patient data to a central database in real time. There is no conclusive evidence that data quality is related to the number of patients enrolled in each centre (Hawkins *et al.*, 1990; Sylvester *et al.*, 1981).

In multicentre trials, randomisation of the patients is generally organised centrally, rather than performed in each centre. Centralised randomisation requires that all centres access a central resource, usually by internet, telephone or fax, to obtain the next treatment allocation. Such centralised control is useful to follow the accrual of patients into the trial and to check eligibility criteria in a uniform way prior to treatment allocation. Centralisation of the randomisation process also guarantees that it cannot be biased by foreknowledge of the next treatment assignment, which could happen in open-label trials with the use of randomisation lists. It is usually desirable to stratify the allocation by centre and more generally by important prognostic factors measured at baseline, such as severity of disease, patient status, age etc. Such stratification can be implemented with permuted lists of treatment allocations or through dynamic allocation using MINIMISATION. Allocation through minimisation has the advantages of being able to take account of many prognostic factors and of being completely unpredictable at any given centre in absence of information on patients already randomised in all other centres.

Multicentre trials are usually designed and their sample size calculated under the assumption that the treatment effect is the same in all centres. Whether this assumption is supported by the data can be tested formally. Assume that in the ith of I centres, the true treatment effect is given by τ_i, and the estimate of τ_i, noted $\hat{\tau}_i$, is asymptotically normally distributed with variance v_i:

$$\hat{\tau}_i \sim N(\tau_i, v_i)$$

The measure of treatment effect is taken such that no treatment effect corresponds to $\tau_i = 0$. Interest focuses first and foremost on whether there is statistical evidence of an overall treatment effect, which can be tested through the test statistic:

$$X^2_{treatment} = \frac{\left(\sum_{i=1}^{I} \hat{\tau}_i w_i\right)^2}{\sum_{i=1}^{I} w_i} \sim \chi^2_1$$

where $w_i = v_i^{-1}$ denotes the inverse of the variance of the treatment effect in the ith centre. Under the null hypothesis of no treatment effect ($\tau_1 = \tau_2 = ... = \tau_I = 0$), this test statistic has an asymptotic χ^2 distribution with one DEGREE OF FREEDOM.

Under the assumption of a common treatment effect in all trials ($\tau_1 = \tau_2 = \ldots = \tau_I = \tau$), the treatment effect is estimated by:

$$\hat{\tau} = \frac{\sum_{i=1}^{I} \hat{\tau}_i \, w_i}{\sum_{i=1}^{I} w_i}$$

In order words, a weighted average of the treatment effects in all centres. The presence of heterogeneity between centres can be tested through the test statistic:

$$X^2_{heterogeneity} = \sum_{i=1}^{I} (\hat{\tau}_i - \hat{\tau})^2 \, w_i \sim \chi^2_{I-1}$$

which has an asymptotic χ^2 distribution with $I-1$ degrees of freedom. In practice, this test for heterogeneity in treatment effects between centres is not very informative, because it lacks power to detect true underlying differences, especially when there are many centres (I large) with few patients per centre. Moreover, when statistical heterogeneity is found between centres, it may be difficult to ascribe it to a well-identified factor and the interpretation of the overall treatment effect may be controversial. The same test for heterogeneity is more useful when centres can be meaningfully combined according to a common characteristic (for instance, all centres that have access to certain equipments or that use certain supportive treatments). When centres are thus combined for the purposes of statistical analysis, the grouping should be defined prospectively and blindly to treatment allocation and results in the various centres. A grouping of centres based solely on their sample sizes is unlikely to be informative. Even when the formal test of heterogeneity fails to reach statistical significance, heterogeneity can be explored through descriptive statistics or graphical displays of the treatment effects in individual centres or groups of centres. Large differences in treatment effects between centres would cause concern, especially if much of the overall effect was attributable to an unexpectedly large effect in a single centre or if treatment had a markedly negative effect in some centres an overall positive treatment effect notwithstanding. Whenever substantial heterogeneity is found, attempts should be made to find an explanation in terms of identifiable features of trial management or subject characteristics. Such an explanation may suggest further analyses or appropriate interpretation. In the absence of an explanation, alternative estimates of the treatment effect may be required in order to substantiate the robustness of the trial results (International Conference on Harmonisation, 1998).

Regardless of the presence of statistical heterogeneity between centres, the statistical model adopted for the estimation and testing of treatment effects may account for centre through stratification or by inclusion of a fixed or random effect for centre in the model. If the number of subjects per centre is limited, centre effects are poorly estimated and the inclusion of centre effects in the model negatively affect the power of the treatment comparisons. In such cases, it is preferable to ignore centre in the analysis.

MB

Hawkins, B.S., Prior, M.J., Fisher, M.R. and Blackhurst, D.W. 1990: Relationship between rate of patient enrolment and quality of clinical center performance in two multicenter trials in ophthalmology. *Controlled Clinical Trials* 11, 374–94. International Conference on Harmonisation 1998: E-9 document: Guidance on statistical principles for clinical trials. *Federal Register* 63, 179, 49583–98. Peto, R., Collins, R., Sackett, D., Darbyshire, J., Babiker, A., Buyse, M., Stewart, H., Baum, M., Goldhirsch, A., Bonadonna, G., Valagussa, P., Rutqvist, L., Elbourne, D., Altman, D., Dalesio, O., Parmar, M., Hill, C., Clarke, M., Gray, R. and Doll, R. 1997: The trials of Dr Bernard Fisher: a European perspective on an American episode. *Controlled Clinical Trials* 18, 1–13. Sylvester, R., Pinedo, H., De Pauw, M., Staquet, M., Buyse, M., Renard, J. and Bonadonna, G. 1981: Quality of institutional participation in multicenter clinical trials. *New England Journal of Medicine* 305, 852–5. Weiss, R.B., Rifkin, R.M., Stewart, F.M., Theriault, R.L., Williams, L.A., Herman, A.A. and Beveridge, R.A. 2000: High-dose chemotherapy for high-risk primary breast cancer: an on-site review of the Bezwoda study. *The Lancet* 355, 999–1003.

multicollinearity A term used particularly in MULTIPLE LINEAR REGRESSION to indicate situations where the EXPLANATORY VARIABLES are linearly related, making where the estimation of regression coefficients in the usual way impossible. Including the sum or average of the explanatory variables as a variable would lead to this problem. For example, in a blood pressure study one cannot include among explanatory variables systolic blood pressure (SBP), diastolic blood pressure (DBP) and, additionally, linear combination of the two such as mean blood pressure without causing the model to break down completely.

Approximate multicollinearity can also cause problems when estimating regression coefficients. In particular, if the multiple correlation coefficient (see CORRELATION) for the regression of one of the explanatory variables on the others is high, the variance of the corresponding regression coefficient estimate will also be high. *BSE*

multidimensional scaling A technique often used in psychology but less often in medicine. The basis of the method is a proximity matrix arising either directly from experiments in which subjects are asked to assess the similarity of pairs of stimuli or, indirectly, as a measure of the correlation or covariance of a pair of stimuli derived from a number of measurements made on each. In some cases, high proximity values correspond to stimuli that are similar (similarities); in others, the reverse is the case (dissimilarities). As an example, the table shows judgements

multidimensional scaling *Dissimilarity data for all pairs of 10 colas for a subject*

Cola number	Subject 1									
	1	2	3	4	5	6	7	8	9	10
1	0									
2	16	0								
3	81	47	0							
4	56	32	71	0						
5	87	68	44	71	0					
6	60	35	21	98	34	0				
7	84	94	98	57	99	99	0			
8	50	87	79	73	19	92	45	0		
9	99	25	53	98	52	17	99	84	0	
10	16	92	90	83	79	44	24	18	98	0

about various brands of cola made by a subject using a visual analogue scale with anchor points 'same' (having a score of 0) and 'different' (having a score of 100). In this example, the resulting rating for a pair of colas is a dissimilarity-low values indicate that the two colas are regarded as alike and vice versa. A similarity measure would have been obtained had the anchor points been reversed, although similarities are usually scaled to lie between zero and one.

Researchers with data in the form of proximity matrices are generally interested in uncovering any structure or pattern they may contain and multidimensional scaling aims to help by representing the observed proximities as a spatial or geometrical model in which the distances between the points (usually taken to be Euclidean) correspond in some way to the observed proximities. In general, this simply means that the larger the dissimilarity (or the smaller the similarity), the further apart should be the points representing them in the final geometrical model.

The required spatial model is defined by a set of d-dimensional points, each representing one of the stimuli of interest and a measure of the distance between these points. The objective of multidimensional scaling is to determine both the dimensionality of the model (i.e. the value of d) and the values of the coordinates. The coordinates of the points in the model that represent the proximities can be found in a variety of ways. One simple approach is to choose the coordinate values (for a given value of d) to minimise S, defined as:

$$S = \sum_{ij} (\delta_{ij} - d_{ij})^2$$

where δ_{ij} is the observed dissimilarity for stimuli i and j and d_{ij} is the distance between the points representing stimuli i and j. Since the distances d_{ij}, are function of the coordinate values, so also is S. For various reasons, S is not generally a suitable function for comparing distances and dissimilarities and full details of more suitable criteria can be found in, for example, Everitt and Rabe-Hesketh (1997). This also includes a discussion of how many dimensions are needed to give an adequate fit of the geometrical model to the observed proximities.

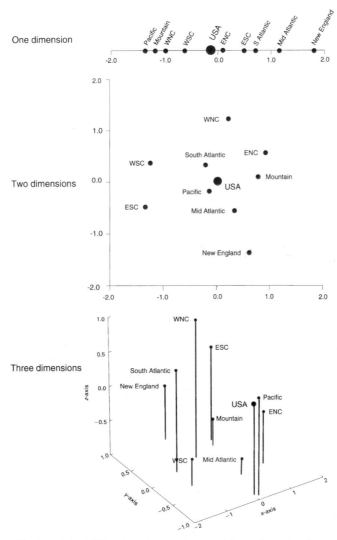

multidimensional scaling *MDS plots of the USA regions in one-, two- and three-dimensional space. Data are from monthly time series of reported measles cases 1960–90. Taken from Cliff et al, 1995*

An illustration how multidimensional scaling has been used in a medical setting is provided in Cliff *et al.* (1995). Here, a matrix of similarities is calculated in which each element is the number of months in which there were reported measles cases/deaths in both of a pair of areas. The greater the value of such a similarity, the greater the similarity of the time series of the occurrence of measles in the two areas. (In this study, the time series for each area considered consisted of monthly totals of measles cases for the 31-year period from January 1960 to December 1990.) The Figure on page 229 shows the multidimensional scaling solutions corresponding to a one-, two- and three-dimensional solution. *BSE*

Cliff, A.D., Haggett, P., Smallman-Raynor, M.R., Stroup, D.F. and Williamson, G.D. 1995: The application of multidimensional scaling methods to epidemiological data. *Statistical Methods in Medical Research* 4, 102–23. **Everitt, B.S. and Rabe-Hesketh, S.** 1997: *The analysis of proximity data.* London: Arnold.

multilevel models Multilevel (also known as random effect, hierarchical and mixed) models are an extensive and flexible class of models for correlated data, which arise widely in medical statistics. For example, adult height or weight may be correlated with those of other family members; chance of post-surgical infection may be correlated with that of other patients with the same surgical team. Further, many studies involve the repeated measurement of subjects' outcomes throughout follow-up (longitudinal data). Such observations are usually quite strongly correlated.

Multilevel models relax the assumption, required for ordinary least squares (OLS) regression, that each response is independent. They have their roots in agricultural experiments; indeed they embrace all the classical analysis of variance models. They have found ready application in social science, medical and economic research. A brief history is given by Kreft and deLeeuw (1998: 16).

The data structure is viewed as a series of levels (or hierarchies). For example, consider a multicentre trial where subjects' quantitative outcomes are recorded repeatedly over time. The first Figure shows a possible data structure. Level 1 has the repeated observations that are nested within subjects at level 2. Subjects are in turn nested within centres at level 3.

A multilevel analysis enables us to allow correctly for, and model, the correlation induced by this structure. If we have longitudinal data, we can investigate how subjects change with time, which could be quite different to the cross-sectional relationship (Diggle *et al.*, 2002: 16). In addition to the usual *fixed parameters* (whose interpretation is similar to their OLS counterparts), RANDOM EFFECTS are introduced to model the correlation structure, as described below. The mix of fixed and random effects gives rise to the term *mixed models*.

Once alerted, we see hierarchical structures everywhere; subjects within wards within counties; patients within hospitals within health authorities, and so on. Thus it is natural to ask what is gained by a multilevel model, and when they are unnecessary.

First, OLS standard errors are wrong when the data are multilevel. For example, subjects within a cluster are often similar to each other, i.e. not independent. They therefore convey less information about the value of a parameter than an independent (unclustered) sample of the same size (Goldstein, 2003: 23).

Secondly, OLS does not permit exploration of the variance structure. For example, we may wish to estimate the proportion of the total variance between subjects [the intra-cluster correlation coefficient (ICC), equation (1) below]. Or we may want to investigate how the variance changes as a function of covariates.

Multilevel models will add little to an analysis when observations are effectively independent so that the ICC is close to zero. However, it is wise to be cautious as even a small ICC can have a non-trivial effect.

The plan of this article is as follows. First, the key ideas of multilevel models are outlined, followed by a discussion of commonly used algorithms for fitting multilevel models. Then extensions to discrete data are described and the relationship to generalised estimating equations is given. Medical applications and further extensions are discussed, then missing data, design and software. Some suggestions for further reading are given at the end.

Consider the multicentre trial of the first Figure. Focusing on levels 1 and 2, we begin by describing the simplest model, which allows for correlation between the observations, before outlining how more flexible models can be built up.

The idea is to generalise OLS regression. An OLS model would have a single regression line relating the average response to time. A multilevel model, however, can be thought of as extending this to include a regression line for each subject.

Thus, whereas in OLS regression the observations are distributed about a single regression line, in multilevel models we can view each subject's responses as distributed about their subject-specific regression line. The subject-specific regression lines are then distributed about the overall average regression line.

This is illustrated in the second Figure (see page 231). Here, the overall average relationship between the response and time is given by the bold line, $Y = \alpha + \beta t$. Five subject specific regression lines are shown, which are parallel to this. Each subject's observations are distributed about their regression line. Five examples of this are given in the top half of the Figure.

In this simple case, each subject's regression line is parallel to the overall average line. The distance between the *j*th subject specific line, $Y = (\alpha + u_j) + \beta t$ and the average line $Y = \alpha + \beta t$ is u_j (in the second Figure, $j = 1, 2, 3, 4$ or 5). These u_j are known as the subject-specific *random effects*, also known as the *level 2 residuals*. They are assumed to be normally distributed about zero.

The vertical distances between each subject's responses and their subject-specific regression line are known as the *level 1 residuals*. These are analogous to the residuals in OLS models, and are likewise assumed to be normally distributed about zero.

Level 3: [**Centres**]

Level 2: [**Subjects**]

Level 1: [**Observations**]

multilevel models *Data structure for a multicentre trial*

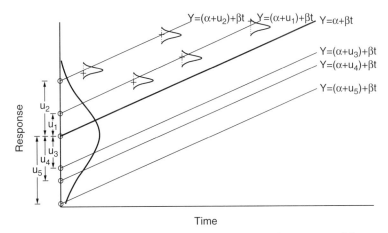

multilevel models *Schematic illustration of random intercepts model*

The normal densities of the level 2 and some level 1 residuals are shown in the second Figure. In the top half, we see five observations, marked '+'. The five vertical distances to their subject-specific regression are five level 1 residuals. The normal distribution of these residuals is illustrated by the five normal densities about the subject-specific regression lines. Then, on the left-hand side, the level 2 residuals, u_1, ..., u_5 are shown. Their normal distribution is sketched at the left-hand side of the Figure.

The parameters α and β in the Figure are known as *fixed* parameters. They have a similar interpretation to their counterparts in OLS models. So α is the average response at time zero, and β is the average change in response per unit change in time. However, we have two new parameters, known as *random parameters*, which are the variance of the level 2 residuals, called σ_u^2, and the variance of the level 1 residuals, called σ_e^2. Thus, in the second Figure, the density of the u_js is sketched on the left and has variance σ_u^2. The five densities of the level 1 residuals have common variance σ_e^2. Often, σ_u^2 is called the between-subject variance and σ_e^2 the within-subject variance.

The second Figure represents the simplest multilevel model. As each u_j can be viewed as a random contribution to the intercept of the jth person's regression line, which is $(\alpha + u_j)$, this is often known as a *random intercepts model*. It is also a simple example of a COMPONENTS OF VARIANCE model, as there is a single variance term corresponding to each level in the model (σ_u^2 for level 2, σ_e^2 for level 1).

The motivation for multilevel models was their ability to model the correlation structure of the data. We therefore consider the correlation structure implied by the random intercepts model. To do this, we have to consider the VARIANCE of each observation, and the covariance between observations.

First consider the variance. In multilevel models, the random component is the residuals. Residuals from different levels are always assumed to be independent. Likewise, residuals corresponding to different units within a level (i.e. different observations within level 1 and different subjects within level 2) are assumed to be independent. The total variance of each observation is thus the sum of the variance of the residuals at each level. Thus, in the random intercepts model, where each observation has

a residual at level 1 and level 2, the variance of an observation is $\sigma_e^2 + \sigma_u^2$.

Secondly, consider the covariance. In the random intercepts model of the second Figure, different observations from the same subject, j, share a common random component, their level 2 residual u_j. Their covariance is therefore $\mathrm{Cov}(u_j, u_j) = (u_j, u_j) = \sigma_u^2$. However, observations from different subjects share no common residuals. Their covariance is therefore zero.

Recalling that $\mathrm{Cor}(A,B) = \overline{\mathrm{Cov}(A,B)/\sqrt{Var\,(A)\,Var\,(B)}}$, we see that the correlation structure implied by the random intercepts model is:

$$\begin{cases} 1 & \text{same subject and time} \\ \rho = \sigma_u^2 / \sqrt{(\sigma_u^2 + \sigma_e^2)(\sigma_u^2 + \sigma_e^2)} = \sigma_u^2/(\sigma_u^2 + \sigma_e^2) & \text{same subject, different time} \\ 0 & \text{different subjects.} \end{cases} \quad (1)$$

Thus the random intercepts model of the second Figure implies a fixed correlation, ρ, among a subject's responses, independent of how far apart in time they are. This is known as a *compound symmetry* or *exchangeable* correlation structure.

The correlation, ρ, in (1) is also known as the *intra level-2-unit* or more commonly ICC; in random intercepts models, ρ measures the proportion of total variance, which is between subjects. If $\rho=0$, then observations are independent.

Consider how the random intercepts model illustrated in the second Figure compares to fitting an OLS line to each subject in turn. Such OLS lines would be unbiased estimates of each subject's true line. However, they might be imprecisely estimated, particularly if a subject has few observations. Conversely, the estimate of the overall average line ($\alpha + \beta t$) is a precise, but biased, estimate of each subject's true line. Both extremes are undesirable. By fitting a multilevel model, we compromise between the two extremes. The estimates of the u_js are known as 'best linear unbiased predictors' (BLUPs) and, as their name suggests, have certain optimality properties (Verbeke and Molenberghs, 2000: 80). The practical effect is that the subject-specific regression lines estimated by the multilevel model are drawn (or shrunk) closer to the mean line than the OLS estimates, and the fewer the observations on a subject, the more their line is drawn toward (borrows strength from) the mean regression line. This is often referred to as *shrinkage* in the literature.

Having fitted the random intercepts model, we should examine the level 1 and level 2 residuals to check they are approximately normal, as the multilevel model assumes, and identify outliers. Level 2 residuals can also be used to distinguish outlying subjects; this has found wide application in medical settings.

For most longitudinal data, the correlation between observations declines as the time between them increases. Thus the fixed correlation structure of the random intercepts model, ρ, is insufficient. A natural extension is to allow subjects to have their own slopes as well as their own intercepts, as illustrated in the third Figure. As before, the overall average regression line is $Y = \alpha + \beta t$. Now, though, the jth subject's regression line is $Y = (\alpha + u_j) + (\beta + v_j)t$. In the random intercepts model the u_js were normally distributed with mean 0 and variance σ_u^2. In the random intercepts and slopes model (u_j, v_j) have a bivariate normal distribution about $(0,0)$.

As before, the level 1 residuals are the vertical distances between a subject's observations and their subject-specific regression line. The level 2 residuals are now (u_j, v_j), so we have two level 2 residuals per subject, representing the random intercept and slope, respectively.

We can calculate the variance and covariance of observations, in a similar way to the random intercepts model, although the algebra is more involved. Then we can derive the correlation structure implied by this model. The variance of the responses is no longer constrained by the model to be constant; it can now increase with time. Further, the correlation between observations on the same subject can decline as the time between them increases. Hence this model is often more appropriate for longitudinal data.

The way the random intercepts and slopes model builds on the random intercepts model suggests many further extensions. To begin with, if we have additional covariates, they too can have random effects. For example, if we include a treatment variable, subject-specific treatment effects can be estimated.

Levels can be added to the model to describe additional levels in the data. For example, the first Figure (see page 230) shows subjects are nested within centres. We can extend the random intercepts model to include a random effect at the centre level. Such a model yields estimates of components of variance at each level (centre, subject and observation), so the proportion of the total variance between centres can be calculated. Further, the level 3 (centre) residuals can be examined to indicate outliers and covariates can be given random centre-level terms as well as random subject-level terms.

The level 1 variance (which is analogous to the residual variance in OLS models) can also be modelled by covariates, e.g. male level 1 residuals may be more variable than those from females. This is known as modelling *complex variation*.

Sometimes the random intercepts and slopes model is not sufficiently flexible to model the correlation structure, particularly if observations are close together in time. Many options are possible; if subjects are observed at identical times then an attractive alternative is an *unstructured* COVARIANCE MATRIX, which imposes no parametric model on the covariance. Much has been written on this; see for example Verbeke and Molenberghs (2000: chap 16) and Diggle *et al.* (2002: chap 5).

Multilevel models for quantitative data are typically based on the multivariate normal distribution. Thus, the likelihood of the data can be written down and maximised using adaptations of Newton-Raphson techniques (for details, see Raudenbush and Bryk, 2002: chap 14). Alternatively, a Bayesian approach can be adopted (see chapter by Clayton, D. G. in Gilks *et al.*, 1996).

If likelihood methods are adopted, restricted maximum likelihood (REML) is usually used (Verbeke and Molenberghs, 2000: 43). This corrects the downward bias of maximum likelihood estimates of variance and requires negligible extra work computationally. However, changes in REML log-likelihoods cannot generally be used to compare nested models; so maximum likelihood may be preferred for model building (Goldstein, 2003: 36) although in uncommon situations with many fixed parameters the two can give quite different answers (Verbeke and Molenberghs, 2000: 198).

GENERALISED LINEAR MODELS (GLMs) extend OLS models to discrete responses. Analogously, *generalised*

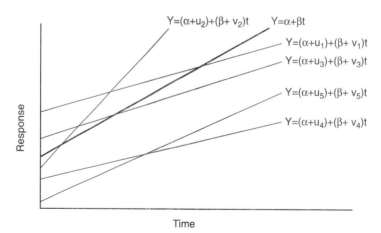

multilevel models *Schematic illustration of random intercepts and slopes model*

linear mixed models (GLMMs), sometimes called *non-linear mixed models*, extend multilevel models to discrete responses.

As with GLMs, we model a function of the probability that the response takes on a particular value. In GLMMs, though, for responses on the same subject, this probability shares a subject-specific term. For example, we can make the random intercepts model, illustrated by the second Figure, a GLMM by letting Y follow a binomial distribution, and writing the overall regression line as $\text{logit}(\text{Pr}\{Y=y\})=\alpha+\beta t$. The subject specific regression line for subject j would be

$$\text{logit}(\text{Pr}\{Y=y\})=(\alpha+u_j)+\beta t, \qquad (2)$$

and, as before, the level 2 residuals, u_j, would be normally distributed about zero with variance σ_u^2. Note that, as in GLMs, in GLMMs the level 1 variance is a fixed function of the mean. Therefore, there is no term corresponding to σ_e^2.

Also, as with GLMs, the function 'logit' in (2) is known as the link function. Alternative link functions (e.g. log, inverse normal) can be used together with other probability models such as Poisson or negative binomial.

Unfortunately, fitting GLMMs is not nearly as straightforward as fitting multilevel models to quantitative data, because the likelihood is much more difficult to compute. Three approaches, all discussed by Goldstein (2003), are commonly adopted.

First, QUASI-LIKELIHOOD. There are two forms of this, penalised quasi-likelihood and marginalised quasi-likelihood. Both methods rely on approximations, which can be made to first or second order. The approximations involved mean that quasi-likelihood methods provide biased parameter estimates; in particular, estimates of variance components tend to be downwardly biased. This bias is most marked in data sets with few level 1 units per level 2 unit or probabilities close to boundaries (e.g. 1 or 0 for binary data). The bias is least for second-order penalised quasi-likelihood. Another drawback is that, with quasi-likelihood, no estimate of the log-likelihood is available for comparing models.

The second approach relies on numerical or Monte Carlo integration methods. This is computationally considerably more intensive if several random effects or levels are involved. Nevertheless, it is becoming increasingly feasible. An additional advantage is that these methods provide an estimate of the log-likelihood, which can be used for hypothesis testing and interval estimation.

The third approach is to adopt a Bayesian formulation with uninformative priors. Many common models are implemented in MLwiN (Rasbash *et al.*, 2000), and several models are described in the WinBUGS manual (Spiegelhalter *et al.*, 1999).

Note that these methods can be extended to provide multilevel versions of more general multinomial models (see chapter by Yang, M. in Leyland and Goldstein, 2001).

Multilevel models are likelihood based. An alternative class of methods, known as GENERALISED ESTIMATING EQUATIONS (GEEs), can also be used for multilevel data (see Diggle *et al.*, 2002: chap. 11). GEEs model the mean and variance of the data only; unlike multilevel models, a probability distribution for the data (e.g. normal) is not specified. Standard errors are often estimated robustly from the sampling variance of the residuals, using the 'Huber-White' sandwich estimator (Diggle *et al.*, 2002: 80).

A theoretical advantage of GEEs is that the fixed parameter estimates are consistent (i.e. reliable if there is sufficient data) even if the covariance structure is wrongly specified; however they may be inefficient if the covariance structure is substantially mis-specified (Goldstein, 2003: 21). The drawback is that variance components are not explicitly modelled, but treated as nuisance parameters, whereas from the multilevel modelling perspective the variance components contain useful insights.

This is directly related to an important, but subtle, difference between the two. Fixed parameter estimates from multilevel models estimate the effect of a covariate on a subject *conditional on the value of their subject-specific effects*. GEE parameter estimates are marginalised over subject-specific effects; they estimate the average effect of a covariate over the population the data are drawn from. For multilevel models for quantitative data, conditional and marginal estimates of fixed parameters coincide. For discrete data they do not; often marginal estimates are markedly smaller in magnitude (compare Tables 11.1 and 8.2 in Diggle *et al.*, 2002).

The appropriate approach adopted depends on the scientific question. If the primary aim is to model the average response as a function of covariates and time, and the correlation is a nuisance, GEEs may be preferred. The resulting parameter estimates are often known as *population averaged*. Conversely, if understanding of the variance structure is important, e.g. in investigating determinants of variation in growth rates, multilevel models are required. A complication with conditional models is that, because the interpretation of the fixed parameters is conditional on the variance model, if this is changed the interpretation is generally altered.

The literature on medical applications of multilevel models is vast and growing. A good starting point is the collection of papers in Leyland and Goldstein (2001), which includes models for growth data, spatial distribution of mortality and morbidity and institutional comparisons. The latter is an important and widespread application of multilevel models.

Applications to meta-analysis are discussed by Hardy and Thompson (1996) (quantitative data) and Turner *et al.* (2000) (binary data); cross-over trials by Jones and Kenward (2003: chaps 5 and 6) and cluster randomised trials by Donner and Klar (2000).

So far, we have assumed that each subject at each time only has one response. However, the covariance model readily extends to allow multivariate responses at each time. For example, a subject's diastolic and systolic blood pressure can be modelled simultaneously (see chapter by McLeod, A. in Leyland and Goldstein, 2001).

The multilevel framework can also be extended to handle time-to-event data, with subjects having repeated events and a common frailty (the commonly adopted term for a subject-specific random effect in survival analysis). Indeed, frailties at different levels of the hierarchy can be fitted (Singer and Willett, 2002).

Another extension is what is termed 'cross-classified' data. Here subjects are members of more than one hierarchy. For example, subjects may be nested within general practices and health authorities, but may also be nested within distinct neighbourhoods, served by a number of general practices. They therefore belong to more than one hierarchy. Parameter estimation is no longer always straightforward (Goldstein, 2003: chap. 11).

Frequently in studies involving longitudinal follow-up, a proportion of the intended responses will be unobserved. An important advantage of multilevel models over classical techniques is that a complete set of observations on each subject included in the analysis is not required; subjects can still be included in the analysis with partially observed response data.

Further, if subjects are missing responses, or drop out, then provided that, given their observed data, the reason for drop-out does not depend on the unseen responses (the missing at random, MAR, assumption), parameter estimates from multilevel models are still valid (Little and Rubin, 2002). Thus, if data are analysed using multilevel models, and response data are MAR, ad-hoc imputation techniques such as replacing a missing observation by the previous seen observation (LOCF) are not required; indeed they will generally introduce bias (Molenberghs et al., 2004). Sensitivity to MAR can be assessed; see e.g. Carpenter et al. (2002).

However, parameter estimates from GEEs are not valid under MAR; to guarantee their validity a stronger assumption, missing completely at random (MCAR) is required. This assumption states that the reason for a subject's unobserved data is independent of both their observed and unobserved data. Although GEEs can be modified to cope with MAR data, to do this efficiently requires a non-trivial multistage estimation process.

The above does not apply to missing covariate information; if a non-trivial degree of covariate information is missing, it usually needs to be recovered using appropriate data imputation methods.

The generality of multilevel models means that the distribution of many test statistics is only known under the null hypothesis, so simulation often has to be employed in sample size calculations. Simplifying assumptions enable progress in special cases (Diggle et al., 2002: 24).

As multilevel models become more mainstream, software to fit the basic models for quantitative data is becoming increasingly available in standard packages. All the models described here can be fitted using MLwiN (Rasbash et al., 2000); many can be fitted using PROCs MIXED, GLMMIX and NLMIXED in SAS version 8.x (SAS, v. 8.1, 2002). For very large datasets, SAS is preferable. A comprehensive review of the capabilities of available packages is given on the MLwiN website, www.mlwin.com.

Bayesian model fitting can be performed with the WinBUGS package (Spiegelhalter et al., 1999). This is very flexible, but the user is required to write the program to fit the model, and a degree of knowledge about Markov chain Monte-Carlo methods is required.

Newcomers to multilevel modelling should start with one of the many excellent books now available. The least technical of these is Kreft and deLeeuw (1998), which gives a basic introduction to models for quantitative data, from a social science perspective. The software MLwiN (Rasbash et al., 2000) also comes with an accessible manual and many examples. Raudenbush and Bryk (2002) give a much more extensive treatment, including discrete response models, with many detailed social science examples.

For the methodologically inclined, Verbeke and Molenberghs (2000) give a comprehensive overview for quantitative data from a longitudinal perspective. Examples are analysed in detail using mostly SAS (SAS, v. 8.1, 2002) and some MLwiN (Rasbash et al., 2000) and SPLUS (SPLUS v. 6, 2003). The latter half is given over to problems with missing data. Less detailed but more general is Diggle et al. (2002), who also come from a longitudinal standpoint, and discuss quantitative and discrete data, multilevel models, GEEs and transition models. Most recently, Goldstein (2003) gives a comprehensive account of the current state of multilevel modelling, including outlines of technical details and many illustrative examples.   *JRC*

[**Acknowledgement:** James R. Carpenter was supported by ESRC Research Methods Programme grant H333250047, titled 'Missing data in multi-level models'.]

Carpenter, J., Pocock, S. and Lamm, C.J. 2002: Coping with missing data in clinical trials: a model based approach applied to asthma trials. *Statistics in Medicine* 21, 1043–66. **Diggle, P.J., Heagerty, P., Liang, K.Y. and Zeger, S.L.** 2002: *Analysis of longitudinal data*, 2nd edn. Oxford: Oxford University Press. **Donner, A. and Klar, N.** 2000: *Design and analysis of cluster randomization trials in health research.* London: Arnold. **Gilks, W.R., Richardson, S. and Spiegelhalter, D.J.** (eds) 1996: *Markov chain Monte-Carlo in practice.* London: Chapman and Hall. **Goldstein, H.** 2003: *Multilevel statistical models*, 2nd edn. London: Arnold. **Hardy, R.J. and Thompson, S.G.** 1996: A likelihood approach to meta-analysis with random effects. *Statistics in Medicine* 15, 619–29. **Jones, B. and Kenward, M.G.** 2003: *Design and analysis of cross-over trials*, 2nd edn. London: Chapman and Hall. **Kreft, I. and de Leeuw, J.** 1998: *Introducing multilevel modelling.* London: Sage. **Leyland, A.H. and Goldstein, H.** (eds) 2001: *Multilevel modelling of health statistics.* Chichester: Wiley. **Little, R.J.A. and Rubin, D.B.** 2002: *Statistical analysis with missing data*, 2nd edn. Chichester: Wiley. **Molenberghs, G., Thijs, H., Jansen, I., Beunkens, C., Kenward, M.G., Mallinkrodt, C. and Carroll, R.J.** 2004: Analyzing incomplete longitudinal clinical trial data. *Biostatistics* 5, 445–64. **Rasbash, J., Browne, W., Goldstein, H., Yang, M., Plewis, I., Healy, M., Woodhouse, G., Draper, D., Langford, I. and Lewis, T.** 2000: *A user's guide to MLwiN (version 2.1).* London: Institute of Education, 20 Bedford Way. **Raudenbush, S.W. and Bryk, A.S.** 2002: *Hierarchical linear models: applications and data analysis methods*, 2nd edn. London: Sage. **SAS, v. 8.1.** 2002: SAS Worldwide Headquarters, SAS Campus Drive Cary, NC 27513-2414, USA, www.sas.com. **Singer, J.D. and Willett, J.B.** 2002: *Applied longitudinal data analysis: modelling change and event occurrence.* New York: Oxford University Press. **Spiegelhalter, D.J., Thomas, A. and Best, N.G.** 1999: *WinBUGS version 1.2 user manual.* Cambridge: MRC Biostatistics Unit. **SPLUS v. 6.** 2003: Insightful Switzerland, Christoph Merian-Ring 11, 4153 Reinach, Switzerland. **Turner, R.M., Omar, R.Z., Yang, M., Goldstein, H. and Thompson, S.G.** 2000: A multilevel model framework for meta-analysis of clinical trials with binary outcomes. *Statistics in Medicine* 19, 3417–32. **Verbeke, G. and Molenberghs, G.** 2000: *Linear mixed models for longitudinal data.* New York: Springer Verlag.

multinomial distribution

A generalisation of the BINOMIAL DISTRIBUTION to the case where more than two outcomes are possible for every 'trial'. Whereas the binomial distribution addresses the number of successes (and thus implicitly the number of failures also) in the case where every event or trial can only result in a success or a failure, the multinomial distribution models the numbers of each outcome in the case where each event or trial can have one of multiple outcomes.

For example, Lossos *et al.* (2000) note that, when modelling genetic mutations in a situation with four rather than two distinct genotypes, it is necessary to extend the usual binomial model to a multinomial one.

In general, for n observations, each of which can independently take one of N mutually exclusive outcomes with probabilities $p_1, p_2, ..., p_N$ (where $p_1 + p_2 + ... + p_N = 1$), then the probability of seeing x_1 observations achieving outcome 1, x_2 observations achieving outcome 2 etc. where $x_1 + x_2 + ... + x_N = n$ is given by:

$$\Pr[(X_1, X_2, ..., X_N) = (x_1, x_2, ..., x_N)] = \frac{n!}{x_1! x_2! ... x_N!} p_1^{x_1} p_2^{x_2} ... p_N^{x_N}$$

where $n!$ (factorial n) is the product of all the integers up to and including n, namely, $n \times (n-1) \times (n-2) \times ... \times 3 \times 2 \times 1$, with 0! defined to be 1.

Note that since the data are multidimensional, there is no single mean value of the distribution as such, although (as for the binomial distribution) the expected number to be seen with outcome k is $p_k n_k$. *AGL*

Lossos, I.S., Tibshirani, R., Narasimhan, B. and Levy R. 2000: The inference of antigen selection on Ig genes. *Journal of Immunology* 165, 5122–6.

multiple comparisons

Procedures for a detailed examination of where differences between a set of means lie, usually applied after a significant F-test in an ANALYSIS OF VARIANCE has led to the rejection that all the means are equal. A large number of multiple comparison techniques have been proposed but no single technique is best in all situations. The major distinction between the techniques is how they control the inflation of the TYPE I ERROR that would occur if, for example, a simple STUDENTS t-TEST was applied to test the equality of each pairs of means.

One very simple procedure for dealing with the inflation procedure is to judge the P-values from each t-test against a significance level of α/m rather than α, the nominal size of the Type I error, where m is the number of t-tests performed – this is known as the BONFERRONI CORRECTION. Many alternatives approaches are available, most of which are based on the usual t-statistic, but which differ in the choice of critical value against which the t-statistic is compared. A comprehensive account of multiple comparisons procedures is given in Hsu (1996). *BSE*

Hsu, J.C. 1996: *Multiple comparisons*. London: Chapman & Hall.

multiple correlation coefficient See CORRELATION

multiple imputation

A method by which missing values in a dataset are replaced by more than one, usually between 3 and 10, simulated versions. Each of the simulated complete datasets is then analysed by the method relevant to the investigation to hand and the results combined to produce estimates, standard errors and CONFIDENCE INTERVALS that incorporate MISSING DATA uncertainty. Introducing appropriate random error into the imputation process makes it possible to get approximately unbiased estimates of all parameters, although the data must be missing at random for this to be the case. The multiple imputations themselves are created by a Bayesian approach (see BAYESIAN METHODS), which requires specification of a parametric model for the complete data and, if necessary, a model for the mechanism by which data become missing. A comprehensive account of multiple imputation and details of associated software are given in Schafer (1997). *BSE*

[See also DROPOUTS]

Schafer, J. 1997: *The analysis of incomplete multivariate data*. Boca Raton: CRC/Chapman & Hall.

multiple linear regression

A technique used to model, or characterise quantitatively, the relationship between a response variable, y, and a set of explanatory variables, $x_1, x_2, ..., x_q$. The explanatory variables are strictly assumed to be known or under the control of the investigator, i.e. they are not considered to be random variables. In practice, where this is rarely the case, the results from a multiple regression analysis are interpreted as being conditional on the observed values of the explanatory variables. The multiple regression model can be written as:

$$y = \beta_0 + \beta_1 x_1 + ... + \beta_q x_q + \varepsilon$$

where β_0 is an intercept and $\beta_1, \beta_2 \cdots \beta_q$ regression coefficients that measure the change in the response variable associated with a unit change in the corresponding explanatory variable, conditional on the other explanatory variables remaining constant. If the explanatory variables are highly correlated such an interpretation is problematic. The residual, ε, is assumed to have a normal distribution with mean zero and variance σ^2. An alternative way of writing the multiple regression model is that y is distributed normally with mean μ and variance σ^2, where $\mu = \beta_0 + \beta_1 x_1 + ... + \beta_q x_q$. This formulation makes it clear that the model is only suitable for continuous response variables with, conditional on the values of the explanatory variables, a normal distribution with constant variance. For a sample of n response values along with the corresponding values of the explanatory variables the aim of multiple regression is to arrive at a set of values for the regression coefficients that make the values of the response variable predicted from the model as 'close' as possible to the observed response values. Estimation of the parameters of the model $(\beta_1, \beta_2 \cdots \beta_q)$ is usually by LEAST SQUARES (see Rawlings, Pantula and Dickey, 1998). The variation in the response variable can be partitioned into a part due to regression on the explanatory variables and a residual. This partition can be set out in an ANALYSIS OF VARIANCE-type table of the form:

Source	df	SS	MS	MSR
Regression	q	RGSS	RGSS/q	RGMS/RSMS
Residual	n – q – 1	RSS	RSS/(n – q – 1)	

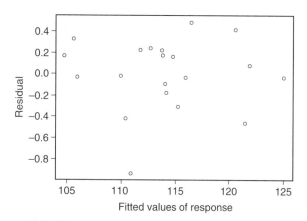

multiple linear regression *Residuals plotted against fitted values*

Under the null hypothesis that all the regression coefficients, $\beta_1, \beta_2 \cdots \beta_q$, are zero, the mean square ratio (MSR) in this table can be tested against an F-DISTRIBUTION with q and $n - q - 1$ DEGREES OF FREEDOM. The residual mean square is an estimator of σ^2 and is used in calculating standard errors of the estimated regression coefficients (see Rawlings, Pantula and Dickey, 1998). The MULTIPLE CORRELATION COEFFICIENT is the correlation between the observed values of the response and the values predicted by the model. The square of the multiple correlation coefficient gives the proportion of the variance of the response that can be explained by the explanatory variables.

The overall test that all the regression coefficients in a multiple regression model are zero is seldom of great interest. The investigator is more likely to be concerned with assessing whether some subset of the explanatory variables might be almost as successful as the full set in explaining the variation in the response variable, i.e. a more parsimonious model is sought. Various procedures have been suggested to help in this search (see ALL SUBSETS REGRESSION, AUTOMATIC SELECTION PROCEDURES).

Once a final model has been settled on, the assumptions of the multiple linear regression approach for the data to hand need to be checked. One way to investigate the possible failings of a model is to examine what are known as *residuals*, defined as:

residual = observed response value – predicted response value

The n sample residuals can be plotted in a variety of ways to assess particular assumptions of the multiple regression model: a HISTOGRAM or STEM-AND-LEAF PLOT of the residuals can be useful in checking for normality of the error terms in the model; plots of the residuals against the corresponding values of each explanatory variables may help to uncover when the relationship between the response and an explanatory variable is more complex than that originally assumed; for example, it may suggest that a quadratic term is needed to model a 'U-shape' or 'J-shape' apparent relationship; a plot of the residuals against the fitted values may identify that for example, the presence of the multivariate OUTLIERS worthy of further investigation and checking or perhaps that the vari-

ance of the response increases with the fitted values, suggesting that a transformation of the response should be considered. There are now many other regression diagnostics available (see, for example, Lovie, 1991).

To illustrate multiple regression we shall use the data shown in the first Table. These data arise from a study of 20 patients with hypertension (Daniel, 1995). In practice, of course, there would be too few patients to allow a sensible analysis with seven explanatory variables. The response variable here is mean arterial blood pressure (mmHg).

The least square estimates of the regression parameters are shown in the second Table. The square of the multiple

multiple linear regression *Data for 20 patients with hypertension*

	BP	Age	Weight	BA	TimeHt	Pulse	Stress
1	105	47	85.4	1.75	5.1	63	33
2	115	49	94.2	2.10	3.8	70	14
3	116	49	95.3	1.98	8.2	72	10
4	117	50	94.7	2.01	5.8	73	99
5	112	51	89.4	1.89	7.0	72	95
6	121	48	99.5	2.25	9.3	71	10
7	121	49	99.8	2.25	2.5	69	42
8	110	47	90.9	1.90	6.2	66	8
9	110	49	89.2	1.83	7.1	69	62
10	114	48	92.7	2.07	5.6	64	35
11	114	47	94.4	2.07	5.3	74	90
12	115	49	94.1	1.98	5.6	71	21
13	114	50	91.6	2.05	10.2	68	47
14	106	45	87.1	1.92	5.6	67	80
15	125	52	101.3	2.19	10.0	76	98
16	114	46	94.5	1.98	7.4	69	95
17	106	46	87.0	1.87	3.6	62	18
18	113	46	94.5	1.90	4.3	70	12
19	110	48	90.5	1.88	9.0	71	99
20	122	56	95.7	2.07	7.0	75	99

BP: Mean arterial blood pressure (mmHg)
Age: Age in years
Weight: Weight in kg
BA: Body surface area (square metres)
TimeHt: Duration of hypertension (years)
Pulse: Basal pulse (beats/mim)
Stress: Measure of stress

multiple linear regression *Results for data in the first Table*

Term	Estimated regression coefficient	Standard error	T-value	P-value
(Intercept)	−12.8705	2.5566	−5.0341	0.0002
Age	0.7033	0.0496	14.771	0.0000
Weight	0.9699	0.0631	15.3691	0.0000
BA	3.7765	1.5802	2.3900	0.0327
TimeHT	0.0684	0.0484	1.4117	0.1815
Pulse	−0.0845	0.0516	−1.6370	0.1256
Stress	0.0056	0.0034	1.6328	0.1265

Residual standard error: 0.4072 on 13 degrees of freedom
Multiple R-Squared: 0.9962

correlation coefficient is 0.99, and the mean square ratio described above takes the value 560.6; tested against an F-distribution with 6 and 13 degrees of freedom the associated P-VALUE is extremely small. Clearly, the hypothesis that all the regression coefficients are zero can be safely rejected. For these data the sample size is too small for residual plots to be particularly informative. But, for interest, the Figure on page 236 shows a plot of residual against fitted values. The plot gives no cause for concern in respect of the constant variance assumption.   *BSE*

[See also GENERALISED LINEAR MODELS, LOGISTIC REGRESSION]

Daniel, W. 1995: *Biostatistics: a foundation for analysis in the health sciences*, 6th edn. New York: John Wiley & Sons. **Lovie, P.** 1991: Regression diagnostics. In Lovie, P. and Lovie, A.D. (eds), *New developments in statistics for psychology and the social sciences*. London: Routledge. **Rawlings, J.O., Pantula, S.G. and Dickey, D.A.** 1998: *Applied regression analysis: a research tool*. New York: Springer.

multiple record systems   See CAPTURE-RECAPTURE METHODS

multiple testing   See ANALYSIS OF VARIANCE, MULTIPLE COMPARISON PROCEDURES, PITFALLS IN MEDICAL RESEARCH

multistage cluster sample   A non-probabilistic method of sampling used when members of a population are arranged in subgroups or clusters. In this method clusters are the sampling unit rather than individuals. Members within a cluster should be as different as possible whereas clusters, by way of contrast, should be as alike as possible. However, this condition is hard to satisfy and since two members of a cluster will be more alike than two from different clusters, it is better to have many small clusters than a few large clusters, as this reduces sampling error. Each cluster should be similar to the total population but on a smaller scale. Clusters must be distinct from each other and every member of the population should fall within a cluster. In some situations, it is necessary for all clusters to be a similar size and this may require the pooling of some clusters. Otherwise, the probability that a cluster is chosen can be made proportional to its size, so that bigger clusters are more likely to be chosen than smaller clusters and the probability of selecting an individual member of the cluster is inversely proportional to the size of the cluster.

For a single-stage cluster sample a list of the clusters is constructed. Then a RANDOM SAMPLE of the clusters is taken. This may be a simple random sample, with each cluster having an equal probability of being included in the sample, or it may be that the probability of being in the sample can be proportional to the size of the cluster. Once the clusters have been selected each member of the cluster is included in the sample.

For a two-stage cluster sample the method is the same as a single-stage cluster sample but once the clusters have been selected then a simple random sample is used to select the members of cluster to be included in the sample. Clusters may also form larger clusters, in which case, multistage sampling would be used. First the clusters would be sampled, followed by the sub-clusters. Depending on the makeup of the population there may be many stages to the multistage sampling.

Multistage cluster sampling was used in a study of violations of the international code of marketing of breast milk substitutes (Taylor, 1998). Here, the capital city of four chosen countries were the main cluster, districts were randomly selected sub-clusters, health facilities were randomly selected from the sub-clusters and mothers were systematically sampled from the health facilities.

The main advantage is that no sampling frame is required. The main disadvantage is that the sampling is non-random and sampling error increases by taking multiple samples, as there is sampling error at each stage.   *SLV*

Crawshaw, J. and Chambers, J. 1994: *A concise course in A level statistics*, 3rd edn. Cheltenham: Stanley Thornes Publishers Ltd. **Taylor, A.** 1998: Violations of the international code of marketing of breast milk substitutes: prevalence in four countries. *British Medical Journal* 316, 1117–22.

multivariate analysis of variance (MANOVA)
See ANALYSIS OF VARIANCE

multivariate normal distribution   A generalisation of the NORMAL DISTRIBUTION to more than one dimension and the probability law that underlies many methods of multivariate analysis.

Any dataset comprises measurements made on a collection of individuals, and all measurements exhibit variation between individuals. A graphical presentation, such as a HISTOGRAM, of all the population values would show the range of variation as well as the relative preponderance of some values over others. Such a histogram would thus allow the calculation of probabilities of observing particular sample values and this in turn would form a quantitative basis for methods of statistical analysis.

However, such histograms can never be obtained and must instead be modelled by theoretical probability distributions. Many such distributions exist, but the one that is used most often in statistical analysis is the normal distribution. Many measurements have been empirically shown to follow normal distributions, while the central limit theorem provides a mathematical justification whenever the measurements represent either sums or means of quantities (see Nolan, 1998).

For a single variable, the normal distribution is characterised by a bell-shaped curve centred at its mean μ and with width governed by its variance σ^2; these are the parameters of the distribution. In the multivariate case, the curve becomes a surface in multidimensional space, while the parameters include not only the means and variances of each variable but also the covariances between all pairs of variables.

The multivariate normal distribution is a relatively simple distribution to handle and it has a number of attractive properties. All marginal and conditional distributions of subsets of a multivariate normal set of measurements are themselves multivariate normal, as are all collections of linear combinations of these variables. In particular, the marginal or conditional distribution of any single such measurement, or the distribution of a single linear combination, is univariate normal. Since many techniques of multivariate analysis involve consideration of either linear combinations or subsets of measurements, these properties make the multivariate distribution a very attractive model to use as a basis for these techniques.

To delve any further into the multivariate normal distribution requires considerable technical mathematics; the interested reader is referred to any standard multivariate text, e.g. Morrison (1990).   *WK*

Morrison, D.F. 1990: *Multivariate statistical methods*, 3rd edn. New York: McGraw-Hill. **Nolan, D.** 1998: Central limit theorem. In Armitage, P. and Colton, T. (eds), *Encyclopedia of biostatistics*. Chichester: John Wiley & Sons.

N

negative binomial distribution The PROBABILITY DISTRIBUTION of the number of events required in order to observe k 'successes'. Contrast this with the BINOMIAL DISTRIBUTION, which models the number of successes that will occur given a fixed number of trials. Also note that, since the GEOMETRIC DISTRIBUTION models the number of events required to observe one success, it is a special case of the negative binomial. An alternative formulation in terms of the number of failures required in order to observe k successes is also common.

If each event independently has a probability of success, p, then the probability mass function for the number of events, x, required before observing k successes is:

$$\Pr(X = x) = \frac{(x-1)!}{(k-1)!(x-k)!} p^k (1-p)^{x-k}$$

where $n!$ (factorial n) is the product of all the integers up to and including n, and $0!$ is defined to be 1. The MEAN of the distribution is k/p and the VARIANCE is $k(1-p)/p^2$.

The distribution can be generalised to the case where the k parameter is not an integer (by replacing the factorial terms with gamma functions as mentioned in GAMMA DISTRIBUTION), which then enables the following interpretation.

Suppose we have observations of count data from a population of size N, where each person's count will be independently distributed as Poisson with some parameter λ. In this case, we would expect the number of people with each value of count to be distributed again as a POISSON DISTRIBUTION.

For example, if we were looking to model the number of injuries per year that resulted in hospitalisation in a sample of 1000 people, we might obtain observations as in the Table. Attempting to fit a Poisson distribution to these data is clearly not satisfactory. This is not surprising, since the variance of the raw data exceeds the mean considerably and the Poisson distribution has the variance equal to the mean. One possible explanation for this is that the value λ is not constant for every individual in the population (i.e. in this example some women are more accident prone than others), but varies according to some distribution. This variation in λ will lead to greater variation in the observed frequencies that a Poisson distribution will not be able to model.

Specifically, if λ varies according to a gamma distribution, then the frequencies will be distributed as a negative binomial distribution. In this example, we can see that the negative binomial provides a much better fit than the Poisson. Further discussion of this phenomenon can be found in Glynn and Buring (1996). *AGL*

Gelman, A., Carlin, J.B., Stern, H.S. and Rubin, D.B. 1995: *Bayesian data analysis*. Boca Rotan: Chapman & Hall/CRC. Glynn, R.J. and Buring, J.E. 1994: Ways of measuring rates of recurrent events. *British Medical Journal* 312, 364–7. Grimmet, G.R. and Stirzaker, D.R. 1992: *Probability and random processes*, 2nd edn. Oxford: Clarendon Press.

negative predictive value (NPV) Defined for a diagnostic test for a particular condition as the PROBABILITY that those who have a negative test do not actually have the condition under investigation as measured by a reference or 'gold' standard. (Contrast with POSITIVE PREDICTIVE VALUE.)

If the data are set out as in the Table, then $NPV = \dfrac{d}{c+d}$.

NPV can also be expressed as a percentage.

negative predictive value *General table of test results among $a + b + c + d$ individuals sampled*

	Present	Disease absent	Total
Positive	a	b	$a + b$
Negative	c	d	$c + d$
Total	$a + c$	$b + d$	$a + b + c + d$

The NPV should be presented with CONFIDENCE INTERVALS (typically set at 95%) calculated using an appropriate method such as that of Wilson that will not produce impossible values (percentages greater than 100 or below 0) when NPV approaches extreme values. *CLC*

[See also FALSE NEGATIVE RATE, FALSE POSITIVE RATE, NEGATIVE PREDICTIVE VALUE SENSITIVITY, SPECIFICITY]

Altman, D.G., Machin, D., Bryant, T.N. and Gardner, M.J. 2000: *Statistics with confidence*, 2nd edn, London: BMJ Books.

negative binomial distribution *Simulated data showing the numbers of people suffering injuries that require hospitalisation*

No. of injuries	Observations	Expected from a Poisson distribution	Fitted via negative binomial distribution
0	735	687	727
1	195	258	198
2	43	49	54
3	18	6	15
4	6	1	4
5	1	0	1
6	2	0	0

nested case-control studies A form of CASE-CONTROL STUDY in which the cases and controls are drawn from within a larger study. In other words, they are nested within a parent study, which is usually a COHORT STUDY but sometimes a cross-sectional or prevalence study. The nested nature of such studies provides the method's strength. One concern in the design of case-control studies is the appropriate choice of controls, all of whom should be eligible to be cases if they were to develop the disease. A case-control study nested within a cohort study overcomes this concern as a control within the cohort who developed the disease would be counted as a case. Usually, but not necessarily, the controls who are chosen are matched to the cases on various confounding factors such as age and sex.

The usual reason for conducting a nested case-control study, rather than analysing data on the entire cohort or survey, is economy. Usually more data are collected on the participants of the nested study than in the main study. Sometimes these data are derived from the analysis of stored samples, blood or urine for example, or from further information being obtained from the participants.

In a study to examine the role of sex steroid hormones in relation to endometrial cancer, Lukanova et al. (2004) nested a case-control study within three large cohort studies from the Italy, Sweden and United States. The cohorts comprised over 65,000 women from whom venous blood samples had been taken at enrolment in the cohorts. From within the cohorts, 124 cases of endometrial cancer were identified and 2 controls per case were chosen from within the same cohort as the case, and matched on various factors including date of and age at blood donation. In this way, they were able to confine the processing of the samples to the 124 cases and corresponding controls, providing a great saving on processing samples from all participants in the three cohorts, yet without major loss of statistical POWER.

While the processing of blood samples is often a component of nested case-control studies, other samples can be the focus. In a study to assess the role of selenium in coronary heart disease in men, toenail clippings were obtained for selenium analysis (Yoshizawa et al. 2003). The study was nested within the Health Professionals' Study in the United States, which is a cohort study of over 50,000 men. Within the cohort 470 participants developed coronary heart disease and a matched control was chosen for each one. Thus, fewer than 1000 toenail samples had to be analysed for selenium.

The cost of sample processing is not the only reason for conducting a nested case-control study. While information collected on the cohort is of interest, sometimes further data collection is required. For example, London et al. (2003) conducted a case-control study of breast cancer nested within a cohort study of more than 50,000 women. Their interest was in residential magnetic field exposure and for this they were able to focus on the 743 cases identified in the cohort as having breast cancer and a comparable number of controls. Detailed assessment of the magnetic field exposure was made in the homes of the selected participants. Data on other risk factors for breast cancer and possible confounding factors were already available in the data that had been collected for the entire cohort.

Case-control studies can also be nested within cross-sectional surveys. Baker et al. (2003) conducted a survey of approximately 3000 men in southern England to ascertain the prevalence of knee disorders in the general population. A nested case-control component considered the cases who had undergone knee surgery. The focus was on occupational and sporting activities. The activities undertaken by the cases at the birthday prior to their reported onset of symptoms were considered. For each case, five controls were selected matched to the case within 1 year of age. The activities undertaken by the controls at the same

birthday as the case were then considered. The nested case-control study thus allowed the investigators to avoid BIAS due to the cases being likely to give up activities at an earlier age than the controls, because of knee pain. A matched analysis was required and thus the entire CROSS-SECTIONAL STUDY was a weaker tool for this particular analysis than the matched nested case-control method.

A further variant on the method is to nest a case-control study within a large routine data collection system. Agerbo (2003) analysed the risk of suicide in relation to spouse's psychiatric illness or suicide. The data were obtained by linking the Danish population registers using the unique personal identification numbers assigned to all people in the country. All suicides were identified, as were 20 matched controls per case. All the spouses and children living with the cases and controls were identified from the registers, along with information on diagnoses from the Danish psychiatric register. The study showed that there was a greater risk of suicide among those whose spouse had been admitted to hospital with a psychiatric disorder or who had died, particularly if the death had been by suicide. Few countries are able to conduct such studies as the linkage between record systems is not possible or is not allowed, but where it is possible, such as in Scandinavia, the opportunities for such epidemiological studies are great.

In a cohort study in which cases are recruited prospectively it is possible that controls identified at one time point become cases later. This is particularly likely to happen if the disease is common. An example of this is a nested case-control study within a birth cohort in Sweden (Emenius et al., 2003). Here the focus was on recurrent wheezing in children in relation to nitrogen dioxide exposure. Wheezing is common in childhood and cases were identified from assessment of the cohort at 1 and 2 years of age. Controls were chosen from within the cohort and matched to the cases on day of birth. Three controls, selected to match cases identified at the age of 1 year, were found to be wheezing at the 2-year assessment and so were also included as cases at that time point. Such nested case-control studies in which controls can become cases are sometimes called case-cohort studies. *HI*

[See also BIRTH COHORT STUDIES, CASE-CONTROL STUDIES]

Agerbo, E. 2003: Risk of suicide and spouse's psychiatric illness or suicide: nested case-control study. *British Medical Journal* 327, 1025–6. **Baker, P., Reading, I., Cooper, C. and Coggon, D.** 2003: Knee disorders in the general population and their relation to occupation. *Occupational and Environmental Medicine* 60, 794–7. **Emenius, G., Pershagen, G., Berglind, N., Kwan, H.-J., Lewné, M., Nordvall, S.L. and Wickman, M.** 2003: NO$_2$ as a marker of air pollution, and recurrent wheezing in children: a nested case-control study within the BAMSE birth cohort. *Occupational and Environmental Medicine* 60, 876–81. **London, S.J., Pogoda, J.M., Hwang, K.L., Langholz, B., Monroe, R., Kolonel, L.N., Kaune, W.T., Peters, J.M. and Henderson, B.E.** 2003: Residential magnetic field exposure and breast cancer risk: a nested case-control study from a multiethnic cohort in Los Angeles County, California. *American Journal of Epidemiology* 158, 969–80. **Lukanova, A., Lundin, E., Micheli, A., Arslan, A., Ferrari, P., Rinaldi, S., Krogh, V., Lenner, P., Shore, R.E., Biessy, C., Muti, P., Riboli, E., Koenig, K.L., Levitz, M., Stattin, P., Berrino, F., Hallmans, G., Kaaks, R., Toniolo, P. and Zeleniuch-Jacquotte, A.** 2004: Circulating levels of sex steroid hormones and risk of endometrial cancer in post-menopausal women. *International Journal of Cancer* 108, 425–32.

Yoshizawa, K., Ascherio, A., Morris, J.S., Stampfer, M.J., Giovannucci, E., Baskett, C.K., Willett, W.C. and Rimm, E.B. 2003: Prospective study of selenium levels in toenails and risk of coronary heart disease in men. *American Journal of Epidemiology* 158, 852–60.

net monetary benefit (NMB) See COST-EFFECTIVE-NESS ANALYSIS

net reproduction rate (NRR) See DEMOGRAPHY

neural networks A general class of algorithms for MACHINE LEARNING. A neural network can be described as a parameterised class of functions, specified by a weighted graph (the network's architecture). The weights associated with the edges of the graph are the parameters. Originally, neural networks were motivated by analogy with the structure of the brain. The nodes of the neural network correspond to the neurons and the edges to neuron interactions.

For directed graphs, we can distinguish recurrent architectures (containing cycles) and feed-forward architectures (acyclic). A very important special case of feed-forward networks is given by layered networks, in which the nodes of the graph are organised into layers such that connections are possible only between elements of two consecutive layers. The weight between the jth unit and the kth unit of successive layers $l-1$ and l in a network is indicated with w_{kj} and it is often assumed that all elements of a layer are connected to all elements of the successive layer (fully connected architecture). In this way, the connections between two layers $l-1$ and l can be represented by a weight matrix W_l, whose entry at row k and column j corresponds to the weight w_{kj} of the edge from node j to node k in the successive layers (see Figure). It is customary to call the first layer the input layer and the last one the output layer. The remaining ones are called hidden layers.

A 'perceptron' can be described as a network of this type with no hidden layers. It can also be seen as the building block of complex networks, in that each unit can be regarded as a perceptron (if instead of the transfer function one uses a threshold function, returning Boolean values). Therefore, layered feed-forward neural networks

as described above are also often referred to as 'multilayer perceptrons'.

In a layered network, the function is computed sequentially, assigning the value of the argument to the input layer, then calculating the activation level of the successive layers as described later, until the output layer is reached. The output of the function computed by the network is the activation value of the output unit.

All units in a layer are updated simultaneously, all the layers are updated sequentially, based on the output of the previous layer. The units of layer l calculate their output values y_l by a linear combination of the values at the previous layer y_{l-1}, followed by a nonlinear transformation $t:R{\rightarrow}R$, as follows: $y_l = t(W_l y_{l-1})$ where W_l is the edge weight matrix between layer $l-1$ and layer l, and where t is called the *transfer function*. A common choice for this transfer function is the logistic function $f(z) = \dfrac{1}{1 + e^{-z}}$.

Notice that each neural network thus represents a class of nonlinear functions parameterised by the weights whose values determine the input/output behaviour of the neural network. Training the network amounts to choosing the values of the weights automatically.

For this, a (labelled) training dataset is needed and an error function for the performance of the network has to be fixed. Training a neural network can then be done by finding those weights that minimise the network's error on such sample (i.e. by fitting the network to the data).

More concretely, in the parameter space the error function evaluated on the training data translates to a cost function that associates each configuration of the edge weights with a given error on the training set. Such function is typically non-convex, so that it can be minimised only locally, which is often done by gradient descent. A technique known as 'back propagation' provides a way to compute the necessary gradients efficiently, allowing the network to find a local minimum of the training error with respect to network weights.

The fact that the training algorithm is thus only guaranteed to converge to a local minimum implies that the solution is affected by the initial estimate for the weights. This is one of the major problems of neural networks. Also problematic is the design of the architecture (for example, the size and the number of hidden layers), often chosen as the result of trial and error. Some such problems have been overcome by the introduction of the related method of SUPPORT VECTOR MACHINES.

Other types of network arise from different design choices. For example, radial basis function networks use a different transfer function; Kohonen networks are used for clustering problems; Hopfield networks for combinatorial optimisation problems. Different training methods also exist. *NC/TDB*

[See also CLUSTER ANALYSIS IN MEDICINE]

Baldi, P. 1998: *Bioinformatics: a machine learning approach.* Cambridge, MA: MIT Press. **Bishop, C.** 1996: *Neural networks for pattern recognition.* Oxford: Oxford University Press. **Cristianini, N. and Shawe-Taylor, J.** 2000: *An introduction to support vector machines.* Cambridge: Cambridge University Press. **Mitchell, T.** 1995: *Machine learning.* Maidenhead: McGraw-Hill.

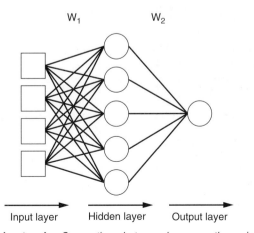

neural networks *Connections between layers on the weight matrix*

W₁   W₂

Input layer   Hidden layer   Output layer

NMB Abbreviation for net monetary benefit. See COST-EFFECTIVENESS ANALYSIS.

N-of-1 trials

An N-of-1 (or single-patient) trial combines clinical practice with the well-established methodology of the randomised controlled trial, to compare the effectiveness of two or more treatment options within an individual. The N-of-1 trial offers a design that facilitates identification of responders and non-responders to treatment and subsequent determination of optimum therapy for the individual. Indeed, within the context of the hierarchy of evidence-based study designs, it has recently been suggested that N-of-1 trials deliver the highest strength of evidence for making individual patient treatment decisions (Guyatt, Haynes *et al.*, 2000).

In clinical practice, the clinician commonly performs a 'therapeutic trial' or 'trial of therapy', in which the individual patient receives a treatment and the subsequent clinical course determines whether treatment is judged effective and is continued. Such an approach has serious potential biases due to the PLACEBO EFFECT, the natural history of the condition and the urge of the patient and clinician not to disappoint one another. The methodology of the N-of-1 trial at least partially overcomes some of these potential biases.

N-of-1 trials generally compare a single new therapy with a current standard therapy or a placebo. However, as with traditional randomised controlled trials it is also possible to compare more than two treatment options. In an N-of-1 trial the individual serves as his or her own control, receiving all treatments under investigation. Ideally, such a trial is conducted as a double-blind (both the individual and outcome assessor blind to allocated treatment in any treatment period), multi-crossover trial with three or more periods for each treatment. Repeated alternations between treatment periods with the new intervention and the control ensure several comparisons between the treatments. The trial design will, however, be tailored to the clinical entity and therapies involved.

The time commitment of such trials by both patients and health professionals is considerable. N-of-1 trials rely on cooperation between individual clinicians and patients. Hence, the patient's (and clinician's) commitment to the trial is essential for it to reach fruition. The duration of an N-of-1 trial will largely depend on the nature of the condition and the treatments under investigation, but is likely to continue for between several weeks and several months if not for longer. Hence, such trials are only effective for chronic and stable conditions where the natural history of the condition is unlikely to change dramatically over the course of the trial. Examples of their use in different clinical areas include osteoarthritis, gastro-esophageal reflux disease, attention deficit hyperactivity disorder and chronic airflow limitation among others (March, 1994).

One problem encountered in N-of-1 trials, as in CROSSOVER TRIALS, is carry-over effects of treatment, which may reduce the estimated treatment effect. The therapies under investigation should therefore have a rapid onset and cessation of effect that will help to minimise any carry-over effects. In addition, a wash-out period between treatments can be incorporated into the trial or a run-in period, where the first few days on each treatment are not evaluated. Because of the expense and time involved, it is important to determine at the outset whether an N-of-1 trial is really indicated for an individual, that is, is the effectiveness of treatment in doubt for this specific individual. Full criteria (summarised earlier) that should be satisfied before an N-of-1 trial is commenced are provided by Guyatt, Sackett *et al.* (1988).

When the individual patient and clinician are in agreement that an N-of-1 trial is justifiable this design provides the additional opportunity to measure the symptoms that matter to the individual concerned. In addition to standardised and validated disease-specific and generic outcome measures, the individual is asked to identify their most troubling symptoms or problems associated with the illness that are important in their everyday lives. These then form the basis of a self-administered diary or QUESTIONNAIRE. It may be a daily diary or weekly summary depending on symptoms and treatment duration, however, where possible several separate measurements should be taken within each treatment period. The opportunity to measure the symptoms that matter to the individual is a unique feature of N-of-1 trials.

In a classical randomised controlled trial the lowest experimental unit is the individual; in an N-of-1 trial it is the treatment period. Therefore the sample size in an N-of-1 trial is the number of treatment periods applied. Sample size or power calculations used with classical randomised controlled trials can also be used for N-of-1 trials. However, they make certain assumptions concerning the independence of data from each treatment period, which may not be reasonable. While a large number of treatment periods would increase the statistical power, the natural course of the clinical entity, therapy characteristics and patient compliance will generally put an upper limit on this number and thus statistical POWER will generally remain low.

Random assignment of subjects to treatments in classical randomised controlled trials is essential in order to obtain comparable groups with respect to explanatory and confounding variables. Correspondingly, random assignment of treatments to treatment periods is essential in N-of-1 trials. Once the number of treatment periods has been determined there are a number of ways of randomising the treatments to periods. The most recommended design when comparing two treatments (as is most commonly the case) is random allocation within pairs of treatment periods. For example, for the comparison of Treatment A versus Treatment B during 8 treatment periods, the following RANDOMISATION schedule might be generated: AB AB BA AB. This approach avoids the possibility of several consecutive treatment periods with the same treatment.

In terms of the analyses of an N-of-1 trial an important first approach is to plot the data and examine the results visually. The more theoretical methods depend heavily on the type of randomisation used. When the paired design is employed, the simplest approach may be to perform a SIGN TEST, which examines the LIKELIHOOD of the individual preferring the same treatment within each pair of treatment periods. However, this does not assess the strength of the treatment effect, only the direction of it. A more powerful alternative is the STUDENT'S t-TEST (either paired or unpaired depending on randomisation). For such analyses the paired design is again preferable since it goes some way to reduce the impact of autocorrelation (that is, the assumption of such a statistical test that observations from one treatment period to the next will be independent). Recording several measurements within each treatment period and comparing averages across the periods can reduce this problem further. Parametric tests also make the assumption of normality and non-parametric tests may alternatively be used. In addition, BAYESIAN METHODS are available (Zucker et al., 1977) for combining information from a series of N-of-1 trials. When an individual's N-of-1 trial has been completed the results will be summarised and disseminated during a feedback session between the clinician and patient to inform future treatment.   *SB*

March, L., Irwig, L., Schwarz, J., Simpson, J., Chock, C. and Brooks, P. 1994: N of 1 trials comparing a non-steroidal anti-inflammatory drug with paracetamol in osteoarthritis. *British Medical Journal* 309, 1041–5. **Guyatt, G.H., Haynes, R.B., Jaeschke, R.Z., Cook, D.J., Green, L., Naylor, D. et al for the Evidence-Based Medicine Working Group** 2000: User's guides to the medical literature XXV. Evidence-based medicine: principles for applying the users' guides to patient care. *Journal of the American Medical Association* 284, 1290–6. **Guyatt, G., Sackett, D., Adachi, J., Roberts, R., Chong, J., Rosenbloom, D. et al.** 1988: A clinician's guide for conducting randomized trials in individual patients. *Canadian Medical Association Journal* 139, 497–503. **Zucker, D.R., Schmid, C.H., McIntosh, M.W., D'Agostino, R.B., Selker, H.P. and Lau, J.** 1997: Combining single patient (N-of-1) trials to estimate population treatment effects and to evaluate individual patient responses to treatment. *Journal of Clinical Epidemiology* 50, 401–10.

non-compliance   See ADJUSTMENT FOR NON-COMPLIANCE IN RCTs

non-ignorable dropout   See DROPOUTS, MISSING DATA

non-inferiority   See ACTIVE CONTROL EQUIVALENCE STUDIES

non-informative censoring   See CENSORED OBSERVATIONS, SURVIVAL ANALYSIS

non-informative censoring/dropout   See CENSORED OBSERVATIONS, DROPOUTS, MISSING DATA

non-parametric methods – an overview   Inferential methods used when the assumptions of parametric methods are violated or the sample size is small, i.e. fewer than 25–30 in each group. Non-parametric methods do not assume that data are normally distributed as parametric methods do, although they usually have their own assumptions. Several situations suggest the use of non-parametric methods, including: when the independent and/or dependent variables are nominal in measurement; when the data are ordered with many ties; when the data are rank ordered; when there is a small sample size or unequal groups; when the dependent variable has a distribution other than a NORMAL DISTRIBUTION; when the groups have unequal variances; when there are unequal pairwise correlations across repeated measurements; when the data has notable OUTLIERS.

Non-parametric methods have common characteristics, including: independence of observations; few assumptions; dependent variable may be categorical; focus on rank ordering or frequencies; hypotheses in terms of rank, medians or frequencies; sample sizes are less stringent.

Most parametric methods have at least one non-parametric alternative. Some may have several and which to choose depends on which assumptions are met and what is to be shown with the data.

There are two non-parametric correlation coefficients; they are non-parametric versions of Pearson's correlation coefficient. These are Spearman's rank correlation, also known as SPEARMAN'S ρ, and Kendall's τ coefficient. There are several different versions of Kendall's τ including a, b and c. Spearman's rank is Pearson correlation calculated on the ranks of the data rather than the raw data. It is therefore often preferred due to its similarity to Pearson, in fact, if the data are normally distributed both coefficients give numerically similar answers. Spearman's rank is difficult to interpret if there are many ties in the data, so in this situation Kendall's τ is often preferred. Kendall's τ can be extended to give a partial correlation coefficient; this finds the correlation between variables while controlling for the effects of a third variable.

Non-parametric methods can also be used to analyse CONTINGENCY TABLES. The most common of these methods is the CHI-SQUARE TEST of independence, which is used if both variables in the contingency table are nominal. If the assumptions of the chi-square test are not met then the FISHER'S EXACT TEST or its extension the Fisher-Freeman-Houlton test can be used instead. Both the chi-square and Fisher's exact tests can only be used if the groups are independent. If there is an ordering in the data within a contingency table then a test for trend may be more powerful than a test of association. In a $2 \times c$ table, the chi-square test for trend can be used to look for a trend in proportions between the two groups. In an $r \times c$ table where both variables are ordered then linear-by-linear association, also known as the Mantel-Haenszel test for trend, can be used (see MANTEL-HAENSZEL METHODS).

McNEMAR'S TEST is used to analyse binary data in two groups where the groups are paired, these can be data before and after some event or matched pairs, McNemar's test takes two different forms depending on the sample size. There are two extensions to the McNemar's test, these are the COCHRAN Q-TEST which is for more than two time points or more than two groups, with a binary outcome, and the Stuart-Maxwell test, which is used when there are two paired groups with more than two outcomes. If agreement rather than association is of interest then the kappa coefficient can be used. Kappa measures agreement while adjusting for chance agreement. There are three forms of kappa, simple or Cohen's kappa for agreement between two raters rating on the same scale, weighted kappa, which takes into account the degree of disagreement and multi-rater kappa, which allows for more than two raters (see KAPPA AND WEIGHTED KAPPA).

Contingency tables can also be analysed using contingency coefficients. The phi coefficient is used to give strength to the association found in a significant chi-square test of association in a 2×2 table. Cramer's V, also called Cramer's C, is the extension of the phi coefficient to an $r \times c$ table and should only be used when the chi-square test has already proved to be significant. If both variables in the contingency table are ordered, the gamma statistic, G, can be used to measure the strength of association. If there is a special distinction between the ordered variables, for example one is the dependent and one is the independent, Somer's D can be used: this is asymmetric and gives a different answer if the variables are interchanged.

Goodness-of-fit tests are usually non-parametric. These tests are used to see if a sample distribution is similar to a pre-specified distribution or not. The binomial test is used for dichotomous data, i.e. data that can only take two outcomes. It sees whether such an extreme split into the two groups is likely to have occurred by chance or not. If there are more than two outcomes then the chi-square goodness-of-fit test could be used instead. The KOLMOGOROV-SMIRNOV TEST takes two different forms the first is the two-sample test. This test compares the distribution of two different groups to see if they are similar or not. This is done by seeing if the largest difference between the distributions of the two groups could have occurred by *chance alone*. The one-sample test compares the observed data to a theoretical distribution to see if the largest differences between the two distributions could have occurred by chance. It is often used to test if data are normally distributed enough to use parametric tests. However, it should only be used if the parameters of the distributions can be specified in advance. If this is not the case then the Lilliefors test, which is similar to the Kolmogorov-Smirnov test but allows the MEAN and STANDARD DEVIATION to be estimated from the data rather than being specified in advance, should be used. The Shapiro-Wilks test is also similar to the Kolmogorov-Smirnov test and is usually used to compare to a normal or EXPONENTIAL DISTRIBUTION. The runs test sees whether the order of occurrence of two values of a variable is random. A run is a sequence of like observations. If a sample contains too many or too few runs then that sample may not be random.

Non-parametric tests for two-samples are non-parametric versions of the t-test. These tests are the MANN-WHITNEY RANK SUM TEST, which tests for a difference in spread and location or medians between two independent groups. The hypothesis tested depends whether the assumption of similarity of distributions is met or not. The SIGN TEST tests for a difference in medians between two paired groups but is less powerful than the WILCOXON SIGNED RANK TEST for doing the same. The Wilcoxon signed rank test can only be used if there is a similarity of difference scores about the true MEDIAN difference.

There are many non-parametric versions of ANALYSIS OF VARIANCE; the most commonly used is the KRUSKAL-WALLIS TEST, which is the extension of the Mann-Whitney rank sum test to more than two groups. The median test can be used when the assumptions of the Kruskal-Wallis test are violated; it compares medians between *k* groups. The JONCKHEERE-TERPSTRA TEST is used when the independent variable is ordinal and looks for an increase in medians rather than a difference in medians, the order of the groups having been specified *a priori*. If there are repeated measures in the independent groups then the Scheirer-Ray-Hare test can be used; this is an extension of the Kruskal-Wallis test to allow for repeated measures within independent groups. The FRIEDMAN TEST is the non-parametric version of repeated measures analysis of variance. It is used for multiple paired samples. There is a multivariate extension of the Friedman test, the Quade test, which is similar to the Friedman test but takes account of the range of the data within a block. If the independent variable is ordinal then the Page test for ordered alternatives is more powerful than the Friedman test, it tests for an increase in medians rather than a difference in medians but the order of the groups must be specified *a priori*.

As the size of the samples used in non-parametric methods increase, the test statistics tend towards a NORMAL or CHI-SQUARE DISTRIBUTION. Therefore, when the sample size is large enough a normal or chi-square approximation to the test statistic is used to calculate the *P*-VALUE. It is important to report this asymptotic *P*-value only when the sample size is large enough. If the sample size is small, the exact *P*-value should be quoted instead since it is more appropriate and more accurate than the asymptotic one. *SLV*

Conover, W.J. 1999: *Practical nonparametric statistics*, 3rd edn. Chichester: John Wiley & Sons. **Pett, M.A.** 1997: *Nonparametric statistics for health care research*. Thousand Oaks: Sage. **Siegel, S. and Castellan, N.J.** 1998: *Nonparametric statistics for the behavioral sciences*, 2nd edn. New York: McGraw-Hill.

non-response bias

This occurs in all types of study when there is a systematic difference between the characteristics of those who choose to participate and those who do not.

In surveys, it is common practice to select a representative sample from the target population and collect data by means of a QUESTIONNAIRE. Some of the sample will not respond, either because they cannot be contacted or because they do not wish to participate. If the non-responders differ in a systematic way in terms of characteristics (such as age, sex or deprivation) that are related to the response variable(s), biased estimates will result. If basic demographic information is available for the entire sample, including the non-respondents, this information may be of use in adjusting estimates to account for the BIAS. However, the best approach is to maximise the response rate by using techniques such as incentives, reminders or enclosing stamped addressed envelopes. Edwards, Roberts *et al.* (2002) summarise the evidence for a range of these techniques.

Non-response bias can also be a problem in comparative studies. For example the classic Salk Polio Vaccine Trial of 1954 was conducted as a randomised, double-blind, placebo-controlled trial (see CLINICAL TRIALS) in some health departments in the USA (Tanur *et al.*, 1989). Parents of almost 750,000 6–7-year-old children were asked for permission to include their child in the randomised trial. Forty five percent refused. Those who consented were randomly allocated to Salk vaccine or placebo. All children, including those who refused inoculation, were followed up for one year. The INCIDENCE rates of polio in the following year were 28 per 100,000 in the vaccinated group, 71 per 100,000 in the placebo group and 46 per 100,000 in those who refused. Although other more subtle biases may be present, the large statistically significant difference in polio incidence between those randomised to placebo and those who refused is largely due to non-response bias. Those who refused were more likely to be from deprived households who were known to have a *lower* incidence of polio in 6–7-year-old children. In this randomised trial, a valid comparison between vaccine and placebo among volunteers is obtained, giving convincing evidence of the effect of the vaccine. The non-response bias here is an interesting side issue, but a non-response bias of this magnitude in an observational study would be a serious problem.

Non-response can also occur among individuals lost from observation in LONGITUDINAL STUDIES. Any resulting bias is known as withdrawal bias or loss to follow-up bias (see DROPOUTS). *WHG*

[See also BIAS]

Edwards, P., Roberts, I., Clarke, M. *et al.* 2002: Increasing response rates to postal questionnaires: systematic review. *British Medical Journal* 324, 1183–91. **Sackett, D.L.** 1979: Bias in analytic research. *Journal of Chronic Diseases* 32, 51–63. **Tanur, J.M.** *et al.* 1989: *Statistics: a guide to the unknown*, 3rd edn. Pacific Grove, CA: Wadsworth and Brooks/Cole.

normal distribution

normal distribution Probably the most important of the PROBABILITY DISTRIBUTIONS, the normal distribution takes the form of the familiar, symmetric, unimodal, bell-shaped curve, as illustrated in the Figure. Indeed, it is often referred to as the *bell-shaped distribution* or *Gaussian distribution*. The normal distribution has a number of properties that are appealing.

First and foremost, there is a mathematical result called the *central limit theorem* that, broadly speaking, tells us that if a sample is taken from a single population and all observations in that sample are independent then the sample mean will be approximately normally distributed, with approximation improving with the size of the sample. It is also the distribution that leads to a statistical model for a regression resulting in the same parameter estimates as a least squares regression. This is the reason for Gauss' interest in the distribution (hence Gaussian).

The normal distribution is related to many others. The F-DISTRIBUTION, CHI-SQUARE DISTRIBUTION, T-DISTRIBUTION and LOGNORMAL DISTRIBUTION can all be derived from it. It is what is known as a limiting distribution for,

and thus can be a good approximation to, the BETA and GAMMA DISTRIBUTIONS and even discrete distributions such as the BINOMIAL and POISSON.

The normal distribution is defined by two parameters: the MEAN, μ, and the STANDARD DEVIATION, σ. The density function for a variable X following a normal distribution with parameters μ and σ is:

$$f(x) = \frac{1}{\sigma\sqrt{2\pi}}\exp\left[-\frac{(x-\mu)^2}{2\sigma^2}\right]$$

By transforming the data X to create $Z = (X - \mu)/\sigma$ one can reduce the data to that with the standard normal density function with mean zero and standard deviation of one:

$$f(z) = \frac{1}{\sqrt{2\pi}}\exp\left(-\frac{z^2}{2}\right)$$

Performing such a transformation is sometimes referred to as calculating the Z-SCORE of the data.

Since it is symmetric and unimodal, the median and the mode of the distribution equal the mean (μ). The distribution can be re-centred by changing μ or rescaled by changing σ, but the shape of the distribution remains unchanged. Because of this, properties of the shape such as SKEWNESS and KURTOSIS are constant for all normal distributions. There is an added benefit that 95% of the density will lie within 1.96 (or approximately two) standard deviations of the mean. This result is invaluable in calculating confidence intervals or performing tests on the mean.

Despite the name, it is not always normal to see a normal distribution! Indeed, there are times when it would be a positively *ab*normal distribution. However, a number of statistical procedures such as ANALYSIS OF VARIANCE (and its variants) and the STUDENT'S t-TEST do assume that data are normally distributed. Other techniques and procedures that might make assumptions of normality include Pearson's correlation coefficient, linear regression, PRINCIPAL COMPONENT ANALYSIS and FACTOR ANALYSIS. This leaves the problem of testing to see if data or residuals are normally distributed.

The normal distribution always stretches from minus infinity to infinity and as such, while it can often provide an adequate approximation to a bounded distribution, if the data have to be positive or between 0 and 1 or are constrained by the inclusion/exclusion criteria of a trial then this might be cause for alarm. Essentially, if there are no observations near the boundary, i.e. the density of the distribution at the boundary is negligible, the approximation may well be fine.

There are a number of tests available to seek evidence of non-normality. One can test the skewness and kurtosis of the sample, but this is not generally advisable. One can conduct the KOLMOGOROV-SMIRNOV TEST, but this can be over-sensitive as can the Shapiro-Wilk W test, another popular alternative. There are few methods more reliable than graphical assessment of the sample in question, either through HISTOGRAMS or quantile-quantile (Q-Q) plots.

If one decides that a sample of data is not normally distributed, one has the choice of using a method that makes no assumption of normality (e.g. a non-parametric method) or performing a TRANSFORMATION of the data so

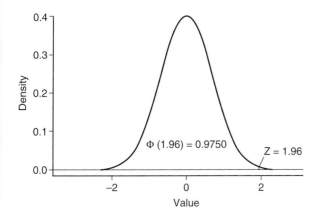

normal distribution *Illustrating the form of the normal (or Gaussian) distribution. Illustrated here is the standard normal distribution with mean zero and variance of one. Marked is the line corresponding to a value for the z-score of 1.96. As can be seen, 97.5% of the distribution lies to the left of 1.96 and 2.5% of the distribution is associated with larger values. The probability of seeing a value greater in magnitude than 1.96 is 2 × 2.5% as the distribution is symmetric about zero*

that they approximate normality. For example, taking the logarithm of ratios often leaves them acceptably approximated by the normal distribution. This is the most common way of estimating confidence intervals for odds ratios and relative risks.

It is not often that one is required to perform a normal test (as opposed to a test for normality), as this requires knowledge of the standard deviation of the distribution. If the standard deviation is to be estimated from the sample, then a t-test should be performed. There are, however, tables of probabilities associated with z-scores in many texts. These are normally the probabilities of a standard normal variable taking a value less than the z-score; a function (the distribution function) usually denoted by the upper case Greek letter phi (Φ). If the z-score is positive, then the probability of observing a score as large in magnitude is $2(1 - \Phi(z))$. Alternatively if the z-score is negative, the probability is $2\Phi(z)$. When the z-score is zero, it is taking the mean value and so $\Phi(0) = 0.5$ as the distribution is symmetric about zero. Note then that $2(1 - \Phi(0)) = 2\Phi(0) = 1$, as the score must always be at least as large in magnitude as zero.

As an example of its use, Kanis (2002) models the density of bone minerals as a normal distribution and by so doing is able to calculate the effect of several variables on fracture risks. *AGL*

[See also MULTIVARIATE NORMAL DISTRIBUTION]

Altman, D.G. and Bland, M.J. 1995: The normal distribution, *British Medical Journal* 310, 298. **Armitage, P. and Colton, T.** (eds) 1998: *Encyclopaedia of biostatistics.* Chichester: John Wiley & Sons. **Kanis, J.A.** 2002: Diagnosis of osteoporosis and assessment of fracture risk. *The Lancet* 359, 1929–36. **Leemis, L.M.** 1986: Relationships among common univariate distributions. *The American Statistician* 40, 2, 143–6. **Lindley, D.V. and Scott, W.F.** 1984: *New Cambridge elementary statistical tables.* Cambridge: Cambridge University Press.

normal probability plot See PROBABILITY PLOT

nQuery Advisor A software package useful for determining sample sizes when planning research studies. Details are available from Statistical Solutions Ltd., 8 South Bank, Crosse's Green, Cork, Ireland. www.statsol.ie/nquery/nquery.htm. *BSE*

nuisance parameter A parameter of a model in which there is little or no scientific interest but whose presence is needed to make valid inferences and estimates of the parameters which are of real interest. An example of a nuisance parameter is the variance of the random effect terms in a random intercept model (see MULTILEVEL MODELS). *BSE*

number needed to treat (NNT) Often a useful way to report the results of a randomised clinical trial, the NNT is the estimated number of patients who need to be treated with the new treatment rather than the standard treatment for one additional patient to benefit. The NNT is calculated as one divided by the absolute risk reduction (ARR), where the latter is simply the absolute value of the difference between the control group event rate and the experimental group event rate. The concept of NNT can equally well be applied to harmful outcomes as well as benefical ones, when instead it becomes the number needed to harm (NNH).

For example, in a study into the effective of intensive diabetes therapy on the development and progression of neuropathy, 9.6% of patients randomised to usual care and 2.8% of patients randomised to intensive therapy suffered from neuropathy. Consequently,

$$ARR = |9.6\%-2.8\%| = 6.8\%,$$

leading to

$$NNT = 1/ARR = 1/6.8\% = 14.7,$$

which is rounded up to 15. This means 15 diabetic patients need to be treated with intensive therapy to prevent one from developing neuropathy. (This example is given on the web site of the Centre for Evidence Based Medicine.)

Altman (1998) shows how to calculate a confidence interval for NNT, although this is not considered helpful if the 95% confidence interval for ARR includes the value zero, as this gives rise to a non-finite confidence interval for NNT. Walter (2001) illustrates some statistical properties of NNT and similar measures, with examples drawn from different types of study design. While there have been a few critics of NNT as an index, most medical statisticians, including Altman and Deeks (2000) defend the concept as a useful communication tool when presenting results from clinical studies. Bandolier, an Oxford-based, independent research group promoting EVIDENCE-BASED MEDICINE, maintain a useful website with further information on NNTs and their applications, www.jr2.ox.ac.uk/bandolier/booth/booths/NNTs.html. *BSE/CRP*

Altman, D.G. 1998: Confidence intervals for the number needed to treat, *British Medical Journal* 317, 1309–12. **Altman, D.G. and Deeks, J.J.** 2000: Comment on the paper by Hutton. *Journal of the Royal Statistical Society, Series A* 163, 415–16. **Walter, S.D.** 2001: Number needed to treat (NNT): estimation of a measure of clinical benefit, *Statistics in Medicine* 20, 3947–62.

number needed to harm (NNH): See NUMBER NEEDED TO TREAT (NNT).

O

observational studies There are situations where medical research has to be conducted using study designs which do not involve randomisation. These observational studies include a range of different study types, four main types of which are described and illustrated briefly below: CASE-CONTROL, COHORT, CROSS-SECTIONAL and ecological (see EPIDEMIOLOGY). Case reports (or case series), which involve only studying patients with specific diagnoses, are sometimes included under this heading. While providing valuable information about characteristics of patients, from the scientific perspective they are limited and, therefore, are considered no further.

Interest in most observational studies typically focuses on studying the relationship between disease and exposure. Exposure data are collected for those diagnosed with a disease and also for those who are disease free. In the absence of RANDOMISATION, observational studies are particularly prone to problems associated with confounding and this needs to be considered at the design and analysis stage of such studies. Sample size considerations for observational studies are described elsewhere.

In *ecological studies*, the unit of analysis is a group of individuals, or 'community', where each community provides its measure of disease outcome and exposure. Examining the strength of association between disease and exposure in these studies is usefully examined graphically using a scatter diagram (see SCATTERPLOT). A study examining the association between incidence of squamous-cell carcinoma of the eye and ambient levels of solar ultraviolet is one such example (Newton *et al.*, 1996). When this suggests a linear relationship between the disease and exposure a regression analysis can be informative. In this example, the incidence of squamous-cell carcinoma was found to decrease by 29% per unit reduction in ultraviolet exposure, a finding that was highly statistically significant ($p < 0.0001$).

Associations observed between disease and exposures in ecological studies may not necessarily reflect the pattern seen when individuals are the unit of analysis. *Cross-sectional studies*, in contrast, provide the opportunity to study data on disease and exposure on individuals at a particular point in time. In a cross-sectional study of elderly women, for example, interest focused on the PREVALENCE of falls (Lawlor, Patel and Ebrahim, 2003). Such disease measures can be examined in relation to one or more exposures also recorded at that time. The effects of chronic diseases and drug use on prevalence of falls were of interest and data on these factors were also recorded at that time. The findings from this study illustrate the importance of considering confounding factors. While the prevalence of falling increased with increasing numbers of simultaneously occurring chronic diseases, no such relation was found with the number of drugs used after adjusting for such factors (Lawlor, Patel and Ebrahim, 2003).

Case-control and *cohort studies* both offer the important advantage of measuring disease and exposure at different points in time. Case-control studies proceed by identifying a representative group of individuals diagnosed with a certain condition ('cases') and a representative group of individuals who are disease free ('controls') (see first Figure). Information regarding specific exposures of interest is collected and compared in cases and controls using odds ratios (see RELATIVE RISK AND ODDS RATIO) that are estimated by dividing the odds of exposure in cases by the odds of exposure in controls. Case-control studies have particular appeal for studying rare diseases and it is noteworthy that this was the study design the first used to demonstrate the link between smoking and lung cancer (Doll and Hill, 1950). They do, however, rely on individuals being able to accurately recall their past exposure histories: RECALL BIAS is a particular problem in case-control studies.

Confounding in case-control studies can be taken into account by matching cases and controls at the study design but allowance must be made for this in subsequent data analyses. The United Kingdom Childhood Cancer Study provides such an example, where interest focused on the relationship between neonatal exposure to vitamin K and childhood cancer (Fear *et al.*, 2003). Here, cases were children diagnosed with cancer and controls were those without cancer. One measure of 'exposure' was whether neonatal vitamin K had been received orally or by the intramuscular (im) route. Cases and controls were matched on sex, month and year of birth and region of residence at diagnosis. The odds ratio for cancer in children who had received vitamin K orally compared to those who received it by the im route was 1.09 (95% CI 0.94 to 1.61) after adjusting for the matching and other confounding factors. This study did not, therefore, provide support for an association between exposure of neonates to vitamin K and subsequent risk of childhood cancer.

When ordered according to the strength of scientific evidence which observational studies have the potential to provide, cohort studies hold the top position. In its simplest form, this involves identifying disease-free individuals, who are classified according to an exposure at a

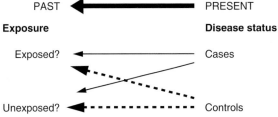

Case-control studies start with the single disease (or outcome) of interest and examine the association with past exposure(s)

observational studies *Principles of a case-control study design*

247

A cohort study starts with a selected group of disease-free people who are classified according to a specific exposure. They are then observed over time to see who develops the disease or outcome(s) of interest

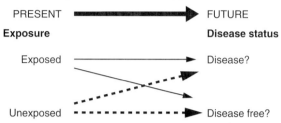

observational studies *Principles of a cohort study design*

particular point in time and followed up to determine which of them develops the disease of interest (see second Figure). In contrast with case-control studies that rely solely on odds ratios, cohort studies provide the opportunity to measure disease in many different ways using absolute (e.g. risks, rates or odds) or relative (risks ratios, rate ratios or odds ratios) measures. Cohort studies also have the important advantage of collecting exposure data prior to disease occurrence, i.e. avoiding recall bias, and studying a range of different health outcomes. Such studies, however, have the disadvantages of requiring larger study size and taking much longer to conduct, particularly for rare diseases.

Studying disease rates in a specific cohort often requires identifying a separate comparison cohort. A cohort study of cancer incidence in 51,721 UK service personnel deployed in the 1991 Gulf war, for example, also involved assembling a cohort of 50,755 active service personnel who were not deployed in that war (era cohort) (Macfarlane *et al.*, 2003). In order to take account of confounding, members of the Gulf war veterans, cohort members were matched to members of the era cohort according to age, sex, rank, service and level of fitness. The main outcome measure here was incidence rate ratio (IRR). After adjusting for confounding factors, this study suggested no different in cancer rates between these two cohorts (IRR = 0.99 95% CI 0.83 to 1.17). When the outcome studied was other symptoms of ill health, however, Gulf war veterans were found to have an excess of illness at follow-up (Hotopf *et al.*, 2003). *LC*

Doll, R. and Hill, A.B. 1950: Smoking and carcinoma of the lung. Preliminary report. *British Medical Journal* ii, 739–48. **Fear, N.T., Roman, E., Ansell, P., Simpson, J., Day, N. and Eden, O.B.** 2003: Vitamin K and childhood cancer: a report from the United Kingdom Childhood Cancer Study. *British Journal of Cancer* 89, 1228–31. **Hotopf, M., David, A.S., Hull, L., Nikalaou, V., Unwin, C. and Wessely, S.** 2003: Gulf war illness – better, worse, or just the same? A cohort study. *British Medical Journal* 327, 1370–2. **Lawlor, D.A., Patel, R. and Ebrahim, S.** 2003: Association between falls in elderly women and chronic diseases and drug use: cross-sectional survey. *British Medical Journal* 327, 712–17. **Macfarlane, G.J., Biggs, A.-M., Maconochie, N., Hotopf, M., Doyle, P. and Lunt, M.** 2003: Incidence of cancer among UK Gulf war veterans: cohort study. *British Medical Journal* 327, 1373–7. **Newton, R., Ferlay, J., Reeves, G., Beral, V. and Parkin, D.M.** 1996: Effect of ambient solar ultraviolet radiation on incidence of squamous-cell carcinoma of the eye. *The Lancet* 347, 1450–1.

odds ratio See RELATIVE RISK AND ODDS RATIO

one-sample t-test See STUDENT'S t-TEST

one-sided tests In hypothesis tests, we try to distinguish between chance variation in a DATASET and a genuine effect. We do this by comparing the null hypothesis, which states that there is no difference between the populations in which the data arose, to the alternative hypothesis, which states that there *is* a difference. For a one-sided test, this alternative hypothesis specifies the direction of the difference, i.e. we wish to distinguish chance variation from a decrease or increase in comparison to the null hypothesis. The *P*-VALUE for a one-sided test is calculated by considering only one side of the test statistic's distribution.

One-sided tests are used in situations where a genuine difference can only occur in one pre-specified direction and any differences seen in the opposite direction are a result of mere chance. For example, in Völzke *et al.* (2002) only increases in cardiovascular risk were looked at, as a lower cardiovascular risk was not biologically plausible for the study group. One-sided tests are also useful in situations where we are only interested in differences in one direction. For example, when introducing a new cheaper and more convenient diagnostic test we might only be interested in whether it is less accurate than the current test.

Tests should never be one-sided unless there is strong evidence present prior to data collection suggesting that any change from the null hypothesis must be in one (specified) direction only. Using one-sided tests makes it easier to reject the null hypothesis when the alternative is true, thus one-sided tests are attractive to those who define success as having a *P*-value less than the significance level. A one-sided test should not be used just because a difference in a particular direction is expected, as things do not always turn out as planned. *MMB*

Bland, J.M. and Altman, D.G. 1994: Statistics notes: one- and two-sided tests of significance. *British Medical Journal* 309, 248. **Völzke, H., Engel, J., Kleine, V., Schwahn, C., Dahm, J.B., Eckel, L. and Rettig, R.** 2002: Angiotensin I-converting enzyme insertion/deletion polymorphism and cardiac mortality and morbidity after coronary artery bypass graft surgery. *Chest* 122, 31–6.

ordered categorical data See ORDINAL DATA

ordinal data Data that have been collected from research studies generally falls into three main categories: (i) nominal; (ii) interval and (iii) ordinal. In the case of ordinal data, the most appropriate methods for analysis are those that take advantage of the ordering of the response categories. These methods are collectively termed ordinal regression models. In the literature, there are six main types of ordinal regression model, including the following: polytomous model; proportional odds model; unconstrained/constrained partial proportional odds model; adjacent category model; continuation ratio model; stereotype model.

Ordinal regression models have been included in the broader category of generalised linear models and therefore consist of the usual components: a *random component*, which identifies the probability distribution of the response variable; a *systematic component*, which specifies a linear function of explanatory variables, and a *link*, which describes the functional relationship between the systematic component and the expected value of the random component. All ordinal regression models can be expressed as:

$$F(\pi) = \alpha_j + X_1\beta_{j1} + X_2\beta_{j2} + \ldots X_p\beta_{jp}, \quad (1)$$

where $F(\pi)$ denotes the link function, also known as the *logit* or *log odds* and this function includes the 'cumulative' logits, the 'continuation ratio' logits, the 'adjacent category' logits and 'generalised' logits. The α_j and $\beta_{j1}, \ldots \beta_{jp}$ are the parameters to be estimated based on the jth cut-point (this is the point at which the scale is dichotomised) and the $X_1, \ldots X_p$ are the covariates measured on the subjects in the study. If we let $\Pr(Y = y_j)$ denote the probability that a subject falls into the y_j category, then using (1) we can express the logit functions for various ordinal regression models. For the purpose of illustration, the 5-point ordinal scale from the health status question on the SF-36 Health Survey (Ware and Gandek, 1998) is used. This question asks: 'In general would you say your health is "*excellent*", "*very good*", "*good*", "*fair*" or "*poor*"?'

The generalised logit or polytomous model is a straightforward extension of the logistic regression model for binary response and accommodates for multinomial responses (Agresti, 1984). It does not, however, take account of the ordering of the categories.

To indicate the form of the polytomous model, let X_1 and X_2 denote covariates of interest and y be the response measured on the ordinal scale of the health status question. Then taking the last category (i.e. '*poor*') as referent, the polytomous model is expressed as:

$$\log\left[\frac{\Pr(Y = y_j)}{\Pr(Y = y_4)}\right] = \alpha_j + X_1\beta j_1 + X_2\beta j_2 \quad j = 1, 2, 3, 4 \quad (2)$$

There are four logits functions based on the cut-points '*excellent*' vs '*poor*', '*very good*' vs '*poor*'; '*good*' vs '*poor*' and '*fair*' vs '*poor*'. The logit functions are expressed in terms of the four cut-point-specific intercept parameters (α_j) and for each of the covariates X_1 and X_2, the four cut-point-specific regression coefficients are β_{j1} and β_{j2} respectively.

For a given covariate, say X_1, the parameters β_{j1} corresponds to the four log-odds of ($Y = y_j$), relative to the referent category ($Y = y_4$). Exponentiating the regression coefficients β_{j1} results in the cut-point-specific odds ratios comparing ($Y = y_j$) versus ($Y = y_c$) for a unit increase in the levels of X_1 having adjusted X_2.

The prime feature of the proportional odds model is that a single summary measure (in terms of an odds ratio) is used to summarise the relationship of the ordinal response and the covariates. The proportional odds model (sometimes known as the *cumulative logit model*) allows for the ordering of the response categories through the use of cumulative probabilities.

The proportional odds model was first introduced by Walker and Duncan (1967) and their model was based on cumulative probabilities. McCullagh (1980) considered their model in great detail and derived from it the *proportional odds model*. For this latter model, it is assumed that one can combine the cut-points of the response into a single model, in which the same slope parameter β is used for each logit. The proportional odds model fitted for the ordinal scale of the health status question would take on the form:

$$\log\left[\frac{\Pr(Y \leq y_j)}{\Pr(Y > y_j)}\right] = \alpha_j + X_1\beta_1 + X_2\beta_2 \quad j = 1, 2, 3, 4 \quad (3)$$

Here the logits are based on the four cut-points: '*excellent*' vs ('*very good*', '*good*', '*fair*', '*poor*'); ('*excellent*', '*very good*') vs ('*good*', '*fair*', '*poor*'); ('*excellent*', '*very good*', '*good*') vs ('*fair*', '*poor*'); ('*excellent*', '*very good*', '*good*', '*fair*') vs '*poor*'. There are four intercept parameters $\{\alpha_j\}$ in this model. As j increases, these parameters increase, reflecting an increase in the logits, as additional probabilities are added into the numerator (i.e. $\alpha_1 \leq \alpha_2 \ldots \leq \alpha_4$). Also the β_1 and β_2 are the common slope parameters over the four cut-points for each covariate respectively.

There are two assumptions of the proportional odds model: (1) the existence of an underlying continuous variable – not all ordinal scales will have an underlying continuum (e.g. the total score). The proportional odds model can still be used in such circumstance, the only drawback being that the interpretation of the parameters becomes difficult; (2) homogeneity in the cut-point-specific regression parameters (known as the *proportional odds assumption*). Prior to fitting the proportional odds model, it is important that the assumption of proportionality be checked, either graphically or formally, for instance, using the score test (Peterson and Harrell, 1990).

An appealing requirement for ordinal data is that the model should in some sense be invariant under a reversal of category order. This implies that the magnitude of the summary estimates does not depend on the direction employed in modelling the outcome, i.e. whether the cutpoints are formed using increasing or decreasing levels of severity. However, the sign of the β parameter is changed and the $\{\alpha_j\}$ reverse sign and order.

The proportional odds model is also invariant under the collapsability of the response categories. Hence, if two adjacent response categories are pooled together and the cut-point removed, the estimates of β should remain essentially unchanged, although the $\{\alpha_j\}$ are affected.

For the covariate, say X_1, the parameter β_1 corresponds to the global log-odds over all the four cut-points. The exponential of the regression coefficients β_1, results in a single estimate of the odds ratios for a unit increase in the levels of X_1 having adjusted X_2.

The proportional odds model and the partial proportional odds models are collectively termed *cumulative logit models*.

In practice, it is often difficult to find data for which a proportional odds model is a plausible description. There is, therefore, a need for a model that permits partial proportional odds, where some explanatory variables may meet the proportional odds assumption and others may not. Thus, the primary reason for the formulation of the 'partial proportional odds models' was to relax the stringent assumption of constant odds ratio presented by the proportional odds model. The assumption that a constant slopes model holds, when in fact, for a given variable a constant log-odds ratio is not representative of all the log-odds ratios over the cut-points, can lead to the formulation of an incorrect model.

The partial proportional odds models were initiated by the work of Peterson and Harrell (1990) and in general there are two types of partial proportional odds model: *the unconstrained partial proportional odds model*, for which no constraints are placed in the estimation of the parameters, and the *constrained partial proportional odds model*, for which a certain relationship may have been observed between the log-odds ratios and *j*, the point of dichotomisation. Such a relationship may be linear, for example, in which case a linear constraint is placed on the parameters of the model.

The cut-points that are used for the partial proportional odds models are the same as for the proportional odds model.

Assuming X_1 has proportional odds and X_2 does not have proportional odds, then the unconstrained partial proportional odds model for the ordinal scale of the health status question takes the form:

$$\log\left[\frac{\Pr(Y \le y_j)}{\Pr(Y > y_j)}\right] = \alpha_j + X_1\beta_1 + X_2\beta_2 + T_2\gamma_{j2}$$

$$j = 1, 2, 3, 4 \tag{4}$$

Here the β_1 and β_2 are the regression coefficients associated with the two covariates of interest. The T_2 is the covariate which is a subset of the X_2 for which the proportional odds assumption either is not assumed or is to be tested and γ_{j2} are the regression coefficients associated with T_2, so that $T_2\gamma_{j2}$ is an increment associated only with the *j*th cumulative logit and $\gamma_{12} = 0$. If $\gamma_{j2} = 0$ for all *j*, then this model reduces to the proportional odds model. Thus a simultaneous test of the proportional odds model assumption is a test of the null hypothesis that $\gamma_{j2} = 0$ for all $j = 2, 3, 4$. Since $\gamma_{12} = 0$, the model uses only $\alpha_1 + X_2\beta_{j2}$ to estimate the odds ratio associated with the dichotomisation of the *y*-response categories into the first category versus the rest of the categories, where the estimation of the odds ratios associated with the remaining cumulative probabilities involve incrementing $\alpha_j + X_2\beta_2$ by $T_2\gamma_{j2}$.

Given the relationship of a covariate and the response is represented with non-proportional odds, then for the individual cut-point-specific odds ratios, often a certain type of trend may be anticipated, e.g. a linear trend may be expected. In such a case, a constraint can be placed on the parameters in the model, so that the trend is taken into account. When the constraints are incorporated into the unconstrained partial proportional odds model, for scale of the health status question, this model takes the form:

$$\log\left[\frac{\Pr(Y \le y_j)}{\Pr(Y > y_j)}\right] = \alpha_j + X_1\beta_1 + X_2\beta_2 + T_2\gamma_2\Gamma_j$$

$$j = 1, 2, 3, 4 \tag{5}$$

Here the Γ_j are fixed pre-specified scalars and $\Gamma_1 = 0$. The new parameter γ_2 is not subscripted by *j*. Although γ_2 depends on *j*, it is multiplied by the fixed constant scalar Γ_j in the calculation of the *j*th cumulative logit.

The underlying assumptions of the partial proportional odds models are as for the proportional odds model.

Given covariate X_2, the test of whether a single γ_2 parameter fits the data as well as 3 (number of categories − 2) γ_{j2} parameters can be obtained by using the LIKELI-

HOOD RATIO test. Here we compare the loglikelihood of unconstrained and constrained models. This gives an approximate chi-square with 2 (number of categories − 2) − 1 df.

The adjacent category model utilises single-category probabilities rather than cumulative probabilities. Agresti (1984) states that when the response categories have a natural ordering, logit models should utilise that ordering. One can incorporate the ordering directly in the way we construct the logits. Like the proportional odds model the adjacent categories logit model implies stochastic orderings of the response distributions for different predictor values.

Agresti (1989) describes the adjacent category logistic model as modelling the ratio of the two probabilities $\Pr(Y = y_j)$ and $\Pr(Y = y_{j+1})$ $j = 1, 2, 3, 4$. The cut-points that are used for the adjacent categories, given the scale of the health status question would be: 'excellent' vs 'very good'; 'very good' vs 'good'; 'good' vs 'fair'; 'fair' vs 'poor'.

There are two types of adjacent category logit model. The constant slope adjacent category model has the following representation:

$$\log\left[\frac{\Pr(Y = y_j)}{\Pr(Y = y_{j+1})}\right] = \alpha_j + X_1\beta_1 + X_2\beta_2 \quad j = 1, 2, 3, 4 \tag{6}$$

Manor, Matthews and Power (2000) described the adjacent category model in a slightly different way. His version of the model is:

$$\log\left[\frac{\Pr(Y = y_j)}{\Pr(Y = y_{j+1})}\right] = \alpha_j + X_1\beta_{j1} + X_2\beta_{j2} \quad j = 1, 2, 3, 4 \tag{7}$$

In model (6), for a given covariate, say X_1, the parameter β_1 corresponds to the log-odds of falling in categories 'excellent' vs 'very good'; 'very good' vs 'good'; 'good' vs 'fair' and 'fair' vs 'poor'. If the exponential is taken, this results in the global odds ratios for the adjacent categories for each unit increase in the levels of X_1.

On a similar note, model (7) provides the cut-point-specific adjacent category odds ratios and for the health status question scale there are four of these, for each unit increase in the levels of a given covariate.

Given an ordinal scale, where one is particularly interested in assessing the relative chance of a given rating, against all more favourable ones, then one would normally consider employing the *continuation ratio logits*. The continuation ratio model is best suited to circumstances in which the individual categories are of particular interest. It is well suited for failure-time data and outcomes that measure threshold points, where individuals at a given level of an outcome must have passed through all previous levels of an outcome.

The logits for the continuation ratio model are based on the cut-points: 'excellent' vs ('very good', 'good', 'fair', 'poor'); 'very good' vs ('good', 'fair', 'poor'); 'good' vs ('fair', 'poor'); 'fair' vs 'poor'. As for the adjacent category models, there are two versions of the continuation ratio model.

The form of the continuation ratio model was initially formulated by Feinberg (1980) and originated from survival time data. Various forms of the model exist and the most common is the forward formulation model and is written as:

250

$$\log\left[\frac{\Pr(Y = y_j)}{\Pr(Y > y_j)}\right] = \alpha_j + X_1\beta_1 + X_2\beta_2 \quad j = 1, 2, 3, 4 \quad (8)$$

Model (8) is described by Cole and Ananth (2001) as a *fully constrained continuation ratio* model. It allows the cut-point-specific continuation ratios to be described by a single regression parameter (in a similar way to the proportional odds model). This model represents the probability of being in category j; conditional on being in category greater than j. The intercept parameters denoted by $\{\alpha_j\}$ and are the same as the cumulative logit model, but are not necessary ordered for the continuation ratio model. Essentially, this model can be viewed as the ratio of the two conditional probabilities, $\Pr(Y = y_j/Y \geq y_j)$ and $\Pr(Y > y_j/Y \geq y_j)$, i.e. one models the odds of falling in category j as opposed to higher than category j, given that one has been in category j or higher.

By viewing the outcome as going from more to less severe, this model can be applied in reverse and forms the backward continuation ratios $\frac{\Pr(Y = y_j)}{\Pr(Y < y_j)}$. Because of the conditioning on adjacent cut-points, the continuation ratio, unlike the proportional odds, is affected by the direction chosen for the response variable and the forward and backward ratios are not equivalent and yield different results. Thus, the continuation ratio model is not invariant under reversal of categories, unless Y is binary, in which case one has to be careful which continuation ratio model one uses.

Another form is the different slopes continuation ratio model and for this model the regression parameters are allowed to vary by the cut-point. This model is written as:

$$\log\left[\frac{\Pr(Y = y_j)}{\Pr(Y > y_j)}\right] = \alpha_j + X_1\beta_{1j} + X_2\beta_{2j} \quad j = 1, 2, 3, 4 \quad (9)$$

In this case, the multinomial likelihood factors into a product of the binomial likelihoods for the separate logits. The continuation ratio model has the advantage that the $c - 1$ logits produced when fitting the ratios in relation to the cut-points are asymptotically independent of each other. Thus, the estimation of the parameters in the each of the $c - 1$ logits can be carried out separately, using the method of maximum likelihood and the summation of the individual chi-square statistics gives the overall goodness of fit statistics for the set of the logit models. In practice, the continuation ratio model can be fitted in any statistical package that includes binary logistic regression, after suitable restructuring of the data. As the fully constrained model is nested within the different slopes continuation ratio model, the difference in –2 loglikelihood (deviance) provides a test of the validity of the assumption that the threshold-specific continuation ratios are equal and is distributed as a χ^2 variate under the null with df equal to the difference in the number of parameters between the nested models.

The odds ratios for the different slopes and fully constrained continuation ratio models can be described in a similar way to those of the adjacent category models, as described earlier.

The stereotype ordinal regression model was introduced by Anderson (1984) as part of a general model for discrete multivariate outcomes and also arises naturally in the context of truly discrete outcomes.

The stereotype model is a derivative of the polytomous logistic model (2). The polytomous model provides the best possible fit to the data, at the cost of a large number of parameters that can be difficult to interpret. The stereotype model aims to reduce the number of parameters by imposing constraints without reducing the adequacy of the model.

For the health status scale, the starting point for the stereotype model is to impose a structure on the β_{j1} and β_{j2} such that:

$$\beta_{j1} = -\phi_j\beta_1 \text{ and } \beta_{j2} = -\phi_j\beta_2 \quad j = 1, 2, 3, 4 \quad (10)$$

Then model (2) becomes:

$$\log\left[\frac{\Pr(Y = y_j)}{\Pr(Y = y_4)}\right] = \alpha_j - \phi_j(X_1\beta_1 + X_2\beta_2)$$
$$j = 1, 2, 3, 4 \quad (11)$$

There are certain features that are specifically relevant to the stereotype ordinal regression model and these include the *dimensionality* of the model, *distinguishable y*-response categories and the *ordering* of the y-response categories with respect to the covariates.

The dimensionality of the model for the y-response and the covariates is determined by the number of linear functions required to describe the relationship. If only one linear function is used to describe the relationship between the ordinal response and a set of predictors, model (11) is a *one-dimensional stereotype model*. One-dimensional relationships are much more common in the literature compared to the higher dimensions.

Having decided on the dimensionality of the model, there are questions about ordering and model simplification, perhaps using distinguishability as a criterion. The concept of *indistinguishability* is described when a given covariate, X_1, affects two response categories y_j and y_{j+1} in an identical manner (thus X_1 is not predictive between the two categories): we then say that these two categories are indistinguishable with respect to X_1. The hypothesis that $y = y_s$ is indistinguishable from $y = y_t$, with respect to the covariates takes the form $H_0: \beta_s = \beta_t$. In the one dimension stereotype model, this is equivalent to asking whether there are differences among the ϕ_js ($H_0: \phi_s = \phi_t$).

In the regression models discussed so far (with the exception of the polytomous model), the regression parameters and consequently the logits are based on the ordering of the y-response categories. Therefore the proportional odds, continuation ratio and adjacent category models assess the association of y-response and the covariates conditional of the order that the categories occur. In this case the ordering is 'inbuilt' and assumed *a priori*.

In many cases, one cannot be too certain about the relevance of the ordering of the response categories. The stereotype model is based on the polytomous model and therefore uses generalised logits. The polytomous model does not have the mechanism to account for the ordering of the y-response categories. Anderson (1984) took the latter model and assessed the relationship of the y-response and a given covariate. If the individual cut-point-specific regression parameters were ordered (leading to the stereotype model), then one could assume that an ordered nature existed in the response categories. This is quite different from the 'ordinality' aspect of the proportional odds, continuation ratio and adjacent category models. For these latter models, the ordered categories are accounted for through the formation of the logits. Therefore they are not necessarily ordered with respect to the covariates and in a sense it is not necessary to have any regressor variables. By contrast, in the stereotype model, the 'ordinality' only reveals itself through assessing the relationship of the y-response and covariates.

If ordering is appropriate, the model orders the β_js (in the polytomous model) instead of ordering the odds or the link function. The 'ordering' is more directly tied to the effects of the explanatory variables and becomes a testable statement. If the dimensionality is one, ordering of the odds ratios is easily verified. If $\beta > 0$ and the odds ratios form a decreasing sequence $e^{\phi_1 \beta} = e^{\phi_1 \beta} = \ldots e^{\phi_5 \beta} = 1$, then:

$$\phi_1 = 1 \geq \phi_2 \ldots \geq \phi_5 = 0 \qquad (12)$$

Note that (12) is not strictly ordinal, as adjoining categories may be indistinguishable. If (12) is satisfied, then the effect of the covariates upon the first odds ratio is greater than its effect on the second and so on.

For the health status scale, model (11) has a standard multinomial intercept with four parameters for a response variable. It estimates three independent scale values of $\{\phi_j\}$ for the response factor and a single beta parameter for each independent variable. The larger the difference between any two ϕ_j values, the more the log odds between the outcomes is affected by the independent variables. The ϕ_1 parameters show how the independent variable, X_1 affects the log odds of higher versus lower scores, where 'higher' and 'lower' is defined by the ϕ_j scale.

Most of the ordinal regression models detailed here can be fitted in well-known statistical software packages. However, there are some models (e.g. the partial proportional odds models) that are not very well accommodated for and in the literature these model cannot be easily fitted and are more computational intensive.

The goodness-of-fit for a c-category model is a natural extension of that for the two categories. However, methods to assess the residual, where there is lack-of-fit are underdeveloped and require further research.

Indices such as AKAIKE'S INFORMATION CRITERIA (AIC) are often used to compare different models from the same data. However, the use of such an index has been rarely cited and it would be worthwhile to exploit and evaluate such an index in the context of ordinal regression models.

RL

Agresti, A. 1984: *Analysis of ordinal categorical data*. New York: John Wiley & Sons. **Agresti, A.** 1989: Tutorial on modelling ordered categorical response data. *Psychological Bulletin* 105, 290–301. **Anderson, J.A.** 1984: Regression and ordered categorical variables (with discussion). *Journal of the Royal Statistical Society Series B* 46, 1–30. **Ashby, D., Pocock, S. and Shaper, A.** 1986: Ordered polytomous regression: an example relating serum biochemistry and haematology to alcohol consumption. *Applied Statistics* 35, 3, 289–301. **Cole, S. and Ananth, C.** 2001: Regression models for unconstrained, partially or fully constrained continuation odds ratios. *International Epidemiological*

Association 30, 1379–82. **Feinberg, B.** 1980: *Analysis of cross-classified data*, 2nd edn. Cambridge, MA: MIT Press. **Manor, O., Matthews, S. and Power, C.** 2000: Dichotomous or categorical response? Analysing self-rated health and lifetime social class. *International Journal of Epidemiology* 29, 149–57. **McCullagh, P.** 1980: Regression models for ordinal data (with discussion). *Journal of the Royal Statistical Society Series B* 42, 109–42. **Peterson, B. and Harrell, F.** 1990: Partial proportional odds models for ordinal response variables. *Applied Statistics* 39, 205–17. **Walker, S. and Duncan, D.** 1967: Estimation of the probability of an event as a function of several independent variables. *Biometrika* 54, 167–79. **Ware, J. and Gandek, B.** 1998: Overview of the SF-36 health survey and the international quality of life assessment (IQOLA) project. *Journal of Clinical Epidemiology* 51, 11, 903–12.

ordinary least squares (OLS) See LEAST SQUARES ESTIMATION

outliers

Observations judged to be too far from their group average. Outliers may genuinely come from long-tailed distributions, but they may also be irrelevant or erroneous observations that need to be expunged from the datasets before analysis, with due precautions.

Outliers in the distribution of a single variable (*univariate* outliers) are defined in terms of the data spread (Ramsey and Schafer, 2002). The Figure shows the BOX-PLOT for some data with MEDIAN value equal to 60, first quartile equal to 40 and third quartile equal to 80.

The INTERQUARTILE RANGE of these data (shown as the central box) is thus equal to 40. Outliers are defined as all observations that are more than 1.5 interquartile ranges away from the box. In the Figure, all values exceeding 140 ($= 80 + 1.5 \times 40$) are outliers (shown as circles).

When the data come from a NORMAL DISTRIBUTION, a test can be used to detect univariate outliers. *Grubbs' test statistic* is defined as the largest absolute deviation from the sample MEAN in units of the sample STANDARD DEVIATION: $max \mid y_i - m \mid /s$, where y_i is the ith observation, m is the sample mean and s the sample standard deviation. Critical values for this test statistic can be computed from the t-distribution with N-2 DEGREES OF FREEDOM, where N is the sample size (Grubbs, 1969).

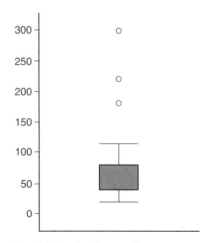

outliers *A boxplot showing three outliers*

Some statistical tests are resistant to outliers, but many are not. The simplest example arises from the calculation of a sample mean: the mean is very sensitive to outliers; in contrast, the median is resistant to outliers. Likewise, the comparison of two sample means through a t-test is sensitive to outliers; in contrast, a test that uses the ranks of the observations, rather than the observations themselves, is resistant to outliers (such a rank test is non-parametric and is also robust to deviations from normality).

Outliers in the distribution of several variables (multivariate outliers) are defined in terms of the distance of each observation to the multivariate mean. The Mahalanobis' distance is computed by standardising the variables of interest (subtracting the mean and dividing by the standard deviation) and summing the squares of these standardised variables. The sum approximately follows a CHI-SQUARE DISTRIBUTION with m degrees of freedom, if m variables are considered.

Multivariate outliers can exert undue influence on the analysis, particularly if multivariate regression is used. Case-influence statistics such as the leverage, COOK'S DISTANCE or studentised residual, are useful to detect influential observations, and assess their impact on the results of the analyses (Ramsey and Schafer, 2002).   *MB*

[See also STUDENT'S t-TEST]

Grubbs, F. 1969: Procedures for detecting outlying observations in samples. *Technometrics* 11, 1–21. **Ramsey, F.L. and Schafer, D.W.** 2002: *The statistical sleuth. A course in methods in data analysis.* Pacific Grove, CA: Duxbury.

overdispersion Overdispersion occurs whenever the outcome (or the response variable in a regression model) has a larger VARIANCE than that predicted by whatever model is being used. It is not usually a problem in regression models with a continuous outcome and a Normally distributed error term, as the NORMAL DISTRIBUTION has separate parameters for the variance and MEAN. Overdispersion arises more commonly in the case of discrete variables - usually either count or binary variables. For the analysis of count variables, a usual assumption is that they follow the POISSON DISTRIBUTION. For binary variables, the binomial distribution is often assumed. In each case, the distribution has only one parameter, so the variance is determined by the mean. The Poisson distribution assumes that the mean and variance of the distribution are equal. The BINOMIAL DISTRIBUTION assumes that the variance is the mean multiplied by (1–the probability of success). Overdispersion occurs when the actual variance seen is greater than that predicted by the Poisson or binomial distributions.

An example in ageing research is the analysis of activities of daily living (ADL) scores in a trial of a prehabilitation program (Byers *et al*, 2003). ADL were scored on a 16-point scale, and had a positively-skewed distribution with a mode of 0 and mean of 2.8. The variance was 16.4, indicating considerable over-dispersion.

There are two common causes of overdispersion (Agresti, 1990). These are:

i) positive correlation (rather than independence) between observations
ii) the true sampling distribution being a mixture of Poisson distributions.

The latter could be caused by heterogeneity among subjects. For example, suppose that the distribution of ADL for women was Poisson with a mean of 9 and for men was Poisson with a mean of 4. For a group of equal numbers of men and women, ADL would have a distribution with a mean of approximately 6.5 but a variance of approximately 13, thus showing overdispersion.

Overdispersion can be examined by comparing the variance of a set of observations to the predicted variance under an assumed distribution (as above). However, overdispersion can also be examined using regression models. For example, using a Poisson regression model, if there is no overdispersion and the model is correctly specified, the DEVIANCE of the model would be expected to equal the number of degrees of freedom (Lindsay *et al*, 2002). If the deviance is larger than the number of degrees of freedom, this is traditionally taken to indicate over-dispersion. For example, in the ADL example (above), the ratio of deviance to number of degrees of freedom was 4. Lindsay *et al* recommend that a deviance greater than twice the number of degrees of freedom be taken as an indication that overdispersion ought to be examined.

Overdispersion can result in under-estimation of standard errors, if the overdispersion is not taken into account. Traditionally, variances have been adjusted by multiplying them by an inflation factor. This inflation factor (or 'heterogeneity factor') is equal to the deviance divided by the number of degrees of freedom. It will thus be greater than 1 if there is overdispersion. Inference is then based on the maximum likelihood estimates obtained by the fitting of the Poisson model to the overdispersed data, but with multiplication of the standard errors by the square root of the inflation factor.

However, in the era of fast statistical programming, overdispersion can be investigated and taken into account using statistical models, rather than merely correcting the standard errors (Lindsay *et al*, 2002). For count data, the standard alternative to the Poisson model is the negative binomial model. This model includes a disturbance or error term, i.e. it assumes that the mean varies randomly in the population. For binary data, the standard alternative to the binomial model is the beta-binomial, which assumes that the probability has a beta distribution. Inclusion of appropriate covariates in a simple Poisson or binomial model may also be a way of accounting for overdispersion.

Lindsay *et al* (2002) examined the presence and effect of overdispersion in data on the annual number of black-grouse, and the effect of climate on this number. Using the Poisson distribution, there was evidence of overdispersion, with the model having a deviance of 29 on 18 degrees of freedom (inflation factor of 1.6). However, allowing for overdispersion using the negative binomial model gave parameter estimates and standard errors which were very close to those from the Poisson model. Another example has an inflation factor of 1.95, and yet the negative binomial model fitted no better than the Poisson model. In this case, from the model-fitting there was no evidence of overdispersion - and yet using the inflation factor would have multiplied the standard errors by 1.4. The recommendation from this paper is that the deviance can be used to indicate possible overdispersion, but this should then be investigated using model-based techniques, rather than merely inflating the standard errors.   *KT*

Agresti, A. 1990: *Categorical data analysis*. New York: John Wiley and Sons. **Byers, A.L., Allore, H., Gill, T.M. and Peduzzi, P.N.** 2003: Application of negative binomial modeling for discrete outcomes: a case study in aging research. *Journal of Clinical Epidemiology* 56(6): 559–64. **Lindsay, J., Laurin, D., Verreault, R., Hebert, R., Helliwell, B., Hill, G.B.** *et al.* 2002: Risk factors for Alzheimer's disease: a prospective analysis from the Canadian Study of Health and Aging. *American Journal of Epidemiology* 156(5): 445–53.

overmatching See CASE-CONTROL STUDIES

P

paired t-test See STUDENT'S t-TEST

partial correlation coefficient See CORRELATION

partial likelihood A function, consisting of a product of conditional LIKELIHOODS, used in certain situations for estimation and hypothesis testing.

The most commonly used partial likelihood is that used in COX's REGRESSION MODEL. In this model, it is assumed that the hazard of failure at time t for an individual with covariates $X = (X_1,...,X_K)$ is $\lambda_0(t) f(X, \beta)$, where $f(X, \beta) = \exp(\sum_{k=1}^{K} \beta_k X_k)$, $\beta = (\beta_1,...,\beta_K)$ are the hazard ratio parameters of interest and $\lambda_0(t)$ is the unknown baseline hazard function. No assumptions are made about the form of $\lambda_0(t)$.

In the full likelihood function for Cox's model, information about β is tied up with information about the nuisance function $\lambda_0(t)$. Cox's partial likelihood sacrifices some of the information about β contained in the data, in order to eliminate this dependence on $\lambda_0(t)$.

Let t_j denote the time of the jth failure and let R_j denote the risk set at time t_j, i.e. the set of individuals who, just before time t_j, remained not failed and not censored. Then, conditional on the risk set R_j and the fact that a failure took place at time t_j, the probability that it was person i who failed is:

$$\frac{\lambda_0(t_j) f(X_i, \beta)}{\sum_{l \in R_j} \lambda_0(t_j) f(X_l, \beta)} = \frac{f(X_i, \beta)}{\sum_{l \in R_j} f(X_l, \beta)}$$

The partial likelihood is the product, over all the failure times, of these conditional probabilities. It uses not the actual failure times, but the ranks of the failure times. Note that it does not depend on $\lambda_0(t)$.

Intuitively, since no assumptions are being made about the form of the baseline hazard and since censoring (see CENSORED OBSERVATIONS) is assumed non-informative, information about the actual times of failure and the censoring events would not be expected to reveal much about the parameters of interest, β; and indeed, this turns out to be the case. Thus, conditioning on these leads to very little loss of information about β.

Less obviously, it also turns out that this partial likelihood function, although not a proper likelihood function, has similar statistical properties. Thus, it may be used to estimate β, to calculate a variance-covariance matrix for β and for likelihood ratio hypothesis testing.

A more general definition of the partial likelihood can be found in, for example, Kalbfleisch and Prentice (2002).

SRS

Clayton, D. and Hills, M. 1993: *Statistical models in epidemiology*. Oxford: Oxford Science Publications. **Collett, D.** 2003: *Modelling survival data in medical research*, 2nd edn. London: Chapman & Hall. **Kalbfleisch, J.D. and Prentice, R.L.** 2002: *The statistical analysis of failure time data*, 2nd edn. Chichester: John Wiley & Sons.

path analysis A tool for evaluating the interrelationships among a set of observed (or latent) variables based on their correlational structure. The postulated relationships between the variables are often illustrated graphically by means of a path diagram, in which single-headed arrows indicate the direct influence of one variable on another, and curved double-headed arrows indicate correlated variables. (For an example of such a diagram see CONFIRMATORY FACTOR ANALYSIS.) Originally introduced for simple regression models for observed variables, the method has now become the basis for more sophisticated procedures such as confirmatory factor analysis and use of structural equation models, involving both manifest and latent variables.

BSE

path diagram See PATH ANALYSIS

pattern recognition See CLUSTER ANALYSIS IN MEDICINE, SUPPORT VECTOR MACHINES

Pearson's contingency coefficient See CONTINGENCY COEFFICIENT

Pearson's correlation coefficient See CORRELATION

per protocol A term used to describe a subset of participants in a randomised CLINICAL TRIAL who complied with the protocol (see PROTOCOLS FOR CLINICAL TRIALS). It is also used to describe an analysis based only on these participants.

The per protocol data set consists of those participants who complied with the protocol sufficiently to ensure that their data would be likely to show the effects of treatment. Aspects of compliance that could be considered include exposure to treatment and violations of the entry criteria. For example, participants could be excluded if they took less than 80% of the prescribed treatment, if they used an additional treatment that could also affect outcome or if retrospective evaluation shows that they did not meet eligibility criteria. The rules for inclusion and exclusion of participants from the per protocol dataset should be carefully specified before treatment allocations are unblinded. Any decisions made after the data are unblinded should be regarded with suspicion.

The rationale for per protocol analysis is to estimate the efficacy of an intervention, undiluted by factors such as non-compliance, lack of eligibility and additional treatments. It is therefore most often used in explanatory trials that aim to measure the efficacy of an intervention under equalised conditions, rather than in pragmatic trials that aim to measure the effectiveness of an intervention policy in routine practice (Roland and Torgerson, 1998).

However, per protocol analysis is subject to SELECTION BIAS because some participants are excluded after RANDOMISATION. Selection bias may be less when the nature

255

and number of exclusions is similar in different randomised groups, but bias can still occur in this situation. Therefore per protocol analysis should only be used when estimating efficacy is more important than avoiding selection bias. When a per protocol analysis is done, other analyses, such as INTENTION-TO-TREAT (ITT), should also be reported.

One specific situation where both per protocol and intention to treat analyses are routinely reported is in EQUIVALENCE STUDIES (ICHE9, 1999). ITT is anti-conservative for equivalence trials because the inclusion of participants who do not comply or switch treatments causes dilution of differences. But since per protocol analysis is always potentially biased, it is best to do both and carefully characterise exclusions from the per protocol analysis (Jones et al., 1996).

Participants without outcome measurements may also sometimes be excluded from a per protocol analysis. However, this may lead to biased results and the potential impact of MISSING DATA should be considered (Shih, 2002). *SH/IW*

International Conference on Harmonisation E9 Expert Working Group (ICH E9) 1999: ICH harmonised tripartite guideline. Statistical principles for clinical trials. *Statistics in Medicine* 18, 15, 1905–42. **Jones, B., Jarvis, P., Lewis, J.A. and Ebbutt, A.F.** 1996: Trials to assess equivalence: the importance of rigorous methods. *British Medical Journal* 313, 36–9. **Roland, M. and Torgerson, D.J.** 1998: Understanding controlled trials: what are pragmatic trials? *British Medical Journal* 316, 285. **Shih, W.J.** 2002: Problems in dealing with missing data and informative censoring in clinical trials. *Current Controlled Trials in Cardiovascular Medicine* 3, 4.

person-years at risk Time in years summed over several individuals. In any COHORT STUDY of incidence rate or rate ratios, different members of the cohort will be at risk for different amounts of time.

Some members may enter the risk set later, because they joined the cohort later, and some will leave earlier, because they were censored or experienced the event of interest. The length of time at risk (measured in years) experienced by each of a set of individuals, summed over those individuals, is the total person-years at risk for that set.

Incidence rates (measured in units of per person-year) are calculated by dividing the number of events occurring in a set of individuals while they are at risk by their total time at risk (measured in person-years).

Notice the implicit assumption being made here: one person at risk for 10 years is equivalent to a group of 10 people at risk for 1 year; both yield 10 person-years at risk. *SRS*

Rothman, K.J. and Greenland, S. 1998: *Modern epidemiology*, 2nd edn. Philadelphia: Lippincott-Raven Publishers.

PEST See SEQUENTIAL ANALYSIS

pharmacovigilance The terms 'post-marketing surveillance' and 'pharmacovigilance' are often used synonymously to refer to monitoring (both actively and prospectively or reacting to spontaneously occurring safety concerns) licensed pharmaceutical and biological medicinal products. At the time a marketing authorisation is granted (see MEDICINES AND HEALTHCARE PRODUCTS

REGULATORY AGENCY) there may have been between a few hundred and a few thousand patients studied. Typically, each of the PHASE III CLINICAL TRIALS may have only randomised a few hundred patients to the new, experimental treatment. It is quite likely, therefore, that rare reactions (perhaps occurring in one in a thousand patients or fewer) may never have been seen in such trials. No medicine is ever completely safe and it is therefore important that once widespread use of a new one has begun, safety signals are monitored and followed up. Rare events may manifest themselves as may adverse interactions with other drugs commonly used but in whom interaction studies were never carried out.

Pharmacovigilance is a relative new science, its grounds perhaps being set out by Finney (1971) who suggested that 'the primary duty of a drug monitoring system is less to demonstrate danger or to estimate incidence than to initiate suspicion'. It might be argued that once 'danger' has been determined, the monitoring process is too late and patients have already been injured (or may have died). What we need is a system than can 'initiate suspicion' so that preventive measures can be taken. Evans (2000) discusses a similar theme.

The great challenge for phamacovigilance is the uncontrolled nature of the data. Marketing authorisations are generally based on randomised, double-blind, PLACEBO (or active) controlled studies. Assessing post-marketing data is much closer to working in EPIDEMIOLOGY. Various national systems for reporting unexpected adverse reactions exist including the 'Yellow Card' system in the United Kingdom and the 'MedWatch' system in the USA. These (and other) systems rely on reports from a variety of sources including doctors, pharmacists, pharmaceutical companies and sometimes from patients themselves. However, they rely on the judgement of whether an adverse reaction needs to be considered. By the very nature of the rarity of the reactions that pharmacovigilance systems are trying to identify, doctors may not realise that an adverse event in a particular patient has anything to do with the medication(s) he or she is receiving. Conversely, reporting any and all adverse events experienced by patients and highlighting a *possible* relationship to any or all of the medications the patient is receiving would overburden any doctor and monitoring system. A middle ground needs to be found. A further problem arises when a 'new' adverse reaction is suspected and reported (in the scientific or lay press) and then the incidence of spontaneous reports often suddenly increases. The system swings from (almost always) under-reporting to (occasionally) over-reporting.

Various methods have been proposed to try to overcome problems of over- and under-reporting. Systems exist to record all medical events (prescriptions, illnesses, etc.) for samples of patients (say, all patients within selected general practitioners). These are better at overcoming selective reporting and, although they are based on samples, they are typically much larger samples than can be recruited into clinical trials. They also represent samples from practical experience in the community, rather than the highly controlled environment of a clinical trial.

For further reading, van der Heijden et al. (2002) proposed statistical methods that use 'all reports of reactions' as a means of adjusting for a general level of under-reporting. Grigg, Farewell and Spiegelhalter (2003) have reviewed statistical methods taken from ideas in quality control to monitor streams of reports (adverse reactions, and others) in 'real time', while Strom (2000) gives an excellent and detailed coverage of issues and methods used in pharmacovigilance.   *SD*

Evans, S.J.W. 2000: Pharmacovigilance: a science or fielding emergencies? *Statistics in Medicine* 19, 3199–209. **Finney, D.J.** 1971: Statistical aspects of monitoring for dangers in drug therapy. *Methods of Information in Medicine* 10, 1–8. **Grigg, O.A., Farewell, V.T. and Spiegelhalter, D.J.** 2003: Use of risk-adjusted CUSUM and RSPRT charts for monitoring in medical contexts. *Statistical Methods in Medical Research* 12, 147–70. **Strom, B. (ed.)** 2000: *Pharmacovigilance*, 3rd edn. Chichester: John Wiley & Sons Ltd. **van de Heijden, P.G.M., van Puijenbroek, E.P., van Buuren, S. and van der Hofstede, J.W.** 2002: On the assessment of adverse drug reactions from spontaneous reporting systems: the influence of under-reporting on odds ratios. *Statistics in Medicine* 21, 2027–44.

Phase I trials   CLINICAL TRIALS carried out in the early development of a drug, after animal toxicology studies have been completed, when the drug will first go into man. They involve human volunteers, healthy or patient, and as such the subject of such trials expects no therapeutic benefit. The focus of Phase I trials is on the safety and tolerability of drugs and pharmacokinetics (i.e. what the body does to the drug) and pharmacodynamics (i.e. what the drug does to the body). Pharmacokinetics involves measurement of drug concentrations in the body, determined by taking blood samples at specific times throughout the study. These are then summarised using such measures as AREA UNDER THE CURVE (AUC – representing total exposure) and maximum drug concentration (C_{max}). Other measures that might be used are time to maximum drug concentration (t_{max}) and elimination half-life. It is not possible to cover these topics in detail here, but Roland and Tozer (1995) give more details and applications for these measurements as well as how to look at the relationships between them, using PK/PD modelling.

Phase I trials can also be carried out prior to drug submission or when a new formulation is being developed. Examples of such studies are bioequivalence, drug interactions (both pharmacokinetic and pharmacodynamic), the effect of food and certain special populations, such as renal or hepatic impairment, elderly or males versus females.

These trials can also be carried out in early development to give a company a general idea of the effect studied, however, a confirmatory study will inevitably be required during submission to a regulatory body. They are highly regulated studies, with design and analysis being very standard. Further details on the studies can be found at the FDA website: www.fda.gov/cder/guidance.

First-into-man studies take place after completion of toxicology tests. The primary objective of Phase I trials should always be the examination of the safety and tolerability; however, pharmacokinetic and pharmacodynamic data are usually collected and analysed.

Since the drug has not been previously administered to humans the doses have to be escalated, meaning that each subject starts on a low dose and proceeds through the doses to progressively higher ones. Obviously, data have to be reviewed prior to any escalation and, if there is any cause for concern over safety, escalation will not occur,

remembering that the safety of subjects is most important.

The table gives examples of dosing escalation schemes showing just single cohorts. In reality, there is likely to be up to 24 subjects in 6 or 8 cohorts, although this depends on how many subjects can be recruited and how many safety data need to be collected.

Notice that both designs incorporate a PLACEBO period for each subject. This is so the measurements from an active period can be put into some context and it can be determined, for example, whether headache is a real drug effect or merely a result of being in a clinical trial.

Much of the analysis for these types of study is likely to be data driven, since they are mainly exploratory. Such things as dose or exposure response curves, with safety and pharmacokinetics, can be examined, as can the determination of a maximum tolerated dose. In addition, Bayesian techniques (see BAYESIAN METHODS) can be used optimally to design and analyse these studies (Whitehead *et al.*, 2001).   *AB*

Rowland, M. and Tozer, T.N. 1995: *Clinical pharmacokinetics – concepts and applications*, 3rd edn. Baltimore: Williams and Wilkins. **Whitehead, J., Zhou, Y., Patterson, S., Webber, D. and Francis, S.** 2001: Easy-to-implement Bayesian methods for dose-escalation studies in healthy volunteers. *Biostatistics* 2, 47–61.

Phase I trials *Examples of a rising dose scheme*

Example 1

Subject	Period 1	Period 2	Period 3	Period 4
1	10 mg	20 mg	30 mg	Placebo
2	10 mg	Placebo	20 mg	30 mg
3	10 mg	20 mg	Placebo	30 mg
4	Placebo	10 mg	20 mg	30 mg

Example 2

Subject	Period 1	Period 2	Period 3
1	10 mg	Placebo	30 mg
2	10 mg	20 mg	Placebo
3	Placebo	20 mg	30 mg

Phase II trials   CLINICAL TRIAL of a new agent or procedure in which the primary objective is typically to determine whether it has sufficient therapeutic efficacy with an acceptable safety profile in patients to warrant further testing and development in additional Phase II trials or large Phase III trials. Before starting a Phase II trial, however, a safe dose and schedule of the new drug or procedure has to be established in earlier dose-finding Phase I trials. As such, Phase II trials are most similar to the therapeutic exploratory studies according to the ICH Harmonised Tripartite Guideline E8 and start with the studies in which the primary objective is exploration of and screening for therapeutic efficacy.

Phase II trials often employ study designs such as historical controlled studies in which comparison is made with the efficacy from the historical controls or self-controlled studies in which comparison is made with the baseline status. Phase II trials are often conducted in patients who meet narrowly defined eligibility criteria in order to ensure homogeneity in patient baseline characteristics. ENDPOINTS of Phase II trials can be biological or a surrogate of clinical outcome and sometimes Phase II trials may be further classified as IIa or IIb accordingly. Also in Phase II trials additional objectives such as exploration of other study endpoints, therapeutic regiments including concomitant medications or target patient populations are evaluated and analyses for these objectives are, by necessity, exploratory and involve many subset analyses.

In the early development of a new therapeutic agent or procedure, the dose and schedule to be used in subsequent trials are determined in Phase I trials. For example, with traditional cytotoxic agents for cancer treatment, this dose is generally known as the maximum tolerated dose (MTD), although other choices, for example, dose level before the MTD, may be used. In subsequent Phase II trials, patients are treated at the dose level established as safe and acceptable in Phase I trials to screen if the treatment has sufficiently promising clinical activity or therapeutic efficacy, usually evaluated by the probability of treatment success, for example, objective response in cancer, for further investigation and development.

Since Phase II trials serve as initial screening, it is desirable to achieve the goals of the study with a minimal number of patients so that as few patients are given inactive treatment as possible. Also it is important to minimise the Type II error probability of reaching a false negative conclusion (see FALSE NEGATIVE RATE). To this end, sequential designs have been proposed in which a fixed number of patients are accrued in each stage and the study is stopped early if the observed number of treatment successes is too small.

Gehan (1961) was the first to propose a two-stage design for screening in Phase II trials in which 14 patients are initially accrued during stage 1 and the study stops if no treatment success is observed and otherwise another cohort of patients are accrued in stage 2. The number of patients during stage 1 is chosen to keep the probability of early termination very small, say < 0.05, when the treatment is active with the probability of treatment success $p \geq 0.20$. The sample size for stage 2 is determined to achieve a specified level of confidence in the estimation of the probability of treatment success with the maximum sample size. Later this notion of two-stage designs was formalised as a test of statistical hypotheses regarding the probability of treatment success as in Simon (1989). Multi-stage designs have also been formalised by Fleming (1982), among others.

In general, a two-stage design is defined by the numbers of patients to be accrued, n_1 and n_2, and the boundary values, r_1 and r, during stages 1 and 2, respectively, and is denoted as $(r_1/n_1, r/n)$ where $n = n_1 + n_2$ is the maximum sample size. During stage 1, n_1 patients are initially enrolled and treated. If the number of treatment successes during stage 1 is less than or equal to r_1, the trial is terminated for lack of therapeutic efficacy and it is concluded that the treatment does not warrant further investigation. Otherwise, the study is continued to stage 2 during which an additional n_2 patients are enrolled and treated. If the total number of treatment successes after stage 2 exceeds r, it is concluded that the treatment has sufficient therapeutic efficacy and it is, therefore, considered for further investigation. Early acceptance of the treatment is not considered here, as there are no ethical reasons to do so when there is evidence of therapeutic efficacy. The ethical imper-

ative for early termination occurs when the treatment has unacceptable therapeutic efficacy. Furthermore, when there is sufficient therapeutic efficacy, there is often interest and desire in studying additional patients to assess the safety of treatment more extensively.

The sample sizes and the boundary values for such two-stage designs can be determined based on a test of hypothesis. Consider testing $H_0 : p \leq p_0$ against $H_1 : p \geq p_1$ with Type I and II error probabilities α and β where p denotes the probability of treatment success. The value of p_0 is chosen to represent the maximally unacceptable level of therapeutic efficacy and the value of p_1 is chosen to represent the minimally acceptable level of therapeutic efficacy. These parameters $(p_0, p_1, \alpha, \beta)$ are the design parameters. Then the probability of early termination because of insufficient therapeutic efficacy indicated by no more than r_1 treatment successes is given by $P_{ET} = B(r_1; n_1, p)$ where B denotes the BINOMIAL DISTRIBUTION function and the expected sample size for the true value of p is determined by:

$$E(N|p) = n_1 + (1 - P_{ET})n_2.$$

The probability of rejecting a treatment with a success probability P is thus given by:

$$B(r_1; n_1, p) + \sum_{x=r_1+1}^{\min|n_1, r|} b(x; n_1, P)B(r - x; n_2, p)$$

where b denotes the binomial probability mass function.

Simon (1989) proposed two-stage designs that are optimal in the sense that the expected sample size $E(N|p)$ is minimised when $p = p_0$ with insufficient therapeutic efficacy subject to the Type I and II error probabilities. Despite the minimum expected sample size, the maximum sample size $n = n_1 + n_2$ for the optimal design can be much larger than other designs, which is undesirable. Therefore, Simon (1989) also suggested the minimax design, which minimises the maximum sample size, again subject to the same Type I and II error probabilities. However, Simon's minimax and optimal designs sometimes result in quite different sample size requirements. For example, the minimax design can have a much larger expected sample size $E(N|p_0)$ than the optimal design and the optimal design can have a much larger maximum sample size n than the minimax design. For example, with the design parameters $(p_0, p_1, \alpha, \beta) = (0.3, 0.5, 0.05, 0.15)$, the minimax design is $(r_1/n_1, r/n) = (14/37, 17/42)$ and the optimal design is $(7/21, 19/48)$ whereas the expected sample size is 37.6 and 28.5 for the minimax and the optimal design, respectively.

Jung et al. (2004) used a Bayesian decision-theoretic criterion of admissibility to define a class of designs based on a loss function which is a weighted average of the maximum sample size and the expected sample size under the null hypothesis, the two criteria used by Simon (1989). The admissible designs include Simon's minimax and optimal designs as special cases and compromises between Simon's minimax and optimal designs. For our earlier example, one can find an admissible design (4/15, 18/45) with a maximum sample size of 45, which is a compromise between the minimax and the optimal designs and an expected sample size of 29.5, which is close to the expected sample for the optimal design. These compromise admissible designs can be found on a convex hull formed by Simon's minimax and optimal designs. The admissible designs of Jung *et al.* (2004) can be easily generalised to any number of stages. *KK*

Fleming, T.R. 1982: One sample multiple testing procedures for Phase II clinical trials. *Biometrics* 38, 143–51. **Gehan, E.A.** 1961: The determination of the number of patients required in a follow-up trial of a new chemotherapeutic agent. *Journal of Chronic Diseases* 13, 346–53. **Jung, S.-H., Lee, T., Kim, K. and Geroge, S.L.** 2004: Admissible two-state designs for Phase II cancer clinical trials. *Statistics in Medicine* 23, 561–9. **Simon, R.** 1989: Optimal two-stage designs for Phase II clinical trials. *Controlled Clinical Trials* 10, 1–10.

Phase III trials

New medicines, in particular new drugs, are generally developed in a phased process. Phase I and Phase II trials are small trials, the former generally in volunteers, the latter in patients and tend to be learning or exploratory trials. In contrast, Phase III trials are larger and are confirmatory. Phase III trials provide confirmation of the properties of the new medicine that have been discovered in early phases of the development programme.

In order to be approved for marketing, a new drug must be shown to constitute a worthwhile contribution to medical treatment. Phase III trials are designed to identify an appropriate population of patients who are better treated with the new drug than with other treatments. Additionally, they should identify those patients who do not benefit from treatment with the new drug and those who may be harmed by its use. The prime goal of such trials is to recommend treatment strategies, including the appropriate dose, or dose titration, for the prescribing physician. This goal is achieved by the detailed label whose content is informed by the results of all three phase of drug development, although primarily Phase III trials.

Phase III clinical trials will generally exhibit all the characteristics that have come to be associated with the 'mythical' gold standard trial. They will generally be randomised, be run double-blind, PLACEBO controlled and conducted in a well-defined population of patients. They will most often be parallel group, fixed sample trials. However, there is a growing appreciation that group sequential, adaptive or flexible designs provide drug sponsors with the opportunity to manage their drug development programmes in a more efficient way. This class of trials is characterised by the ability to make changes to the initial setting of the trial, in such a way as protect the TYPE I ERROR. The changes include the dropping of treatment arms for inefficacy (futility) including the stopping of the trial; resample sizing based on learning about either the variability in the trial and/or the estimated effect; early stopping because of mounting evidence of a large beneficial effect. The ability of drug sponsors to stop individual trials early because of evidence of a large beneficial effect may be restricted by the requirement for a prescribed level of exposure of patients to the exploratory medicine. For example, it may be that a drug sponsor is required to have 500 patients exposed to the exploratory medicine for at least 12 months. Phase III trials are normally conducted in parallel groups and while it is not unknown for a trial to include more than one dose of the experimental medicine, such trials are not the norm since the appropriate dose will normally have been chosen in Phase II.

Generally, two Phase III trials are required for the registration of new medicine. One reason for this is that to require two trials each to be significant at the one-sided 0.025 level corresponds to an overall Type I error of 0.000625 corresponding to a FALSE POSITIVE RATE of 1/1600. The use of a one-sided SIGNIFICANCE LEVEL is necessary since we clearly require both tests to be positive, that is the treatment effects are in the same direction. It can be shown that if this is the only requirement, then there are more efficient ways to ensure its achievement other than requiring the individual trials to be separately significant. More recently, the Federal Drugs Administration (FDA) in the USA has set conditions under which it is possible to register a new medicine on the basis of a single, large clinical trial with a smaller than usual Type I error. The circumstances tend to be when there is a critical need among seriously ill patients. In such circumstances it is not unusual for standard practices to be relaxed. One well-known example is in the development of treatment for HIV and AIDS in which regulators, under pressure from patient, relaxed standard clinical practice.

The choice of control in Phase III trials is a matter of considerable debate. It was noted earlier that Phase III trials are generally placebo controlled. There are, however, circumstances in which it is not possible ethically to require patients to be treated with a placebo. Such circumstances typically, although not exclusively, arise when the disease under investigation is associated with a mortality outcome. The recent International Conference on Harmonization (ICH) guideline (E10), entitled 'Choice of control group and related issues in clinical trials', addresses a number of important issues when an active control group is chosen and the primary aim of the study is to demonstrate non-inferiority. Of prime importance in this context is what E10 terms *assay sensitivity*. Assay sensitivity is the ability of a clinical trial to differentiate between effective, minimally effective and ineffective treatments. Assay sensitivity is important in all trials, but has particular implications in trials whose prime purpose is to demonstrate non-inferiority. If a drug sponsor intends to claim effectiveness of a new medicine by showing it to be non-inferior to a active control, but the trial lacks assay sensitivity, it is possible that an ineffective treatment will be found to be non-inferior and thereby lead to an erroneous conclusion of efficacy.

The E10 guideline points to a number of issues that need to be addressed: Was the appropriate patient population chosen? Was the appropriate dose of the active comparator used? Was treatment with the active comparator of the appropriate duration? How was the non-inferiority margin, which defines non-inferiority, chosen? Is there historical evidence that the design has in the past shown itself to be capable of distinguishing effective from ineffective treatments?

After the conclusion of the experiment, the guideline requires a demonstration that the results obtained on the active comparator are similar to those obtained in previous trials. *AG*

Phase IV trials

No totally adequate definition has yet been arrived at. One working definition, however, is that these types of trial encompass all the studies undertaken after the obtaining of a marketing licence. While studies conducted in the run-up to the registration process are regarded as adequate for the purpose of determining whether a new drug is efficacious and in large part safe, they do, by their very nature, leave important questions unanswered. As an example, during the pre-registration phase, the toxicity of a drug could not have been accurately assessed in a Phase III clinical trial if the incidence of agranulocytosis was 1 in 20,000 or less. In general, Phase II and Phase III studies are restricted because they are based on limited numbers of patients, a limited duration of patient exposure and a restricted population of patients.

Phase IV trials are designed to answer detailed questions about the practical use of a drug. There are many different aspects of this, not all of which will be studied at the same time. Such trials may be conducted to investigate other doses or the scheduling of a new treatment; they may be used to look at side-effects in more detail, particularly in long-term chronic usage; they can be used to investigate drug efficacy in long-term usage where, for example, the course of a disease may be modified over a period of months or years; they can be used to collect comparative data of a long term usage if the original studies were restricted to a comparison against placebo; they can be used to investigate new uses and indications leading, potentially, to a new submission; or to investigate alternative populations.

Phase IV trials are usually conducted after a drug has already been through the full trial process and has already got a licence from the authorities for general use, although Phase IV trials can also be run during the registration process itself. In many aspects, Phase IV trials are similar to Phase III trials. They will, in the main, be randomised and controlled, although not generally placebo controlled; furthermore, some of their objectives may be investigated by *uncontrolled* studies.

It is important to distinguish between Phase IV trials and post-marketing surveillance (PMS) or monitored release studies (MRS). A PMS trial will tend to be observational and non-interventional and will be conducted primarily to monitor safety in a new medicine shortly after it has begun to be prescribed in daily practice. While there may be simple measures of efficacy included so that additional risk/benefit judgements may be made, this is not the prime purpose of the trial. A further type of study that may be conducted post registration is a so-called 'seeding' study. A 'seeding study' involves the drug sponsor providing a new medicine to physicians in order to familiarise them with its use and to encourage them to prescribe it. In such studies there is neither intention nor attempt to gather data that could provide useful scientific or medical information.

More recently Phase IV trials have been used in order to collect health economics, also known as outcome research, data concerning resource utilisation. Such data are required in order to provide information on the cost-effectiveness of new medicines for reimbursement agencies. Although this information may be required at, or shortly after, registration of a new medicine, forcing its collection during Phase II and Phase III trials – so-called piggybacking – may not be appropriate. Phase II and Phase III trials are highly controlled scientific experiments designed to minimise variation and to make it possible to detect small, but clinically relevant, treatment effects. In one sense, therefore, they are artificial and do not represent the environment in which new medicines will ultimately be prescribed.

This has a number of consequences. First, protocols in Phase III trials may include investigations that are non-standard in the clinical treatment of patients but are entirely appropriate in a clinical trial to monitor the safety of patients. If these 'extra' investigations are allocated against the new medicine their cost may bias the overall evaluation of its cost and hence its cost-effectiveness. Second, health outcomes may be more variable than the clinical ENDPOINTS studied in Phase III trials. If, therefore, health economic outcomes are piggybacked on a Phase II trial this is likely to increase the sample size and lead to an even greater cost of drug development than hitherto. Ideally, health economic studies should be conducted in a more naturalistic setting. They will tend to be large trials, using endpoints that are patient centric so that quality of life outcomes (see QUALITY OF LIFE MEASUREMENT) may predominate over clinical outcomes and they will tend to be simple with the minimum of information being collected. Such trials may more appropriately be carried out in a Phase IV programme.   *AG*

phenotype This term refers to the observable characteristics of an individual or organism, as distinct from its GENOTYPES, which, before modern molecular genetics, were not observable. Although many genotypes are also now measurable, the distinction is still useful.

Phenotype covers a wide range of possibilities, including diseases (affected or not affected), quantitative traits (for example, blood pressure or height) and biological measurements (for example, blood glucose levels). In some cases, there is a close relationship between a particular gene and a particular phenotype. For example, in the ABO example, there are four main blood groups, as measured by serology, determined by the ABO gene: A, B, AB and O. These phenotypes are determined by the genotypes: individuals with genotypes (A,O) and (A,A) are group A; genotypes (B,O) and (B,B) give rise to group B; (A,B) gives rise to group AB; and (O,O) to group O.

Most phenotypes are, however, related to genotype in a more complex fashion – most diseases and other common phenotypes are related to genotypes at many genetic loci and are also influenced by environmental or lifestyle factors.

The probabilities with which particular genotypes are associated with particular phenotypes are referred to as *penetrances*.   *DE*

[See also GENETIC EPIDEMIOLOGY, TWIN ANALYSIS]

Balding, D.J., Bishop, M. and Cannings, C. (eds) 2001: *Handbook of statistical genetics.* Chichester: John Wiley & Sons. **Sham, P.** 1998: *Statistics in human genetics.* London: Arnold.

pie chart A graphical display in which a series of frequencies or percentages are represented by sections of a circle having areas proportional to the observed values. An example is given in the Figure on page 261.

Although very popular in the media, both the general and scientific use of pie charts has been severely criticised (see Tufte, 1983; Wainer, 1997) and tables are preferable for most small datasets. Among particular dangers to be

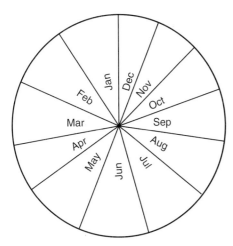

pie chart *Frequencies of first births in each month in a Swiss town*

aware of concerning pie charts are the following: distortion of the basic shape from a circle; misleading use of 3-dimensionality; detaching of slices from the pie; rotation to promote of hide a given slice; and failure to show sample size on which the proportions are based.   *BSE*

[See also BAR CHART, DOTPLOT, HISTOGRAM, STEM-AND-LEAF PLOT]

Tufte, E.R. 1983: *The visual display of quantitative information.* Cheshire, CT: Graphics Press. **Wainer, H.** 1997: *Visual revelations.* New York: Springer.

pilot studies Small-scale research experiments primarily undertaken to inform or improve the conduct of related future research. In general, pilot studies do not in themselves aim to generate scientifically useful evidence. Instead, pilot studies are conducted for a variety of reasons, including: testing feasibility and appropriateness of data collection (e.g. are sufficient manpower and time resources planned to gather required information?); identifying problems with QUESTIONNAIRE wording, if extracting information in this manner (e.g. do patients' responses indicate that questions have been properly understood and answered?); identifying problems with data processing (e.g. does a null, or a blank, response mean answer is missing, or not asked, or no response, or an unknown answer?); training observers or interviewers to equally high standards to help ensure uniformity of data quality, whenever multiple individuals are involved in data collection and processing as in most large or multicentre studies (e.g. is there a learning curve in how data are extracted, and do all attain a sufficient level of expertise?); assessing, at least initially, anticipated variation of responses for this can help sample size estimation for the main study (e.g. when such information is either not available or not applicable from the published literature, being better than relying on 'educated guesswork' alone); estimating main study duration and cost (e.g. if uncertain, both time and money estimates may need to be firmed up before submitting a realistic budget to potential sponsors).

Although often on a hidden agenda, a well-conducted pilot study can also help serve to convince potential sponsors of the main study to follow that the research team is indeed capable of performing their intended study, once awarded the necessary funding. Pilot studies do not need to be large to serve their purposes. There may be the need for several drafts before the final version of a questionnaire is deemed most suitable, although one pilot is generally sufficient and its cost and effort are usually well rewarded.

On the negative side, pilot studies can cause results from an investigation to be delayed, a classic case of the compromise between speed and quality. (This is reminiscent of the service salesperson's banter: 'You can have it fast, cheap or reliable – pick any one!') However, various attempts to circumvent this problem have been proposed that involve internal pilot studies. These are study designs that seek to incorporate a seamless transition from pilot to main study, in which initial information arising helps dictate the choice of overall study sample size, a similar motivation to some DATA-DEPENDENT DESIGNS for CLINICAL TRIALS. See, for instance, contributions by Burkett and Day (1994), Wittes *et al.* (1999) and Zucker *et al.* (1999) for a flavour of these developments.

One warning about running a pilot study is the potential for BIAS brought about by inappropriately combining results from pilot and main study, especially if changes occur after the pilot phase. This is so even if these changes are as innocuous looking as rephrasing questions from positive to negative or from open to closed (see QUESTIONNAIRES). Pilot patients will be in a different timeframe, so beware any temporal or seasonal variation in response. Furthermore, eligibility criteria for inclusion in the main study and in the pilot study may differ in important ways, meaning it would not be obvious to which population (if any) inferences from such a hybrid sample might apply.

In conclusion, pilot studies are well worth the initial effort involved. Too few are undertaken in advance of major studies. This may be attributable in part to too much research occurring on a tight timescale to accommodate individuals' medical career steps. Also, it is more than a pity that much published research is labelled as a 'pilot' as if this were somehow a post-experimental justification for inadequate, or worse still, absent, design planning. For one's own research, always run a pilot study unless there is sound reason not to do so. Expect to discard its results from the main analysis, unless it causes nothing to change and it was pre-planned as an internal pilot study.   *CRP*

Burkett, M.A. and Day, S.J. 1994: Internal pilot studies for estimating sample size. *Statistics in Medicine* 13, 2455–64. **Wittes, J.T., Schabenberger, O., Zucker, D.M., Brittain, E. and Proschan, M.** 1999: Internal pilot studies I: Type I error rate of the naïve t-test. *Statistics in Medicine* 18, 3481–91. **Zucker, D.M., Wittes, J.T., Schabenberger, O. and Brittain, E.** 1999: Internal pilot studies II: comparison of various procedures. *Statistics in Medicine* 18, 3493–509.

pitfalls in medical research Many people working in healthcare become involved in the design, execution, analysis and dissemination of medical research at some point in their careers. Doctors are taught about medical research and in the course of their professional training may well be expected to be actively involved in research. Other health professionals and even managers are also likely to be required to be active researchers. Consumers (that band of once passive recipients of healthcare formerly known as patients) are also increasingly contributing to the commissioning and design of research. There will always be those for whom research is at the centre of their professional lives and those for whom it is at the periphery, but many individuals are expected at some point to be researchers. Research, however, presents many pitfalls for the inexperienced, some of which are described here in the hope that this may assist future researchers to avoid them.

Research and clinical audit are sometimes confused and the novice researcher may be uncertain what kind of activity it is they are undertaking. The UK NHS working definition of research is 'the attempt to derive generalisable new knowledge by addressing clearly defined questions with systematic and rigorous methods' (Department of Health, 2001), while clinical audit can be defined as 'a quality improvement process that seeks to improve patient care and outcomes through systematic review of care against explicit criteria and the implementation of change' (NICE, 2002).

The distinction is not an academic one, as research has wider ethical and governance implications than audit, as patients must be protected and the scientific quality of the research guaranteed (World Medical Association, 2002). For example, access to confidential patient information for research purposes requires independent ethical review and generally the informed consent of the patient, access for an audit activity aimed at improving patient care does not. Appropriate review for research should be obtained, including scientific review, ethical review from a research ethics committee or institutional review board and other approvals. For example, in England and Wales, approval must be sought from each NHS trust hosting the research (see ETHICAL REVIEW COMMITTEES). Hence the first pitfall may sometimes be not to recognise research activity, thus denying participants the protection offered by ethical and scientific review.

Many individuals are involved in and contribute to research, but they do not all have the same experience or expertise. It follows that researchers who do not seek out the range of skills needed for their projects are likely run into problems. Successful medical research no longer involves a single scientist working in isolation, if, indeed, it ever did. Major grant-awarding bodies look not only for individuals with research track records, but also for a research team with appropriate clinical and other collaborators, including explicitly identified statistical expertise. Even a relatively junior and isolated researcher should seek to identify a research team that will support her project. This should include ideally senior clinicians and investigators with deeper knowledge of the research area, statistical support and advice (often available in research active institutions). Peer support enables researchers to benefit from shared experience.

Essential though it may be, collaboration, or, more particularly, *academic supervision*, can cause difficulties for researchers. Collaborators and supervisors may have over-ambitious views of what their researchers can achieve and may underestimate the time required. Supervisors may have their own special interests that are not shared by students or that do not constitute appropriate research for the students' objectives, particularly academic ones. Indeed, more than one supervisor may have conflicting special interests. There are no easy answers, but early

development of an agreed protocol for the research and a project plan for student's time offers some protection against conflicting interests and changes of direction.

Why might failing to seeking statistical collaboration be a pitfall? This can be answered by considering what a statistician can contribute to a research project. Researchers whose memory of learning basic statistics consists of a succession of hypothesis tests might be surprised to find that a consultation with a statistician is unlikely to focus on the statistical tests required in the proposed research. Discussions will focus on, first, the question that the research will address, moving on to the appropriate research design to answer that question and the data to be collected. Only then can the proposed analysis and the required sample size be considered. The statistician contributes to the whole research design, not merely the statistical analysis (see CONSULTING A STATISTICIAN).

If the role of statistics in research is about design as much as it is about analysis, what problems are encountered where the research design is inadequate? The pitfalls involved in proceeding with research without a clearly thought-out research design are several: the finished research may answer no clear question; although the researcher had a clear question, an inappropriate design that cannot give a clear answer has been used; some of the information needed properly to answer the question was not collected; the study size may be too small to answer the researcher's question.

Why does it matter that a research proposal should address a clear question? Medical research progresses by framing hypotheses and addressing answerable questions and patient involvement in research cannot be justified when this does not apply. Without a research question, a statistician cannot develop a research design, just as an architect cannot develop a drawing unless he knows whether a house or a railway station is required. Research questions and research designs are so closely linked that once a researcher has framed a clear question, the appropriate design often becomes apparent. Without an *a priori* answerable question, the data collected may well be inadequate to provide the answer to any useful question. Some researchers might find an evidence-based approach to medicine (see EVIDENCE-BASED MEDICINE) helpful in thinking through clinical research questions. Different types of clinical question, for example concerning treatment, prognosis or diagnosis can be framed, and then a research protocol with the appropriate design to answer the question can be developed (Sackett *et al.*, 2000). For example, a question concerning a medical intervention needs to define the population to be studied, an intervention and a comparator and an outcome.

The design most likely to control for confounding in an intervention study and thus provide high-quality evidence is a randomised controlled trial (see CLINICAL TRIALS). In specifying the question, the preferred research design has also been determined. Not all research has a clinical focus – it might be epidemiological or laboratory research – but the researcher will still need to have clearly formulated, refutable hypotheses, if a protocol designed to test them is to be developed.

A researcher may have developed a question, but is it the right question? A further pitfall is that the research question may already have been adequately answered. Would the proposed research add anything new to the existing literature? Once the component parts of an initial question, e.g. the patient population, the precise intervention, the most valid comparators and outcomes, are clearly defined, they can be turned into search terms to be used in reviewing the medical literature, perhaps to be used in a formal systematic review (see SYSTEMATIC REVIEW AND META-ANALYSIS) (Chalmers and Altman, 2001). If the question has been answered or there is a good-quality study in progress likely to give a definitive answer, then continuing to plan a new study is neither ethical nor cost-effective. Even where a thorough literature search confirms that the research question has not previously been adequately answered, it may be that the literature or contact with experts, clinical colleagues and patients suggests that the initial question was not clinically relevant or has already been partially answered and thus the question may need to be modified before developing a research protocol.

Once the research question has been framed, inappropriate research design presents the next pitfall. It is possible for a researcher to have a clear research question, but to have chosen a research design that cannot answer it. An epidemiologist evaluating the results of a study will consider whether they are a chance finding, are explained by confounding (when more than one factor are associated both with each other and the outcome so that it is impossible to say what the true effect of each is on the outcome) or by BIAS (Rothman 2002). The research design must answer the research question in a way that minimises the influence of chance, bias and confounding.

Bias is any process that causes the study results systematically to depart from the true result. The selection of participants can be biased, perhaps because the sample is drawn from a highly selected hospital population but the intention is to generalise the results to the whole population (see SELECTION BIAS). The measurement of outcomes can be biased by poor ascertainment or poor response, by bias in the recording of information or by inadequate follow-up. Sometimes proposed research has a biased design because the researcher starts with the data that are most easily available, not with the data that can answer the question. Suppose the accuracy of a blood test is under consideration and a researcher has access to test results and associated patient records. Suppose that diagnosis requires expensive tests. It is likely only the most severe and quite probably only those with positive test results will have the expensive investigations and the results will reflect this bias inflating the apparent accuracy of the test. If the researcher had started by considering an optimal design, then a COHORT STUDY including a representative sample of patients all of whom receive both tests would be the preferred design. Underpinning clearly framed research questions there should be an understanding of how research design can as far as possible avoid bias and confounding, whether that understanding is mediated through a traditional approach to epidemiology or to the design of experiments or by evidence-based medicine.

A further pitfall in the design of a research study is that the data collected may be inadequate for the purpose. The chosen outcome measures may not adequately measure the chosen outcome. Standardised instruments (including QUESTIONNAIRES and psychological tests) with known validity and reliability should be used where possible (see MEASUREMENT ERROR AND RELIABILITY). If researchers are developing their own outcome measures, whether laboratory tests or questionnaires, they should investigate the proposed outcome's properties. All questionnaires should be piloted, preferably using the target population (see PILOT STUDIES). Investigators should be wary of confusing process with outcomes. Some potential outcome measures will not be available for all patients, for example, the gold standard for clinical diagnosis may depend on histological confirmation of disease that can only be obtained in the most ill patients. Hence, protocol outcome definitions may need to be pragmatically adapted to the realities of the clinical setting.

Important data items may be omitted, for example, it is not unknown for inexperienced researchers interested in the survival of their patients carefully to collect information about deaths among their patients, but not explicitly to record the last date living patients were seen, without which SURVIVAL ANALYSIS is impossible. Important confounding factors (age and sex should almost always be recorded) may be omitted. Consultation with clinical and statistical collaborators and careful reading of previous relevant studies will prevent some of these mistakes.

It is equally possible to collect far more data than is necessary, particularly when many tests are repeated as part of clinical care or research is designed by large, multidisciplinary committees comprised of specialists, where each wants to promote his or her own area of clinical interest. Decisions should be made at the outset on at which time points data will be collected and what will be measured. A researcher might, for example, want to know the lowest white cell count following a bone marrow transplant or the time point at which the white cell count recovered, but will certainly not need the results of daily blood tests. All of this should be specified in the research protocol, not after the end of data collection (see PROTOCOLS FOR CLINICAL TRIALS).

Researchers are often disappointed when their apparently interesting data do not show statistically significant results and thus may have occurred simply by chance. To avoid this disappointment, a researcher must before the research starts calculate what sample size is required in order to be reasonably certain that, if the desired results are obtained, they are precise enough to be convincing, as demonstrated by narrow CONFIDENCE INTERVAL or by the result of a hypothesis test that is statistically significant at a pre-specified level. To estimate how many patients are needed (a sample size calculation) the researcher must typically specify what the researcher expects to find, e.g. outcome in control group and what the researcher hopes to detect, e.g. a clinically important difference that might be achieved with a new treatment. The researcher also needs to specify acceptable statistical power so that there is a reasonable chance of detecting such a difference if it does exist (minimum acceptable is 80%, which will detect a true result in 80% of samples with a given level of statistical significance) and the significance level (typically $\alpha = 0.05$) or precision (that is, confidence interval, typically 95%).

Statistical aspects of sample size calculations are straightforward, given appropriate reference books, tables (e.g. Machin *et al.*, 1997) or software (e.g. NQUERY ADVISOR), but deciding what is a worthwhile outcome is not (see various SAMPLE SIZE DETERMINATION entries). It is easy to manipulate the inputs to the calculation by adjusting the researcher's expectations and the statistical power required. All too often a researcher approaches a statistician for a sample size calculation in the expectation the answer will be precisely the number of patients available. It is important, however, to explore what the sample size requirements would be if the initial assumptions were wrong. Researchers should aim for samples larger than the minimum necessary to identify a substantial improvement over standard treatment.

There may be few data to inform calculations and the temptation is to under-estimate sample size (e.g. by assuming implausibly small standard deviations). As an illustration of what can go wrong, consider a placebo-controlled trial where there is good reason to expect a 60% response with the intervention and where $\alpha = 0.05$ and power is 90%. Placebo response rates are notoriously variable. If an overoptimistic researcher assumes a 30% placebo response and the actual rate is only 5% higher, then 50% more patients will be required (see Figure).

Determination of sample size is not simply a statistical calculation. Researchers often overestimate the availability of patients. In practice, patients do not always consent to take part, default from clinics, drop out, move house and even die at inconvenient times (see DROPOUTS). Medical records are often indefinitely unavailable if not explicitly lost. A generous allowance should be added to the sample size to allow for such contingencies.

What can be done if the researcher cannot recruit enough patients to meet a realistically estimated sample size? If a proposed study cannot answer the proposed question, it would be unethical to ask patients to take part and the study should not go ahead. If a single-centre study had been proposed, it might be possible to find collaborators in other centres in order to obtain sufficient numbers, although MULTICENTRE TRIALS have further potential pitfalls compared to single-centre studies.

After careful consideration of the research question and the design, the researcher should have developed a research protocol. This should be sufficiently detailed to provide a clear picture of what the study will involve. Studies based on inadequate or even non-existent protocols are likely to fail to provide data that match the researcher's objectives. If the study aims are unclear in the protocol, if it does not clearly specify which patients are to be recruited, what is to happen to them and what data are to be collected, then everyone involved in carrying out the study will share the same uncertainties. While not all studies need the detailed protocols of commercial drug trials, the protocol should describe the research aims and lay out the activities necessary to achieve them. The researcher might ask the question: 'Is there enough information in the protocol for someone from outside the research team to understand why the study is being carried out and what would be needed to replicate it?' If the answer is no, there is the danger that the research project will not follow the research design and will provide meaningless or biased results. The research protocol is at the heart of good clinical practice (GCP) in research, the code of conduct that aims to protect the rights and safety of research subjects and to ensure the scientific quality of the research. While some aspects of GCP are specific to drug trials (ICH, 1996), most of it applies to all clinical studies (MRC, 1998; 2000). Scientific and ethical review of the protocol ensures that the research design is valid and ethical. Adherence to the protocol while the research is in progress should ensure that the study aims are met.

Many novice researchers have little awareness of GCP, but adhering to its principles would avoid many pitfalls for the research project in progress. The principal investigator and other suitably qualified personnel involved in the research should be identified and, particularly in drug trials, responsibilities should be explicitly delegated in writing. In commonsense terms, this means that all members of the research team should understand their role in the project and should receive adequate training. The scientific quality of the study is assured by adherence to the protocol, but this is only meaningful if it is possible to monitor that adherence. This is done (extensively in commercially sponsored trials) by comparing the study documentation, the 'case report forms', against the source documentation, for example, patient notes and laboratory records. Thus, not only should the study be meticulously documented, but also patients' records need to be maintained to high standards.

Even where a study is not likely to be audited in any detail, adherence to the protocol, careful study documentation and maintenance of high-quality patient records will help ensure that all subjects successfully complete the study and will contribute to the quality of the data collected. Conversely, in studies where standards of record keeping are low, even the investigators will find it difficult

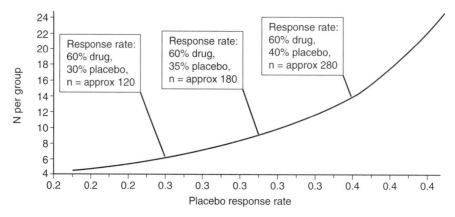

pitfalls in medical research *Impact of different levels of placebo response on sample size*

to find out what was actually done, should they need to go back to the study records and raw data. Study records must be kept securely and, in clinical research, separately from the patient record, which should contain all important information, including that the patient has given informed consent. Study records should be archived after completion of the study, so that there is an audit trail should there be any queries concerning the way the study was carried out or the accuracy of the data.

A researcher will not be able to start a project as soon as the protocol is finalised. Enough time must be allowed at the start of the project to obtain research ethics approval, any institutional approvals required and any regulatory approvals required, for example, a clinical trial authorisation for a trial of a medicinal product in the UK (see MEDICINES AND HEALTHCARE PRODUCTS REGULATORY AGENCY (MHRA)). The time required should not be underestimated, as research ethics committees generally have queries that must be answered before final approval is given. Often these queries concern incomplete application forms or badly drafted patient information and might have been avoided if guidance on drafting forms and leaflets had been followed. Never allow only the minimum possible time for approvals to be obtained.

Even after all the data have been collected, some further pitfalls remain. Before preparing the data for analysis, the coding of data items should be considered, as tidying up a messy dataset can add considerably to the time needed for data analysis. Codes should be allocated for MISSING DATA, taking care to distinguish genuine missing data from 'unknown' and zero entries. Each patient should be allocated a study number, so that individuals can be easily identified in data analysis if necessary. The use of a database with an appropriate form for DATA ENTRY incorporating checks on the data entered can facilitate quick and accurate data entry. Databases are preferred to spreadsheets as it is easier to ensure the correct data are entered for a particular case. If, however, a spreadsheet is used, one row should be used for all the information on a single patient and care should be taken when sorting the data to ensure that the correct data remains attached to the correct patient. At least a sample of data should be checked by double data entry or proofreading (see DATA MANAGEMENT).

Data should be kept securely and password protected to protect patient confidentiality, should always be anonymised and should be backed up regularly so that at worst only the last few cases entered are lost. Data protection is a legal requirement as well as good practice: losing precious data when a portable computer is stolen is bad enough; it is worse if the back-up copies were in the computer bag; it is far more serious if confidential personal information is lost or revealed.

Where available, statistical packages offer more flexibility and speed in statistical analysis than spreadsheets and databases and, an important factor, the statistical calculations made have been checked. Data can be imported from databases, spreadsheets and other formats. Menu-driven STATISTICAL PACKAGES are easy to use and offer extensive help files, but that can in itself present a hazard. A statistical method should only be used if the assumptions underlying it are met by the data to which it is applied. Advice should be sought if a researcher does not understand the application of assumptions behind the

statistical methods they are using else the researcher risks presenting superficially sophisticated but meaningless results.

Poor or non-existent planning often means that a research project is never successfully completed. Good project management from the outset, however, increases a project's chance of successful completion. Research projects which have received substantial funding would be expected to have project plans monitored by a management committee to help ensure the project achieves its aims on time and within budget. This approach can be usefully applied to smaller scale projects. The quality of the desired outcome should be specified and the time and other resources available (or else which must be obtained) must be identified. For example, a doctor in a training post planning some research might have a project plan that specifies: the quality of the research must be at least adequate for a conference presentation; the resources available are the researcher's time, some input into the research design from others, a little local funding and some secretarial time; and the time constraints are that sufficient results must be available by the conference abstract deadline and the project must be completed by the conference.

It is important to be realistic when considering both the resources and the time available. A project completed over a year should allow a realistic amount of time for Christmas and other public holidays, vacations and illness (the researcher's, their supervisor's and the patients'), as well as building in some time for unexpected contingencies. Once these constraints have been identified, the researcher should plan backwards from endpoint. He or she should ask the questions: Is there enough time and resources to achieve quality? If not, can the timescale be adjusted or further resources sought (which will itself take time)? Would a less ambitious project meet quality standard?

The timelines can be plotted and an analysis made of the critical pathways where delay might occur: what steps will hold everything up (e.g. obtaining research ethics approval, retrieving records)? Once this has been identified the researcher should focus on how to achieve those steps in a timely fashion. Milestones critical to the success of the project should be identified and targets set for achieving them. A management committee can be set up to monitor progress against targets.

The researcher who wishes to avoid pitfalls will have clearly specified research questions, appropriate research designs, adequately detailed protocols and well-planned projects carried out in line with good practice. Statisticians contribute to all of these objectives. Statisticians, like doctors, are most effectively consulted in the earliest stages and the consequences of not taking this advice are well known. Perhaps, then, the biggest pitfall in medical research is to forget that statistical collaboration should start at the beginning and last throughout the life of a research project.   *CLC*

Chalmers, I. and Altman, D.G. (eds) 2001: *Systematic reviews in health care: meta-analysis in context.* London: BMJ Books. **Department of Health** 2001: *Research governance framework for health and social care.* London: Department of Health. **International Conference on Harmonization** 1996: E6 document: Guideline for good clinical practice. ICH harmonised tripartite guideline. *Federal Register.* **Machin, D., Campbell, M.,**

Fayers, P. and Pinol, A. 1997: *Sample size tables for clinical studies*, 2nd edn. Oxford: Blackwell Sciences Ltd. **MRC** 2000: *MRC ethics series. Good research practice.* London: Medical Research Council. **MRC** 1998: *MRC guidelines for good practice in clinical trials.* London: Medical Research Council. **National Institute for Clinical Excellence** 2002: *Principles for best practice in clinical audit.* Oxford: Radcliffe Medical Press. **Rothman, K.J.** 2002: *Epidemiology.* Oxford: Oxford University Press. **Sackett, D.L., Straus, S.E., Richardson, W.S., Rosenberg, W. and Haynes, R.B.** 2000: *Evidence-based medicine: how to practice and teach EBM*, 2nd edn. London: Churchill Livingstone. **World Medical Association** 2002: Declaration of Helsinki: Ethical principles for medical research involving human subjects (amendment). 52nd WMA General Assembly: Edinburgh.

placebo Consists of a treatment that mimics a potentially active treatment in every respect except the ingredient or other feature through which the treatment is assumed to exert its effects. A placebo can be pharmacological (e.g. a tablet or an injection), physical (e.g. a manipulation) or psychological (e.g. a conversation). The ideal placebo is indistinguishable from its active counterpart in all respects other than its effects (appearance, taste, etc.). Placebos should avoid any risk inherent in the active intervention. For instance, in ophthalmology, a trial of intraocular injections of a new drug could use 'sham' subconjunctival injections of saline as the appropriate placebo.

Randomised clinical trials in which a placebo is used can be conducted with blinding or masking of the treatments. In a single-blind trial, the investigator is aware of the treatment but the subject is not or vice versa. In a double-blind trial neither the subject nor the investigator is aware of the treatment received. Blinding limits the occurrence of conscious and unconscious BIAS arising from the influence that the knowledge of treatment may have on the recruitment and allocation of subjects, their subsequent care, the response of subjects to treatment, the assessment of ENDPOINTS, the handling of withdrawals and so on (International Conference on Harmonization, 1998).

Placebos can sometimes be useful even in so-called active control trials, i.e. trials comparing two or more active treatments, say A and B. A first situation requiring use of placebos is when blinding of treatment is deemed essential but A and B cannot be made identical. In this case, each subject can be allocated randomly to two sets of treatment ('double-dummy'): either A and placebo for B or B and placebo for A. Another use of placebos in active control trials is when two active treatments A and B must be compared, but a placebo arm can also reasonably be contemplated. In that case, the treatment contrast of interest is A versus B and the placebo group is of little use if A differs from B. However, if A does not differ from B, the contrasts of A or B versus placebo may suggest whether A and B are equally active or equally inactive.

The Declaration of Helsinki states that: 'The benefits, risks, burdens and effectiveness of a new method should be tested against those of the best current prophylactic, diagnostic and therapeutic methods. This does not exclude the use of placebo, or no treatment in studies where no proven prophylactic, diagnostic or therapeutic method exists' (World Medical Association, 2002). The appropriateness of placebo control vs active control should be considered on a trial-by-trial basis. For serious illnesses, when a therapeutic treatment has been shown to be efficacious, a placebo-controlled trial is unethical. A placebo may also be less necessary in these cases because the assessment of 'hard' endpoints such as death or a major clinical event are unaffected by knowledge of treatment.

In a placebo-controlled trial, the estimated treatment effect represents any effect of the active treatment A over and above that of the placebo (δ_A on the Figure). This is generally the effect of interest. In contrast, if the active treatment is compared to an untreated control group, the estimated treatment effect includes any placebo effect ($\delta_A + \delta_P$ on the Figure). If there is interest in estimating the placebo effect on its own (δ_P on the Figure), the trial should randomise patients between an untreated control group and a placebo group as shown on the Figure, in order to control for the natural evolution of the disease (e.g. spontaneous regressions).

Is there such a thing as a placebo effect? A seminal paper on placebos (Beecher, 1955), largely responsible for the general adoption of the double-blind study design, reported an average placebo response rate of about one-third in 26 studies. Another paper (Roberts *et al.*, 1993) suggested that the effects of placebos could be much greater 'under conditions of heightened expectations'. This claim is not supported by a recent systematic review of 130 clinical trials in which patients were randomly assigned to either placebo or no treatment. Outcomes were binary in 32 trials and continuous in 82 trials. As compared with no treatment, placebo had no significant effect on binary outcomes, regardless of whether these outcomes were subjective or objective. For the trials with continuous outcomes, placebo showed a statistically significant beneficial effect on subjective outcomes, but the effect decreased with increasing sample size, indicating a possible bias in small trials.   *MB*

Beecher, H.K. 1955: The powerful placebo. *JADA* 159, 1602–6. **Hrobjartsson, A. and Gotzsche, P.C.** 2001: Is the placebo powerless? An analysis of clinical trials comparing placebo with no treatment. *New England Journal of Medicine* 344, 1594–60. **International Conference on Harmonization** 1998: E9 document: Guidance on statistical principles for clinical trials. *Federal Register* 63, 179, 49583–98. **Roberts, A.H., Kewman, D.G., Mercier, L. and Hovell, M.** 1993: The power of nonspecific effects in healing: implications for psychosocial and biological treatments. *Clinical Psychology Review* 13, 375–91. **World Medical Association** 2002: Declaration of Helsinki. Ethical principles for medical research involving human subjects (amendment). 52nd WMA General Assembly: Edinburgh.

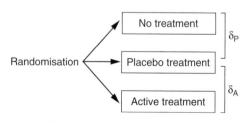

placebo *A trial design randomising patients to a no treatment control group, a placebo treatment group or an active treatment group*

placebo run-in In some CLINICAL TRIALS, especially trials of preventive (rather than therapeutic) interventions, the enrolled subjects go through a run-in placebo period prior to RANDOMISATION. The run-in period is useful to screen the subjects who are likely to comply with the intervention and to avoid randomising subjects who are unlikely to do so, thereby diluting any benefit of the intervention being tested. Run-in periods allow investigators to document why eligible subjects refuse trial enrolment or fail to be randomised at the end of the run-in period. They may also be used to evaluate the feasibility of strategies designed to promote trial enrolment and adherence. The disadvantage of selecting good compliers in a run-in period is that these subjects are not representative of the targeted population, thereby compromising the external validity of the trial.

For instance, a chemoprevention trial in patients at high risk of a recurrence of a head and neck cancer included an 8-week placebo run-in period (Hudmon, Chamberlain and Frankowski, 1997). Of 391 former cancer patients who entered the run-in period, 356 were randomised; the others were no longer interested in trial participation (n = 20), did not return within 10 weeks of enrolment date (n = 3), did not achieve a drug adherence level of at least 75% (n = 9) or were not randomised for another reason (n = 3). The most significant predictors of run-in outcome (randomised or not randomised) were education level and Karnofsky performance score. The odds of randomisation were more than twice higher in subjects with a good Karnofsky performance score and those with more than a high school education.   *MB*

Hudmon, K.S., Chamberlain, R.M. and Frankowski, R.F. 1997: Outcomes of a placebo run-in period in a head and neck cancer chemoprevention trial. *Controlled Clinical Trials* 18, 228–40.

point-biserial correlation coefficient See CORRELATION

Planning and Evaluation of Sequential Trials (PEST) See SEQUENTIAL ANALYSIS

Poisson distribution The PROBABILITY DISTRIBUTION of the number of (rare) events occurring in a fixed time or area. Whereas the BINOMIAL DISTRIBUTION is used to model the number of 'successes' observed given the number of 'trials' taking place (and the independent probability of success in any one trial), the Poisson distribution has the advantage that the number of trials need not be known (although it still needs to be large).

For example, Armitage *et al.* (1999) model the numbers of cases of juvenile-onset Crohn's disease in Scotland as being Poisson random variables. This is a typical example of its use as the risk for an individual is small, but the population of at-risk individuals, while unknown, can be presumed to be large.

Named after (but not originating from) the great French mathematician Siméon Denis Poisson (hence 'Poisson' is always capitalised), the Poisson distribution is defined by a single parameter (here we use λ) that represents both the MEAN and the VARIANCE and hence *must* be positive. If X is a random variable taking a Poisson distribution with parameter λ, then the probability that we will observe X taking the value x, the probability mass function of X, is:

$$\Pr(X = x) = \frac{\lambda^x e^{-\lambda}}{x!}$$

for non-negative integer values of x.

The fact that the mean and variance are the same is one of the signatures of the Poisson distribution and of use in identifying the correct model when we have several observations from the distribution. Note that:

$$\Pr(X = x) = \frac{\lambda}{x} P(X = x - 1)$$

and so the mode of the distribution is the largest integer value smaller than λ (since this is the last value for which λ/x is greater than one and thus the last value for which the probability is increasing) or, if λ is an integer, λ and $\lambda - 1$ are both modal values.

The Poisson distribution is the limiting distribution for a binomial distribution, i.e. as n increases in the binomial distribution and p decreases to keep np constant, then the Poisson distribution provides an increasingly better approximation. As λ increases in the Poisson distribution, then the NORMAL DISTRIBUTION provides a better and better fit. It is of no surprise then to learn that the Poisson distribution is skewed, but that this SKEWNESS decreases as λ increases.

While the normal distribution may provide a good approximation to the Poisson data, techniques such as the t-test may often not be valid for comparing two groups because the assumption of equal variances only holds under the *null hypothesis*. In this case, a square-root TRANSFORMATION of the data can equalise the variances while leaving a distribution that is still reasonably approximated by the normal.

In practice, the data may suffer from overdispersion, that is, there is more variation in the data than would be anticipated from a Poisson model. This may be a result of heterogeneity in the population; the probability of a 'success' may not be constant. Such variation may be accounted for by using a NEGATIVE BINOMIAL DISTRIBUTION or if the sources of variation are known it can be modelled via Poisson regression (see GENERALISED LINEAR MODEL).   *AGL*

Altman, D.G. and Bland, M.J. 1995: Transforming data. *British Medical Journal* 312, 770. **Armitage, P. and Colton, T. (eds)** 1998: *Encyclopaedia of biostatistics.* Chichester: John Wiley & Sons. **Armitage, E., Drummond, E.H., Ghosh, S. and Ferguson, A.** 1999: Incidence of juvenile-onset Crohn's disease in Scotland. *The Lancet* 353, 1496–7. **Leemis, L.M.** 1986: Relationships among common univariate distributions. *The American Statistician* 40, 2, 143–6.

Poisson regression See GENERALISED LINEAR MODEL (GLM)

population projection See DEMOGRAPHY

positive predictive value (PPV) Defined for a diagnostic test for a particular condition as the probability that those who have a positive test actually have the condition as measured by a reference or 'gold' standard. (Contrast with NEGATIVE PREDICTIVE VALUE.)

If the data are set out as in the Table, then $PPV = \frac{a}{a + b}$.

positive predictive value *General table of test results among* a + b+ c + d *individuals samples*

	Disease Present	Disease Absent	Total
Positive	a	b	a + b
Negative	c	d	c + d
Total	a + c	b + d	a + b + c + d

PPV can also be expressed as a percentage. PPV depends on the prevalence of disease in the target population and this has important consequences in the context of population screening. In contrast, test SENSITIVITY and SPECIFICITY often remain the same when a test is applied in different populations. For example, suppose that test sensitivity and test specificity both equal 95% and 1,000,000 people are tested in a screening programme: If the prevalence of the disease in the population is 10%, i.e. 1 in 100, then 95,000 out of the 140,000 with positive tests would have the disease and PPV = 68%. If the prevalence of the disease in the population, however, is only 0.1%, i.e. 1 in 1000 then 950 out of the 50,900 with positive tests would have the disease and PPV = 1.86%.

Thus even with a relatively high prevalence of the condition in the population, many false positive test results may be generated, with the attendant harm to the patient from anxiety and further investigations. Hence the usefulness of a diagnostic test depends not only on the test characteristics, that is, the test's sensitivity and specificity, but also on the prevalence of the condition in the population in which the test is used. As disease prevalence is likely to be lower in community populations than in hospital populations, a diagnostic test may be useful in a hospital setting where there is a high prior probability that a patient has the disease, but may not be useful as population screening test.

The PPV should be presented with confidence intervals (typically set at 95%) calculated using an appropriate method such as that of Wilson that will not produce impossible values (percentages greater than 100 or below 0) when PPV approaches extreme values. *CLC*

[See also FALSE POSITIVE RATE, POPULATION SCREENING, PREVALENCE, TRUE POSITIVE RATE]

Altman, D.G., Machin, D., Bryant, T.N. and Gardner, M.J. 2000: *Statistics with confidence*, 2nd edn. London: BMJ Books.

posterior distribution A PROBABILITY DISTRIBUTION that represents the information, or beliefs, associated with

a parameter of interest after data are collected or an experiment conducted. The posterior distribution is produced by combining the PRIOR DISTRIBUTION, which represents information about the parameter before the collection of data, with the likelihood function, which represents the information about the parameter contained in the experimental data, by the use of BAYES' THEOREM.

Formally the posterior distribution is derived as follows:

$$p(\theta|\text{Data}) \propto p(\text{Data}|\theta)p(\theta)$$

in which $p(\theta)$ is the prior distribution expressing initial beliefs in the parameter of interest, θ, $p(\theta|\text{Data})$ is the corresponding posterior distribution of beliefs and $p(\text{Data}|\theta)$ is the LIKELIHOOD. The posterior distribution provides the full information concerning the parameter of interest. It is often useful to display the posterior on the same plot as the prior distribution and likelihood, in a so-called triplot. This allows the reader to understand to what extent the prior distribution is contributing to the overall inference. Examples of these plots are shown in the Figure. In Figure (a) an example is shown in which the prior distribution dominates the likelihood and almost fully determines the posterior. Figure (b), in contrast shows an example in which the prior distribution is weak and the posterior is essentially determined by the likelihood.

It is sometimes convenient to represent this posterior information by summaries. As posterior estimates the posterior mean and posterior mode are most often used and the uncertainty in the estimate is often reported by a posterior CREDIBLE INTERVAL.

An important consideration following a Bayesian analysis is the reporting of the results. The statistician's job is not over when the analysis is completed and a report written, because it is at this stage that thought needs to be given to the transmission of information to diverse groups of remote customers. For example, in the context of a pharmaceutical drug trial, there are at least three groups of individuals who interact with each other during the drug development process. These groups are the experimenters, the reviewers and the consumers. The aim of the experimenters, among whom are individual pharmaceutical companies, research organisations and clinicians, is to influence the customers, who are the doctors treating patients. They do this by providing them with information that has, in a sense, been 'sanitised' to ensure objectivity by the reviewers, who are the editors of journals and regulatory authorities. Because they each have different motivations it is not at all clear that there will be a single

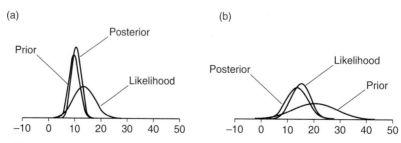

(a) (b)

posterior distribution *Examples of triplots of prior distribution, likelihood and posterior distribution*

'parcel of information' appropriate for each customer group.

One approach is to provide a range of posterior distributions based on a 'community of priors'. This approach works well if the community is broad enough to cover many different prior beliefs about treatment effects. Alternatively, the likelihood function can be reported allowing remote customers to input their own prior distributions to derive the appropriate posterior distribution. This approach will only work if the remote customers are able to carry out the calculations, which may limit its use to only the simplest cases.   *AG*

post-hoc analyses   Analyses that were not specified in advance of data collection. Such analyses tend to be regarded with suspicion, because of the possibility that an observed association may have been selected from among a large number of potential associations that were examined but not reported ('data dredging'). Such multiple comparisons can lead to inflation of TYPE I ERROR rates. If the number of associations tested is known then formal procedures such as the BONFERRONI CORRECTION may be used to correct P-VALUES (SIGNIFI- CANCE LEVELS). However, these methods have substantial disadvantages, one in particular being that they are highly conservative.

Unfortunately, the notion that the formulation of prior hypotheses is a guarantor against being misled is itself misleading. If we do 100 randomised trials of useless therapies, each testing only one hypothesis and only performing one statistical test, all statistically significant results will be spurious. Furthermore, it is impossible to police claims that reported associations were examined because of existing hypotheses. This notion has been satirised by Cole (1993), who announced that, using a computer algorithm, he had generated every possible hypothesis in epidemiology so that all statistical tests are now of *a priori* hypotheses. In practice, the best approach is to report accurately the context in which an association was examined and to regard findings selected from among many comparisons as requiring confirmation by further research.   *JS/GDS*

Cole, P. 1993: The hypothesis generating machine. *Epidemiology* 4, 3, 271–3.

power   See SAMPLE SIZE DETERMINATION IN CLINICAL TRIALS

P-P plots   See PROBABILITY PLOTS

prevalence   The prevalence, or point prevalence, of a disease is the number of cases of a disease that exist at a specified point in time in a defined population. It is generally presented as a rate. Thus:

$$\text{Prevalence} = \frac{\text{Number of cases of a disease at a particular point in time}}{\text{Number in the population at that point in time}}$$

This results in a number between 0 and 1, but for ease of presentation it is often expressed as a rate per 1000, per 100,000 or per 1,000,000 depending on rarity of the disease. As an example, the number of males living with colorectal cancer in Scotland on 31 December 1998 was reported as 7712, giving a prevalence rate of 310 per 100,000 Scottish males (Scottish Health Statistics).

Care should be taken to distinguish between prevalence and INCIDENCE. Although the definitions appear similar at first sight, they are used for different purposes and it is essential to distinguish between them correctly.

The prevalence of a disease clearly depends on the incidence and also on the duration of the disease. A disease with a high incidence rate, from which most sufferers die very quickly, will have a low prevalence at any point in time. Conversely, a chronic disease with a low incidence rate may have a high prevalence if the duration is long. If the incidence and average duration of the disease remain approximately constant over time the prevalence and incidence will be related by:

$$\text{Prevalence} = \text{Incidence} \times \text{Duration}$$

Prevalence is of most use in determining the burden of chronic disease in the population and therefore is useful in allocating resources and planning healthcare services. It is of limited use in epidemiological studies of disease aetiology because it does not measure RISK (Woodward, 1999). Using prevalence to assess disease burden requires care when dealing with curable diseases. The prevalence rate quoted previously for colorectal cancer in Scottish males (310 per 100,000) includes cases first diagnosed up to 20 years ago. A more realistic assessment of current burden for males is obtained from the number of prevalent cases diagnosed within the previous year, which was 1415 (57 per 100,000 Scottish males) on 31 December 1998 (Scottish Health Statistics).

Paradoxically, some important advances in treatment can lead to an increase in prevalence of a disease. For example, the introduction of insulin as a treatment for diabetes resulted in a reduction in the number of deaths and an increase in the prevalence of diabetes in the population.

A more detailed discussion of prevalence and the relationship between prevalence, incidence and disease duration is given in Rothman and Greenland (1998).   *WHG*

Rothman, K.J. and Greenland, S. 1998: *Modern epidemiology*, 2nd edn. Philadelphia: Lippincott Wilkins and Williams. Scottish Health Statistics: www.isdscotland.org. Woodward, M. 1999: *Epidemiology: study design and data analysis*. Boca Raton: Chapman & Hall.

primary endpoint   See ENDPOINT

principal component analysis   An exploratory technique, mainly used in partitioning the variation present in a quantitative multivariate dataset and in examining the data to highlight their important patterns or features.

Suppose that *p* observations have been taken on each of *n* individuals and the values have been collected into a data matrix having *n* rows and *p* columns. For example, Jackson (1991: 107–9) provides a dataset on hearing loss as assessed by audiometry for 100 males aged 39. Each subject had decibel loss measured at 4 frequencies for each of two ears, yielding a 100×8 data matrix with values between −10 and 99 in each cell. Other instances of multivariate medical datasets might arise when screening patients, for example when a variety of measurements are routinely taken on all individuals signing up for a health centre, or in disease characterisation, where measurements are taken on variables that should distinguish sufferers from healthy individuals.

One of the main stumbling blocks in trying to assimilate a multivariate data matrix is the fact that ASSOCIATIONS exist between the columns. For quantitative data, VARIANCE measures scatter while covariance or correlation measures association. The Table illustrates such associations for the audiometry data. The variables are denoted by ear (L/R) plus frequency (500, 1000, 2000, 4000 Hz); the values down the left-to-right diagonal give the variances of the variables; the entries below the diagonal give the covariances between pairs of variables; and the entries above the diagonal give the corresponding correlations.

In essence, principal component analysis simply transforms the p measured variables $x_1, x_2, ..., x_p$ into a set of linear combinations $y_1, y_2, ..., y_p$ (i.e. $y_i = a_{i1}x_1 + a_{i2}x_2 + ... + a_{ip}x_p$ for all i, where the coefficients a_{ij} are suitable constants), which are mutually uncorrelated and which successively maximise the variance of such linear combinations. In other words, y_1 is the linear combination of the xs that has the greatest possible sample variance among all linear combinations for the given dataset, y_2 is the linear combination of the xs that has the next largest variance and so on. Technically, the variances of the ys are given by the eigenvalues of the covariance matrix of the original xs, and the coefficients a_{ij} are given by the elements of the corresponding eigenvectors. These quantities are obtainable from the raw data in all standard statistical software packages; the ys are known as the *principal components* of the data.

Principal components are useful for multivariate data exploration in various ways. It is often the case that each y can be interpreted by relating the size of the coefficients a_{ij} to the variables that they multiply and hence a substantive meaning can be attached to the component. Since the components are arranged in decreasing order of variance, such interpretation will therefore identify the main sources of variation among the sample members. Second, by considering the variance of each component in relation to the total variance of all components, it is often apparent that just a few components account for most of the variability in the sample and the remaining components can be ignored as essentially representing the 'noise' in the system. A typical rule of thumb employed by practitioners is to retain only as many components as account for around 75% to 80% of the total variance. Each sample individual's value (or *score*) is easily obtained on each principal component by applying the definition of the component to the original sample data. Taking the scores on the first two principal components and plotting the individuals in a SCATTERPLOT from these two sets of values then gives the best two-dimensional view of the data. This

enables any OUTLIERS or groupings of individuals to be identified and other patterns in the data can also be readily discerned. Finally, since the principal components are uncorrelated, the scores on the ys can form useful input to further statistical analysis.

However, forming a linear combination of the xs only really makes sense if they are all similar entities. So if they are all different (e.g. a height, a weight, and a count, say) or if they are similar but of very varying magnitudes (e.g. height of individual, length of leg, length of arm and head circumference) then it is preferable to *standardise* the variables before analysis. In this case, the *correlation* rather than the covariance matrix should form the basis of the calculations. It is important to be aware that analysis of the standardised data gives different results from analysis of the unstandardised data, so careful consideration is needed at the outset to decide which analysis is the more appropriate.

To illustrate these ideas, consider a principal component analysis of the audiometry data. First, although all units of the eight variables are the same (Hz), it is evident from the diagonal elements of the table that the variances of the two highest frequencies (384.78, 373.66) are nearly ten times the size of those of some lower frequencies (e.g. 40.92, 41.07). Hence standardisation is warranted and the analysis should be conducted on the correlation matrix. The eigenvalues of this matrix, i.e. the variances of the principal components, are found to be 3.93, 1.62, 0.98, 0.47, 0.34, 0.31, 0.20 and 0.15. The first four components have combined variance 6.0, which is 75% of the overall variance of 8.0, so we can effectively replace the 8 original variables by the first four principal components.

How might we interpret these components? The first one is:

$$y_1 = 0.40x_1 + 0.42x_2 + 0.37x_3 + 0.28x_4 + 0.34x_5 + 0.41x_6 + 0.31x_7 + 0.25x_8,$$

where the numbering is from L500 for x_1 through to R4000 for x_8. The coefficients are all positive and of approximately the same size, so the component is approximately proportional to the sum of the xs. This represents the overall hearing level of an individual and implies that individuals who suffer loss at some frequencies are likely to suffer loss at the other frequencies also. The main source of variation among the sample is thus in terms of the individual's overall hearing level. The second component is:

$$y_2 = -0.32x_1 - 0.23x_2 + 0.24x_3 + 0.47x_4 - 0.39x_5 - 0.23x_6 + 0.32x_7 + 0.51x_8$$

principal components analysis *Variances, covariances and correlations for audiometry data*

	L500	L1000	L2000	L4000	R500	R1000	R2000	R4000
L500	41.07	0.78	0.40	0.26	0.70	0.64	0.24	0.20
L1000	37.73	57.32	0.54	0.27	0.55	0.71	0.36	0.22
L2000	28.13	44.44	119.70	0.42	0.24	0.45	0.70	0.33
L4000	32.10	40.83	91.21	384.78	0.18	0.26	0.32	0.71
R500	31.79	29.75	18.64	25.01	50.75	0.66	0.16	0.13
R1000	26.30	34.24	31.21	33.03	30.23	40.92	0.41	0.22
R2000	14.12	25.30	71.26	57.67	10.52	24.62	86.30	0.37
R4000	25.28	31.74	68.99	269.12	18.19	27.22	67.26	373.66

The coefficients are similar between left and right ear for each frequency but now show a 'contrast' – negative coefficients attached to low frequencies (500 and 1000 Hz), positive coefficients attached to high frequencies (2000 and 4000 Hz). It is known that hearing loss as individuals age is first noticeable at high frequencies, so the second most important source of variation among sample members is in terms of this form of hearing loss. The third component is:

$$y_3 = 0.16x_1 - 0.05x_2 - 0.47x_3 + 0.43x_4 + 0.26x_5 - 0.03x_6 - 0.56x_7 + 0.43x_8$$

'Small' coefficients correspond to 'unimportant' variables, so we can conclude that the third most important source of variation among sample members is a contrast between just the two higher frequencies. Finally, the fourth component has negative coefficients for the first four variables and positive coefficients for the other four variables and is therefore a contrast between left and right ears. Thus we have been able to characterise the main sources of variability among sample members. A scatterplot of the scores on the first two components reveals three potential outliers in the sample, which should be checked for aberrant values and possibly removed from further analysis, but no other structure of interest.

In addition to its role in multivariate exploration and description, principal component analysis is often also used either as a prelude to, or in conjunction with, a range of other techniques such as variable selection or orthogonal regression. (See Jackson, 1991 and Jolliffe, 2002.)

WK

[See also CORRESPONDENCE ANALYSIS, FACTOR ANALYSIS]

Jackson, J.E. 1991: *A user's guide to principal components*. New York: John Wiley & Sons. **Jolliffe, I.T.** 2002: *Principal component analysis*, 2nd edn. New York: Springer.

prior distribution

A PROBABILITY DISTRIBUTION that represents the information, or beliefs, associated with a parameter of interest before data are collected or an experiment conducted. The prior distribution is an essential component of a Bayesian analysis (see BAYESIAN METHODS) and differentiates it from traditional, so-called frequentist, analysis. The prior distribution is used together with the LIKELIHOOD function, which represents the information about the parameter contained in the experimental data, to produce the POSTERIOR DISTRIBUTION from BAYES' THEOREM. Formally, a Bayesian analysis proceeds from the following formula:

$$p(\theta|\text{Data}) \propto p(\text{Data}|\theta)p(\theta)$$

in which $p(\theta)$ is the prior distribution expressing initial beliefs in the parameter of interest, θ, $p(\theta|\text{Data})$ is the corresponding posterior distribution of beliefs and $p(\text{Data}|\theta)$ is the likelihood.

There are many types of prior distribution and many ways to derive them. Prior distributions can be based on information available in the literature – historical data – and quantified through a formal process of meta-analysis (see SYSTEMATIC REVIEWS AND META-ANALYSIS). In the pharmaceutical industry, prior distributions about potential treatment effects can be determined from existing clinical databases of similar drugs from the same class of compounds. Where existing data are not available, experts can be used to elicit prior distributions by a process of questioning and refinement. Formalistic prior distributions can be determined to represent cases in which there is little or no relevant prior information. Such prior distributions are normally called non-informative and a Bayesian analysis with a non-informative prior will usually give very similar conclusions to those obtained using a frequentist analysis. However, the output and presentation of the analysis will be very different from standard approaches and is often found to be more intuitive and helpful by non-statisticians. Finally, a set of prior distributions may also be used in order that a range of assumptions may be tested against their subsequent conclusions. For example, a community of priors could consist, in addition to a neutral uninformative prior, of priors that represent both 'pessimistic' and 'optimistic' scenarios. A 'pessimistic' prior would be one in which, for example, there would be considerable doubt about the effectiveness of a treatment, an 'optimistic' prior, in contrast, would represent strong prior belief that the treatment is effective.

The use of prior distributions in a Bayesian analysis is not without controversy. From one perspective, their use is a strength in that it allows the scientist to access more information and thereby produce stronger inferences. This strength, however, can also be regarded as a weakness and gives rise to any number of questions. First, if the prior is based on historical data, is it relevant to the current investigation? If it is elicited from experts to what extent are the resulting inferences subjective and hence of less credibility than inferences based on data alone? In practice, the influence of the prior distribution may be minimal if the information contained in experimental data outweighs that contained in the prior, which will generally be the case if the experimental study has a large sample size

AG

probability

The notion of probability has two connotations: (1) as a mathematical discipline concerning the study of uncertainty; and (2) as a numerical scale from zero to one to describe the frequency of occurrence, or degree-of-belief in, a given event.

The first definition is akin to statistics as a discipline, with broad distinction between the two being that whereas probability seeks to learn about the sample given characteristics of the population, statistics seeks to learn about the population given characteristics of the sample. Their interrelationship is such that the theory of probability is the backbone of statistics. However, the second connotation of probability will be our focus here.

Any chance event happens according to some numerical measure between zero and one, with these extremes representing the probability of impossible and certain events, respectively. In practice, most probabilities lie between these extremes (see first Figure). Sometimes, probability is expressed on an entirely equivalent 0–100% scale, conventionally known as *chance*, if so.

Usual notation to describe the probability of an event is to write the event in brackets or parentheses, namely {...}, [...] or (...), immediately after an abbreviation of probability to P, Pr or Prob, with no consensus about capitalising the initial letter. Thus:

Pr{a male is pregnant} = 0
P[a coin lands heads uppermost] = 0.5
prob(baby is either male or female) = 1

are just some of the many ways that simple probability statements can be written. For the sake of brevity, the event being considered is often reduced to a single letter, so for example when considering the coin-tossing scenario, one might say Pr{H} = Pr{T} = 0.5, where H and T are shorthand for landing heads and tails, respectively, it being understood from context that only one toss of a fair coin at a time is being considered. (Note that a generalisation to describe chances of sequences of events when tossing a coin three times, say, could be Pr{HHH} or Pr{2H, 1T}, although one has to be mindful to distinguish whether one means in the latter case the ordered sequence H, H, then T or *any* sequence with two Hs and one T.)

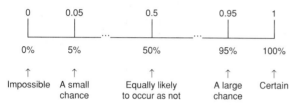

probability *Probability quantifies the scale of uncertainty. Note that probabilities of 0.05 and 0.95 are simply convenient round numbers towards the ends of the scale, with 'small' and 'large' being just (non-standard) descriptive labels*

It is important to know there are two ways of interpreting probability, as follows: (1) long-run average proportion or 'frequentist' view; and (2) degree-of-belief or 'subjective' view.

The first type applies strictly only to those events that are repeatable, under assumed identical conditions, such as idealised coin tossing or die rolling, whereas the second applies universally, even to one-off events. Arguably, in medicine, all events are one-offs as they refer to individual patients with their own unique set of symptoms and treatments, genetic and environmental backgrounds and occur in particular places and times. Incidentally, statisticians need reminding from time to time there is no such thing as an average patient! (See CONSULTING A STATISTICIAN.) Largely due to mathematical convenience and history (see HISTORY OF MEDICAL STATISTICS), it is the frequentist definition that is by far the more commonly used in statistics, dominating almost all courses, textbooks and software.

However, there is a growing tendency among biostatisticians nowadays to favour the subjective formulation of probability, being the cornerstone of the Bayesian approach (see BAYESIAN METHODS). While some may criticise this approach for being too subjective and somehow less scientific than the frequentist approach, others argue that the ability to tailor results to one's own beliefs is actually advantageous and especially beneficial for applications in medical research.

At least the two philosophical approaches do not lead to conflicting results, even though the subjective approach is undoubtedly more intuitively appealing and more obviously applicable. It is helpful to bear in mind both definitions when thinking about probabilities and their interpretation. To illustrate, one can say Pr{H} = 0.5

either because the long-run ratio of number of heads to number of tosses approaches the value one-half as the number of tosses increases indefinitely *or* because in a single toss you reckon it is 50:50, being equally likely to fall tails as heads. Thus, a statement such as Pr{a person's blood group is type O} = 0.47 can, and does, mean both that in a large random sample of the population we can expect 47 in every 100 people to have blood group O and that, in the absence of further information, one's degree-of-belief about an individual patient being type O is 0.47.

How are probabilities assigned numerically? In simple situations, they are enumerated by appealing to the somewhat circular notion of 'equally likely' outcomes. Thus, for example, a standard die of six sides is equally likely to land any side facing upwards, hence the deduction Pr{getting a 6 on a single roll} = 1/6. This line of reasoning is unrealistic in medical applications, however. In practice, we assign probabilities by gathering (preferably large amounts of) data from random samples, in order to compute the average frequencies. For instance, it may be that based on a large, national, randomly selected cohort that the proportions of blood types O, A, B and AB are, respectively, 0.47, 0.42, 0.08 and 0.03, leading to the earlier pair of statements about type O blood group.

Notice in this simple example the proportions representing the probabilities sum to one. This is no surprise given that the list of ABO types was exhaustive. A PROBABILITY DISTRIBUTION more generally describes the theoretical distribution of the total probability of one. These can be either for discrete values (some classic examples being BINOMIAL, POISSON and GEOMETRIC DISTRIBUTIONS) for which respective formulae for probability density function sum to one or else continuous distributions (e.g. NORMAL, UNIFORM, CHI-SQUARE DISTRIBUTIONS) for which area under probability distribution curve integrates to one. A HISTOGRAM can be thought of as pictorial representation of a probability distribution. The larger the sample on which it is based, the closer the histogram's shape approximates the underlying population probability distribution.

Next consider the combining of probabilities to quantify chances of more complex interactions of events. There are two rules that apply for special types of events that are said to be 'mutually exclusive' or 'independent', respectively, as follows:

1. *Addition rule.* The probability that any of two or more mutually exclusive events occurs is given by the sum of their individual probabilities.

For example:

Pr{person is type B *or* type AB}
= Pr{person is type B} + Pr{person is type AB}
= 0.08 + 0.03 = 0.11

Mutual exclusivity, or incompatibility, of events simply means that if one event occurs, then other events are precluded (e.g. if someone is of blood type B, they cannot also be simultaneously of type AB).

2. *Multiplication rule.* The probability that two (or more) independent events both (or all) occur together is given by the product of their individual probabilities. For example:

Pr{two unrelated people are both type A}
= Pr{first is type A} × Pr{second is type A}
= 0.42 × 0.42 = 0.176

Independence of events means the outcome of one has no bearing on the other(s), such as here the blood types of unrelated individuals.

Note that the concept of independence or dependence of events plays a fundamental role in EPIDEMIOLOGY. In CASE-CONTROL STUDIES, patients with a disease (the 'cases') are compared with disease-free individuals (the 'controls') with respect to some possible risk factor. For instance, men with testicular cancer might be compared with controls regarding, say, milk consumption during adolescence. If more cases were 'exposed to the risk' of high milk consumption than controls, then the probabilities of exposure being different might suggest a possible causative link. In other words, the events {having the disease} and {having had the exposure} would not be independent events.

Thus, an observational study can be thought of in probabilistic terms as seeking to demonstrate whether these two events are dependent or independent of one another. If deemed to be dependent, there is an ASSOCIATION (note, not the same as *causation* (see CAUSALITY)) linking the exposure to the disease, a matter of central importance.

To explore this further, one needs to introduce the concept of CONDITIONAL PROBABILITY. In brief, probabilities of events can change in the light of unfolding information, in particular whether or not another event is known to have occurred. To illustrate this, consider that the probability someone has tuberculosis is no longer the same if it is known that their skin test for tuberculosis was positive. Letting D denote the event {person has disease} and T+ denote the event {skin test is positive}, then interest focuses on the probability of {D given T+}, which is written $\Pr\{D \mid T+\}$ for short. The '|' sign is read as 'given', meaning events written after it are already known to have occurred. Now $\Pr\{D \mid T+\}$ is not equal to $\Pr\{D\}$, since the skin test result, obviously, is not independent of the presence of the disease. Equally, no test is 100% accurate, for if it were in this example, knowledge of skin test result would be equivalent to knowing tuberculosis status, but in reality no test is this reliable (see POSITIVE PREDICTIVE VALUE).

In general, the conditional probability of any one event A given another (non-impossible) event B, is defined as $\Pr\{A \mid B\} = \Pr\{A \text{ and } B\}/\Pr\{B\}$, where '/' represents division. If it is the case that A and B are independent, then the multiplication rule says that the numerator, $\Pr\{A \text{ and } B\} = \Pr\{A\} \times \Pr\{B\}$ and so it follows that $\Pr\{A \mid B\} = \Pr\{A\}$. Indeed, this is an alternative definition of independence of events, namely that the conditional probability of an event, A, on another, B, is the same as the unconditional probability of event A. (See related and important result known as BAYES' THEOREM.)

An application of probability is in the use of the summary measure odds ratio (OR) or relative risk (RR (see RELATIVE RISK AND ODDS RATIOS)). Odds is simply an alternative way of expressing probability, adopted and favoured by bookmakers perhaps to make it less obvious their total probabilities within a given horse race, say, sum to more than one in order to guarantee themselves a long-run profit margin. If a probability of an event is denoted by p, then the odds for the same event equal $p/(1 - p)$.

The odds of an event having probability 1/2 is quoted as evens. Probabilities below one-half are quoted as number of chances of failing to number of chances of occurring,

for a suitable total number of chances to avoid fractions. For example, a probability 1/8 is the same an odds 7 to 1; probability 2/5 is odds 3 to 2; probability 1/21 is odds 20 to 1. Probabilities of events greater than one-half are expressed with larger number first and then 'on' (instead of 'against', the default assumption), e.g. odds of '2 to 1 on' means a probability of 2/3, whereas 2 to 1 against is the complementary probability of 1/3. Odds are virtually never used in health applications by themselves, but do occur in the context of odds ratios when it is convenient especially when analysing case-control studies to have a comparative measure of relative probabilities across two groups, typically cases versus controls. When using LOGISTIC REGRESSION models also, computer output usually displays odds ratios and their confidence intervals in association with categorical variables.

The RR is defined as the ratio of two conditional probabilities:

$$RR = \Pr\{\text{disease} \mid \text{exposed}\}/\Pr\{\text{disease} \mid \text{not exposed}\}$$

If disease status and exposure to risk factor are independent, as when there is no causal link between them, then $RR = \Pr\{\text{disease}\}/\Pr\{\text{disease}\} = 1$, whereas if exposure and disease are dependent the RR will not equal 1.

Finally, there are two further rules for handling probability one can consider. The first of these, referring to any events A and B, regardless of whether independent or not, mutually exclusive or not, says:

$$\Pr\{A \text{ or } B\} = \Pr\{A\} + \Pr\{B\} - \Pr\{A \text{ and } B\}$$

This rule is best visualised with a Venn diagram showing overlapping events, A and B (see second figure). Notice it reduces to the addition law just given if A and B happen to be mutually exclusive, for then $\Pr\{A \text{ and } B\} = 0$, being impossible to occur together, so that a Venn diagram representation would show no overlap between sets representing A and B.

The second general rule for combining probabilities is as follows:

$$\Pr\{A \text{ and } B\} = \Pr\{A\} \times \Pr\{B \mid A\}$$

Note, by symmetry, this can equivalently be stated as:

$$\Pr\{A \text{ and } B\} = \Pr\{B\} \times \Pr\{A \mid B\}$$

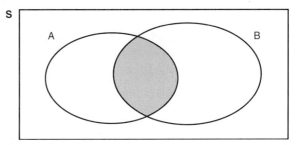

probability *Venn diagram depicting two general events A and B among all those possible within 'state space' S. The general rule says the probability of lying within the region covered by A or B is that of the two individual regions minus the double-counted shaded region where A and B overlap*

Examples of the application of this rule are found in SCREENING STUDIES, where it is useful to consider SENSITIVITY and SPECIFICITY as well as false positive and false negative rates.

Other common uses of probability abound, for instance in the summary measures of incidence and prevalence, survival rates within life tables and applications in genetic epidemiology to mention but a few. The most common sighting of probability in medical journals, for better or worse, is due to the preference to summarise evidence from studies in terms of *P*-VALUES, measures of probability used to assess plausibility of the null hypothesis of chance variation.

For further reading at a recreational level, Everitt (1999) provides an accessible account of the role of probability including health and research applications, while more formal accounts can be found in just about any textbook of medical statistics.   *CRP*

Everitt, B.S. 1999: *Chance rules: an informal guide to probability, risk and statistics*. New York: Springer.

probability distribution A statement of all the outcome values that a variable can take, and the individual probabilities of obtaining those values. If outcomes are discrete (as in categorical variables, or variables that can only take integer numbers), we have two paired lists; one of outcomes, and one of probabilities. For example when interested in the number of heads achieved when tossing four fair coins, we have outcomes and probabilities:

Outcome (x)	Probability $\Pr(X = x)$
0	0.0625
1	0.2500
2	0.3750
3	0.2500
4	0.0625

This list of probabilities defines our probability distribution. Note that the list of probabilities must sum to one. However, even with five possible outcomes such an approach is becoming cumbersome, and we prefer to relate the outcome and probability mathematically. For our example we note that the outcome, x, and probability, $\Pr(X = x)$, are related as

$$\Pr(X = x) = \frac{3}{2x!(4-x)!}$$

where $x!$ (x factorial) is the product of all the integers up to and including x, and 0! is defined to be one. We refer to $\Pr(X = x)$ as the probability mass function. To define our probability distribution, we can just provide the mass function (if one exists). Note that in our example the distribution is an example of a BINOMIAL DISTRIBUTION. Other discrete examples are the POISSON, GEOMETRIC and NEGATIVE BINOMIAL distributions.

If the outcomes are on a continuous scale, for example the length of a tumour, then there are an infinite number of possible outcomes. Since the total probability must be equal to one, then generally, the probability of the outcome being exactly a particular value is 0. In this case, rather than defining a distribution function, we define a probability density function (pdf). This is a curve, the area under which represents probabilities. The total area under the curve represents the total probability and therefore must be equal to one. In general, the area under the curve between any two values gives the probability that the outcome will lie between those two values.

It is often the case that we will work with the distribution function (or cumulative distribution function), which gives the probability of being less than a particular value and so equates to the area under the curve to the left of a particular value. As an example consider the success rate of a new type of operation. Suppose that it is equally likely to be anywhere from 0 (never successful) to 1 (always successful). Our probability density function will be a horizontal line (at $y = 1$ since the area under the curve must be equal to one). See Figure. The probability that the operation is successful more than 80% of the time is the area under the curve between 0.8 and 1, which is equal to 0.2. Note that our example is an example of the beta distribution. Other continuous probability distributions include the CHI-SQUARE, EXPONENTIAL, F, GAMMA, LOGNORMAL, T and (most importantly) NORMAL distributions.   *AGL*

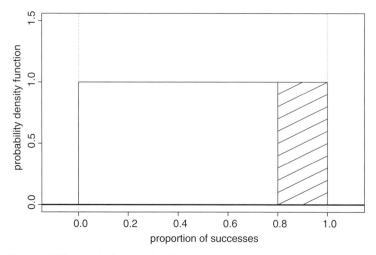

probability distribution *The probability density function for the success rate of an operation, when all rates are equally likely. Note that the area under the curve is equal to one, and the area under the curve between 0.8 and 1 is 0.2.*

probability plots Plots for comparing two probability distributions or for assessing assumptions about the probability distribution of a sample of observations. There are two basic types, the *probability–probability plot* (P-P plot) and the *quantile-quantile plot* (Q-Q plot). Each type is illustrated in the first Figure.

A plot of points whose coordinates are the cumulative probabilities $\{p_x(q), p_y(q)\}$ for different values of q is a probability–probability plot, whereas a plot of the points whose coordinates are the quantiles $\{q_x(p), q_y(p)\}$ for different values of p is a quantile–quantile plot. As an example, a quantile–quantile plot for investigating the assumption that a set of data is from a NORMAL DISTRIBUTION would involve plotting the ordered sample values $y_{(1)}, y_{(2)}, \ldots, y_{(n)}$ against the quantiles of a standard normal distribution, i.e.:

$$\Phi^{-1}[p_i]$$

where usually:

$$p_i = \frac{i - \frac{1}{2}}{n} \text{ and } \Phi(x) = \int_{-\infty}^{x} \frac{1}{\sqrt{2\pi}} e^{-\frac{1}{2}u^2} du$$

This is usually known as a *normal probability plot*. Two such plots are shown in the second Figure: the first (a) is

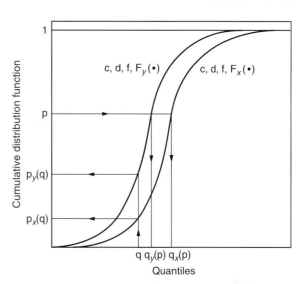

probability plots *Diagram illustrating P-P and Q-Q plots*

the probability plot for 100 points generated from a normal distribution and the second (b) is the corresponding plot for 100 points generated from an EXPONENTIAL DISTRIBUTION. *BSE*

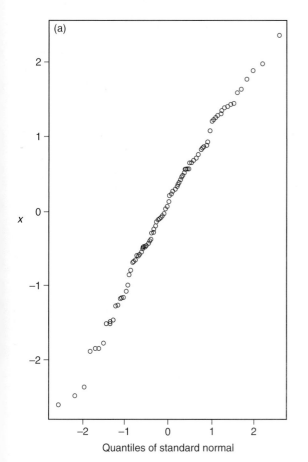

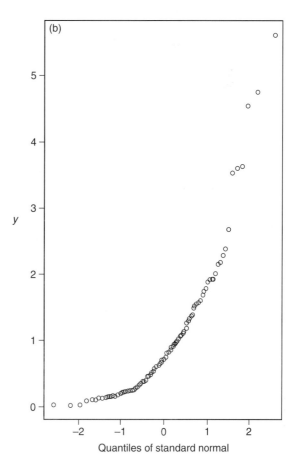

probability plots *Two normal probability plots (a) 100 observations from a normal distribution and (b) 100 observations from an exponential distribution*

probit model A model for dichotomous or ordinal responses that can be defined either as a GENERALISED LINEAR MODEL or by using a latent response formulation. In a generalised linear model, the expectation μ_i of the response for unit i given covariates x_i is modelled as $g(\mu_i) = \beta_0 + \beta_1 x_1 + \ldots + \beta_k x_k$ (also written, for brevity, as $x_i'\beta$), where $g(\cdot)$ is a link function and β are regression parameters. In a binary probit model (for dichotomous responses), a probit link $\Phi^{-1}(\cdot)$ is specified:

$$\Phi^{-1}(\mu_i) = x_i'\beta \text{ or } \mu_i = \Phi(x_i'\beta) \qquad (1)$$

where $\Phi(\cdot)$ is the standard normal cumulative distribution function. The distribution of y_i is then specified as Bernoulli with MEAN μ_i. Proportions out of a total of n_i trials can be modelled using the same link function by specifying a BINOMIAL DISTRIBUTION with binomial denominator n_i.

The same model can be formulated by specifying a linear regression model for an underlying latent (unobserved) continuous response y_i^*:

$$y_i^* = x_i'\beta + \varepsilon_i$$

with ε_i having a standard NORMAL DISTRIBUTION written as:

$$\varepsilon_i \sim \mathrm{N}(0, 1) \qquad (2)$$

The observed dichotomous response y_i then represents an indicator for y_i^* exceeding zero:

$$y_i = \begin{cases} 0 \text{ if } y_i^* \leq 0 \\ 1 \text{ if } y_i^* > 0 \end{cases} \qquad (3)$$

It can be shown that this latent response formulation is equivalent to a generalised linear model with a probit link and Bernoulli distribution:

$$\begin{aligned} \mu_i \equiv \mathrm{E}(y_i|x_i'\beta) &= \Pr(y_i = 1|x_i'\beta) = \Pr(y_i^* > 0|x_i'\beta) \\ &= \Pr(x_i'\beta + \varepsilon_i > 0) = \Pr(\varepsilon_i > -x_i'\beta) \\ &= \Pr(\varepsilon_i \leq x_i'\beta) = \Phi(x_i'\beta) \end{aligned}$$

where the penultimate equality hinges on the symmetry of the normal density of ε_i.

An ordinal probit model can be specified using the latent response formulation by extending the threshold model in (3) to $S + 1 > 2$ ordered categories:

$$y_i = \begin{cases} 0 & \text{if} & -\infty < & y_i^* & \leq \kappa_1 \\ 1 & \text{if} & \kappa_1 < & y_i^* & \leq \kappa_2 \\ \vdots & \vdots & \vdots & \vdots & \vdots \\ S & \text{if} & \kappa_S < & y_i^* & \leq \infty \end{cases}$$

where κ_s, $s = 1, \ldots, S$ are threshold parameters.

Binary and ordinal logit models can be defined in the same way as their probit counterparts by replacing the link in equation (1) by a logit link and the distribution in (2) by a logistic distribution. LOGIT MODELS are more popular than probit models because the regression parameters can be interpreted as log odds ratios and because the models can be used for CASE-CONTROL STUDIES. One advantage of probit models is that they can easily be extended to the multivariate case by using several latent responses having a MULTIVARIATE NORMAL DISTRIBUTION. *SRH/AS*

Finney, D.J. 1971: *Probit analysis.* Cambridge: Cambridge University Press.

product-limit estimator See KAPLAN-MEIER ESTIMATOR

product-moment correlation coefficient A synonym for Pearson's correlation coefficient. See CORRELATION

proportional hazards When comparing two groups with time-to-event data the summary statistic that is usually employed is the hazard rate in one group compared to the hazard rate in the other group, which is usually called the *hazard ratio*. If the hazard ratio is constant over time, i.e. it is *independent* of time, then the hazards in the two groups are said to be proportional – there is a constant multiplicative relationship between the two hazard rates.

Mathematically, this relationship takes the form

$$h_1(t)/h_0(t) = \exp(\beta_1 X_1 + \beta_2 X_2 + \ldots)$$

where $h_0(t)$ and $h_1(t)$ are the hazard functions in the two groups (which may vary over time), X_1, X_2 ... are the explanatory variables and β_1, β_2, ... are the coefficients estimated from the data.

The assumption of proportional hazards underlies the inclusion of any variable in a COX'S REGRESSION MODEL. Therefore, it is usually important to assess that the hazards are approximately proportional across different groups before including a variable in a Cox model. There is, however, no unique or completely satisfactory way in which to test this assumption. Many approaches have been suggested and here we present one numerical and one graphical approach that seem to perform as well as most others (Persson, 1991).

A numerical approach was introduced by Cox himself in his original paper introducing the model. It involves including a time-dependent covariate in the model. Thus for one variable, the model would look like $h_1(t)/h_0(t) = \exp(\beta_1 X_1 + \gamma X_1(t))$, with a simple extension for more variables. The null hypothesis of proportional hazards, i.e. $\gamma = 0$ is tested by fitting the model and assessing this null hypothesis in the usual way.

One simple approach to assess this assumption graphically is to use a complementary log plot. This is a plot of log t against log$\{-\log[S(t)]\}$ where t is time from baseline in whatever unit is being used and $S(t)$ is the surviving proportion at time t (see Figure on page 277). If the assumption of proportional hazards holds true then the curves for each group should be approximately parallel (i.e. the curves will be identical but vertically shifted by a constant). One may formally test that the 'slopes' of these curves do not differ, but this is not usually very helpful or informative (for example, assuming that the curves are approximately linear) and thus usually we are left with visual inspection alone, to assess whether the curves are indeed parallel. This is true of all graphical methods. Except for gross departures from proportional hazards or as a supplement to numerical methods, these methods cannot be widely recommended. *MS/MP*

Cleves, M.A., Gould, W.W. and Gutierrez, R.G. 2003: *An introduction to survival analysis using Stata®,* rev edn. Texas: Stata Press. **Machin, D. and Parmar, M.K.B.** 1995: *Survival analysis: a practical approach.* Chichester: John Wiley & Sons. **Persson,**

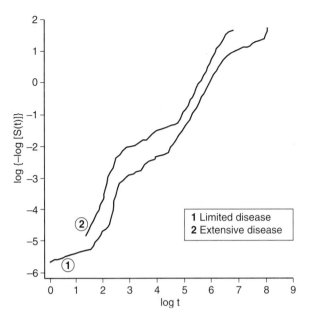

proportional hazards *Graph of log {–log [S(t)]} against log t in patients treated with ECMV chemotherapy with limited and extensive small cell lung cancer (from Machin and Parmar, 1995)*

I. 1991: Essays on the assumption of proportional hazards in Cox's regression. *Acta Universitatis Upsalaiensis.* Uppsala: Comprehensive Summaries of Uppsala Dissertations from the Faculty of Social Sciences. **Piantodosi, S.** 1997: *Clinical trials.* New York: Wiley Interscience.

protocols for clinical trials   Formal documents outlining proposed procedures for carrying out a CLINICAL TRIAL. Protocols for clinical trials serve a variety of masters; consequently, a well-constructed protocol discusses a range of issues relevant to the trial it describes. The principal investigator uses the protocol as a tool to describe the scientific rationale behind the study and the goals of the trial. The study staff depends on the protocol for operational guidance on whom to recruit, what study procedures to perform and how and when to perform them. The protocol must include information about safeguards planned for the participants so that institutional boards and ETHICAL REVIEW COMMITTEES can assess the appropriateness of the plans to protect the participants in the research. If the trial is to be used as part of a regulatory submission, the protocol should include enough information so that when the trial is complete and the final results presented, the regulators will be able to assess the quality of the study, the results and the statistical interpretation. Finally, in anticipation of eventual publication of the results, the investigators, in writing the protocol, should consider the types of data they expect to include in publications.

An ideal protocol addresses these multiple masters in a way that is well organised, easily readable, unambiguous and internally consistent. Several guidelines are available to help the writer construct a protocol that covers all important aspects, notably those produced by the International Committee of Harmonization (in particular E3, E9 and E10) (www.ich.org), the various guidances and the 'points to consider' documents provided by the United States Food and Drug Administration on disease-specific protocols (www.fda.org), as well as the CONSORT statement on recommendations for reporting parallel-group randomised trials (Moher, Schultz and Altman, 2001). All of these provide useful advice to the constructors of clinical protocols. These documents are guidelines; a specific protocol should incorporate the relevant features described in these and related documents, individually tailored to the study at hand. A protocol that reads as if it were constructed of boilerplate sections from various previous protocols, or uncritically edited versions of standard templates, is not only boring to read but, worse, may lead to faulty compliance to its procedures.

Most well-constructed protocols share similar structure. They begin with a section discussing the disease under study. Next comes a description of the context of the particular trial including information on the intervention under study. Depending on the nature of the study, this section might describe the pharmacology of the product and the justification for the particular dose or doses under study, the mechanism and structure of the device or the justification for the particular behavioural intervention. Another section describes the aims and goals of the study. The remainder of this entry assumes that the interventions under study will be drugs or biologics; however, the general considerations apply also to trials of devices and behavioural interventions.

The protocol will carefully define the population of interest, specify the entry criteria and delineate the important facets of the study design. The heart of the protocol will contain a description of the procedures for screening, enrolment and subsequent visits. The actual content of these sections will depend on the design and purpose of the study. PHASE I TRIALS or dose escalation studies, which are typically not hypothesis-driven, aim to provide evidence that the product is sufficiently safe to allow administration to more people. Consequently, the section describing the design of this type of study should address the considerations, statistical and otherwise, that led to the particular sample size and to the choice of criteria for dose escalation. The protocol will describe the criteria by which the various doses under consideration will be evaluated and the methods by which dose escalation will proceed.

Typical PHASE II TRIALS studying non-clinical END-POINTS as well as both PHASE III and later PHASE IV confirmatory trials studying clinical endpoints aim to test hypotheses. A protocol for such a trial should unambiguously describe the primary endpoint, the primary hypothesis and the statistical methods planned to test that hypothesis. A section on statistical power should justify the sample size. If the study has a control group, the protocol should describe its nature and should defend its choice. If the study is testing equivalence or non-inferiority, the protocol should specify the appropriate equivalence or non-inferiority margin (see ACTIVE CONTROL EQUIVALENCE STUDIES). A section on secondary endpoints should present a cogent rationale for each with a discussion of how each one will yield information that augments the data provided by the primary endpoint.

All protocols should contain a statistical section that specifies which participants the primary analysis will include, how missing data will be handled and the planned statistical methods. Early phase studies typically use descriptive and exploratory statistical methods, for such studies aim to produce data relevant to the design of subsequent trials. In Phase III or later trials, however, where the purpose is to test hypotheses, the statistical section should describe a rigorous approach to analysis that preserves the TYPE I ERROR rate. Failure to define the primary endpoint clearly, to select a rigorous statistical approach and to specify statistical analyses unambiguously jeopardises the ultimate validity of the inference from the trial.

Protocols for randomised clinical trials should describe the methods of RANDOMISATION and, if relevant, the nature of any stratification. If randomisation is blocked, the protocol should not include the block size because making that information available can potentially lead the investigator to deduce the treatment given to some participants. For studies involving blinding, a section should describe the methods used to conceal treatment allocation. Generally, protocols should discuss the methods planned for ensuring unbiased assessment of outcome.

The final sections of the protocol provide rules for drug disposition, handling unexpected adverse events, monitoring safety, adhering to regulatory guidelines and administrative matters essential to the conduct of the study. (These sections, unfortunately, sometimes read as if the writers had become tired by the time they reached them. If the trial is studying ovarian cancer, for instance, the use of the pronoun 'he', or even the more politically correct 'he or she', clearly indicates that the writer simply pasted the material from another protocol!)

The protocol must describe the plans for monitoring the safety of the participants during the study, the methods of follow-up and the way in which the investigators plan to protect the participant's rights and confidentiality.

The protocol should be clear enough that the designers of the case report forms can use it to construct the forms.

The inclusion of all this necessary material makes many protocols very long. To ensure that the clinic staff implementing the protocol understands the purpose of the trial and the procedures, the document should contain two summaries. One, which generally comes at the beginning of the document, is a two- to (approximately) four-page synopsis briefly describing the product or other intervention, the objectives, the study design, the study population, the dosing and dosing regimen, the primary and secondary endpoints and the statistical plans for these endpoints along with a discussion of the power. The second summary is a one- or two-page flowchart listing the procedures to be performed at each visit. A helpful aid to accurate implementation of the protocol is a laminated pocket-sized card containing a miniature, but legible, version of this flowchart.

In summary, the protocol for a clinical trial should

justify the study and describe its procedures, hypotheses, statistical plans and administrative guidelines. A clearly written protocol with close connection between the trial's goals, design and analysis plays a crucial role in implementing a study that is likely to result in a correct inference.   *JW*

Moher, D., Shultz, K.F. and Altman, D.G. 2001: The CONSORT statement: revised recommendations for improving the quality of reports of parallel-group randomized trials. *Annals of Internal Medicine* 134, 7–622.

publication bias   See SYSTEMATIC REVIEWS AND META-ANALYSIS

P-values

Introduced by R.A. Fisher (1925) as a means of assessing the evidence against a null hypothesis. Often, such a null hypothesis states that there is no association between two variables, for example between hypertension and subsequent heart disease. The *P*-value is defined as the probability, if the null hypothesis were true, that we would have observed an association as large as we did by chance. If this probability is small we have evidence *against* the null hypothesis, in other words, the smaller the *P*-value, the stronger the evidence against the null hypothesis.

To illustrate the calculation of a *P*-value consider the results, displayed in the Table, of a study to investigate whether smoking reduces lung function. Forced vital capacity (FVC – a test of lung function), was measured in 100 men aged 25–29, of whom 36 were smokers and 64 non-smokers. (For simplicity we will use large-sample formulae.)

The mean FVC in smokers was 4.7 litres compared with 5.0 litres in non-smokers. The difference in mean FVC, $\bar{x}_1 - \bar{x}_0$, is therefore $4.7 - 5.0 = -0.3$ litres. The SD in both groups was 0.6 litres.

If the null hypothesis is true, then the mean of the sampling distribution of $(\bar{x}_1 - \bar{x}_0)$ is zero. The large-sample formulae state that the sampling distribution of $(\bar{x}_1 - \bar{x}_0)$ is normal: its standard error is derived from the standard errors of $\bar{x}_1$ and $\bar{x}_0$) as:

$$SE = \sqrt{\left(s.e._0^2 + s.e._1^2\right)} = \sqrt{0.1^2 + 0.075^2} = 0.125 \text{ litres}$$

The *test statistic* $z = (\bar{x}_1 - \bar{x}_0)/SE$ measures by how many standard errors the mean difference $(\bar{x}_1 - \bar{x}_0)$ differs from the null value of 0. In this example

$$z = (-0.3)/0.125 = -2.4.$$

The difference between the means is therefore 2.4 standard errors below 0. The Figure on page 279 shows that the probability of getting a difference of -2.4 standard errors or fewer (the area under the curve to the left of -2.4) is 0.0082 (this can be found using a computer or statistical tables). This probability is known as the *one-sided P-value*.

P-values *Results of a study to investigate whether smoking reduces lung function*

Group	Number of men	Mean FVC	Standard deviation	Standard error of mean FVC
Non-smokers (0)	$n_0 = 64$	$\bar{x}_0 = 5.0$	$s_0 = 0.6$	$SE_0 = 0.6/\sqrt{64} = 0.075$
Smokers (1)	$n_1 = 36$	$\bar{x}_1 = 4.7$	$s_1 = 0.6$	$SE_1 = 0.6/\sqrt{36} = 0.100$

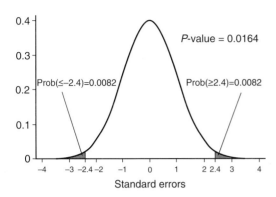

P-values *Using test statistic z to determine probability of getting a difference of −2.4 standard error or fewer*

By convention, we usually use *two-sided* P-*values*. The justification for this is that our assessment of the probability that the result is due to chance should be based on how extreme is the *size* of the departure from the null hypothesis and not its direction. We therefore include the probability that the difference might (by chance) have been in the opposite direction: mean FVC might have been greater in smokers than non-smokers. Because the normal distribution is symmetrical, this probability is also 0.0082. The 'two-sided' P-value – the probability of observing a difference at least as extreme as 2.4, if the null hypothesis of no difference is correct – is thus found to be 0.0164 (= 0.0082 + 0.0082). Such a P-value provides evidence *against* the null hypothesis and suggests that smoking does, indeed, affect FVC.

While most standard statistical computer packages include P-values as part of their standard output, the interpretation of P-values causes confusion. For the reasons discussed in the section on *hypothesis tests*, there is little justification for dividing results into 'significant' and 'non-significant' according only to whether the P-value is less than 0.05 (or on the basis of any other threshold).

Three errors common in the interpretation of P-values are as follows.

First, potentially clinically important associations observed in small studies, for which the P-value is more than 0.05, are denoted as non-significant and ignored. To protect ourselves against this error, we should always consider the range of possible values for the association shown by the CONFIDENCE INTERVAL as well as the P-value.

Second, statistically significant ($P < 0.05$) findings are assumed to result from real associations, whereas by definition an average of 1 in 20 comparisons in which the null hypothesis is true will result in $P < 0.05$.

Third, statistically significant ($P < 0.05$) findings are assumed to be of clinical importance, whereas given a sufficiently large sample size, even an extremely small association in the population will be detected as different from the null hypothesis value of zero.

Based on considerations of the power of studies and the proportion of null hypotheses that are, in fact, false, Sterne and Davey Smith (2001) adapted the work of Oakes (1986) to suggest that in situations typical of medical statistics P-values less than 0.001 could be considered to provide strong evidence against the null hypothesis. However the interpretation of P-values will always depend on the context in which they were generated. For example Wacholder and Chanock (2004) suggested that in the context of molecular epidemiological studies, in which many thousands or even millions of single-nucleotide polymorphisms (SNPs) may be tested for associations with a disease outcome, it may be appropriate to consider only P-values less than 10^{-4}, or even 10^{-6}, as providing evidence of a real ASSOCIATION. *JS*

Fisher, R.A. 1925: *Statistical methods for research workers.* Edinburgh: Oliver and Boyd. **Oakes, M.** 1986: *Statistical inference.* Chichester: John Wiley & Sons. **Sterne, J.A. and Davey Smith, G.** 2001: Sifting the evidence – what's wrong with significance tests? *British Medical Journal* 322, 226–31. **Wacholder, S. and Chanock, R.M.** 2004: Assessing the probability that a positive report is false: an approach for molecular epidemiology studies. *Journal of the National Cancer Institute* 96, 434–42.

Q

Q-Q plots See PROBABILITY PLOTS

quality of life measurement A measurement that decides a patient's subjective reactions to perceptions of his or her environment. Quality of life (QoL) measures are becoming more frequently used in CLINICAL TRIALS and health services research, both as primary and secondary ENDPOINTS. However, despite this increased use, the concept of QoL is still an ill-defined term and there is no universally accepted definition. The World Health Organization (WHO, 1948) attempted to define 'health' as a: 'A state of complete physical, mental and social well-being, and not merely the absence of disease and infirmity.'

QoL means different things to different people and takes on different meanings according to the area of application. Therefore, to distinguish between QoL in its more general sense and the requirements of clinical medicine, the term health-related quality of life (HRQoL) is used to remove ambiguity.

However, HRQoL is still a vague concept. Most investigators generally agree that relevant concepts (sometimes referred to as domains or dimensions) of HRQoL can include: cognitive functioning; emotional functioning; general health; physical functioning; physical symptoms and toxicity; role functioning; sexual functioning; social well-being and functioning; spiritual/existential issues.

Clearly, HRQoL is a multidimensional construct. With the lack of any formally agreed definition of HRQoL, most investigators get around this problem by describing what they mean by HRQoL and then letting the items (questions) in their QUESTIONNAIRE speak for themselves. Some HRQoL instruments focus on a single concept (or dimension), such as physical functioning. Other HRQoL instruments have several dimensions such as physical, emotional and social functioning. Since there are many potential dimensions of HRQoL, it is impractical to assess all these concepts simultaneously in one instrument. Furthermore, HRQoL is a subjective concept, because the individual patient experiences symptoms, such as pain or depression and even physical functioning, and therefore they cannot entirely be assessed by 'objective' measures. So how do we actually measure HRQoL?

Simplistically, HRQoL measures represent a standardised approach to assessing a patient's perception of their own health using numerical scoring and can include symptoms, function and well-being. The concepts forming the various HRQoL dimensions are subjective measures and should best be evaluated by asking the patient.

The Medical Outcomes Study (MOS) *Short Form* (SF)-36 is the most commonly used HRQoL measure in the world today. It originated in the USA (Ware and Sherbourne, 1992), but it has been validated for use in the United Kingdom (Brazier *et al.*, 1992). It contains 36 questions measuring health across eight dimensions: physical functioning (PF) 10 items; role limitation because of physical health (RP) 4 items; social functioning (SF) 2 items; vitality (VT) 4 items; bodily pain (BP) 2 items; mental health (MH) 5 items; role limitation because of emotional problems (RE) 3 items and general health (GH) 5 items. (The first Figure, on page 281, shows the 10 questions that make up the physical function dimension of the SF-36.)

The responses to the 36 individual questions are classified into a mixture of binary (yes/no) and three-, five- and six-point ordered response categories. In planning and analysis, the question responses are often analysed by assigning equally spaced numerical scores to the ordinal categories (e.g. 1 = 'Yes, limited a lot', 2 = 'Yes, limited a little' and 3 = 'No, not limited at all', for the 10 items in the first figure). The raw scores across similar questions (e.g. the 10 physical functioning items shown in the Figure) are summed to generate a raw dimension score. Thus the 10-item physical function scale of the SF-36, with items scored 1 to 3, would yield a raw score ranging from 10 to 30. Finally, these raw dimension scores are then transformed to generate an HRQoL score from 0 to 100, where 100 indicates 'good health'. In our PF dimension example this transformation is achieved by:

$$\left[\frac{\text{Raw score} - \text{Lowest possible score}}{\text{Range of possible scores}} \right] \times 100,$$

$$\text{i.e.} \left[\frac{\text{Raw score} - 10}{20} \right] \times 100$$

Fayers and Machin (2000) term this procedure the 'standard scoring method' and this basic procedure is used to score many HRQoL instruments besides the SF-36.

The SF-36 is an example of an HRQoL instrument that is intended for general use, irrespective of the illness or condition of the patient. Such instruments are often termed *generic* measures and may often be applicable to healthy people too, hence their use in population surveys. The second Figure (on page 282) shows the distribution of the eight main dimensions of the SF-36 from a general population survey of United Kingdom residents (Brazier *et al.*, 1992), while the third Figure (on page 283) shows how physical functioning in the general population (Walters, Munro and Brazier, 2001) declines rapidly with increasing age.

The SF-36 is also an example of a *profile* HRQoL measure since it generates eight separate scores for each dimension of health (see fourth Figure, on page 283). Other generic profile instruments such as the Sickness Impact Profile (SIP) and Nottingham Health Profile (NHP) are described in Bowling (1997) and Fayers and Machin (2000). Conversely, some other HRQoL measures generate a single summary score or *single index*, which combine the different dimensions of health into a single number. An example of a single-index HRQoL outcome is the EuroQol, or EQ-5D as it is now named (Fayers and Machin, 2000).

Generic instruments are intended to cover a wide range of conditions and have the advantage that the scores from

HEALTH AND DAILY ACTIVITIES

The following questions are about activities that you might do during a typical day. Does your health limit you in these activities? If so, how much?

Activity	Yes, limited a lot	Yes, limited a little	No, not limited at all
a. **Vigorous activities**, such as running, lifting heavy objects, participating in strenuous sports	1	2	3
b. **Moderate activities**, such as moving a table, pushing a vacuum cleaner, bowling or playing golf	1	2	3
c. Lifting or carrying groceries	1	2	3
d. Climbing **several** flights of stairs	1	2	3
e. Climbing **one** flight of stairs	1	2	3
f. Bending, kneeling or stooping	1	2	3
g. Walking **more than a mile**	1	2	3
h. Walking **half a mile**	1	2	3
i. Walking **100 yards**	1	2	3
j. Bathing and dressing yourself	1	2	3

quality of life measurement *The 10 questions that make up the SF-36 physical function dimension (Brazier et al., 1992)*

patients with various diseases may be compared against each other and against the general population. For example, the fourth figure compares the mean SF-36 dimension scores of a group of patients six-months post-acute myocardial infarction (AMI) with an age- and sex-matched general population sample (Lacey and Walters, 2003). The AMI sample has lower HRQoL on all eight dimensions of the SF-36 than the general population sample. Contrariwise, generic instruments may fail to focus on the issues of particular concern to patients with disease and may often lack the SENSITIVITY to detect differences that arise as a consequence of treatments that are compared in clinical trials. This has lead to the development of *condition-* or *disease-specific* questionnaires. Disease-specific QoL measurement scales are comprehensively reviewed by Bowling (1995). Examples of disease-specific HRQoL questionnaires described in Fayers and Machin (2000) include the cancer-specific 30-item European Organisation for Research and Treatment of Cancer (EORTC) QLC-30 questionnaire and the cancer-specific 30-item Rotterdam Symptom Checklist (RSCL).

The instruments described here claim to measure general HRQoL and usually include at least one question about overall QoL or health. Sometimes investigators may wish to explore particular aspects or concepts in greater depth. There are also instruments for specific aspects of HRQoL. These specific aspects may include anxiety and depression, physical functioning, pain and fatigue. Examples of instruments which evaluate specific aspects of HRQoL are again described in Fayers and Machin (2000) and include: the Hospital Anxiety and Depression

Scale (HADS) and the Beck Depression Inventory (BDI) instruments for measuring anxiety and depression; the McGill Pain Questionnaire (MPQ) for the measurement of pain; the Multidimensional Fatigue Inventory (MFI) for assessing fatigue and the Barthel Index of Disability (BID) for assessing disability and functioning.

The historical development of QoL assessment is briefly discussed in Fayers and Machin (2000). One of the first instruments that broadened the assessment of patients beyond physiological and clinical examination was the Karnofsky performance scale, proposed in 1947 for the use in clinical settings. Over the following years a number of other scales were developed to assess functionally ability, such as the Barthel index. The next generation of questionnaires from 1980 onwards, such as the SIP and NHP, attempted to quantify general health status and not just functional ability.

The functional ability dimensions of the generic instruments may not be responsive enough to detect the 'small' changes in physical functioning experienced by patients undergoing treatment. For example the least 'difficult' item of the SF-36 physical function dimension (first Figure) is question 3j, *'Bathing or dressing yourself'*. Older adults with functioning problems may even have difficulty completing this item. For example, a general population survey of older adults aged 65 or more (Walters, Munro and Brazier 2001) found that 6.5% of respondents were at the 'floor' (i.e. scored 0) on the original 10-item PF dimension.

There are several solutions to this problem of unresponsive HRQoL measures, including extending the scales (by adding extra questions), computer-adaptive testing (CAT) and patient-generated measures (PGM).

With the increasing use of information technology we could use computer-adaptive testing (CAT) to assess HRQoL. This would involve the use of 'tailored' or adapted tests. For example, to assess physical functioning (using the SF-36 say), if a patient cannot manage a short walk, why ask questions about long walks or running?

With the use of CAT, the computer software can select questions of appropriate difficulty on the basis of earlier responses. This can result in more precise grading of ability and fewer questions put to each person.

A simpler solution to the problem of non-responsive generic HRQoL instruments is to use patient-generated measures (PGMs). These are a set of HRQoL instruments that ask patients to select their own dimensions and/or items. PGMs have the advantages that they are more relevant to the patients and likely to be more sensitivity to change. The disadvantages of PGMs are the reduced comparability between patients, the dimensions may change before and after treatment and they are more complex to administer. Fayers and Machin (2000) give two examples of PGMs: the patient-generated index (PGI) and schedule for the evaluation of individual quality of life (SEIQOL).

There is a continuing philosophical debate about the meaning of QoL and about what should be measured. Despite this, it is still important to measure health-related quality of life (HRQoL) as well as clinical- and process-based outcomes. This is because 'all these (QoL) concepts reflect issues that are of fundamental importance to patients' well-being. They are all worth investigating and quantifying' (Fayers and Machin, 2000).

Most investigators treat the 'summated scores' from the

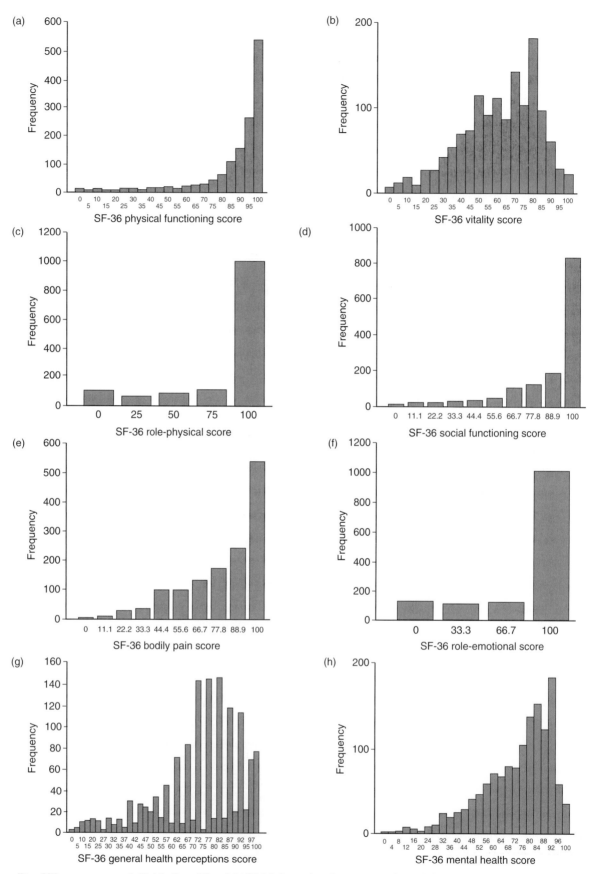

quality of life measurement *Distribution of the eight SF-36 dimensions from a general population survey (n = 1372), a score of 100 indicates 'good health'*

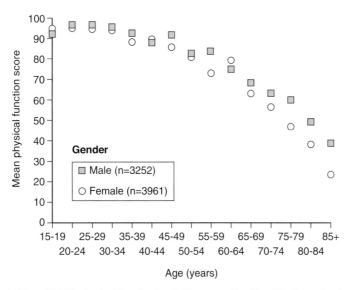

quality of life measurement *Mean SF-36 physical functioning (PF) age profile. The PF dimension is scored on a 0 to 100 (good health) scale*

HRQoL instruments as if they are from a continuous distribution. This is probably not an unreasonable assumption, particularly if we believe that there exists an underlying continuous latent variable that measures HRQoL and that the actual measured outcomes are ordered categories that reflect contiguous intervals along this continuum.

Most HRQoL outcome measures, such as the SF-36, which use the standard scoring method described previously, generate data with discrete, bounded and non-standard distributions (see second Figure). The scaling of HRQoL measures such as the SF-36 may lead to several problems in determining sample size and analysing the data (Walters, Campbell and Lall, 2001; Walters, Campbell and Paisley, 2001).

The apparent continuum hides the fact that only a few discrete values are possible. For example, the role physical (RP) dimension of the SF-36 is scored on a 0 to 100 scale but there are only five possible categories/scores, e.g. 0, 25, 50, 75 and 100 (see c in the second Figure). Furthermore, the scale may not be linear. For example,

using the SF-36 RP dimension, is a change of score from 0 to 25 the same as a change from 75 to 100?

There can often be a floor or ceiling effect. Patients cannot be worse than the worst category or better than the best category. (In the case of the SF-36 score either 0 or 100). For some populations the level is wrong and most people score on either the best category or the worst category. Floor and ceiling effects are more likely to be a problem in longitudinal studies because they limit the ability of the instrument to detect an improvement or deterioration in a patient's HRQoL over time (c in the second Figure shows that for the RP dimension of the SF-36 over 72% (1000/1372) of the general population sample had scored 100 and were at the ceiling of the distribution).

Methods based on the NORMAL DISTRIBUTION (such as MULTIPLE LINEAR REGRESSION) assume that the outcome variable has a constant variance. The variances of changes may depend on initial values. This is a common problem with range-limited values. Patients may enter the study with a wide variety of scores, but tend always to increase

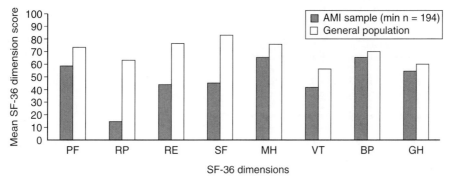

quality of life measurement *Profile of mean SF-36 scores for an acute myocardial infarction patient sample (6 weeks post-MI) compared with age- and sex-matched general population sample (contains data from Lacey and Walters, 2003)*

283

their scores. Thus patients who score lower at the start of the study have more range to improve than those who are already close to the maximum.

Yet again, normal approximations may not apply. Since the data are, in fact, categorical, they may require different techniques of analysis. By definition, no ordinal variable can be normally distributed, although in some cases a normal approximation will suffice.

MISSING VALUES are likely, for example in questionnaires that ask '*How far can you walk?*' when the patient is in a wheelchair. And then, it can be difficult to quantify an effect size (e.g. a desirable difference in mean score between groups) in advance.

The advantages in being able to treat HRQoL scales as continuous and normally distributed are simplicity in sample size estimation and statistical analysis. Therefore, it is important to examine such simplifying assumptions for different instruments and their scales. Since HRQoL outcome measures may not meet the distributional requirements (usually that the data have a normal distribution) of parametric methods of sample size estimation and analysis, non-parametric methods are often used to analyse HRQoL data.

Conventional methods of analysis of HRQoL outcomes are extensively described in Fayers and Machin (2000) and Fairclough (2002). Papers by Walters and colleagues (Walters, Campbell and Lall, 2001; Walters, Campbell and Paisley, 2001) discuss alternative ways of determining sample size and analysing HRQoL outcomes including the use of the proportional odds model for ORDINAL DATA and the non-parametric BOOTSTRAP computer simulation method.

In summary, there are numerous HRQoL instruments now available (and these are extensively described in Bowling 1995, 1997). By far the easiest way to assess HRQoL is to use an 'off-the-shelf' instrument rather than designing one's own. But, how to choose between the various HRQoL instruments? This fundamentally depends on the purpose of the study and the reliability, validity, responsiveness and practicality of the instrument. A 'belt and braces' approach is recommended for the assessment of HRQoL, i.e. both a generic and condition-specific instrument should be used.   *SJW*

Bowling, A. 1995: *Measuring disease: a review of disease-specific quality of life measurement scales.* Buckingham: Open University Press. **Bowling, A.** 1997: *Measuring health: a review of quality of life measurement scales,* 2nd edn. Buckingham: Open University Press. **Brazier, J.E., Harper, R., Jones, N.M.B., O'Cathain, A., Thomas, K.J., Usherwood, T. and Westlake, L.** 1992: Validating the SF-36 health survey questionnaire: new outcome measure for primary care. *British Medical Journal* 305, 160–4. **Fairclough, D.L.** 2002: *Design and analysis of quality of life studies in clinical trials.* New York: Chapman & Hall. **Fayers, P.M. and Machin, D.** 2000: *Quality of life assessment, analysis and interpretation.* Chichester: John Wiley & Sons. **Lacey, E.A. and Walters, S.J.** 2003: Continuing equality: gender and social class influences on self-perceived health after a heart attack. *Journal of Epidemiology and Community Health* 57, 622–7. **Walters, S.J., Campbell, M.J. and Lall, R.** 2001: Design and analysis of trials with quality of life as an outcome: a practical guide. *Journal of Biopharmaceutical Statistics* 11, 3, 155–76. **Walters, S.J., Campbell, M.J. and Paisley, S.** 2001: Methods for determining sample sizes for studies involving health-related quality of life measures: a tutorial. *Health Services & Outcomes Research Methodology* 2, 83–99. **Walters, S.J., Munro, J.F. and**

Brazier, J.E. 2001: Using the SF-36 with older adults: cross-sectional community based survey. *Age & Ageing* 30, 337–43. **Ware, J.E. Jr and Sherbourne, C.D.** 1992: The MOS 36-item short-form health survey (SF-36). I. Conceptual framework and item selection. *Medical Care* 30, 473–83. **World Health Organization** 1948: *Constitution of the World Health Organization.* Geneva: WHO Basic Documents.

quantile–quantile (Q-Q) plots See PROBABILITY PLOTS

quantitative trait loci (QTL)

The chromosomal locations of functional variants that affect continuous characteristics (e.g. height, blood pressure) or common diseases that are thought to have an underlying continuous liability (e.g. hypertension). The mode of inheritance of such traits is usually consistent with a polygenic model that assumes multiple small genetic and environmental effects. The term QTL is sometimes used to describe all the constituent loci in the polygenic model, but more often restricted to the loci that have relatively major and therefore potentially detectable effects, while the rest are known collectively as the *residual polygenic background.* Recent developments in molecular genetics have made available multiple genetic markers throughout the genome and enabled the localisation and detection of individual QTL by linkage and association strategies.

The most popular method of QTL linkage analysis is based on an extension of the variance components model for partitioning phenotypic variance into genetic and environmental components. Traditional variance components models in genetics rely on different genetic relationships having different extents of genetic sharing and therefore different magnitudes of correlation for the genetic component of the trait. For example, monozygotic twins share all their genes and have a genetic correlation of 1, whereas dizygotic twins share half their genes and have a genetic correlation of 0.5, so that a greater trait similarity between monozygotic twins than between dizygotic twins would suggest the presence of a genetic component.

The extension involves introducing a COMPONENT OF VARIANCE that is correlated between relatives to the same extent as the proportion of alleles they share at the QTL (in the identity-by-descent sense). In other words, relatives who share both alleles at the QTL will be completely correlated for the effects of the QTL and similarly those sharing one or none of the alleles will have correlations of 0.5 and 0, respectively, for the effects of the QTL. A genome scan for QTL linkage would involve estimating the extent of allele sharing between family members in a sample, from marker genotype data, and systematically testing each chromosomal location for a significant QTL component.

Another approach to QTL linkage analysis is based on linear regression of some measure of trait similarity on the proportion of allele sharing, for the relative pairs in a sample of families. The original method, proposed by Haseman and Elston, uses the square of the trait difference between relatives as the measure of trait similarity, but more recent work has shown that another definition based on a weighted sum of the squared difference and squared sum (of the mean-centred variables) is more powerful. The original regression approach (see ORDINAL DATA) was restricted to sibling pairs but it has been extended to general pedigrees.

A major problem of QTL linkage analysis is that the power to detect a QTL decreases rapidly with decreasing QTL effect size. If random population samples are studied, a sample size of tens of thousands is required for adequate power to detect a QTL that accounts for as much as 10% of the trait variance. Selective genotyping on the basis of informativeness has been proposed as a method for reducing the cost of linkage studies; typically families are selected for genotyping only if they contain individuals at the extreme of the trait distribution. Both variance components and regression methodologies can be modified to deal with samples with selective genotyping.

Association analysis is complementary to linkage analysis for the localisation and identification of QTL. Both family and unrelated designs are used for QTL association studies, the former providing for the possibility of a within-family test that is robust to population stratification. Typically, QTL association data are analysed by linear regression or an extension of linear regression to family data that makes allowance for correlated data. A popular method assumes that the trait has a MULTIVARIATE NORMAL DISTRIBUTION within a family, where the means are determined by a linear function of allelic effects and the covariance structure is determined by degree of genetic relationship, and possibly local allele sharing, between relative pairs. *PS*

[See also GENETIC EPIDEMIOLOGY, TWIN ANALYSIS]

Sham, P. 1997: *Statistics in human genetics*. London: Arnold.

quasi-likelihood

quasi-likelihood A generalisation of the GENERALISED LINEAR MODELS approach. In GENERALISED LINEAR MODEL (GLM) methods, such as Gaussian, Poisson and LOGISTIC REGRESSION, the distribution of the response variable is assumed to be one of the EXPONENTIAL FAMILY of distributions. The unknown parameters of the model are estimated by maximising the LIKELIHOOD function. This likelihood function is based on a specification of the whole distribution of the response variable conditional on the covariates.

However, it turns out that the MAXIMUM LIKELIHOOD ESTIMATES and the estimated variance-covariance matrix (and so standard errors) depend only on the first two moments (the mean and variance) of the distribution of the response conditional on the covariates. The quasi-likelihood approach makes use of this property of GLMs. Models are fitted in which only the link and variance functions (the functions that determine how the mean and variance of the response depend on the covariates) are specified, rather than the whole distribution of the response. This may be done even if the link and variance functions do not correspond to a member of the exponential family.

An example may make this clearer. Suppose that $Y_1, ..., Y_N$ are the numbers of tumours induced in N mice. We might model the association between the expected number of tumours, $E(Y)$, and some covariate of interest, X, using Poisson regression with log-link function. So, log $E(Y) = \alpha + \beta X$, where α and β are unknown parameters. This model includes the assumption that $Var(Y) = E(Y)$.

In many experiments, however, there is overdispersion, i.e. the variance of the response is greater than its expected value. This will lead to the standard errors of α and β being underestimated and the TYPE I ERROR rate of any hypothesis test being inflated.

So instead, one might adopt a quasi-likelihood approach. One possibility would be to assume again that log $E(Y) = \alpha + \beta X$, but that $Var(Y) = \phi E(Y)$, where ϕ is some unknown parameter. If $\phi = 1$, we have the POISSON DISTRIBUTION; if $\phi > 1$, there is OVERDISPERSION. Also, note that if $\phi > 1$, the response distribution does not belong to the exponential family.

A generalisation of quasi-likelihood are GENERALISED ESTIMATING EQUATIONS (GEEs). Whereas quasi-likelihood is for independent responses, GEEs allow responses to be correlated. This might be of use, for example, for repeated-measures data (see REPEATED MEASURES ANALYSIS OF VARIANCE). *SRS*

Diggle, P., Heagerty, P., Liang, K.-Y. and Zeger, S. 2002: *Analysis of longitudinal data*, 2nd edn. Oxford: Oxford University Press. **McCullogh, P. and Nelder, J.A.** 1983: *Generalised linear models*. London: Chapman & Hall.

questionnaires

questionnaires A means of collecting information from participants in a study. They are useful in many research settings and good design is paramount to ensure that results are informative.

Questionnaires can be self-administered or interviewer-administered, in which case this might be done face to face or over the telephone. Information gained from interviewer-administered questionnaires is more complete and is usually thought to be more accurate, because the interviewer is able to provide additional guidance to the respondent. Interviewer-administered questionnaires must be used with respondents who are illiterate or semiliterate in the language of the questionnaire. Self-administered questionnaires, by way of contrast, are cheaper to use and are generally quicker for the respondent to complete. Self-administered questionnaires are often considered a more appropriate technique when questions are of a very sensitive nature, such as enquiries about illegal drug use.

When developing a questionnaire the precise issues of interest should be considered carefully and numbers of questions apportioned correspondingly. Time spent conducting a PILOT STUDY on a small sample from the target population is rarely wasted; analysis of the process and responses will highlight problems with timing, omission of questions, or misunderstanding of instructions.

There are two major types of question that can be included in any questionnaire: open and closed. Open questions ask respondents to reply in their own words. For example, the following open question could be included in a survey about children's attitudes to smoking: '*How did you feel when you had your first cigarette?*'

Such questions have the advantage that the respondent is not influenced by the researcher's suggestions and is able to provide a more detailed reply. However, supplying such answers takes more time and effort on the part of the respondent and the process of coding answers is time consuming and can be complex.

Closed questions provide a set of responses from which the individual chooses their answer(s). For example, the open question from earlier could be made into a closed question by supplying the following list of possible responses.

- ☐ I felt grown up
- ☐ I enjoyed it
- ☐ I was disappointed
- ☐ I felt ill
- ☐ I felt guilty
- ☐ Other ....

When using a closed question in a face-to-face interviewer-administered questionnaire, it is helpful to list possible responses on a flashcard so that the participant can easily see all the options. Closed questions must provide all possible responses or include a category entitled 'other', as shown here. Note that a question that includes the 'other' category (as in this example) is sometimes deemed 'semi-open'. A pilot study can be useful to determine popular responses in the 'other' category, which can then be included as defined options on the final questionnaire.

To standardise responses, categories should be qualified as far as possible. For example, use the descriptions on the right of the following frequencies, rather than those on the left, in response to the question 'How often do you eat chocolate?'

☐ Not often	☐ Less than once a week
☐ Fairly often	☐ Between one and seven times a week
☐ Very often	☐ More than once a day

A further possible mistake to avoid is to have categories that are not mutually exclusive, for example, by asking a participant to indicate their age by ticking a box below:

- ☐ Under 18
- ☐ 18–25
- ☐ 25–30
- ☐ 30–40
- ☐ 40–55
- ☐ 55 or older

When deciding on categories it can be helpful to ensure that they will be comparable with external data, such as ethnic groupings used by government bodies.

Scales are a specific type of closed question. Two commonly used scales are the LIKERT SCALE and the VISUAL ANALOGUE SCALE. The Likert scale requires a participant to choose a response indicating their level of agreement with a statement. For example, the participant might be asked whether they agree with the statement 'I am restricted in my activities because of pain'. He or she would have to choose one of the responses that follow.

- ☐ Strongly agree
- ☐ Agree
- ☐ Neither agree nor disagree
- ☐ Disagree
- ☐ Strongly disagree

The visual analogue scale requires participants to indicate their response on a continuous scale, marked at either end. For example, the respondent might be asked to indicate their level of pain following an operation with a cross on the following scale.

Worst pain imaginable   No pain

Once the data have been collected the researcher must measure the distance from the lower end of the scale to convert the response into a score. For convenience, the scale is often 10 cm long and measurements are taken to the nearest millimetre.

It is helpful if questions are as specific as possible, so that instead of asking 'Do you have a car?' ask 'Is there a car or van available for private use by you or a member of your household?' It is also important that the wording of questions is not ambiguous. For example, the question 'Where do you live?' might elicit responses about geographical locations or types of accommodation.

Hedges (1979) describes other ways in which the wording of questions affects responses. In answering question (a) in the following questionnaire, 82% of respondents replied that they take enough care of their health, whereas only 68% gave this response to question (b).

(a) Do you feel you take enough care of your health or not?

(b) Do you feel you take enough care of your health or do you think you could take more care of your health?

The description of the alternative to taking enough care of your health may have influenced respondents. However, it is also notable that the two options in question (b) are not necessarily mutually exclusive: a respondent may be aware that he or she could take *more* care of his or her health, but at the same time considers that he or she takes *enough* care.

A respondent must only be asked one question at a time. The enquiry 'Were you satisfied with the treatment you received in hospital and at home?' would be better split into two separate questions. Difficulties also arise when respondents are asked questions that are irrelevant to them. If a questionnaire distributed to an elderly population asks whether they get breathless when doing housework, an individual who never does any housework might answer 'no' for this reason.

For some measurements, such as birth weight, both imperial and metric units are in common use. More accurate responses will result if the respondent is allowed to report on either scale and the conversion done at the analysis stage.

The layout of questionnaires is also important. The form should be easy to read, particularly for self-administered questionnaires; it helps if there is plenty of white space on each page. Questions on the same topic are best grouped together and 'transitions' such as 'We would now like to find out about the health of your family' are useful. If sections on a questionnaire are to be skipped by some respondents, then this should be made as clear as possible, perhaps by the use of arrows.

Sampling considerations are as important in questionnaire-based studies as in any others and as such it is vital to use a representative sample from the population to whom the results are to be applied. Non-response often introduces bias (see NON-RESPONSE BIAS) and this can be a considerable problem when using self-administered questionnaires, particularly postal questionnaires. To minimise non-response, questionnaires should be kept concise, easy to read and should not begin with personal or difficult questions that discourage the participant from starting. A covering letter explaining the reason for the research and the investigator's credentials may also help motivate the respondent. Pre-paid return envelopes should be included with postal questionnaires and one or preferably two reminders sent to those who do not respond, enclosing further copies of the questionnaire and pre-paid return envelopes. The investigator must make every effort to ensure that names and addresses used are current.

Before a questionnaire is used the issues of validity and reliability should be addressed (see MEASUREMENT PRECISION AND RELIABILITY). Validity assesses whether a questionnaire measures what it intends to measure, while reliability evaluates the consistency of the questionnaire when it is administered repeatedly to the same individual. It is therefore important that the questionnaire is known to be valid and reliable before time and resources are invested in the study. McDowell and Newell (1996) give information on how validity and reliability can be assessed.

An important consideration before writing a new questionnaire is whether a suitable instrument already exists. The use of an existing questionnaire saves time in writing and piloting. Also, information may be available regarding validity and reliability, and results could be more comparable with those from other studies. Again, McDowell and Newell (1996) provide detailed descriptions of existing questionnaires for measuring aspects of health such as depression, pain and quality of life.   *SRC*

Hedges, B.M. 1979: Question wording effects: presenting one or both sides of a case. *The Statistician* 28, 83–99. **McDowell, I. and Newell, C.** 1996: *Measuring health: a guide to rating scales and questionnaires*, 2nd edn. Oxford: Oxford University Press.

quota sample Quota sampling is a non-random SAMPLING METHOD. Before the sample is chosen, the population is divided into groups according to certain characteristics, for example, age, sex or smoking status. The interviewer is then told to interview a specified number of people within each group, but is given no instructions on how to find the people to interview. Quota sampling is often used in opinion polls and in market research surveys.

Quota sampling has the advantage that it is quick and easy to do. Any member of the sample can be replaced with another member with the same characteristics, which is not the case in random sampling.

A major disadvantage of quota sampling is that, as it is completely non-random, there is likely to be a great deal of BIAS in the selection process. The interviewer is more likely to approach people who are easy to question or who appear cooperative. It is also difficult to find out about those who do not cooperate, since they are replaced in the sample. However, if no sampling frame exists then quota sampling maybe the only practical method of obtaining a sample.

As an example, in a paper assessing the priorities for allocation of donor liver grafts (Neuberger *et al.*, 1998), quota sampling was used to choose members of the general public to be included. The quota was designed so that the sample would be 'nationally representative' and included 1000 people aged 15 or above. It was based on 10-cell quota for sex, household tenure, age and work status. Quota sampling was also used to choose the regions from which the family doctors came, quotas being based on region, with one practitioner per practice. Within regions the selection of practices was random.   *SLV*

Crawshaw, J. and Chambers, J. 1994: *A concise course in A level statistics*, 3rd edn. Cheltenham: Stanley Thornes Publishers. **Neuberger, J., Adams, D., MacMaster, P., Maidment, A. and Speed, M.** 1998: Assessing priorities for allocation of donor liver grafts: survey of public and clinicians. *British Medical Journal* 317, 172–5.

R

R Free statistical software that offers extensive data analysis and graphics facilities. R runs on many different computer operating systems (including Windows, Macintosh and various forms of UNIX) and provides a wide range of statistical analyses and has very powerful facilities for producing publication-quality graphics.

In addition to the predefined statistical analyses and graphics capabilities, R provides a fully featured programming language for manipulating data and for creating new analysis and graphics functions. This programming language is based on the S language, so functions written for S-PLUS will often run in R without modification. The basic functionality of R can be extended by loading add-on packages, of which there are over 400 available.

The default user interface for R is a command line, but a number of GUI interfaces are available via related software projects and add-on packages.

For more information on R, see the R homepage (www.r-project.org/), which has links to download sites, mailing lists, documentation, add-on packages and related software projects. The documentation on this website includes several book-length introductions to using R. For published books, Dalgaard's *Introductory statistics with R* provides an entry-level statistical context and Venables and Ripley's *Modern applied statistics with S* provides a more sophisticated treatment. Some of Everitt and Rabe-Hesketh's *Analyzing medical data using S-Plus* also applies to R. *PM*

Becker, R.A., Chambers, J.M. and Wilks, A.R. 1988: *The new S language*. London: Chapman & Hall. **Dalgaard, P.** 2002: *Introductory statistics with R*. New York: Springer. **Everitt, B. and Rabe-Hesketh, S.** 2001: *Analyzing medical data using S-Plus*. New York: Springer. **Venables, W.N. and Ripley, B.D.** 2002: *Modern applied statistics with S*, 4th edn. New York: Springer.

random effect One of a set of effects on a response variable corresponding to a set of values taken by an explanatory variable. Random effects are included in a regression model to acknowledge that response tends to differ between the groups defined by the explanatory variable. By including random effects, the investigator can estimate the mean level of response across groups and the extent to which response varies between groups or estimate the effect of another variable of interest while controlling for the differences between groups.

Typical examples of explanatory variables include indicator variables for hospitals in a national survey, centres in a multicentre study, patients in a longitudinal dataset or studies in a meta-analysis. If the variable defines k distinct groups in the dataset, for example if k hospitals are recruited for a survey, the k random hospital effects in the present survey are assumed to be drawn from a distribution of effects associated with the population of hospitals in general. It is common to assume random effects to be drawn from a NORMAL DISTRIBUTION. The variance of this distribution is estimated in the analysis and represents the extent of variation between the groups. For example, researchers may be interested in the variability between hospitals in admission rates or the variability between family doctors in prescribing of lipid-lowering drugs.

Random effects are appropriate when the investigator wishes to estimate or control for the distribution of the group effects defined by the explanatory variable over the population of possible groups. When fitting random effects, the groups are assumed to be exchangeable, which means that the investigator has no reason to distinguish one group from another and would (in principle) be prepared to mix up the names of the groups in the dataset before carrying out the analysis. An alternative approach to modelling the differences between groups is to model these as FIXED EFFECTS. This is appropriate when the focus is on the group effects for the k specific groups included in the dataset, for example when estimating the response of patients to each of three treatments compared in a CLINICAL TRIAL. *RT*

random effects models
Essentially a synonym for MULTILEVEL and LINEAR MIXED EFFECTS MODELS. This term is commonly used to represent regression models that include both fixed effects and random effects. *RT/BSE*

[See also RANDOM EFFECT, MULTILEVEL MODELS]

random effects models for discrete longitudinal data
Discrete responses include categorical responses (e.g. dichotomous or ordinal) and integers (e.g. counts). We can use well-known models such as LOGISTIC REGRESSION and Poisson regression (see GENERALISED LINEAR MODEL) to model the effects of covariates on the responses. However, an extra complication with longitudinal data is that the responses on the same subject tend to be dependent over time. For instance, in the example considered later, some subjects are consistently more prone to thought disorder than others. While some of this dependence is due to subject-specific covariates that we can include in the model, some extra dependence usually remains even after controlling or adjusting for the covariates. This extra dependence, which may be due to omitted covariates, can be modelled using random effects. Our focus here is on random effects models for dichotomous responses but we briefly consider random effects model for counts or incidence rates later.

For dichotomous and ordinal responses the most popular models are logistic regression and probit regression (see PROBIT MODELS). Let y_{ij} be the measurement at occasion $i = 1,...,n_j$ for a subject $j = 1,...,N$. The simplest random effects logistic regression model includes a subject-specific random intercept ζ_{0j} to model the dependence among the repeated measurements. Here the log of the odds of a '1' response versus a '0' response is modelled as:

$$\ln\left(\frac{\Pr(y_{ij} = 1 | \mathbf{x}_{ij}, \zeta_{0j})}{\Pr(y_{ij} = 0 | \mathbf{x}_{ij}, \zeta_{0j})}\right) = (\beta_0 + \zeta_{0j}) + \beta_1 x_{1ij} + ... + \beta_p x_{pij},$$

where $x'_{ij} = (x_{1ij}, \ldots, x_{pij})$ are covariates with regression co-efficients β_1 to β_p, β_0 is the mean intercept and ζ_{0j} is the deviation of subject j's intercept from the mean. The covariates typically include time or functions of time to model changes in the log odds over time. The random intercept ζ_{0j} is assumed to be normally distributed with zero mean. Inclusion of ζ_{0j} allows the overall log odds of the response to vary between subjects, even after controlling for the covariates. Since ζ_{0j} remains constant over time, the log odds and therefore the probability of a '1' response for a given subject is either greater than expected given the covariates at all occasions (if $\zeta_{0j} > 0$) or smaller than expected (if $\zeta_{0j} < 0$), producing the required within-subject dependence. The random intercept can be interpreted as the effect of all omitted subject-specific covariates that are constant over time on the log odds.

The random intercept logistic regression model can equivalently be expressed in terms of a latent (unobserved) response y_{ij}^* (see LATENT VARIABLES) underlying the observed response y_{ij}, where $y_{ij} = 1$ if $y_{ij}^* > 0$ and $y_{ij} = 0$ otherwise. The logistic regression model becomes a linear regression model for the latent response:

$$y_{ij}^* = \beta_0 + \beta_1 x_{1ij} + \ldots + \beta_p x_{pij} + \zeta_{0j} + \varepsilon_{ij}$$

where ε_{ij} is independent of ε_{0j} and has a logistic distribution with mean zero and variance $\pi^2/3$.

The strength of the residual within-subject dependence can be expressed by the intraclass correlation for repeated latent responses y_{ij}^* and $y_{i'j}^*$:

$$\rho = \text{Cor}(y_{ij}^*, y_{i'j}^* | x_{ij}, x_{i'j}) = \text{Cor}(\zeta_{0j} + \varepsilon_{ij}, \zeta_{0j} + \varepsilon_{i'j})$$
$$= \frac{\text{Var}(\zeta_{0j})}{\text{Var}(\zeta_{0j}) + \pi^2/3}.$$

The random intercept model assumes that the log odds change in the same way over time for all subjects with the same covariate values. Since this may be unrealistic, we can allow the linear growth or rate of change of the log odds to vary randomly between subjects by including a random slope ζ_{1j} of time in the model, giving the random coefficient model:

$$\ln\left(\frac{\Pr(y_{ij} = 1 | x_{ij}, \zeta_{0j}, \zeta_{1j})}{\Pr(y_{ij} = 0 | x_{ij}, \zeta_{0j}, \zeta_{1j})}\right)$$
$$= (\beta_0 + \zeta_{0j}) + (\beta_1 + \zeta_{1j})x_{1ij} + \beta_2 x_{2ij} + \ldots + \beta_p x_{pij},$$

where x_{1ij} represents the time at measurement occasion i for subject j. β_1 is the mean slope and ζ_{1j} is the deviation of subject j's slope from the mean slope. The random intercept ζ_{0j} and slope ζ_{1j} are typically assumed to have a bivariate normal distribution with zero means. The model can be extended by including further random effects for other variables, for instance polynomials in time to model variability in nonlinear growth.

MAXIMUM LIKELIHOOD ESTIMATION is the state-of-the-art method for estimating random effects models for discrete data. The marginal likelihood is obtained by 'integrating out' the random effects. When the random effects are multinormal, the integration is typically performed using Gaussian quadrature or the superior adaptive quadrature approach (e.g. Rabe-Hesketh, Skrondal and Pickles, 2002). Computationally efficient but rather crude approximations such as penalised QUASI-LIKELI-HOOD or marginal quasi-likelihood are commonly used. Sometimes the distribution of the random effects is left unspecified and nonparametric maximum likelihood used (e.g. Aitkin, 1999).

The Madras Longitudinal Schizophrenia Study followed up patients monthly after their first hospitalisation

random effects models for discrete longitudinal data *Data on thought disorder*

j	early	y_0	y_2	y_4	y_6	y_8	y_{10}	j	early	y_0	y_2	y_4	y_6	y_8	y_{10}
1	0	1	1	1	0	0	0	52	0	1	1	1	0	1	0
6	1	0	0	0	0	0	0	53	0	1	0	0	0	0	0
10	0	1	1	0	0	0	0	56	1	1	0	1	0	0	0
13	0	0	0	0	0	0	0	57	0	0	0	1	0	0	0
14	0	1	1	1	1	1	1	59	0	1	1	0	0	0	0
15	0	1	1	0	0	0	0	61	0	0	0	0	0	0	0
16	0	1	0	0	1	0	0	62	1	1	1	1	0	0	0
22	0	1	1	1	0	0	0	65	1	0	0	0	0	0	0
23	0	0	0	0	1	0	0	66	0	0	0	0	0	0	0
25	1	0	0	0	0	0	0	67	0	0	1	0	0	0	0
27	1	1	1	1	1	0	1	68	0	1	1	1	1	1	1
28	0	0	0					71	0	1	1	0	1	0	0
31	1	1	1	1	0	0	0	72	0	1	0	0	0	0	
34	0	1	1	0	0	0	0	75	1	1	0	0	0		
36	1	1	1	0	0	0	0	76	0	0	1				
43	0	1	1	0	1	0	0	77	1	0	0	1	0	0	0
44	0	0	1	0	0	0	0	79	0	1					
45	0	1	1	1	0	1	0	80	0	1	1	1	0	0	0
46	0	1	1	1	1	0	0	85	1	1	1	1	1	0	0
48	0	0	0	0	0	0	0	86	0	0	1				
50	0	0	0	0	1	1	1	87	0	1	0	0	0	0	
51	1	0	1	1	1	0	0	90	0	1	1	1	0	0	0

for schizophrenia. We will use random effects logistic regression to investigate whether the course of illness differs between patients with early and late onset. The variables considered are: [Month]: number of months since first hospitalisation; [Early]: early onset (1: before age 20, 0: at age 20 or later); [y]: repeated measures of thought disorder (1: present, 0: absent)

The first Table, on page 289, contains a subset of the data, namely on whether thought disorder [y] was present or not for 44 female patients at 0, 2, 4, 6, 8 and 10 months after hospitalisation.

Maximum likelihood estimates based on adaptive quadrature are given in the second Table (estimates were obtained using gllamm: www.gllamm.org). For the random intercept model the odds of thought disorder decrease over time in late-onset women with an estimated odds ratio of $\exp(-0.40) = 0.67$ per month. Early onset patients do not seem to have a higher odds of thought disorder at first hospitalisation (odds ratio $\exp(0.05) = 1.05$). Early-onset patients appears to have a greater decline in their odds of thought disorder over time. The intraclass correlation of the latent responses was estimated as $\hat{\rho} = 0.46$.

Estimates for the random coefficient model are also reported in the second Table. The random slope variance is estimated as 0.14 and the covariance between intercept and slope as –0.71, corresponding to a correlation of –0.70. Therefore those at higher risk of thought disorder at the time of hospitalisation experience a greater reduction in their risk over time than those at lower risk. It is important to note that the random intercept variance and the correlation between the random intercept and coefficient are interpreted at [Month] = 0. (Subtracting 5 months from [Month] yields an estimated correlation close to zero.)

To gain more insight into the model, we have plotted the conditional or *subject-specific* probabilities of thought

random effects models for discrete longitudinal data
Repeated measurements of thought disorder: estimates for dichotomous logistic regressions with random intercept and with random intercept and random slope for [Month]

	Random intercept model	Random coefficient model
	Est (SE)	Est (SE)
Fixed part		
β_0 [Cons]	1.01 (0.46)	1.36 (0.66)
β_1 [Month]	–0.40 (0.08)	–0.51 (0.13)
β_2 [Early]	0.05 (0.88)	0.04 (1.21)
β_3 [Early]×[Month]	–0.07 (0.14)	–0.06 (0.21)
Random part		
$\mathrm{Var}(\zeta_{0j})$	2.76 (1.24)	7.17 (4.03)
$\mathrm{Var}(\zeta_{1j})$		0.14 (0.09)
$\mathrm{Cov}(\zeta_{1j}, \zeta_{0j})$		–0.71 (0.53)
Loglikelihood	–124.75	–121.20

disorder given various values of the random intercept (±3) and slope (±0.4) for women with early onset. These are shown as dashed curves in the Figure where the dotted curve is the conditional probability for random intercept and slope both equal to their population means of zero, thus representing a 'typical' individual. Also shown as a solid bold curve is the *population average* or marginal probability of thought disorder obtained by integrating the conditional probability over the random effects distribution.

Note that the population average curve is considerably flatter than that of a typical patient. Such attenuation of the effects of covariates in marginal models compared

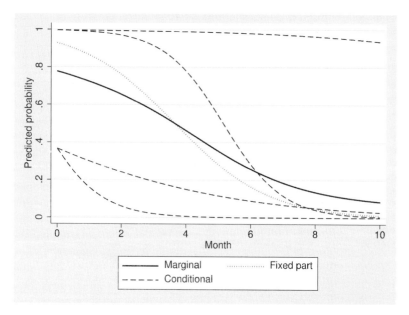

random effects models for discrete longitudinal data *Conditional and marginal predicted probabilities of thought disorder for women with early onset. Dotted curve for conditional probability from random coefficient model when both random intercept and slope are zero*

with conditional models is a well-known phenomenon for dichotomous responses (see GENERALISED ESTIMATING EQUATIONS).

For counts or incidence rates, the most common model is Poisson regression. As for the random effects logistic model, random intercept models and different kinds of random coefficient models can be specified. Note that the marginal effects equal the conditional effects for the random intercept Poisson model. Random effects models for discrete longitudinal data can also be used for truly multilevel designs, for instance where repeated measures are nested in patients who are nested in hospitals. Skrondal and Rabe-Hesketh (2004) give a general treatment of random effects models and other latent variable models for discrete data. *SRH/AS*

Aitkin, M. 1999: A general maximum likelihood analysis of variance components in generalised linear models. *Biometrics* 55, 117–28. **Rabe-Hesketh, S., Skrondal, A. and Pickles, A.** 2002: Reliable estimation of generalized linear mixed models using adaptive quadrature. *The Stata Journal* 2, 1–21. **Skrondal, A. and Rabe-Hesketh, S.** 2004: *Generalized latent variable modelling: multilevel, longitudinal and structural equation models.* Boca Raton: Chapman & Hall/CRC.

random intercept model See LINEAR MIXED EFFECTS MODEL

random intercept and slope model See LINEAR MIXED EFFECTS MODEL

randomisation The process by which patients should be assigned to treatments in a CLINICAL TRIAL. At the outset we should contrast random assignment (randomisation) with random sampling: the latter is the process by which we select individuals to take part in our experiment and forms the basis of our concluding that the results apply to a broad population (see SAMPLING METHODS – AN OVERVIEW). If we were to recruit only young healthy males to a clinical trial or any other form of research, it would be unreasonable to expect our results to apply to a broad population of men, women, adults and children.

Unfortunately, random sampling is almost never possible in the context of medical research although we may still be able to make reasonable reference to a future population to which our results may apply. Little more will be said here about random sampling.

The key reason for using randomisation to decide which patient receives which treatment is to eliminate BIAS (Altman and Bland, 1999). Bias may obviously be introduced deliberately but it can also be introduced inadvertently. Selecting healthier patients or those with fewer – or less severe – symptoms to receive one treatment rather than another would probably influence the outcome from a clinical trial such that we might incorrectly infer that one treatment were better at relieving symptoms than another.

From this it should be clear that not only must the sequence be random but those responsible for recruiting patients must not know what the sequence is – otherwise it would still be possible to enrol the 'milder' patients onto one treatment arm and the 'more severe' patients onto the other. This is also a reason against 'alternate' allocation of one treatment followed by the other (Chalmers, 1999). The strength of a clinical trial should be that causality can be inferred because the two (or more) treatment groups

are balanced – at least in the probabilistic sense – for all factors except the treatment received.

The Table contains an extract of the table of random digits published by Altman (1991: 540).

There are many ways of using such a table to assign patients randomly to two treatment groups. The simplest approach might be to assign even numbers to receive treatment and odd numbers to receive placebo, or control. Reading across the first row the 1st patient is assigned number 47 and so receives placebo; the 2nd patient assigned number 44 would receive active treatment; the 3rd, 4th, 5th and 6th (assigned 76, 60, 72, 56, respectively) all receive active treatment; the 7th patient (99) receives placebo and so on. We could split the numbers up so that the 1st patient is assigned number 4 and the 2nd number 7 (receiving active and placebo treatments respectively), the next patients are assigned 4, 4, 7, 6, 6 etc.

Alternatively, we could choose to read down the columns instead of across the rows. Any one of these procedures is perfectly valid and will result in an unbiased and (in the long run) balanced assignment between the two treatment groups provided that the rule for using the random number digits is set out in advance. If we had three treatment groups then we could use the same tables but use the numbers 1, 2, 3, for assignment to treatment one; 4, 5, 6 for assignment to treatment two; and 7, 8, 9 for assignment to treatment three or placebo. An occurrence of a zero is ignored and the next digit used instead. Other rules can be established for assignment to any number of treatments. This is referred to as 'simple randomisation'. We shall make reference to this Table of random digits later to illustrate different forms of randomisation.

Reference was made earlier to 'balanced' treatment groups. Balance is one of the most important aspects of a clinical trial because it ensures that we are making a fair comparison between the treatments and neither one nor the other is predisposed to showing a better or worse response.

There are three different aspects to balance that are useful to discuss: ensuring the same number of patients receive each of the treatments; ensuring that demographic data and disease severity data are similar between the two treatment groups and ensuring that factors unknown to the experimenter but that may nevertheless influence outcome are also balanced between the treatment groups. Randomisation is quite a remarkable tool – not only does it balance the treatment groups for all the known important prognostic factors, it also balances for any factors that may be important but that we may not know about.

randomisation *Random numbers*

47	44	76	60	72	56	99	20	20	52
31	60	26	13	69	74	80	71	48	73
72	89	83	91	86	62	78	86	95	07
31	40	99	54	61	99	32	30	43	80
03	49	79	75	46	76	56	99	54	46
36	61	26	31	49	40	74	86	32	36
91	72	12	92	31	66	91	99	48	42
42	73	76	68	86	75	21	91	72	38
32	95	21	17	27	63	06	14	24	05
57	24	32	29	46	60	82	90	81	31

In the example given using line 1 of the table, among the first 10 patient assignments only two of them are odd numbers and so would receive the placebo (patient numbers 1 and 7). Superficially, this seems to be a concern although, in fact, if we randomise a sufficiently large number of patients using the full random number table then we should – on average – assign an equal number of patients to each of the treatment arms. Trials of only 10 patients are extremely rare and would probably not be very convincing whatever the results. However, in a relatively small study, perhaps of some complex surgical technique requiring a lot of skill on the part of the surgeon, we might be concerned if so few of the early patients were assigned to placebo (or *sham* treatment).

It is quite possible that the skills of the surgeon might improve over time and so the overall outcome (regardless of treatment group) might tend to improve as the trial progresses. Therefore having an imbalance in the number of patients assigned to one or other treatment very early on could introduce a bias between the treatment groups. For this reason, we often use blocking to ensure that at regular intervals the number of patients assigned to each treatment group is the same.

In the simplest case of two treatment groups, we may use block sizes of 4. This would mean that within every group of four patients, two are assigned to treatment and two are assigned to placebo. We would not know which two patients receive either treatment or placebo, neither would it be the same two in every block of four treatment assignments. When we have two treatments (call them A and B) and assignment is in blocks of size four, there are six possible configurations of each block: AABB, ABAB, ABBA, BBAA, BABA and BAAB. Each of these blocks should be equally likely to occur. With two treatments, the block size does not have to be four but it could be any multiple of the number of treatments. Similarly, if there are four or more treatments then the block size might be anything from twice the number of treatments upwards.

The advantage of using blocks should be quite clear – not only will the total number of patients assigned to each treatment be the same at the end of the study but also, on a regular basis (perhaps once every four patients), the number assigned to each treatment will also be the same. These types of processes are referred to as 'blocked randomisation' or 'restricted randomisation'.

There can be disadvantages to blocking since it can compromise blinding and so allow bias to be introduced. Consider an extreme situation where there are two treatments and the block size is two. If, for some reason, the assignment of the first patient were to be known (possibly because of typical adverse reactions or even some inadvertent unblinding of the treatment) then the identity of the next treatment is necessarily known. This is typically why a block size equal to the number of treatments would not be used. Even if the block size is twice the number of treatments, if one of the early patients in the block is unblinded, then still the probability of future assignments will not be 0.5. Such potential unblindings are arguments against blocking – or at least in favour of longer blocks, but the longer the block the less the balance on a regular basis and so a compromise has to be found. One strategy that is sometimes used is to vary the block length, perhaps between blocks of four treatments and blocks of six treatments. If the fifth patient were to be unblinded then the

investigator would not know if this is the penultimate patient in a block of size six or if it were the first patient following a block of size four. This strategy can greatly help to eliminate possible biases due to unblinding but does increase complication in packing treatment.

This strategy of blocking ensures that there is balance on a regular basis through the duration of the trial but a further feature upon which balance may be desired is that of demographic or disease severity factors. In the simplest case, consider that gender is a factor highly prognostic of treatment outcome so that it is important to ensure that there is not an imbalance of men or women assigned to one or other treatment. Simple randomisation as just described should ensure that this is the case but only in a long term or probabilistic sense and in any particular trial, if there were some imbalance, then this might bring into questions the validity or reliability of the results.

Stratification is a very simple mechanism that uses different randomisation sequences for the different strata on which treatment balance is necessary. Using the random digits in the table, we may decide that the first five rows should be used for assigning men to either treatment (even numbers) or control (odd numbers) and that the second five rows should be used for similarly assigning women to either treatment or control. A common misconception is that stratification ensures equal numbers of men and women on each treatment but considering random sampling, described at the beginning of this section, this is not necessarily the case. The proportion of men and women in the target population with the disease that is being studied may not be equal. The proportion of men and women in the target population who are prepared to take part in the clinical trial may not be equal. Stratification ensures that *of the men* who take part in the trial, half of them will be assigned to treatment and half to control and that *of the women* who take part in the trial, similarly, half will receive treatment and half will receive control. Considering our earlier discussion concerning blocking, it will be evident that the equal allocation to treatment and placebo of the men (and of the women) will only be the case in the long term and it is quite common within stratified randomisation to also include blocking. This introduces very little extra complexity.

One practicality of preparing stratified randomisation sequences is that, instead of one sequence being prepared for the entire trial, two or more sequences are prepared (one for each stratum). The methods used to introduce blocking into the single sequence used for a trial without stratification is simply replicated in each of the stratum-specific randomisation sequences. In multicentre trials, the most common feature of the randomisation scheme is stratification by investigator or centre. This ensures that each centre uses all of the treatments and there is no risk that within any particular centre, all patients might receive only one of the treatments.

It is quite possible to stratify on more than one factor. The simplest approach where this applies is in a multicentre study where there is one (non-centre) factor on which stratification is needed. Different randomisation sequences are prepared for each centre so that we have stratification by centre. In fact, each centre would be given two randomisation sequences, for example one to be used for males and one to be used for females. Such a study then has two stratification factors (centre and gender), although, in practice, each investigator would only see and use one stratification factor, that of gender. When there are two or more important prognostic factors but both needs to be balanced for, then stratification begins to become rather more complex.

Consider the case where we wish to stratify by gender (male and female) and also stage of disease (early or advanced). We now need four randomisation sequences: the first can be used for females with early stage disease, the second for females with advanced stage disease, the third for males with early stage disease and the fourth for males with advanced stage disease. The potential for using the wrong randomisation sequence obviously becomes higher in this situation and if any of the factors has more than two levels or if there are more than two or three factors then the number of sequences usually becomes prohibitively large.

The logistics of randomly assigning patients to treatment can be eased by central (often telephone, or web-based) randomisation schemes where the investigator does not have to concern himself or herself with using different randomisation sequences for different types of patients. If medication is supplied to the investigational site in sequentially numbered packages then a central randomisation system, if given details of the levels of the stratum for any particular patient, can simply inform the investigator which treatment pack to assign to that patient. The details of multiple randomisation sequences need not then concern the investigator.

Despite the fact that the investigator does not need to concern himself or herself with the multiple randomisation schemes, somebody does! The additional complexities of treatment packaging and assignment should not be underestimated and the potential for errors in randomising patients to treatments must be considered. The risk of introducing errors can become quite high. Also, it is quite possible with many strata and relatively few patients that some of the combinations of strata values may occur only very infrequently or not at all. Because of the desire to try to balance within these stratification factors there can sometimes be a problem that the overall balance between the treatment groups (that is, the *total* number of patients on each treatment) may now become unbalanced. Methods exist to try to find a compromise between balancing individual factors and balancing the total treatment assignment.

Most trials are arranged such that the sequence of randomisation codes is established before patients are recruited to the trial and medication is then pre-packed and despatched to investigators. In this case, although the sequence is unknown to the investigators and the patients it is fixed and potentially known to the study statistician or those responsible for packing the medication. Provided patients are assigned sequentially, balance (on average) will be maintained. ADAPTIVE DESIGNS change the randomisation sequence as the trial progresses. One method is called MINIMISATION, which helps to solve the problem discussed earlier of multiple factors on which balance is required when stratified randomisation becomes too complex.

Another type of adaptive randomisation is that called 'response-adaptive randomisation' (see Wei and Durham, 1978). These methods are rarely used but they have an intriguing and appealing ethical basis. They can be used when the response to treatment for each patient is known relatively quickly and the recruitment of patients is relatively slow. Such a design would start with a traditional, equally balanced, randomisation scheme and the first 20 or 30 patients may be assigned randomly to each of the treatment groups. Thereafter if one treatment is appearing to be superior to the other then the randomisation probabilities begin to change in favour of the most advantageous treatment. Early results from trials can be very unreliable and it is quite possible that the treatment appearing to be beneficial early on may subsequently appear less good than the alternative treatment. In this case, the allocation probabilities would then change back through 0.5 to again favour the treatment that is emerging as 'best'. (See DATA-DEPENDENT DESIGNS for further discussion.)

A particular application of randomisation in the design of clinical trials is the randomised consent design proposed by Zelen (1979; 1990). Such designs are used in highly pragmatic trials – that is, those that are intended to mimic, as closely as possible, true clinical practice. They encompass the constraint that some patients may not wish to receive certain treatments so that even if the physician might prescribe a particular treatment, the patient may wish not to take it.

Subjects are randomised to one of two treatment groups and those who are randomised to receive standard therapy then receive that therapy. Those who are randomised to receive the new, experimental treatment are asked to consent to receive that treatment or, if they prefer, they can receive the standard treatment. Their preference is respected and they receive the treatment of their choice.

It is absolutely critical that such trials are analysed by the INTENTION-TO-TREAT principle, so that patients are analysed according to which treatment they were randomised and not which treatment they actually received. Such a trial is then intended to answer the question about what would happen if patients are *prescribed* a particular treatment, considering the inevitable problem that some patients prescribed a particular treatment will choose not to take it.

A related type of trial is called *Wennberg's design* where patients are randomised to receive either the treatment of their own choice or a standard, specified experimental treatment. Such a design is, again, highly pragmatic but it is very difficult to judge the benefit of one treatment strategy over another for future patients since the results of the study are highly dependent on the preferences of the patients who take part.

Another use of randomisation is in testing treatment policies following an existing treatment regime. Examples typically include answering the question: 'If patients do not respond to a low dose, are they likely to respond to a higher dose?' Very commonly this question is addressed as follows: patients are randomised to treatment or control and efficacy assessments made at an appropriate follow-up time after randomisation. Treatment may have been shown to be, on average, superior to control, yet not all patients will have responded to the new active treatment. Those who have not responded are now treated with a higher dose (or some other modification of the treatment regime) and subsequent efficacy or response rates are recorded.

The criterion for being included in such a follow-up is that the patient has not responded to the initial treatment and so any response at all is considered indicative of an additional benefit of the additional treatment regime. The question, of course, remains as to what would have happened to these patients had they either continued with the existing medication or followed some other course of treatment instead. The appropriate means of evaluating such a question is illustrated in the Figure.

Patients who are to be included in this follow-up regime should be randomised to either receive the new modified treatment (perhaps a dose increase) or to continue on existing treatment (usually meaning at the same dose). Again, note the criterion for being included in this follow-up study is that the patient has not responded to the initial treatment and in such a design it is not unusual to see some of the patients who continue on the identical treatment to respond now. This design, however, allows us to see possibly differential response rates in the patients who have continued on exactly the same treatment as those who have been randomised to receive the modified treatment. This then allows a proper assessment of the beneficial effects of changing the treatment regime as oppose to continuing with the same regime.

An ethical debate often arises around randomisation (see ETHICS AND CLINICAL TRIALS). How can it be right to choose treatment for a patient based on chance alone (or the 'throw of a die', to use a more emotional phrase)? This is an important consideration but many counter with the argument that it can be unethical *not* to randomise patients into clinical trials.

The ethics of clinical trials is a very broad subject and cannot be fully covered here. Where genuine doubt exists, however, as to the relative benefits of one treatment over another (a state often called 'equipoise'), then not randomising patients into trials can lead to misleading or even false judgements about the relative efficacy of different therapies.

Even where no alternative treatment exists for life-threatening conditions and a new potential therapy might offer the 'only hope' for a patient, without randomising patients between this new (possible) treatment and placebo, we can never get a true understanding of the risks and benefits of the new treatment.

Folklore often then suggests that the new treatment is, in fact, better than placebo when it has never been properly tested and it then becomes impossible (even if still not unethical) to carry out a randomised trial. Randomised consent designs and some of the adaptive designs discussed in this section can help balance the

ethical arguments. Using 'unequal' randomisation (assigning more patients to some treatment arms than to others – or to placebo) can also help.

Randomisation is one of the most fundamental and one of the most important considerations in the design of a clinical trial. In contrast to observational research and epidemiology, randomisation provides the basis for assigning CAUSALITY of response to the assigned treatment. For a much fuller discussion of randomisation, readers are referred to Rosenberger and Lachin (2002).   *SD*

Altman, D.G. 1991: *Practical statistics for medical research.* London: Chapman & Hall. **Altman, D.G. and Bland, M.** 1999: Treatment allocation in controlled trials: why randomise? *British Medical Journal* 318, 1209. **Chalmers, I.** 1999: Why transition from alternation to randomisation in clinical trials was made (letter to the editor). *British Medical Journal* 319, 1372. **Rosenberger, W.F. and Lachin, J.M.** 2002: *Randomization in clinical trials.* New York: Wiley. **Wei, L.J. and Durham, S.D.** 1978: The randomized play-the-winner rule in medical trials. *Journal of the American Medical Association* 73, 840–3. **Zelen, M.** 1979: A new design for randomized clinical trials. *New England Journal of Medicine* 300, 1242–5. **Zelen, M.** 1990: Randomized consent designs for clinical trials: an update. *Statistics in Medicine* 9, 645–6.

randomised controlled trials (RCT)   See CLINICAL TRIALS

randomised-response technique

A technique that aims to get accurate answers to a sensitive question that respondents might be reluctant to answer truthfully, for example, '*Have you ever had an abortion?*' The randomised response technique protects the respondent's anonymity by offering both the question of interest and an innocuous question, which has a known probability (α), of yielding a 'yes' response, for example;

1. [Flip a coin.] Have you ever had an abortion?
2. [Flip a coin.] Did you get a head?

A random device is then used by the respondent to determine which question to answer. The outcome of the randomising device is seen only by the respondent not by the interviewer. Consequently, when the interviewer records a 'yes' response, it will not be known whether this was a yes to the first or second question (Warner, 1965). If the probability of the random device posing question one, (p) is known, it is possible to estimate the proportion of yes responses to question one, (π), from the overall proportion of yes responses ($P = n_1/n$), where n_1 is the total number of yes responses in the sample size n:

$$\hat{\pi} = \frac{P - (1 - p)\alpha}{p}$$

So, for example if $p = 0.60$ (360/600), $p = 0.80$ and $\alpha = 0.5$ then $\hat{\pi} = 0.125$. The estimated variance of $\hat{\pi}$ is:

$$\text{Var}\,(\hat{\pi}) = \frac{\hat{\pi}(1 - \hat{\pi})}{n}$$
$$+ \frac{(1 - p)^2\,\alpha(1 - \alpha) + p(1 - p)[p(1 - \alpha) + \alpha(1 - p)]}{np^2}$$

For the example here, this gives $\hat{\pi} = 0.0004$.

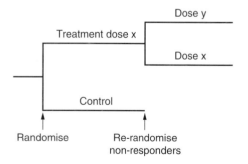

randomisation *Example of re-randomising 'non-responders'*

Further examples of the application of the technique are given in Chaudhuri and Mukerjee (1988). *BSE*

Chaudhuri, A. and Mukerjee, R. 1988: *Randomized response: theory and techniques.* New York: Marcel Dekker. **Warner, S.L.** 1965: Randomized response: a survey technique for eliminating evasive answer bias. *Journal of the American Statistical Association* 60, 63–9.

range The range is simply the interval between the minimum and maximum values in a set of observations. The range is a MEASURE OF SPREAD, although it is of limited use because it is dependent only on the extreme (and possibly unusual) observations, and not on the majority of the values. For this reason, the INTERQUARTILE RANGE is often a preferred measure. However, if the sample size is very small the range may be considered to be a useful summary statistic. It is more informative if the minimum and maximum are both quoted (e.g. 21 to 54), rather than merely the difference between the two (e.g. 33). *SRC*

reading the medical literature See CRITICAL APPRAISAL

recall bias A bias that can occur in CASE-CONTROL STUDIES due to cases being more likely to recall having been exposed than are controls. In some case-control studies retrospective data on exposure are obtained from historical records.

However, in most situations such data are not available and data are instead obtained by interviewing cases and controls (or their relatives). When this is done there is a chance that cases may be more likely to remember having been exposed than are controls. Even where there is no genuine difference in frequency of exposure between cases and controls, this differential recall may cause an apparent difference, so that the exposure appears to be associated with disease.

For example, in a case-control study of congenital malformations, mothers are asked about prior exposures to infectious diseases, drugs, environmental pollutants etc. It is quite plausible that a mother who has given birth to a malformed child will be more interested in the study and make more effort to remember instances of past exposure. It is also possible for recall bias to operate in the opposite direction: for example, if, through shame, cases were less likely than controls to admit exposure. *SRS*

Hennekens, C.H. and Buring, J.E. 1987: *Epidemiology in medicine.* New York: Little, Brown and Company. **Rothman, K.J. and Greenland, S.** 1998: *Modern epidemiology*, 2nd edn. Philadelphia: Lippincott-Raven Publishers.

[See also BIAS IN OBSERVATIONAL STUDIES]

receiver operating characteristic (ROC) curve Diagnostic testing plays an increasingly important role in modern medicine and the ROC curve is a common graphical tool for displaying the discriminatory ability of a diagnostic marker (test) in distinguishing between diseased and healthy subjects. The outcome of a diagnostic test can be dichotomous (positive, negative), ordinal (e.g. normal, questionable, abnormal) or continuous (e.g. PSA measurements). The ROC curve arises only for ordinal and continuous outcomes.

A diagnostic marker is generally evaluated by comparison to a definite gold standard procedure/test. Such gold standards are often complicated to conduct, intrusive, not sufficiently timely or expensive. This motivates the search for inexpensive, easily measurable and reliable alternatives.

A subject is assessed as diseased or healthy depending on whether the corresponding marker value is above or below a given threshold. Associated with any threshold value are the probability of a true positive (SENSITIVITY) and the probability of a true negative (SPECIFICITY). The ROC curve presents graphically the trade-off between sensitivity and specificity for every possible threshold value. By convention, the plot displays the specificity on the y-axis and 1 – sensitivity on the x-axis.

Consider for example ORDINAL DATA arising in the context of medical imaging. A reader is presented with images from diseased and healthy subjects and is required to rate each image on a discrete ordinal scale (1–5): (1) definitely normal, (2) probably normal, (3) questionable, (4) probably abnormal, (5) definitely abnormal. Suppose the results are as shown in the first Table or equivalently expressed as cumulative percentages, as in the second Table.

If we use a threshold of (1), we would have a specificity of 56% and a sensitivity of 96% (100% – 4%). For a threshold of (2), the specificity is 84% while the sensitivity is 88% (100% – 12%). If we ignored the test and called everyone diseased then the specificity is 0% with a corresponding sensitivity of 100%. This gives rise to the specificity/sensitivity pairs in the third Table. The Figure on page 296 shows the plot of specificity versus 1 – sensitivity, the ROC curve or plot.

A diagnostic marker shows good discriminatory ability if both sensitivity and specificity are high for a reasonable range of threshold values. In terms of the ROC plot, this means that the closer the curve comes to the left-hand border and then the top border the better the marker. The closer the curve is to the diagonal (45°) line the worse the discriminatory accuracy of the marker.

receiver operating characteristic (ROC) curve *Ordinal data results from a medical imaging study*

True disease status	(1)	(2)	(3)	(4)	(5)	**Total**
Healthy	28	14	5	2	1	50
Diseased	2	4	10	14	20	50
Total	**30**	**18**	**15**	**16**	**21**	**100**

receiver operating characteristic (ROC) curve *Cumulative percentages results from a medical imaging study*

True disease status	(1)	(2)	(3)	(4)	(5)
Healthy	56%	84%	94%	98%	100%
Diseased	4%	12%	32%	60%	100%

receiver operating characteristic (ROC) curve *Specificity and sensitivity pairs*

True disease status		(1)	(2)	(3)	(4)	(5)
Specificity	0%	56%	84%	94%	98%	100%
Sensitivity	100%	96%	88%	68%	40%	0%

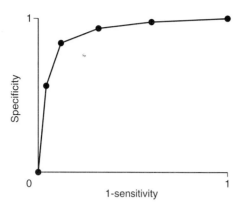

receiver operating characteristic (ROC) curve *A typical ROC curve*

For continuous data, the calculations are carried out similarly. However, for this situation the number of outcome values will be much larger and usually only one of the sensitivity and specificity will change when the threshold value is increased to its next observed value. Consequently, for data arising from a continuous scenario, the resulting ROC plot will tend to look like a step function. Both for the continuous case and the ordinal situation that has arisen from an underlying continuous mechanism, the *true* underlying ROC curve is a smooth function. Many methods, nonparametric, semi-parametric and parametric have been developed to provide smooth estimation procedures for the ROC curve. In addition, methodology for adjusting the ROC curve for covariate information and selection bias has been proposed. In certain situations the diagnostic markers are not measured directly on each subject but are taken on pooled groups of subjects. Faraggi *et al.* (2003) describe estimating the ROC curve for such pooled data.

The discriminatory power of the diagnostic marker that is indicated graphically by the ROC curve is often summarised by a one-number index. The AREA UNDER THE ROC CURVE (AUC) is the most commonly used index. Sometimes, only a particular range of sensitivity values is of interest and a partial area is computed as the area under the curve over the range of sensitivities considered important. An alternative index due to Youden is to compute the max{sensitivity+specificity} – 1 where the maximisation is carried out over all pairs of sensitivity and specificity values.

The ROC curve is also useful in assessing the discriminatory power of statistical models and classifiers for binary outcomes.   *DF/BR*

Faraggi, D., Reiser, B. and Schisterman, E.F. 2003: ROC curve analysis for biomarkers based on pooled assessments. *Statistics in Medicine* 22, 2515–27. **Greiner, M., Pfeiffer, D. and Smith, R.M.** 2000: Principles and practical application of the receiver-operating characteristic analysis for diagnostic tests. *Preventive Veterinary Medicine* 45, 23–41. **Pepe, M.S.** 2003: *The statistical evaluation of medical tests for classification and prediction.* Oxford: Oxford University Press. **Shapiro, D.E.** 1999: The interpretation of diagnostic tests. *Statistical Methods in Medical Research* 8, 113–34. **Zhou, X.H., Obuchowski, N.A. and McClish, D.K.** 2002: *Statistical methods in diagnostic medicine.* New York: Wiley.

regression dilution bias The term applies to any setting where one wishes to assess the relationship between a variable X that is measured with error and an outcome variable Y. When observed values of X are used as estimates of true values, the true relationship between X and Y is underestimated; this is regression dilution bias. In epidemiology, the term is often used to describe the situation where relationships between risk exposures of interest (such as blood pressure) and the risk of a particular disease occurring (such as a heart attack) are underestimated because of the use of single 'baseline' measurements of the risk exposure as estimates of the true underlying level.

The situation arises because studies that aim to identify risk factors for a particular disease usually take 'baseline' assessments of individuals and relate these measurements to disease events observed over a particular follow-up period. However, BASELINE MEASUREMENTS often do not reflect the patient's true usual level during the period of follow-up because of MEASUREMENT ERRORS, short-term 'random' fluctuations from the individual's average level and longer term true changes. Although these effects are random, meaning that the baseline measurement is just as likely to over- as underestimate the patient's true level, the differences between patients estimated from a baseline sample (the between-person variation) exaggerate the true differences that really exist between those patients over a period of time (because the estimated variance consists of both within- and between-person variation). In other words, the differences in the level of the risk exposure between the study participants are not as large as one would estimate from the baseline sample alone.

The effect of this on the estimated relationship between the risk exposure and the risk of disease is shown in the Figure where, for the sake of illustration, it assumed that the risk exposure is positively associated with the risk of disease and that a unit increase in the exposure leads to a proportional increase in the risk of disease (a log-linear relationship).

The solid line in the Figure shows the 'apparent' relationship between the risk exposure and the risk of disease obtained when using the baseline measurement levels as estimates of true usual levels. However, as already described, the true differences in exposure levels between the individuals are not likely to be as great as it would seem, in which case the difference in disease risk between

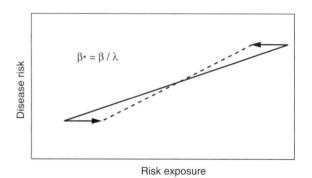

regression dilution bias *Effects of regression dilution bias*

those at the top and those at the bottom of the risk exposure distribution should correspond to a narrower range of values on the horizontal axis than suggested.

The true relationship between the usual risk exposure level and disease risk may therefore be obtained by 'shrinking' the line towards the middle by some predetermined amount (as indicated), so that the true relationship (shown by the dashed line) may be obtained. This line indicates the relationship between usual levels of the risk exposure and the risk of disease and, as can be seen, its slope (the strength of association) is greater than would otherwise be estimated. The extent of regression dilution bias (the difference between the two slopes) can usually be estimated by taking repeated measurements on individuals at various periods throughout the follow-up period, thus enabling estimation of the amount of within-person variation likely to be present. Thus, the apparent regression slope β may be appropriately corrected by a factor λ (the regression dilution ratio that may be estimated by the intraclass correlation) in order to obtain the true slope $\beta^* = \beta / \lambda$.

The concept of regression dilution bias is a very general one and is likely to apply in any setting where interest lies in the association between usual or average exposure levels over an exposure period and disease risk over that period. In situations where the interest is not in assessing relations with usual exposure levels, however, or where the outcome of interest is not determined by usual levels, correction for regression dilution bias would not be appropriate.

For a practical example, see the study into blood pressure differences conducted by MacMahon, Peto *et al.* (1990) that adjusted for the effects of regression dilution bias. *RM/JE*

[See also REGRESSION TO THE MEAN]

MacMahon, S., Peto, R., Cutler, J., Collins, R., Sorlie, P., Neaton, J. *et al.* 1990: Blood pressure, stroke and coronary heart disease. Part 1, Prolonged differences in blood pressure: prospective observational studies corrected for the regression dilution bias. *Lancet* 335, 765–74.

regression to the mean A phenomenon where an unusual or extreme value for a given variable is followed by a much less extreme value when re-measurement takes place. The phenomenon is an inevitable consequence of MEASUREMENT ERROR. A particularly well-known scenario concerns apparent hypertension in a subject who records a very high blood pressure reading. Re-measurement is very likely to result in a lower blood pressure reading, even if the subject has not been treated. The blood pressure has 'regressed' (gone back) towards the true underlying MEAN for that subject.

The phenomenon was first noted by Francis Galton in the 19th century when he compared the heights of parents with those of their children. Galton demonstrated that the children with tall parents tended to be *smaller* than the parents, while children with small parents tended to be *taller* than the parents. Yet the phenomenon also worked the other way round: parents of tall children tended to be smaller than the children and parents of small children tended to be taller. Consequently, when Galton plotted the heights of children against the heights of parents, he observed that the line that best fitted the data had a slope

less than one. Indeed, that is how the 'regression line', nowadays used more widely for relating any pair of continuous variables, obtained its name.

The extent of regression to the mean may be estimated by measuring a group of individuals twice. The Pearson correlation coefficient will estimate the extent to which single individual values would be expected to regress to the mean. Another method involves dividing the distribution of the first measurements on the individuals into fifths (MacMahon, Peto *et al.*, 1990). We calculate the means for those in the top fifth and those in the bottom fifth. For these two extreme groups of individuals, we then calculate the mean of their measurements on the *second* occasion. The means for the two groups on the second occasion will be more similar than on the first occasion. Indeed, the ratio of the difference in means on the second occasion, to the difference in means obtained for the first occasion, has been recommended as a good method of correcting for REGRESSION DILUTION BIAS.

Many examples have been provided about regression to the mean in various branches of medicine (see, for example, Bland and Altman, 1994a; 1994b; Morton and Togerson, 2003). Individual patients, when treated for unusually high blood pressure, will be likely to improve; the mistake is to attribute such improvement to the treatment rather than regression to the mean. Similarly, public health action to prevent a given disease may be targeted at a geographical area where incidence of a given disease has been observed as unusually high. Incidence of the disease will be likely to decline subsequently, but that may have happened even in the absence of the public health intervention.

In both these examples, the true test of the intervention involves an experiment that compares the change following intervention with that seen in a control group who, despite having unusually high initial values observed, are not subjected to the intervention. If the improvement observed in the intervention group was greater than that seen in the control group, then regression to the mean was not the solely responsible factor.

Because of regression to the mean, the British Hypertension Society recommends at least two readings on each of several occasions (Ramsay, Williams *et al.*, 1999). This is partly to address the possibility of poor measurement technique for single readings. However, the blood pressure at the time of the reading may have been genuinely higher than that normally experienced by the individual. The actual clinical objective is to ascertain the individual's true underlying mean value and repeating the measurement a week later may help to address this. *RM/JE*

Bland, J.M. and Altman, D.G. 1994a: Regression towards the mean. *British Medical Journal* 308, 1499. **Bland, J.M. and Altman, D.G.** 1994b: Some examples of regression towards the mean. *British Medical Journal* 309, 780. **MacMahon, S., Peto, R., Cutler, J., Collins, R., Sorlie, P., Neaton, J.** *et al.* 1990: Blood pressure, stroke, and coronary heart disease. Part 1, Prolonged differences in blood pressure: prospective observational studies corrected for the regression dilution bias. *Lancet* 335, 765–74. **Morton, V. and Torgerson, D.J.** 2003: Effect of regression to the mean on decision making in health care. *British Medical Journal* 326, 1083–4. **Ramsay, L.E., Williams, B., Johnston, G.D., MacGregor, G.A., Poston, L., Potter, J.F.** *et al.* 1999: British Hypertension Society guidelines for hypertension management: summary. *British Medical Journal* 319, 630–5.

regulatory statistical matters National and international guidances have been written to set out (in greater or lesser levels of detail) how CLINICAL TRIALS should be planned, executed, analysed and reported for regulatory submissions. The earliest documents were national or regional: FOOD AND DRUG ADMINISTRATION (1988), Ministry of Health and Welfare (1992), CHMP Working Party on Efficacy of Medicinal Products (1995). Later, the International Conference on Harmonization (ICH) began to coordinate guidance in all areas of the regulated pharmaceutical industry (not just statistics and not just clinical trials). They produced the guidance known as 'ICH E9' (see ICH E9 Expert Working Group, 1999) that was adopted by the ICH Steering Committee in February 1998.

The guidance is focused on statistical principles and not on specific methods. It is also aimed at a target audience of non-statisticians as well as statisticians and so should be mostly understandable to the target audience of the current volume. It is the responsibility of a sponsor company to produce convincing evidence of quality, safety and efficacy of a new medicinal product. While the convincing nature of such evidence may be influenced by the specific method of analysis used in a clinical trial, it is more likely to be influenced by the more fundamental issues of design and conduct of the studies. Trials submitted for regulatory submission have to be described and reported in great detail (see MEDICINES AND HEALTHCARE PRODUCTS REGULATORY AGENCY). ICH E9 explains that it is important that all the key features relating to the design, monitoring and analysis of a trial (and sets of trials) should be set out in detailed study protocols (see PROTOCOLS FOR CLINICAL TRIALS). There should then be a traceable record of any changes made to the original protocol, including when the decisions were made and when the changes were implemented. In this way, the protocol, its documented changes and the final clinical study report should all link together.

The ICH E9 document is mostly aimed at confirmatory PHASE III trials, although much of its content may be thought of as good statistical practice and applicable more widely. However, within the context of Phase III trials, the INTENTION-TO-TREAT principle (and, therefore, 'pragmatic' trials) is stressed in preference to 'explanatory' trials where a PER PROTOCOL design and analysis may have a greater part to play. The document introduced a new term, 'full analysis set' referring to the data that are used to try to address the intention-to-treat question. This was a compromise situation, recognising that it is often not possible to include every patient in the analysis for a true intention-to-treat answer. This term 'full analysis set' has not really caught on as a concept outside of the regulatory field and perhaps not within it either; 'intention-to treat', however, is firmly fixed in the language.

The definition (and specification) of primary and secondary ENDPOINTS is clearly important and covered in detail but further consideration is also given to 'composite variables' and 'multiple primary' (now more usually called 'co-primary') endpoints. Many trials use composite variables as primary (or secondary) endpoints – examples include psychiatry where rating scales are used, dermatology (lesion counts), arthritis (total joint scores), dentistry (number of eroded surfaces) and so on. 'Global assessment scores' are widely used in many therapeutic areas and are a clear example of a composite endpoint (even though it may not be clear what the components are). It is important that endpoints (particularly primary endpoints and, more especially, composite endpoints) are well validated both for statistical properties but also for face validity. Co-primary endpoints present further difficulties but obvious examples exist – particularly in cardiology studies. Reduction in 'all cause mortality, recurrent myocardial infarction, and stroke' is an endpoint often used in myocardial infarction treatment trials. While there may be a hierarchy to such endpoints (death being worse than MI and stroke) there are also elements that are not hierarchical (recurrent MI is not necessarily 'better' or 'worse' than having a stroke).

The fundamental techniques to avoid BIAS are considered to be blinding and RANDOMISATION. Each of these is covered in some detail. Fair consideration is given to the difficulties (in some circumstances) of designing trials to be double-blind or of maintaining the blind through the course of the study – but limitations of studies that are not blinded are outlined. Randomisation, including stratified and adaptive (such as MINIMISATION), methods are discussed. Their benefits are explained although some concern is raised about the use of adaptive designs. If such methods are used, it remains for the sponsor to produce convincing evidence that the analysis is adequate to account for the assignment method. Sensitivity analyses (used here and in other contexts) may help to address this.

Basic design issues (parallel groups, cross-over and factorial designs) are described and the relative advantages and disadvantages discussed. CROSS-OVER TRIALS, in particular, can be a very efficient method of experimentation but are highly prone to difficulties in the face of carryover effects between periods. This issue was particularly highlighted by Freeman (1989) but seemed to struggle to become recognised. The ICH E9 document clearly states in relation to carryover and the necessary chronic and stable nature of the disease: 'The fact that these conditions are likely to be met should be established in advance of the trial by means of prior information and data.' This was a significant step forward in the use of (or restriction of) cross-over trials in regulatory work.

Another substantive step was in the explicit recognition and contrast between trials to show superiority (which are what most people think of when discussing clinical trials) and trials to show non-inferiority or equivalence. Much has been written on this subject recently; although some was written before ICH E9 was published, until then it was still rather a new and unclear concept. Within the same section is comment on trials to show a dose–response relationship, another area previously suffering from lack of clear consideration.

A whole raft of other issues is also discussed such as handling MISSING VALUES and OUTLIERS, data transformations, estimation versus hypothesis testing, multiplicity, subgroup analyses and interactions, use of baseline covariates and so on. The document is wide in its scope, covering safety as well as efficacy.

Overall, the ICH E9 guidance has been highly influential both within and outside the pharmaceutical industry. However, as some problems begin to be solved, others come to the forefront and it is now recognised that further guidance on topics covered, perhaps rather sparingly, is necessary. To this end, the European Committee on Human Medicinal Compounds (CHMP) has set up various subcommittees, notably its Efficacy Working Party, which has identified various areas that need further explanation or clarity. This group has developed a number of 'points to consider' documents (not just in statistical areas). Currently, there are five agreed documents relating specifically to statistical/methodological issues: switching between superiority and non-inferiority (August 2000); applications with meta-analyses and one pivotal study (May 2001); MISSING DATA (November 2001); multiplicity issues in clinical trials (September 2002); and adjustment for baseline covariates (May 2003).

They have all been written to help clinical assessors to evaluate applications for marketing authorisations: they have not been written to guide statisticians; they have not been written to guide pharmaceutical companies. However, it is clear that they receive plenty of attention from this latter group and worthily so. They are all freely available on the EMEA website at www.emea.eu.int. More 'points to consider' documents are being drafted and yet more topics are being considered. These are European documents and have no formal status outside the EU, but they are widely recognised as valuable and important guidances. In parallel, the US FDA is currently preparing extensive guidance on the use of INTERIM ANALYSES and DATA AND SAFETY MONITORING COMMITTEES.

SD

CHMP Working Party on Efficacy of Medicinal Products 1995: Biostatistical methodology in clinical trials in marketing authorizations for medicinal purposes. *Statistics in Medicine* 14, 1659–82. **Food and Drug Administration** 1988: *Guideline for the format and content of the clinical and statistical sections of new drug applications.* Rockville, Maryland: FDA US Department of Health and Human Services. **Freeman, P.R.** 1989: The performance of the two-stage analysis of two-treatment, two-period crossover trials. *Statistics in Medicine* 8, 1421–32. **ICH E9 Expert Working Group** 1999: Statistical principles for clinical trials: ICH harmonised tripartite guideline, *Statistics in Medicine* 18, 1905–42. **Ministry of Health and Welfare** 1992: *Guideline for the statistical analysis of clinical trials.* Tokyo: MHW Pharmaceutical Affairs Bureau (in Japanese).

relative risk and odds ratio Two approaches to measuring the effect of a risk factor. The way in which RISK is presented can have an influence on how the associated risks are perceived. For example, one might be worried to hear that occupational exposure at one's place of work doubled the risk of a serious disease compared to some other occupation. However, the statement that the risk had increased from one in a million to two in a million might be less worrisome. In the first case, it is a *relative* risk that is presented, in the second, an *absolute* risk.

Both the relative risk and the odds ratio are measures of relative risk/chance. They measure how the chance of an event, typically of getting a disease, varies between two categories, typically a group that is exposed to a risk factor and one that is not. Explicit definitions are most easily understood in terms of a 2×2 table of exposure by disease as shown in the table. Therein, N denotes the population size and a, b, c and d the absolute frequencies of the respective combinations of the levels of the risk factor (exposed or not exposed) and the disease factor (present or absent).

The (absolute) risk of the disease within a subpopulation

relative risk and odds ratio *Two-way classification of exposure by disease*

		Disease		
		Present	*Absent*	**Total**
Risk factor	Exposed	a	b	$a + b$
	Not exposed	c	d	$c + d$
	Total	$a + c$	$b + d$	$N = a + b + c + d$

is defined as the proportion of subjects within the group that have the disease, i.e. r(Disease present | Exposed group) $= a/(a + b)$ and r(Disease present | Non-Exposed group) $= c/(c + d)$. As a result the risk ratio or relative risk, RR, of disease comparing the exposed with the non-exposed subpopulation is given by the ratio $\text{RR} = \dfrac{a/(a + b)}{c/(c + d)}$.

For example, a relative risk of lung cancer comparing smokers with non-smokers of 2 would be interpreted as doubling the risk of lung cancer when smoking.

In contrast, the ODDS of the disease within a subpopulation is defined as the ratio of subjects within the group that have the disease to those that do not, i.e. o(Disease present | Exposed group) $= a/b$ and o(Disease present | Non-Exposed group) $= c/d$. As a result the odds ratio, OR, of disease comparing the exposed with the non-exposed subpopulation is given by the ratio $\text{OR} = \dfrac{a/b}{c/d}$.

For example, an odds ratio of high blood pressure comparing treatment A with treatment B of 0.8 would be interpreted as a 20% reduction in the odds of high blood pressure under treatment A.

One can evaluate, say, 95%, CONFIDENCE INTERVALS for the population OR or RR by first transforming into the natural (base e) log scale, then exponentiating the lower and upper limits. The formula for the standard error of the log (OR) is memorable as the square root of the sum of the reciprocals of the entries in the 2×2 table of disease and risk factor. (The formula is given explicitly in the entry on CASE-CONTROL STUDIES.)

Usually, the preferred choice of expressing the effect of exposure on disease is the RR. However, not all study designs allow the estimation of this parameter. A CROSS-SECTIONAL STUDY might fix the sample size and in a COHORT STUDY the sizes of the cohorts of exposed and non-exposed subjects (the row totals in the table) are under the control of the investigator. Both these restrictions allow the risk of disease within the exposure groups and hence the RR to be estimated.

In contrast, in a CASE-CONTROL STUDY the number of subjects with the disease and the number of subjects without the disease (the column totals in the table) are chosen by the investigator making it impossible to estimate any risk of disease from the sample data. However, since the odds ratio of disease comparing an exposed with a non-exposed population is the same as the odds ratio of having been exposed to a risk factor comparing cases with controls, the odds ratio can be estimated from all the designs mentioned above. Case-control studies are frequently carried out in practice and this explains the widespread use of the OR as a measure of effect size. In addition, if a disease is relatively rare in the population (say below 5%) the OR can be used as an approximation to the RR.

SL

[See also CONTINGENCY TABLES, EPIDEMIOLOGY, LOGISTIC REGRESSION, MANTEL-HAENSZEL TEST]

Dunn, G. and Everitt, B.S. 1995: *Clinical biostatistics: an introduction to evidence-based medicine.* London: Arnold.

reliability   See MEASUREMENT PRECISION AND RELIABILITY

repeated measures analysis of variance   A test to see if the MEAN varies with either (or both) of a categorical factor and time. The TWO-WAY ANALYSIS OF VARIANCE seeks to partition the variation in a sample into that due to one factor, that due to a second factor and the residual variation that cannot be explained by either factor. The repeated measures analysis of variance (ANOVA) is a special case of the two-way analysis of variance, where one of the categorical factors is the time at which the measurement is taken.

As with other versions of the analysis of variance, the repeated measures ANOVA is usually employed following a designed experiment. If an experimental design decrees that measurements will be taken at baseline, after 3 months, after 7 months and after a year then it is sensible to view time as a factor of four levels. Contrariwise, if we have naturally arising times (e.g. times at which patients choose to visit their GP) then viewing them as categorical will be difficult and repeated measures ANOVA will probably not be appropriate.

Cadogan *et al.* (1997) investigate the effect of increasing milk consumption on the mean bone density in adolescent girls. Measurements were taken at 0, 6, 12 and 18 months and the treatment was a two-level factor. For these reasons, the repeated measures ANOVA was the choice of analysis technique.

As for the other analysis of variance techniques, repeated measures ANOVA can be extended to more complicated situations and for greatest flexibility can be viewed from within a regression framework.   *AGL*

[See also LINEAR MIXED-EFFECTS MODELS]

Altman, D.G. 1991: *Practical statistics for medical research.* London: Chapman & Hall. **Cadogan, J., Eastell, R., Jones, N. and Barker, M.E.** 1997: Milk intake and bone mineral acquisition in adolescent girls: randomised, controlled intervention trial. *British Medical Journal* 315, 1255–60.

replicate designs   See CROSS-OVER TRIALS

re-randomisation designs   See RANDOMISATION

resampling   See BOOTSTRAP

research ethics board (REB)   See ETHICAL REVIEW COMMITTEES

research ethics committee (REC)   See ETHICAL REVIEW COMMITTEES

residual confounding   See MEASUREMENT ERROR

residuals   See MULTIPLE LINEAR REGRESSION

response feature analysis   See SUMMARY MEASURE ANALYSIS

response variable   See ENDPOINT

restricted maximum likelihood (REML)   See LIKELIHOOD, MULTILEVEL MODELS

robustness   A property of statistical procedures that implies that they continue to work well even when there are departures from the assumptions on which they were based.

Many standard statistical procedures require that certain assumptions hold for the underlying theory to be applicable. For example, the two-sample t-test requires that the data are normally distributed with the same variance. In general, statistical procedures are considered to be robust if they are insensitive to small deviations from the underlying assumptions. If the optimal procedure requires the assumption of normality, then the corresponding robust procedures would not be influenced by departures from normality arising from slightly longer or shorter tails or slight SKEWNESS in the underlying distribution, which could result from the presence of a small proportion of OUTLIERS or spurious values. Robust procedures are ones such that these outliers, if they occurred, would have little effect on the analysis of the data.

Perhaps the most common estimator of the population MEAN is the sample mean, but this is not robust against quite small departures from the assumption of normality, being particularly sensitive to outliers. The MEDIAN, by way of contrast, although less efficient than the sample mean when the assumptions hold, is much more robust since it is hardly affected by the presence of outliers. A 'good' estimator is one that combines the properties of high efficiency and robustness.

One of the major problems in the development of robust procedures concerns the appropriate set of criteria that the procedure should satisfy; different criteria have led to different robust methods. Procedures that maintain the Type I error (declared significance level) or the confidence level are known as *validity robust*, while those that maintain high power or size of confidence interval are known as *efficiency robust*. Even within these broad categories there might be different kinds of departure from the assumptions that could be considered. These competing influences have resulted in a wide range of robust estimation methods being developed; these include M-estimators (based on MAXIMUM LIKELIHOOD ESTIMATION), L-estimators (based on linear functions of order statistics) and R-estimators (based on ranking methods).

The M-estimators (which include the sample mean and median as special cases) are based on bounded or re-descending weight functions, which give lower (or even zero) weight to extreme observations and usually involve iterative solution of the resulting likelihood equations. The L-estimators include trimmed means and Winsorised means (and, again, the sample mean and median as special cases), while the R-estimators lead to Wilcoxon and Mann-Whitney procedures based on signed ranks. Generally all these alternative robust methods lead to reasonably high efficiency and wider applicability than the 'optimal' procedures. These ideas have been extended to multivariate data and to regression problems. There is now an extensive literature on robust regression, robustness in scientific modelling and in experimental design.   *PP*

Davies, P.L. 1993: Aspects of robust linear regression. *Annals of Statistics* 21, 1843–99. **Rousseeuw, P.J. and Leroy, A.M.** 1987: *Robust regression and outlier detection.* New York: John Wiley & Sons. **Staudte, R.G. and Sheather, S.J.** 1990: *Robust estimation and testing.* New York: John Wiley & Sons. **Wilcox, R.** 1998: Trimming and Windorisation. In Armitage, P. and Colton T. (eds), *Encyclopedia of biostatistics.* Chichester: John Wiley & Sons.

ROC curves   See RECEIVER OPERATING CHARACTERISTIC (ROC) CURVE

S

sample size determination in clinical trials One hallmark of a well-designed study is to have a formally estimated required sample size before the study commences. Awareness of the importance of this has led to increasing numbers of medical journals demanding that full justification of the sample size chosen is published with reports of trials. The *British Medical Journal*, the *Journal of the American Medical Association* and numerous other journals issue checklists for authors of papers on CLINICAL TRIALS, in which there is a question relating to sample size justification. Investigators, grant-awarding bodies and biotechnology companies all wish to know how much a study is likely to cost them. They would also like to be reassured that their effort (and money) is well spent, by assessing the likelihood that the study will give unequivocal results.

Providing a sample size is not simply a matter of providing a single number from a set of tables but is a two-stage process. At the preliminary stages, 'ballpark' figures are required that enable the investigator to judge whether or not to start the detailed planning of the study. If a decision is made to proceed, then a subsequent stage is to refine the calculations for the formal study protocol itself (see PROTOCOLS FOR CLINICAL TRIALS).

When a clinical trial is designed, the investigator must make a realistic assessment of the potential benefit (the anticipated effect size) of the proposed test therapy. The history of clinical trials research suggests that, in certain circumstances, rather ambitious or overoptimistic views of potential benefit have been claimed at the design stage. This has led to trials of inadequate size for the questions posed.

If too few subjects are involved, the trial may be a waste of time because realistic medical improvements are unlikely to be distinguished from chance variation. A small trial with no chance of detecting a clinically meaningful difference between treatments is unfair to all the subjects put to the risk and discomfort of the clinical trial. Too many subjects is a waste of resource and may be unfair as a larger than necessary number of subjects receive inferior treatment if one treatment could have been shown to be more effective with fewer patients.

The traditional approach to sample size determination is by consideration of significance or hypothesis tests. Suppose we wish to compare two groups with a continuous outcome variable. We set up a null hypothesis that the two population means μ_0 and μ_1 are equal. We carry out a significance test to test this hypothesis. We calculate the observed difference in means $\bar{d}$. This significance test results in a P-VALUE, which is the probability of getting the observed result, $\bar{d}$, or one more extreme, if the null hypothesis is true, by chance. If the P-value obtained from a trial is less than or equal to α, then one rejects the null hypothesis and concludes that there is a statistically significant difference between treatments. The value we take for α is arbitrary, but conventionally either 0.05 or 0.01. Contrariwise, if the P-value is greater than α, we do not reject the null hypothesis.

Even when the null hypothesis is, in fact, true there is still a risk of rejecting it. To reject the null hypothesis when it is true is to make a TYPE I ERROR. Plainly the associated probability of rejecting the null hypothesis when it is true equals α. The quantity α is interchangeably termed the test size, SIGNIFICANCE LEVEL or probability of a Type I (or false-positive) error.

The left-hand curve in the Figure shows the expected distribution of the observed difference $\bar{d}$ under the null hypothesis, centred at zero. If $\bar{d}$ is greater than some value d_α, which is determined so that the shaded area to the right is equal to α, then H_0 is rejected.

The clinical trial could yield an observed difference $\bar{d}$ that would lead to a P-value above α, even though the null hypothesis is not true, that is, μ_0 is indeed not equal to μ_1. In such a situation, we then accept (more correctly phrased as 'fail to reject') the null hypothesis although it is truly false. This is called a TYPE II (false-negative) error and the probability of this is denoted by β.

The probability of a Type II error is based on the assumption that the null hypothesis is not true, that is, $\delta = \mu_0 - \mu_1 \neq 0$. There are clearly many possible values of δ in

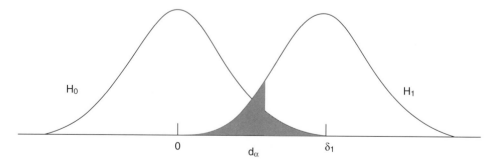

sample size determination in clinical trials *The left-hand curve shows the distribution of $\bar{d}$ under the null hypothesis. If $\bar{d} > d_\alpha$ then H_0 is rejected. The vertically hatched area represents the Type I error α. The right-hand curve shows the distribution of $\bar{d}$ under the alternative hypothesis that the difference in means is δ_1 and the horizontal hatched area represents the Type II error, β*

this instance and each would imply a different alternative hypothesis, H_1 and a different value for the probability β.

The power is defined as one minus the probability of a Type II error, thus the power equals $1 - \beta$. That is, the *power* is the probability of obtaining a 'statistically significant' P-value if the null hypothesis is truly false.

The right-hand curve of the Figure illustrates the distribution of $\bar{d}$ under the alternative hypothesis H_1, centred on the expected difference in means $\delta_1 = \mu_0 - \mu_1$.

If δ, α and β are all fixed, it would appear there is nothing left to vary. However, the distribution of $\bar{d}$ depends on the numbers of subjects in the two groups. With more subjects the standard error decreases, so the curves become narrower and so for a fixed α the value of β decreases. The sample size calculation is a compromise between the power $(1-\beta)$ the effect size δ and the sample size n.

A key element in the design is the 'effect size' that it is reasonable to plan to observe – should it exist. Sometimes there is prior knowledge, which then enables an investigator to anticipate what effect size between groups is likely to be observed and the role of the study or trial is to confirm that expectation. In some situations, it may be possible to state that, for example, only a doubling of MEDIAN survival would be worthwhile to demonstrate in a planned trial. This might be because the new treatment, as compared to standard, is expected to be so toxic that only if substantial benefit could be shown would it ever be used. In such cases the investigator may have definite opinions about the difference that it is pertinent to detect.

In practice, a range of plausible effect size options are considered before the final effect size is agreed. For example, an investigator might specify a scientific or clinically useful difference that it is hoped could be detected and would then estimate the required sample size on this basis. The calculations might then indicate that an extremely large number of subjects is required. As a consequence, the investigator may next define a revised aim of detecting a rather larger difference than that originally specified. The calculations are repeated and perhaps the sample size now becomes realistic in that new context.

One additional problem when planning comparative clinical trials is that investigators are often optimistic about the magnitude of the improvement of new treatments over the standard. This optimism is understandable, since it can take considerable effort to initiate a trial and, in many cases, the trial would only be launched if the investigator is enthusiastic about the new treatment and is sufficiently convinced about its potential efficacy. However, experience suggests that as trials progress there is often a growing realism that, even at best, the initial expectations were optimistic. There is ample historical evidence to suggest that trials that set out to detect large treatment differences nearly always result in 'no significant difference was detected'. In such cases, there may have been a true and worthwhile treatment benefit that has been missed, since the level of detectable differences set by the design was unrealistically high and hence the sample size too small to establish the true (but less optimistic) size of benefit.

The way in which possible effect sizes are determined will depend on the specific situation under consideration. For example, if a study is repeating one already conducted then very detailed information may be available on the options for the effect size suitable for planning the new

study. Estimates of the anticipated effect size may be obtained from the available literature, formal META-ANALYSES of related studies or may be elicited from expert opinion. For clinical trials, in circumstances where there is little prior information available, Cohen (1988) has proposed a standardised effect size, Δ. In the case when the difference between two treatments 1 and 2 is expressed by the difference between their means $(\mu_1 - \mu_2)$ and σ is the standard deviation (SD) of the ENDPOINT variable, then $\Delta = (\mu_1 - \mu_2)/\sigma = \delta/\sigma$. A value of $\Delta \leq 0.2$ is considered a small standardised effect, $\Delta \approx 0.5$ as moderate and $\Delta \geq 1$ as large. Experience has suggested that, in many clinical areas, these can be taken as a good practical guide for design purposes.

In intermediate situations for clinical trials at least, Bayesian approaches to obtaining a distribution of effect size have been suggested by Spiegelhalter Freedman and Parmar (1994) (see BAYESIAN METHODS). These involve obtaining views on likely effect size from a survey of relevant experts and combining their responses into a PRIOR DISTRIBUTION of plausible effect sizes from their responses. Subsequently, this prior distribution is then combined with the data obtained from the trial once conducted to give a POSTERIOR DISTRIBUTION concerning the true effect size from which conclusions with regard to efficacy are then drawn. This approach has also been advocated by Tan *et al.* (2003) who suggest how information, from whatever source, may be synthesised into a prior distribution for the anticipated effect size that is then utilised for planning purposes.

Next, some theory and formulae are presented to show their derivation. In practice, one can refer in simple situations to a graphical approach that yields a suitably approximate sample size (see Altman's nomogram) (Altman, 1991). In a trial comparing two groups, with n subjects per group, if we assume that the outcome variable is continuous, $\bar{x}_1$ and $\bar{x}_2$ summarise the respective means of the observations taken. Further, if the data are normally distributed with equal (population) SDs, σ, then the standard errors (*SE*) are $SE(\bar{x}_1) = SE(\bar{x}_2) = \sigma/\sqrt{n}$. The two groups are compared using $\bar{d}_1 = \bar{x}_1 - \bar{x}_2$ with $SE(\bar{d}) = \sigma\sqrt{\dfrac{2}{n}}$.

Here we assume that $SE(\bar{d})$ is the same when the null hypothesis, H_0, of no difference is true and when the alternative hypothesis, H_A, that there is a difference of size δ_1 is true.

Under the null hypothesis, H_0, the critical value d_α is determined by:

$$\frac{d_\alpha - 0}{\sigma\sqrt{\dfrac{2}{n}}} = z_{1-\alpha}. \tag{1}$$

In contrast, under the assumption that the alternative hypothesis, H_1, is true, $\bar{d}$ now has mean δ_1 but the same $SE(\bar{d}) = \sigma\sqrt{\dfrac{2}{m}}$. In this, case the probability that $\bar{d}$ exceeds d_α must be $1 - \beta$ and this implies that:

$$\frac{d_\alpha - \delta}{\sigma\sqrt{\dfrac{2}{n}}} = -z_{1-\beta}. \tag{2}$$

303

Solving the two expressions (1) and (2) for d_α and re-arranging, we obtain the sample size for each group in the trial as:

$$n = 2\frac{\sigma^2}{\delta^2}(z_{1-\alpha} + z_{1-\beta})^2 = \frac{2(z_{1-\alpha} + z_{1-\beta})^2}{\Delta^2} \quad (3)$$

This is termed the *fundamental equation* as it arises, in one form or another, in many situations for which sample sizes are calculated.

The use of equation (3) for the case of a two-tailed test, rather than the one-tailed test, involves a slight approximation since $\bar{d}$ is also statistically significant if it is less than $-d_\alpha$. However, with $\bar{d}$ positive the associated probability of observing a result smaller than $-d_\alpha$ is negligible. Thus, for the case of a two-sided test, we simply replace $z_{1-\alpha}$ in equation (3) by $z_{1-\alpha/2}$.

For the commonly occurring situation of $\alpha = 0.05$ (two-sided) and $\beta = 0.2$ we find that equation (3) simplifies to:

$$n = \frac{16}{\Delta^2}. \quad (4)$$

This basic equation has to be modified to adapt to the specific experimental design, the allocation ratio (that is the possibility of the design stipulating unequal subject numbers in each group), the particular type of endpoint under consideration as well as for clinical trials the type of RANDOMISATION involved.

Viljanen *et al.* (2002) specified $\alpha = 0.05$, $\beta = 0.2$ and the anticipated effect size, $\delta = 1$ unit with standard deviation 2 units. From this, the standardised effect size is $\Delta = 0.5$ and from equation (4) we find $n = 64$ patients per group are required.

When dealing with binary outcome variables the sample size derivations for binary data are similar to that for continuous data but one has to specify two proportions π_1 and π_2 and the effect size is the difference $\delta = \pi_1 - \pi_2$. Campbell, Julious and Altman (1995) give tables for the sample sizes required for the comparison of two binomial proportions and this is shown in the Table below.

As an example of use of the table, we consider the trial by Viljanen *et al.* (2003). They showed that the proportion of people in their control group with neck pain who had been on sick leave over 12 months was 15%. Suppose we wished to design a trial that proposed to reduce this to 10%. Then from the Table below we would require 686 (say 700) people per group with 80% power at 5% significance.

sample size determination in clinical trials *Components necessary to estimate the size of a study*

Effect size, δ	Anticipated (planning) size of the difference between the two groups
Type I error, α	Equivalently, the test size or significance level of the statistical test to be used in the analysis
Type II error, β	Equivalently, the power, $1 - \beta$

The point to note here is that although this is a 33% reduction in the rate, it still requires a large trial. In general, the binary outcomes will often require large trials because they contain much less information than a continuous outcome. For example, suppose the body mass index (BMI) in a population was about 28 kg/m^2, with a standard deviation 2 kg/m^2. This means that about 16% of the group are defined as obese (BMI > 30 kg/m^2). Suppose a trial tried to reduce this absolute proportion by 5%, to about 11%. Then from the Table below we would need about 686 people to detect this with 5% significance and 80% power.

However, to obtain about 11% obese persons in the population we would have to reduce the mean BMI to 27.54. Thus the standardised effect size is 0.23 = (28 − 27.54)/2 and from equation (4) we would require about 300 patients per group for 80% power at 5% significance level or less than half the equivalent sample size required for the binary outcome. The moral of the story is to try and have continuous outcome variables if possible.

Commonly, the number of patients that can be included in a study is governed by non-scientific forces such as time, money and human resources. Thus with a predetermined sample size, the researcher may then wish to know the probability of detecting a certain effect size with a study confined to this size. If the resulting power is small, say less than 50%, then the investigator may decide that the study should not go ahead. A similar situation arises if the type of subject under consideration is uncommon as would be the case with a clinical trial in rare disease groups. In either case, the sample size is constrained and the researcher is interested in finding the size of effects that could be established for a reasonable power, say, 80%.

Thus the output from a sample size calculation should

sample size determination in clinical trials *Sample sizes to detect a difference in two proportions, π_1 and π_2, at a 5% significance level with 80% power*

π_1	π_2																			
	0.05	0.10	0.15	0.20	0.25	0.30	0.35	0.40	0.45	0.50	0.55	0.60	0.65	0.70	0.75	0.80	0.85	0.90	0.95	1.00
0.00	152	74	48	35	27	22	18	15	13	11	10	8	7	6	6	5	4	4	3	2
0.05		435	141	76	49	36	27	22	18	15	12	11	9	8	7	6	5	4	4	3
0.10			686	199	100	62	43	32	25	20	16	14	11	10	8	7	6	5	4	4
0.15				906	250	121	73	49	36	27	22	17	14	12	10	8	7	6	5	4
0.20					1094	294	138	82	54	39	29	23	18	15	12	10	8	7	6	5
0.25						1251	329	152	89	58	41	31	24	19	15	12	10	8	7	6
0.30							1377	356	163	93	61	42	31	24	19	15	12	10	8	6
0.35								1471	376	170	96	62	43	31	24	18	14	11	9	7
0.40									1534	388	173	97	62	42	31	23	17	14	11	8
0.45										1565	392	173	96	61	41	29	22	16	12	10

be a range of possible sample sizes against the effect sizes detectable with a number of levels of power.

In order to calculate the sample size of a study one must first have suitable background information together with some idea as to what is a realistic difference to seek. Sometimes such information is available as prior knowledge from the literature or other sources; at other times, a PILOT STUDY may be conducted.

Traditionally, a pilot study is a distinct preliminary investigation, conducted before embarking on the main trial. However, Wittes and Brittain (1990) have explored the use of an internal pilot study. The idea here is to plan the clinical trial on the basis of best available information, but to regard the first patients entered as the internal pilot. When data from these patients have been collected, the sample size can be re-estimated with the revised knowledge so generated.

Two vital features accompany this approach: first, the final sample size should only ever be adjusted *upwards*, never down; and, second, one should only use the internal pilot in order to improve the estimation factors that are independent of the treatment variable. This second point is crucial. It means that when comparing the means of two groups, it is valid to re-estimate the planning SD, σ_{Plan} but not δ_{Plan}. Both these points should be carefully observed to avoid distortion of the subsequent significance test and a possible misleading interpretation of the final study results.

The advantage of an internal pilot is that it can be relatively large – perhaps half of the anticipated patients. It provides an insurance against misjudgement regarding the baseline planning assumptions. It is, nevertheless, important that the intention to conduct an internal pilot study is recorded at the outset and that full details are given in the study protocol.

In studies involving a single group, sample size calculations are couched in terms of the CONFIDENCE INTERVAL. Thus for a given study endpoint, for example, the mean systolic blood pressure (SBP), the proportion hypotensive or the median duration of fever, calculated from the subjects in a case-series or a cross-sectional survey, it is usual also to quote the corresponding confidence interval (CI). Thus, when planning a case-series survey, it would be appropriate to define, ω, the width of the desired CI. This width will depend on the variability from subject to subject (which we cannot control) and the number of subjects in the case series. We assume the object of the study is to estimate a population mean μ, and this is thought to be close to μ_{Plan}. Further if the data can be assumed to follow a NORMAL DISTRIBUTION, then provided we choose a relatively large sample size n, the $100(1 - \alpha)\%$ CI for the population mean μ is likely to be close to:

$$\mu_{Plan} - z_{1-\alpha/2}\sqrt{\frac{\sigma^2}{n}} \quad \text{to} \quad \mu_{Plan} + z_{1-\alpha/2}\sqrt{\frac{\sigma^2}{n}} \quad (5)$$

Here σ is the standard deviation which summarises the subject-to-subject variation.

The width, ω, of this CI is obtained from the difference between the upper and lower limits of equation (5) as:

$$\omega = 2 \times z_{1-\alpha/2} \times \sqrt{\frac{\sigma^2}{n}} \quad (6)$$

Thus for a planning value ω, the number of subjects n required is obtained by reorganising equation (6) to give the required study size as:

$$n = 4\left[\frac{\sigma^2}{\omega^2}\right]z_{1-\alpha/2}^2 \quad (7)$$

In practice, to calculate n_{Plan}, a value of σ_{Plan} as well as ω_{Plan} or a value for their ratio has to be provided. The actual value of μ_{Plan} does not feature in this calculation. Once the study is completed, the sample mean $\bar{x}$ replaces μ_{Plan} and the sample standard deviation, s, replaces σ_{Plan} in the calculation of the CI of equation (5).

For example, Weir, Fiaschi and Machin (1998) give the mean latency of the auditory P300 measured in 19 right-handed patients with schizophrenia as 346 ms with SD = 27 ms. Using equation (5), the corresponding 95% CI is from 334 to 358 ms. The width of this CI is $\omega = 358 - 334 = 24$ ms.

If the study were to be repeated but in (say) left-handed patients how many would be required to obtain a narrower width of the CI set at 20 ms? In this case, $\omega_{Plan} = 20$ ms and assuming the same SD of 27 ms, and so equation (7) suggests $4 \times (27/20) \times (1.96)^2 = 28.1$ or approximately 30 patients.

Many clinical trials are designed to show that treatments are effectively equivalent, rather than different (see EQUIVALENCE STUDIES). In Phase II trials one might like to show that a generic drug is equivalent to a standard one in terms of its pharmacokinetics. This *bioequivalence* is often phrased in terms of the AREA UNDER CURVE of the serum levels of the drug after consumption. Since it is impossible to prove equivalence, one has to specify in advance a difference, δ, within which one is willing to concede that there is, in fact, no difference. For bioequivalence, the convention is to accept that two drugs are equivalent if their AUCs are within 20% of each other, or the ratio is between 0.8 and 1.25. Further details are given in Diletti *et al.* (1991).

Cohen (1988) is the classical reference for sample size calculations. The book by Machin *et al.* (1997) gives details of sample size calculations for a large number of other designs, such as studies with more than 2 groups, with ordinal or survival outcomes and for paired data and hints are given by Lenth (2001). Nowadays there is much software, both commercial and freely available on the web, for performing sample size calculations, see for example www.stat.uiowa.edu/~rlenth/Power/.   *MJC*

Altman, D.G. 1991: *Practical statistics for medical* research. London: Chapman & Hall/CRC. **Campbell, M.J., Julious, S.A. and Altman, D.G.** 1995: Sample sizes for binary, ordered categorical and continuous outcomes in two group comparisons. *British Medical Journal* 311, 1145–8. **Cohen, J.** 1988: *Statistical power analysis for the behavioral sciences*, 2nd edn. Mahwah: Lawrence Erlbaum. **Diletti, E., Hauschke, D. and Steinijans, V.W.** 1991: Sample size determination for bioequivalence assessment by means of confidence intervals. *International Journal Clinical Pharmacology, Therapy and Toxicology* 29, 1–8. **Lenth, R.V.** 2001: Some practical guidelines for effective sample size determination. *The American Statistician* 55, 187–93. **Machin, D., Campbell, M.J., Fayers, P.M. and Pinol, A.P.Y.** 1997: *Sample size tables for clinical studies*. Oxford: Blackwell Science. **Spiegelhalter, D.J., Freedman, L.S. and Parmar, M.K.B.** 1994: Bayesian approaches to randomized trials (with discussion). *Journal of the Royal Statistical Society Series A* 157, 357–416. **Tan, S.-B., Dear, K.B.G., Bruzzi, P. and Machin, D.** 2003: Towards a strategy for randomised clinical trials in rare cancers. *British Medical Journal* 327, 47–9. **Viljanen, M., Malmivaara, A., Uitte, J., Rinne, M., Palmroos, P. and Laippala, P.**

2003: Effectiveness of dynamic muscle training, relaxation training or ordinary activity for chronic neck pain: randomised controlled trial. *British Medical Journal* 327, 475–7. **Weir, N.H., Fiaschi, K. and Machin, D.** 1998: The distribution of latency of the auditory P300 in schizophrenia and depression. *Schizophrenia Research* 31, 151–8. **Wittes, J. and Brittain, E.** 1990: The role of internal pilot studies in increasing the efficiency of clinical trials. *Statistics in Medicine* 9, 65–72.

sample size determination in cluster randomised trials

When designing cluster randomised trials, the sample size should be carefully chosen, as when designing conventional CLINICAL TRIALS which randomise individual patients. The use of cluster randomisation must be taken into account at the design stage of the trial; the total number of patients required is larger under cluster randomisation than under individual randomisation, so a trial which randomises clusters without increasing the sample size will lack power. In a cluster randomised trial, the responses of patients from the same cluster cannot be assumed to be independent, because patients within a cluster are more similar than patients from different clusters.

Standard formulae for SAMPLE SIZE DETERMINATION assume the outcomes for patients in the planned study to be independent and this assumption is invalid in a cluster randomised trial. The size of a cluster trial has two components: the number of clusters recruited and the number of patients recruited from each cluster, which is referred to as the cluster size (not usually equal to the population size for each cluster, e.g. the number of patients in a hospital catchment area). To calculate how many patients are required in a cluster randomised trial, sample sizes given by standard formulae should be inflated by a factor known as the design effect. The design effect is equal to $[1 + (\bar{n} - 1)\rho]$, where $\bar{n}$ is the average cluster size and ρ is the INTRA-CLUSTER CORRELATION COEFFICIENT (ICC), which represents the anticipated extent of similarity within clusters. For a cluster trial employing paired or stratified randomisation rather than simple randomisation, more complicated formulae are needed to calculate the sample size (Donner and Klar, 2000).

Deciding to randomise clusters rather than individual patients can have a substantial impact on the sample size required. Consider, for example, designing a trial to detect a difference of 0.25 standard deviations in total cholesterol at a (two-sided) 5% significance level. If the trial were to randomise individual patients, a total of 504 patients would provide 80% power to detect this difference. If choosing to randomise general practices (for example), the sample size required to provide the same level of power depends heavily on the anticipated value for the ICC, as shown in the Table.

Even when the ICC is expected to be small, cluster randomised trials can require considerably increased numbers of patients in comparison with individually randomised trials, especially when cluster sizes are large. This demonstrates the flaw of an approach occasionally used in the past, in which researchers who anticipated a small ICC neglected to allow at all for the use of cluster randomisation in their design. The desired level of power for a cluster trial is more easily achieved through raising the planned number of clusters than through raising the planned average cluster size. In some settings, however, the number of clusters available for recruitment may be

sample size determination in cluster randomised trials
Sample sizes that provide 80% power to detect the specified difference in a cluster randomised trial, at different levels of ICC

Total sample size	Average cluster size	ICC
752	50	0.01
1004	100	0.01
998	50	0.02
1502	100	0.02
1740	50	0.05
2974	50	0.1

limited or fixed in advance because of administrative or financial constraints. The occurrence of DROPOUTS in clinical trials is always undesirable, but in a cluster randomised trial there is the possibility that entire clusters will drop out. Because loss of clusters can seriously reduce the power of a trial, every attempt must be made to retain all clusters recruited and some authors recommend identifying a reserve of potential substitutes before starting the trial (Donner and Klar, 2000).

The value assumed for the ICC when calculating the sample size for a cluster randomised trial is usually based on available estimates for ICC values in similar settings. For example, in designing the hypothetical trial discussed above, the ICC value ρ used in the formula for the design effect would ideally be based on ICC estimates representing similarity of total cholesterol measurements within general practices. In order that researchers planning trials have a good chance of locating relevant information on likely values for the ICC in their trial, it has been recommended that completed cluster trials publish the ICC estimates for all outcomes collected. In addition, some research groups are collating published and unpublished estimates into ICC databases such as Ukoumunne *et al.* (1999). Even when completely relevant information exists, available ICC estimates tend to be imprecise, that is the CONFIDENCE INTERVAL associated with the estimate tends to include a wide range of ICC values. The table demonstrates that if the ICC value in the future trial is higher than the value allowed for at the design stage, there could be a serious loss of trial power. For this reason, several researchers have recommended using a conservative value for the ICC or taking into account the uncertainty in the ICC estimates used (Feng and Grizzle, 1992; Turner *et al.*, 2004). Alternatively, an internal PILOT STUDY design could be used, in which the sample size is recalculated some way into the trial on the basis of the current ICC estimate (Lake *et al.*, 2002). *RT*

Donner, A. and Klar, N. 2000: *Design and analysis of cluster randomisation trials in health research.* London: Arnold. **Feng, Z. and Grizzle, J.E.** 1992: Correlated binomial variates: properties of estimator of intraclass correlation and its effect on sample size calculation. *Statistics in Medicine* 11, 1607–14. **Lake, S., Kammann, E., Klar, N. and Betensky, R.** 2002: Sample size re-estimation in cluster randomization trials. *Statistics in Medicine* 21, 1337–50. **Turner, R.M., Prevost, A.T. and Thompson, S.G.** 2004: Allowing for imprecision of the intracluster correlation coefficient in the design of cluster randomized trials. *Statistics in Medicine* 23, 1195–214. **Ukoumunne, O.C., Gulliford, M.C., Chinn, S., Sterne, J.A.C. and Burney, P.G.J.** 1999: Methods for evaluating area-wide and organisation-based interventions in health and health care: a systematic review. *Health Technology Assessment* 3, 5.

sample size determination in observational studies

Consideration of sample size is as important for OBSERVATIONAL STUDIES as it is for randomised controlled trials (see CLINICAL TRIALS), the crucial issue being whether the study will be large enough to answer the research question (or questions) with sufficient statistical precision or power. As with randomised controlled trials, the degree of statistical uncertainty decreases with increasing sample size and, in general, sample size requirements are substantially greater when studying rarer diseases or less common exposures. Observational studies that are too small may fail to detect important effects or produce estimates too imprecise to be useful, while those that are too large can waste resources and take too long to produce results. At the same time, it should be noted that study size guidelines are not intended as rigid rules. It may be, for example, that the research question is of sufficient importance to outweigh an inadequate, yet unavoidable, sample size (e.g. research into a rare cancer). Although a single study may be too small to provide definitive results, if well designed it will still have the potential to make an important contribution to existing evidence. In contrast, a poorly designed study will be at high risk of producing biased results. The problem of bias will not diminish by increasing the sample size.

Sample size requirements for observational studies should be critically assessed at the study design stage. Regardless of the type of study being planned, the first step involves identifying the primary health outcome of interest and the primary exposure. Sample size calculations should then be carried out for a range of different scenarios. Particular consideration here should be given to the extent of MISSING DATA to be expected. Individuals selected for interview in a CASE-CONTROL STUDY using hospital records, for example, may not all be traced and some of those successfully traced may refuse to take part. In COHORT STUDIES, individuals may be lost to follow-up, particularly when the study period extends over several years. Sample size calculations should be adjusted to take account of the likely effect of these possibilities. If there is more than one outcome measure or more than one exposure being studied, these should be ordered in terms of priority. Once the sample size required to achieve the needs for the primary research question has been determined, this can subsequently be used to examine its adequacy for additional research questions.

The specific type of outcome measure(s) to be studied is an important determinant of sample size requirements for observational studies. Outcome measures in CROSS-SECTIONAL STUDIES, for example, can range from binary proportion or PREVALENCE (e.g. obesity) to those that are continuous where interest may focus on means (e.g. mean systolic blood pressure). In general, sample size requirements will be much larger when the outcome measure is binary.

Sample size requirements can be addressed from two different perspectives: the statistical power to be achieved from a test of statistical significance or the level of precision to be attained from estimation. Standard formulae required when estimating a single prevalence rate or mean, or comparing prevalence (or means) in two groups, are provided elsewhere (Kirkwood and Sterne, 2002). Computer programs required to perform these calculations are also available (Statcorp, 2003).

For brevity, the remainder of this entry considers certain issues associated with sample size requirements for case-control studies and cohort studies only where interest focuses on a binary exposure. Consideration of more advanced issues for these studies, such as tests for trend or interaction, is addressed elsewhere (Breslow and Day, 1987; Smith and Day, 1984).

Sample size requirements in case-control studies depend on the expected magnitude of the odds ratio and the prevalence of exposure in the controls. In order to determine the study size required to achieve adequate statistical power, the number required in each group (cases and controls) can be determined from the formula used for comparing two proportions (Kirkwood and Sterne, 2003; Statcorp, 2003). In general, the closer the odds ratio to be detected is to the null value (1.0) the larger the sample size required, while the closer the prevalence is to 0.5 (or 50%) the smaller is the required sample size.

When the number of cases is fixed, as often occurs in very rare diseases, statistical precision (and power) can be improved by increasing the number of controls per case. The study size required to achieve a certain level of precision can be assessed by examining the width of 95% confidence intervals (95% CIs) for the *odds ratio*. The first Figure shows the effect of increasing the number of controls per case on precision where the expected odds ratio is 2.0, the prevalence of exposure in controls is 25% and the number of cases is fixed at 100. As may be seen, the precision of the estimate increases with the number of controls per case, but little gain is observed beyond 4 controls per case. In general, unless the odds ratio is substantially different from unity there is little advantage in having more than 4 controls per case (Breslow and Day, 1987).

One potential route for improving the efficiency of a case-control study can be achieved at the design stage by matching cases and controls in relation to one or more specific confounders. Matching cases and controls on the basis of strong confounding factors can increase the precision (and power) of a study and also offers the potential of a smaller study size requirement. However, it should be noted that matching does not always yield such gains. In particular, unless the confounding factor is strongly related to the disease there may be little benefit from matching (Smith and Day, 1984).

Unlike case-control studies, cohort studies provide the opportunity to estimate the absolute magnitude of disease

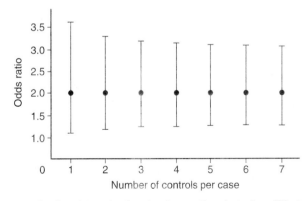

sample size determination in observational studies *Effect of increasing number of controls per case on 95% confidence intervals for odds ratio of 2.0 with 25% of controls exposed*

risks, rates or odds as well as the corresponding measures of effect (risk ratios, rate ratios or odds ratios). As a result, when considering the study size requirements in cohort studies it is particularly important to decide on the primary outcome measure in advance. When planning to compare disease occurrence in two groups (e.g. exposed and unexposed individuals) using a test of statistical significance, sample size requirements depend on: the magnitude of the ratio of (or difference in) disease outcomes to be detected; the level of disease occurrence expected in the unexposed group; the level of statistical significance; and the statistical power required. The required formulae for these calculations are provided elsewhere (Kirkwood and Sterne, 2003).

Alternatively, the level of statistical power can be determined for a variety of different study sizes. The second Figure shows power curves obtained for a cohort study where the rate in the unexposed is 10 per 1000 person-years at risk and the two-sided level of statistical significance is 5%. Two different scenarios are shown. The lower curve shows the power to detect a rate ratio of 1.5 and the upper curve a rate ratio of 2.0. If the true rate ratio is 2.0, and the aim is achieve a minimum of 90% power, this suggests that a study size of 3000 will be required in each group, i.e. a total study size of 6000. This could be achieved by studying 3000 individuals in each group for 1 year or 1500 in each group for 2 years and so on. Similar study sizes will only achieve 40% power, however, if the true rate ratio is only 1.5.

Sample size requirements for cohort studies can also be considered from the perspective of precision of estimates, as addressed in case-control studies above. Again, consideration should also be given to the need to adjust for confounding factors, as this will tend to increase study size requirements (Breslow and Day, 1987). Assessing the effect of exposure on disease experienced by a cohort of individuals exposed to a particular substance may involve comparing the events observed in the cohort with those expected on the basis of rates in a 'standard' population. Sample size requirements for this scenario are provided elsewhere (Breslow and Day, 1987).   *LC*

Breslow, N.E. and Day, N.E. 1987: *Statistical methods in cancer research*. Vol. II. The design and analysis of cohort studies. Lyon: International Agency for Research on Cancer. **Kirkwood, B.R.**

and Sterne, J.A.C. 2003: *Essential medical statistics*. Oxford: Blackwell. **Smith, P.G. and Day, N.E.** 1984: *The design of case-control studies: the influence of confounding and interaction effects*. International Journal of Epidemiology 13, 356–65. **Statcorp** 2003: *Statistical software: release 8*. Vol. 4 (Sampsi program). College Station, TX: Stata Corporation.

sampling distributions Probability distributions of statistics calculated from random samples of a particular size. When we draw a sample from a population, it is just one of the many samples we could take. If we calculate a statistic from the sample, such as a mean or proportion, this will vary from sample to sample. The means or proportions from all the possible samples form the sampling distribution. To illustrate this with a simple example, we could put lots numbered 1 to 9 into a hat and sample by drawing one out, replacing it, drawing another out, and so on. Each number would have the same chance of being chosen each time and the sampling distribution would be as (a) in the Figure on page 309. Now we change the procedure, draw out two lots at a time and calculate the average. There are 36 possible pairs, and some pairs will have the same average (e.g. 1 and 9, 4 and 6 both have average 5.0). The sampling distribution of this average is shown in (b) in the Figure. Notice that it has a different shape to (a). The sampling distribution of a statistic does not necessarily have the same shape as the distribution of the observations themselves, which we call the parent distribution.

If we know the sampling distribution it can help us draw conclusions about the population from the sample, using CONFIDENCE INTERVALS and significance tests. We often use our sample statistic as an estimate of the corresponding value in population, for example using the sample mean to estimate the population mean. The sampling distribution tells us how far from the population value the sample statistic is likely to be.

In most circumstances, we do not know what the sampling distribution is. However, we do not need to take many samples to estimate it. We can do this from a single sample only. Theory tells us what general family of distributions the sampling distribution will fall and we can estimate which member of this family the sampling distribution is. For example, if we follow a case series of 100 patients and find that 89 of them have a satisfactory outcome, we would expect the sampling distribution from which the statistic 89 comes to be a member of the binomial family. The particular member of that family is estimated to be the BINOMIAL DISTRIBUTION with parameters $n = 100$ and $p = 89/100 = 0.89$. For the mean of a large sample, we would expect a normal sampling distribution and we estimate the mean and variance of this NORMAL DISTRIBUTION from the mean and variance of the sample.

If the sample statistic is used as an estimate, we call the standard deviation of the sampling distribution the *standard error*. Rather confusingly, we use this term both for the unknown standard deviation of the sampling distribution and for the estimate of this standard deviation found from the data.   *JMB*

sampling methods – an overview Sampling is a way of choosing a subset of the population of interest, within which it is easier to study the properties that are of interest within the main population. The population is the group of people or items under investigation. The popula-

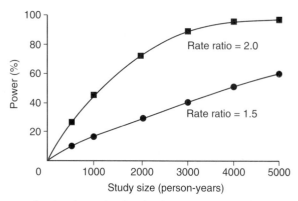

sample size determination in observational studies *Power to detect rate ratio in cohort studies with rate in unexposed = 10 per 1000, with 5% level of statistical significance (two-sided)*

(a) Single digit

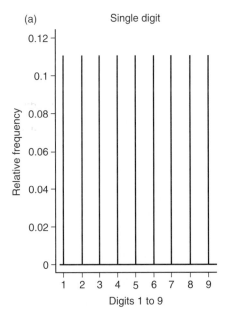

(b) Mean of two digits

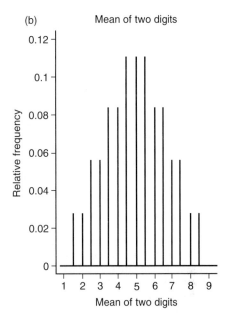

sampling distributions *Sampling distribution for a single digit drawn at random and for the mean of two digits drawn together*

tion may be small, large or infinite. The population is the entire set of units to which the results will be extrapolated. Once the precise purpose of a study has been defined then the target population should be decided. The aim of the process of data collection is to draw conclusions about this population. A sample from the population is the set of all units about which information is collected during the investigation.

The sampling units are the individual members that make up the population. It is important that the sampling units are clearly defined and care must be taken to choose the correct sampling unit to answer the question under consideration. A sampling frame is a list of all sampling units in the target population. It may not be possible, or indeed be too expensive or time consuming, to obtain a complete sampling frame for the population. It is important that if one is used it is as accurate and up to date as possible. It should be as free as possible from omissions and duplications. If MULTISTAGE CLUSTER SAMPLING is being used, then more than one sampling frame will be needed. In this case one sampling frame will be needed for each stage of sampling. The sampling units for the first stage of sampling are called the primary sampling units. Those for the final stage of sampling are called the listing units.

Information is collected using a survey; there are two different forms of survey: a census and a sample survey. A census is a survey that includes every member of a population. A census is often carried out if the population is small enough. In many countries, a population census is carried out every 10 years. When populations are large then a census may be very expensive and time consuming. If the population is very large it might not be possible to survey every member. In some circumstances it may not be sensible to carry out a census.

When a census is not possible or is too difficult then a sample survey can be used instead. This is where less than the entire population is included in the survey. If a repre-

sentative sample is taken then an accurate picture of the overall population can be obtained. Valid inferences can only be made from randomly selected sub-samples. BIAS contaminates the study if the samples are chosen non-randomly. SELECTION BIAS is the most common form of bias in samples.

The statistical objectives of an investigation are: to make inferences about a population by analysing sample data, to make assessments of the extent of uncertainty in these interferences and to design the process and extent of sampling to form a basis for valid and accurate inferences.

Samples can be chosen in two ways, by probability/random sampling or by non-probabilistic/non-random sampling. Random sampling is where the probability of getting any particular sample can be calculated from a probability model. Usually each unit has a known, possibly equal, probability of being chosen to be included in the sample. In non-probability sampling there is an uneven and unknown chance of being included in the sample. Non-probability sampling should only be used with caution when making inference to a general population. Non-probability sampling is often used, as it can be less expensive and time consuming than probabilistic sampling.

There are several examples of non-probabilistic sampling. CONVENIENCE SAMPLES are chosen for ease of access. They might be patients within a clinic or doctors that work in the same hospital. Snowball sampling is where the first respondent recommends a personal contact or a friend and so on until no new members of the sample are found. Purposive or judgement sampling is where the investigator decides who should be included in the sample; they are usually selected to be representative of the population. For example, to estimate the number of blood samples drawn in a year in a clinic, then a few typical days could be chosen and the records reviewed. The main problem with this sort of sampling is that there is no insight into the reliability of the estimates. If only a few days could be looked at then non-random sampling might include some atypical days that would make the estimate inaccurate. A case study is limited to one group or, in the case of N of 1, to one individual. In a QUOTA SAMPLE, the sample is chosen so that there are a certain number of units or individuals in each category. This is often used with convenience samples, the person carrying out the convenience sample maybe told to interview a certain number of, say, males under 25, usually with no instruction on how to select those to be included.

The simplest type of random sampling is the SIMPLE RANDOM SAMPLE this can be carried out in two ways, with or without replacement. Simple random sampling is equivalent to putting all the units in a hat and drawing one out. When the second selection is made there is a choice of replacing the first unit first or not. In the former case each item can be drawn more than once, this is sampling with replacement. In the latter case each unit can be chosen once at the most and this situation is sampling without replacement. Sampling without replacement is more precise than sample with replacement.

SYSTEMATIC SAMPLING is similar to simple random sampling with each unit having an equal and known probability of being chosen to be included in the sample. In systematic sampling a random starting point is chosen and then every kth unit is chosen to be included. It should be ensured that this does not hide a pattern in the data, for example if every $(k-1)$st element has a fault then it is possible that this could be hidden by choosing every kth element.

If there are obvious subgroups or 'strata' within the population then STRATIFIED SAMPLING may be more efficient than simple random sampling. In this case the population is separated into the strata and simple random samples taken in each of the strata. Each stratum is then represented proportionately in the sample. If the population forms distinct strata then stratified sampling may give more precise information than a simple random sample and therefore, maybe more efficient.

If the population is arranged in a hierarchical structure then multistage cluster sampling could be used. In a single stage cluster sample, a sample of the clusters is chosen at random and then a random sample of units is chosen from within this selection of clusters. In a multistage sample then a random sample of clusters are chosen, then a random sample of clusters within these clusters are chosen. This is repeated and eventually a random selection of units is chosen within a cluster.

If a probabilistic sample can be obtained, it is better to do this than a non-probabilistic sample, as a probabilistic sample should be less biased. A probabilistic sample is representative of the population and can therefore be extrapolated to the population from which it was drawn. This is not the case with a non-probabilistic sample. There is no way of knowing how representative a non-probabilistic sample is of the population.

The main sources of bias in sampling are, lack of a good sampling frame, the wrong choice of sampling unit, non-response by chosen units, those that are introduced by the person gathering the data and self-selection bias. It is important if a sampling frame is to be used that it is a good one and is up to date and free from duplications and omissions. If this is not the case, then the probability that each unit be included in the sample will not be equal, as some units will have a probability of 0 of being included in the sample, as they are not in the frame. If for example the telephone directory is used as the sampling frame then all those who are ex-directory or do not have a phone will not be included. The electoral register also misses people. Some units may have more than double the chance of another of being included in the sample, as they are included more than once in the sampling frame.

If the wrong sampling unit is used then the correct inferences might not be drawn from the results as a slightly different question might be being answered, for example if individuals are sampled instead of households, then the same event or experience might be referred to by two individuals and counted twice instead of once. Non-response by particular units maybe due to being unable to locate the particular unit chosen, the person may refuse to respond or the question maybe misunderstood. QUESTIONNAIRES should be worded clearly, be unambiguous and easy to understand; they should also be neutrally worded to avoid pointing towards a particular response. The interviewer can introduce bias by not interviewing people who look uncooperative or the way in which a question is asked may influence the answer given to the question. Self-selection bias is due to those volunteering to be selected to be in the sample being systematically different to those who have not volunteered. Self-selected samples are unlikely to be representative of the population.

The size of a sample to be taken is a very important consideration (see SAMPLE SIZE DETERMINATION). There are many formulae in existence to calculate the correct size for a sample. It is important to make sure that the sample is large enough to make the inferences required from the sample. However, being unbiased is more important than the size of the sample and any sample is only representative of the population from which it was drawn and only with caution should any extrapolations be made beyond that population.   *SLV*

Crawshaw, J. and Chambers, J. 1994: *A concise course in A level statistics*, 3rd edn. Cheltenham: Stanley Thornes Publishers Ltd.
Levy, P.S. and Lemeshow, S. 1999: *Sampling of populations: methods and applications*, 3rd edn. Chichester: John Wiley & Sons.

SAS   See STATISTICAL SOFTWARE

saturated model   See LOG-LINEAR MODELS

scatterplot   An xy plot of the values of two, usually continuous, variables that have been recorded on a sample of individuals. A typical example from medicine is shown in Figure (a) on page 311. Such a plot links the two variables, allows any relationship between them to be visually assessed and may help in identifying OUTLIERS or distinct groups of observations ('clusters'). In many cases, scatterplots can be made more useful by adding the estimated regression line of the two variables or a locally weighted regression fit (see SCATTERPLOT SMOOTHERS). Both possibilities are illustrated in Figure (b) on page 311.

Many other examples of interesting scatterplots are given in Tufte (1983).   *BSE*

[See also SCATTERPLOT MATRIX]

Tufte, E.R. 1983: *The visual display of quantitative information.* Cheshire, CT: Graphics Press.

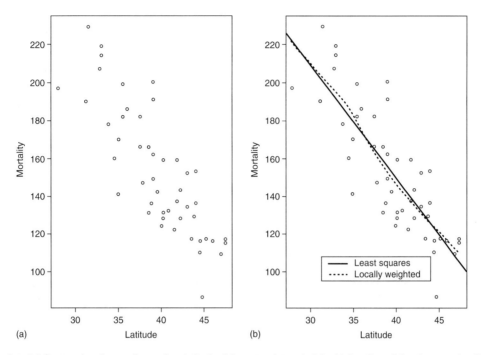

scatterplot *(a) Scatterplot of mortality against latitude, (b) scatterplot as in (a) with locally weighted regression fit added*

scatterplot matrices A convenient arrangement of pairwise SCATTERPLOTS of a set of variables that aids both in understanding the relationships between the variables and in uncovering any unusual features of the data, for example, possible OUTLIERS (Cleveland, 1994). In a scatterplot matrix the separate scatterplots are arranged in the form of a square grid with the same number of rows and columns as the number of variables. Each panel of the grid contains a scatterplot of one pair of variables. The upper left-hand triangle of the grid contains all pairs of scatterplots as does the lower right-hand triangle. The reason for including both the upper and lower triangles in the diagram, despite the seeming redundancy, is that it enables a row and columns to be visually scanned to see one variable against all others, with the scale for the one variable lined up along the horizontal or the vertical. Each panel of the basic scatterplot matrix can often be usefully enhanced with linear regression fits and/or other fitted curves for the pair of variables involved. An example of a basic scatterplot matrix for a set of data obtained in health survey of factory workers is shown in the first Figure on page 312.

The six variables in these data are as follows: HAEMO: haemoglobin concentration; PCV: packed cell volume; WBC: white blood cell count; LYMPHO: lymphocyte count; NEUTRO: neutrophil count; and LEAD: serum lead concentration.

It is often useful to enhance each panel in a scatterplot matrix with some fitted function of the relationship between the corresponding two variables: the second Figure, on page 313, shows the scatterplot in the first Figure, with the panels now showing the linear regression and locally weighted regression fits (see SCATTERPLOT SMOOTHERS). *BSE*

[See also TRELLIS GRAPHICS]

Cleveland, W.S. 1994: *Visualizing data.* Summit, NJ: Hobart Press.

scatterplot smoothers Smooth, generally nonparametric curves added to a SCATTERPLOT to aid in understanding the relationships between the two variables forming the plot. Often a useful alternative to the more familiar parametric curves such as simple linear or polynomial regression fits when the bivariate data plotted is too complex to be described by a simple parametric family.

The simplest scatterplot smoother is a locally weighted regression or *loess fit*, first suggested by Cleveland (1979). In essence, this approach assumes that the variables x and y are related by the equation:

$$y_i = g(x_i) + \varepsilon_i$$

where g is a 'smooth' function and the ε_i are random variables with mean zero and constant scale. Values $\hat{y}_i$ used to 'estimate' the y_i at each x_i, are found by fitting polynomials using weighted least squares with large weights for points near to x_i and small weights otherwise. So, smoothing takes place essentially by local averaging of the y-values of observations having predictor values close to a target value.

Two parameters control the shape of a loess curve: the first is a smoothing parameter, α, with larger values leading to smoother curves – typical values are ¼ to 1. The second parameter, λ, is the degree of certain polynomials that

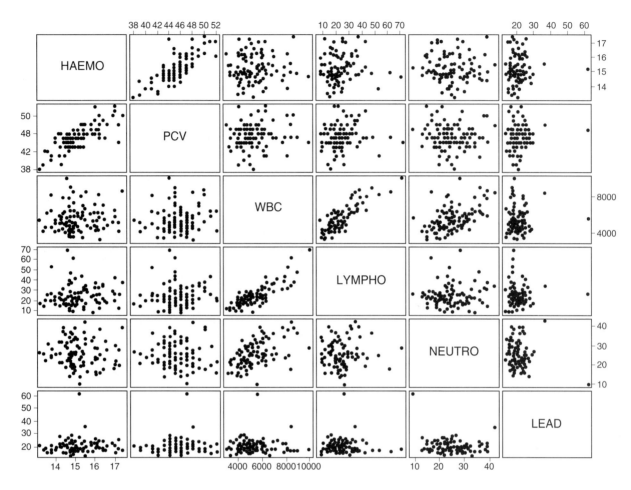

scatterplot matrices *Scatterplot matrix of six variables*

are fitted by the method; λ can take values 1 or 2. In any specific application, the choice of the two parameters must be based on a combination of judgement and of trial and error. Residual plots may however be helpful in judging a particular combination of values.

The use of locally weighted regression is demonstrated in the first Figure on page 314 for data collected on the oxygen uptake and the expired ventilation of a number of subjects performing a standard exercise task. In this Figure, (a), (b), (c) and (d) show plots of the data with added locally weighted regression fits with different values of λ and α. Here the four fitted curves are very similar and, in this relatively simple case, each of them is almost identical to a fitted polynomial containing a quadratic term in oxygen uptake – see (e) in the Figure.

An alternative smoother that can often usefully be applied to bivariate data is some form of *spline function*. (In its non-technical use, a spline is a term for a flexible strip of metal or rubber used by a draftsman to draw curves.) Spline functions are polynomials within intervals of the x variable that are connected across different values of x. The second Figure, on page 314, for example,

shows a linear spline function, i.e. a piecewise linear function, of the form:

$$f(x) = \beta_0 + \beta_1 X + \beta_2 (X - a)_+ + \beta_3 (X - b)_+ + \beta_4 (X - c)_+$$

where $(u)_+ = u \quad u > 0$
$\qquad\quad = 0 \quad u \le 0$.

The interval endpoints, a, b and c are called *knots*. The number of knots can vary according to the amount of data available for fitting the function.

The linear spline is simple and can approximate some relationships, but it is not smooth and so will not fit highly curved functions well. The problem is overcome by using piecewise polynomials, in particular cubics, which have been found to have nice properties with good ability to fit a variety of complex relationships. The result is a *cubic spline*, which arises formally by seeking a smooth curve $g(x)$ to summarise the dependence of y on x, which minimises the expression:

$$\sum [y_i - g(x_i)]^2 + \lambda \int g''(x)^2 dx \qquad (3)$$

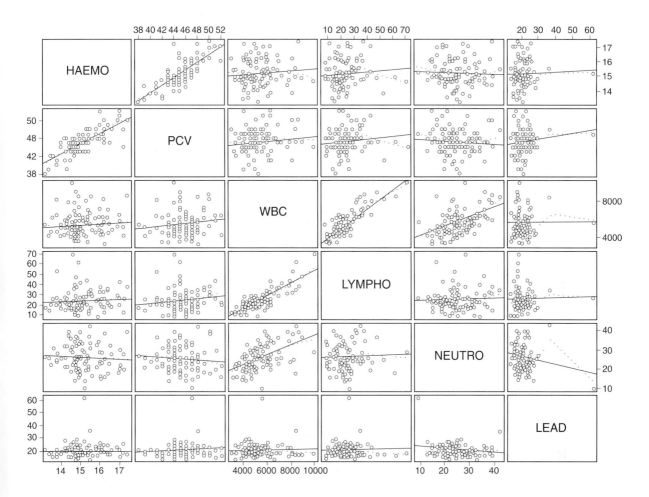

scatterplot matrices *Scatterplot matrix of six variables with individual panels showing linear regression (continuous line) and locally weighted regression fits (dotted line)*

where $g''(x)$ represents the second derivative of $g(x)$ with respect to x. Although when written formally this criterion looks a little formidable, it is really nothing more than an effort to govern the trade-off between the goodness-of-fit of the data (as measured by $\sum [y_i - g(x_i)]^2$) and the 'wiggliness' or departure of linearity of g as measured by $\int g''(x)^2 dx$; for a linear function, this latter part would be zero. The parameter λ governs the smoothness of g, with larger values resulting in a smoother curve. The solution is a cubic spline, that is a series of cubic polynomials joined at the unique observed values of the explanatory variable, x_i. (For more details, see Friedman, 1991.)

The 'effective number of parameters' (analogous to the number of parameters in a parametric fit) or degrees of freedom of a cubic spline smoother is generally used to specify its smoothness rather than λ directly. A numerical search is then used to determine the value of λ corresponding to the required degrees of freedom. The complexity of a cubic spline is approximately the same as a polynomial of degree one less than the DEGREES OF FREE-DOM. But the cubic spline smoother 'spreads out' its para-

meters in a more even way and hence is much more flexible than polynomial regression.

We shall illustrate the use of cubic splines by fitting such a curve to the monthly deaths from bronchitis, emphysema and asthma in the UK from 1974 to 1979 for men and women. A scatterplot of the data and the fitted cubic spline is shown in the third Figure, on page 315.

For these data, locally weighted regression is not so successful in representing the data. The fourth Figure, on page 315, shows a number of plots of the data with added locally weighted regression fits again with different values of λ and α. Here the characteristic cyclical nature of the data is only picked up with $\lambda = 2$ and $\alpha = 0.25$. In the other three diagrams the amount of smoothing is too great to reveal the structure in the data. *BSE*

Cleveland, W.S. 1979: Robust locally weighted regression and smoothing scatterplots. *Journal of the American Statistical Association* 74, 829–36. **Friedman, J.H.** 1991: Multiple adaptive regression splines. *Annals of Statistics* 19, 1–67. **Harrell, F.E.** 2001: *Regression modelling strategies with applications to linear models, logistic regression and survival analysis.* New York: Springer.

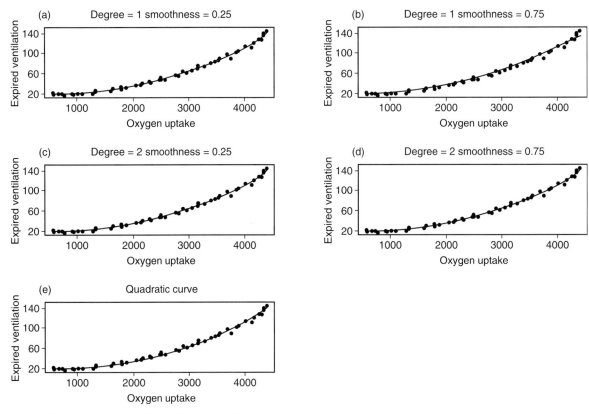

scatterplot smoothers *Locally weighted regression fits for oxygen uptake data*

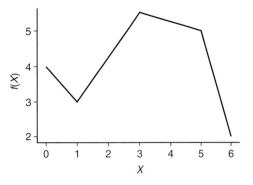

scatterplot smoothers *A linear spline function with knots at a=1, b=3, c=5.*

scree plot A SCATTERPLOT of the variances of the factors in a factor analysis or the components in a PRINCIPAL COMPONENT ANALYSIS against their ranks in terms of magnitude. The plot can be used to provide an informal estimate of the number of factors (components) by retaining as many factors (components) as there are variances that fall before the last large drop on the plot. An example of such a plot that suggests three factors is shown in the Figure, on page 316. Other examples are given in Preacher and MacCallum (2003). *BSE*

[See KAISER'S RULE]

Preacher, K.J. and MacCullum, R.C. 2003: Repairing Tom Swift's electric factor analysis machine. *Understanding Statistics* 2, 13–44.

screening studies Planned investigations to determine the effect of administering a diagnostic test to detect the presence or absence of preclinical disease in asymptomatic individuals (screening). The encounter is initiated by the health professional, rather than by the patient, since no clinical symptoms are apparent that otherwise would drive the patient to seek medical diagnosis. The goal of screening is to separate the population into two groups: those with a high versus low probability of the given disorder, usually one that is perceived to be a serious public health condition. Implicit to screening is the assumption of a clearly recognisable outcome that is indicative of preclinical disease and the assumption that early diagnosis is beneficial in some way, such as better prognosis, safer treatment, less invasive medical procedures, higher 'quality of life' or reduced chances of mortality. Examples of diagnostic tests used in screening are (1) mammography, to detect preclinical breast cancer disease in women; (2) a blood test to detect prostate specific antigen (PSA), as high levels in men are thought to be associated with preclinical disease of prostate cancer; (3) blood pressure and cholesterol levels, as high levels of both are associated with

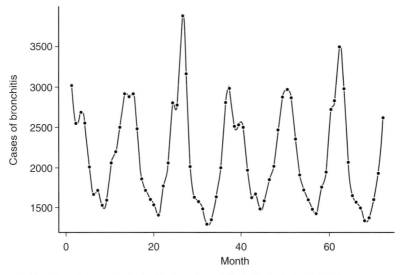

scatterplot smoothers *Cubic spline fit for monthly deaths from bronchitis in the UK, 1974–1979*

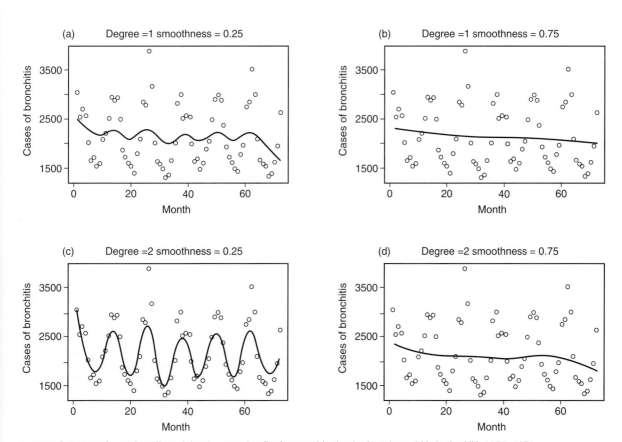

scatterplot smoothers *Locally weighted regression fits for monthly deaths from bronchitis in the UK, 1974–1979*

cardiac disease. Screening tests are not without costs (cost of examination; costs of false positive results arising from follow-up laboratory procedures; costs of false negative results arising from false hope of disease-free status).

Screening studies are designed to quantify: the nature of the 'benefit' (e.g. reduction in mortality, extended survival time, measures of quality of life); the target population that is expected to benefit from screening (in terms of age/gender/ethnic groups); and the error rates (false positives and false negatives). The FALSE POSITIVE RATE is the

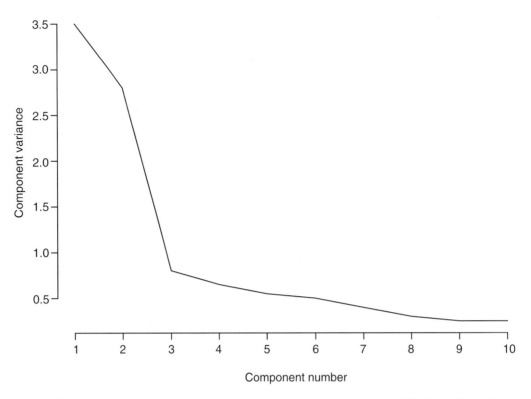

scree plot *A scree plot for a principal component analysis of a correlation matrix of 10 observed variables*

probability that the test asserts 'disease' when, in fact, no disease is present (conversely, SPECIFICITY, or the probability of obtaining a negative result when disease is absent); the FALSE NEGATIVE RATE is the probability that the test asserts 'no disease' when in fact disease is present (conversely, SENSITIVITY, or the probability of obtaining a positive result when disease is present). For diagnostic purposes, sensitivity should be high, while, for screening purposes, specificity should be high, to avoid unnecessary follow-up testing of disease-free individuals. Screening tests are indicated when the benefits are judged to outweigh the potential drawbacks (costs, risks of false positives and false negatives etc.).

Because non-randomised trials are subject to self-selection bias, randomised screening trials offer the best and most reliable mechanism for evaluating the potential benefit from screening. In randomised screening trials, study arm participants are offered screening at regular intervals and the control arm participants follow their 'usual medical care'. Due to the cost of screening, such trials are usually conducted using a 'stop-screen design,' in which screening is offered for a limited time only (e.g. annual screens for 3 to 5 years).

Several important differences between screening studies, used to evaluate the potential benefit of a screening intervention, and CLINICAL TRIALS, for the evaluation of a specific therapeutic intervention, make the design and analysis of screening studies very challenging. In clinical treatment trials, the cases are specified in the protocol to

be comparable in both the study and control arms of the trial; in screening trials, participants are initially asymptomatic and are randomised to the study ('offered screening') or control ('follow usual medical care') arms of the trial and cases evolve as the study progresses. If the screening test is successful, then cases will arise sooner in the study arm than in the control arm, so survival times (time of endpoint minus time of diagnosis) will be longer in the study arm than in the control arm, even in the absence of a screening benefit. This bias in the evaluation of screening is known as 'lead time bias'. Also, because cases with longer preclinical disease durations are more likely to be detected by screening than cases with shorter preclinical durations, the cases that arise in the study arm of a screening trial are more likely to be less aggressive and hence have more favourable prognosis, even in the absence of a screening benefit. This phenomenon is known as LENGTH-BIASED SAMPLING. Study arm participants also experience 'over-diagnosis bias or the tendency of the screening test to suggest apparent but truly non-threatening disease. (In an ideal world, this bias would not affect the results, if further diagnostic tests later eliminate these individuals as cases of disease.) Finally, non-compliance in both arms is inevitable: some participants in the study arm may refuse screening, while some in the control arm may seek screening. Thus, the cases that arise in the two arms of a screening trial may not be comparable as they are in a treatment trial. Randomisation ensures that the participant characteristics are the same in both arms, including those that lead to non-compliance of either type in either arm, arguing for an intention-to-treat analysis (Byar, Simon *et al.*, 1976).

The most common measures used to evaluate screening are *reduction in mortality* (comparison of death rates) and *mean benefit time* (difference in the mean survival time between time of entry into the trial and case endpoint). Randomisation ensures that (1) the participant characteristics are the same in the two trial arms, including those that lead to non-compliance of either type in either arm and (2) the elimination of bias due to lead time, when survival is measured from time of entry into trial.

Statistical methods to estimate the benefit (reduction in mortality, or extended survival time), lead time, and the effect of length-biased sampling, have been proposed. For overviews of the issues related to screening and for statistical methodology of design and analysis of screening studies, see Connor and Prorok (1994), Shapiro *et al.* (1988), Prorok and Connor (1986), Baker, Kramer and Prorok (2002), Goldberg and Wittes (1981), Gastwirth (1987), Kafadar and Prorok (1994; 1996; 2003; 2004), Prorok, Connor and Baker (1990), Zelen (1976) and Zelen and Feinleib (1969).

Screening studies are also used to evaluate the outcomes of designed trials to screen drug compounds for their potential to be biologically active. A typical drug screening protocol may involve several stages based on the response of the compound to various reactions: e.g. 'Conduct experiment 1; if the energy from the reaction is less than a specified level, reject the compound; otherwise, conduct experiment 2; if the second reaction is less than a second specified level, reject; otherwise, submit the compound for further testing.' The evaluation of such drug-screening designs involve the same sorts of consideration as the evaluation of randomised screening trials used on human subjects described earlier. See Roseberry and Gehan (1964) and Schultz *et al.* (1973) for designs and analysis of drug-screening trials, as well as related articles in the literature on screening designs to detect unacceptable products in manufacturing.   *KKa*

Baker, S.G., Kramer, B.S. and Prorok, P.C. 2002: Statistical issues in randomised trials of cancer screening. *British Medical Council Medical Research Methodology* 2, 11 (www.biomedcentral.com/1471-2288/2/11). **Byar, D.P., Simon, R.M., Friedewald, W.T. et al.** 1976: Randomized clinical trials: Perspectives on some recent ideas. *New England Journal of Medicine* 295, 74–80. **Connor, R.J. and Prorok, P.C.** 1994: Issues in the mortality analyses of randomized controlled trials of cancer screening. *Controlled Clinical Trials* 15, 81–99. **Gastwirth, J.L.** 1987: The statistical precision of medical screening procedures. *Statistical Science* 2, 213–38. **Goldberg, J.D. and Wittes, J.T.** 1981: The evaluation of medical screening procedures. *The American Statistician* 35, 4–11. **Kafadar, K. and Prorok, P.C.** 1994: A data-analytic approach for estimating lead time and screening benefit based on survival curves in randomised trials. *Statistics in Medicine* 13, 569–86. **Kafadar, K. and Prorok, P.C.** 1996: Computer simulation experiments of randomized screening trials. *Computational Statistics and Data Analysis* 23, 263–91. **Kafadar, K. and Prorok, P.C.** 2003: Alternative definitions of comparable case groups and estimates of lead time and benefit time in randomized cancer screening trials. *Statistics in Medicine* 21, 83–111. **Kafadar, K. and Prorok, P.C.** 2004: Computational methods in medical decision making: to screen or not to screen? *Statistics in Medicine* (forthcoming). **Prorok, P.C. and Connor, R.J.** 1986: Screening for the early detection of cancer. *Cancer Investigations* 4, 225–38. **Prorok, P.C., Connor, R.J. and Baker, S.G.** 1990: Statistical considerations in cancer screening programs. *Urologic Clinics of North America* 17, 699–708. **Roseberry, T.D. and Gehan, E.A.** 1964: *Biometrics* 20, 73–84. **Schultz, J.R., Nichol, F.R., Elfring, G.L. and Weed, S.D.** 1973: Multiple-stage procedures for drug screening. *Biometrics* 29, 293–300. **Shapiro, S., Venet, W., Strax, P. and Venet, L.** 1988: *Periodic screening for breast cancer: the health insurance plan project and its sequelae, 1963–1986.* Baltimore: Johns Hopkins University Press. **Zelen, M.** 1976: Theory of early detection of breast cancer in the general population. In Heuson, J.C., Mattheiem, W.H. and Rozenweig, M. (eds), *Breast cancer: trends in research and treatment.* New York: Raven Press, 287–301. **Zelen, M. and Feinleib, M.** 1969: On the theory of screening for chronic diseases. *Biometrika* 56, 601–13.

secondary endpoints   See ENDPOINTS

segregation analysis   The observation of characteristic segregation ratios among the offspring of particular parental crosses was first made by Austrian monk Gregor Mendel in his experiments on the garden pea. These observations enabled him to formulate the theory of genetic transmission.

Mendel studied discrete traits (called PHENOTYPES) in the garden pea (e.g. smooth versus wrinkled seed) and, after many generations of inbreeding, obtained pure lines for each trait. When two pure lines are crossed, all the offspring (called the *F1 generation*) were of the same phenotype (e.g. all smooth). The trait that is uniformly present in the F1 generation is said to be *dominant*, while the absent alternative is said to be *recessive*. When F1 individuals are crossed with the recessive pure line (a 'back-cross'), half the offspring had the dominant phenotype and the other half the recessive phenotype. When two F1 individuals were crossed (an 'inter-cross'), three-quarters of the offspring had the dominant phenotype and one-quarter has the recessive phenotype. These characteristic 1:1 and 3:1 ratios are called *segregation ratios*.

Segregation ratios are explained by the fact that each individual receives a complete set of genes from both parents, so that each gene is present in duplicate. When there are different forms of the same gene, each form (or *allele*) may correspond to a different phenotype, but when an individual has two different alleles (i.e. is *heterozygous*), the phenotype of one of the allele (the recessive allele) is completely masked by the phenotype of the other allele (the dominant allele). Thus the F1 generation from two pure (i.e. *homozygous*) lines will be all heterozygous and therefore display the dominant phenotype. A back-cross will result in half the offspring having the heterozygous genotype and the other half having the homozygous recessive genotype. An inter-cross will result in half the offspring being heterozygote, one-quarter being homozygous dominant and one-quarter homozygous recessive.

Classical segregation analysis is the examination of the offspring of different mating types to see if Mendelian segregation ratios are present. When such ratios are observed, the inference that the phenotype in question is determined by a single underlying genetic locus can be made. Complex segregation analysis is a further development of this method for traits in which Mendelian segregation ratios may be masked by complexities such as the involvement of background genetic or environmental factors in addition to a locus of major effect. *PS*

[See also ALLELIC ASSOCIATION, GENETIC EPIDEMIOLOGY, GENETIC LINKAGE, GENOTYPE]

selection bias Selection bias occurs when there are systematic differences between those who are selected for study and those who are not selected, so that the selected sample is not representative of the target population. For example, in a survey of the smoking habits of 14 year olds, a convenient sampling frame would be children attending schools in a defined geographical area. However, not all 14 year olds will be included in this sampling frame and if the reasons for exclusion are associated with smoking habit a biased estimate of the prevalence of smoking will be obtained. Another area where the choice of sampling frame might lead to BIAS is in telephone sampling, where households without telephones would be systematically excluded.

Even when an appropriate sampling frame is used for a survey, non-random sampling can lead to biased estimates. For example, in a study of overcrowding, an appropriate sampling frame might be all households in an electoral ward or postcode sector, listed in order of postal address. However, a systematic sample of every eighth household might over-represent certain types of accommodation, such as flats on a particular floor (e.g. ground floor or top floor) in tenement blocks of eight. If the average number of people per household differs systematically between floors, this is likely to lead to a biased estimate of overcrowding. Ideally, probability sampling methods should be used to avoid selection bias in surveys (see SAMPLING METHODS – AN OVERVIEW).

One type of study that is almost never carried out on a random sample of the target population is a randomised CLINICAL TRIAL. Trials rely on random allocation to treatment groups for their internal validity but, because of tight eligibility criteria for patient selection, those in the trial may not be representative of all patients with the condition being treated.

Epidemiological studies, especially CASE-CONTROL STUDIES, are susceptible to selection bias. In case-control studies it can be extremely difficult to obtain a control group that is representative of all non-cases in the same target population that the cases arise from. This can result in biased estimates of the odds ratio in either direction, depending on the form of selection bias. These issues are discussed in detail in Sackett (1979) and Ellenberg (1994). Even in carefully designed observational studies it can be difficult or impossible to rule out selection bias as a possible explanation for an observed association (Boydell, van Os *et al.*, 2001, and resulting correspondence). *WHG*

Boydell, J., van Os, J., McKenzie, K. *et al.* 2001: Incidence of schizophrenia in ethnic minorities in London: ecological study into interactions with environment. *British Medical Journal* 323, 1336–8. **Ellenberg, J.H.** 1994: Selection bias in observational and experimental studies. *Statistics in Medicine* 13, 557–67. **Sackett, D.L.** 1979: Bias in analytic research. *Journal of Chronic Diseases* 32, 51–63.

sensitivity A measure of how well an alternative test performs when it is compared with the reference or 'gold' standard test for the diagnosis of a condition.

Sensitivity is the proportion of patients who are correctly identified by the test as having the condition out of all patients who have the condition. Sensitivity may also be expressed as a percentage and is the counterpart to SPECIFICITY.

The reference standard may be the best available diagnostic test or may be a combination of diagnostic methods, including following up patients until all with the disease have presented with clinical symptoms. For example, in a study of mammography, the reference standard for breast cancer would include all women who went on to develop breast cancer, whether they were first diagnosed radiologically, histologically or symptomatically. Thus, the best design when a diagnostic test is evaluated against a reference standard is a COHORT STUDY with complete follow-up.

When the data are set out as in the Table,

$$sensitivity = \frac{a}{a + c}.$$

sensitivity *General table of test results among a + b + c + d individuals sampled*

		Disease		
		Present	Absent	Total
Test	Positive	a	b	$a + b$
	Negative	c	d	$c + d$
	Total	$a + c$	$b + d$	$a + b + c + d$

Sensitivity should be presented with CONFIDENCE INTERVALS, typically set at 95%, calculated using an appropriate method such as that of Wilson (described in Altman *et al.*, 2000) that will produce asymmetric confidence intervals without impossible values, i.e. that will not give values for the upper confidence interval >1 when sensitivity approaches 1 and the sample size is small.

Where a test result is a continuous measurement, for example, liver enzymes in serum, a cut-off point for abnormal values is chosen. If a lower value is chosen, then sensitivity will be relatively high, but specificity relatively low.

The impact of all possible cut-off points can be displayed graphically in a RECEIVER OPERATING CHARACTERISTIC (ROC) CURVE by plotting sensitivity at each cut-off point on the y axis against $1 -$ specificity at each cut-off point on the x axis. The choice of cut-off point is not, however, solely a statistical decision, as the balance between the FALSE POSITIVE RATE and the FALSE NEGATIVE RATE should be related to the clinical context and consequences of wrong diagnosis for the patient and healthcare system.

A sample size calculation for sensitivity can be made by specifying a confidence interval (for example, 95%) and an acceptable width for the lower bound of the confidence interval. Where the anticipated sensitivity is high and the sample size small, a 'small sample' method should be used: a sample size table can be found in Machin *et al.* (1997). *CLC*

[See also LIKELIHOOD RATIO, NEGATIVE PREDICTIVE VALUE, POSITIVE PREDICTIVE VALUE, TRUE POSITIVE RATE]

Altman, D.G., Machin, D., Bryant, T.N. and Gardner, M.J. 2000: *Statistics with confidence*, 2nd edn. London: BMJ

Books. **Machin, D., Campbell, M., Fayers, P. and Pinol, A.** 1997: *Sample size tables for clinical studies*, 2nd edn. Oxford: Blackwell Sciences Ltd.

sequential analysis A method allowing hypothesis tests to be conducted on a number of occasions as the data accumulate through the course of a CLINICAL TRIAL. A trial monitored in this way is usually called a sequential trial. This approach is in contrast to the use of a standard fixed sample size trial design, in which a single hypothesis test is conducted at the end of a trial, usually when some specified sample size has been attained, with no allowance to collect further data and repeat the test. Sequential analysis methods are attractive in clinical trials since, for ethical reasons, it is often important to analyse the data as they accumulate and to stop the study as soon as the presence or absence of a treatment effect is indicated sufficiently clearly. Although the total sample size for a sequential trial is not fixed in advance – it depends on the observed data – an additional advantage of sequential methodology is that trials may be constructed so that the expected sample size is smaller than that for a fixed sample size trial with the same Type I error rate and power.

Suppose that in a clinical trial we wish to compare two groups of patients, with one receiving the experimental treatment and the other the control treatment. Formally, we define some measure of the treatment difference between the experimental and control groups, which we will denote by θ. This treatment difference may, for example, be measured by the difference between the mean response for a normally distributed ENDPOINT, the log-odds ratio for a binary endpoint, or the log-hazard ratio for a survival time endpoint. We generally wish to test the null hypothesis that there is no difference between the treatment groups, that is that $\theta = 0$.

In a standard fixed sample size test, some test statistic is obtained and compared with a critical value. The critical value is chosen so as to give a specified Type I error rate; that is to ensure that the risk of concluding that there is a treatment difference when, in fact, the treatments are identical is controlled, usually to be no more than 5%. If this standard hypothesis test is repeated at a number of INTERIM ANALYSES, there are a number of opportunities to conclude that the treatments are different. The risk of doing so on at least one occasion therefore increases above 5%, so that the overall Type I error rate thus exceeds 5% and a valid test is no longer provided. This problem is addressed by sequential analysis, in which the repeated hypothesis tests are conducted in such a way as to maintain an overall Type I error rate for the sequential trial as a whole.

Although sequential monitoring methods have been proposed based on a range of possible test statistics (see, for example Jennison and Turnbull, 2000, for a discussion of possible methods) a general sequential approach is based on the use of the efficient score statistic (see Whitehead, 1997), as a measure of the treatment difference. Large positive values correspond to an indication of superiority of the experimental treatment, large negative values to an indication of superiority of the control treatment while values close to zero indicate little difference between the treatments. The exact form of the score statistic depends on the type of data used and the way in which the treatment difference is measured. As an example, for binary data, with the treatment difference measured by the log-odds ratio, if equal numbers of patients have received the experimental and control treatments, the score statistic is half of the difference in observed numbers of successes on the experimental and control arms. For survival data, with the treatment difference measured by the log-hazard ratio, the score statistic is the log-rank statistic (see SURVIVAL ANALYSIS).

In a sequential trial, a number of interim analyses are conducted. The value of the score statistic is calculated at each interim analysis together with the observed Fisher's information, a quantity related to the sample size summarising the amount of information available. If, at any interim analysis, the value of the score statistic is sufficiently large, the trial is stopped and it is concluded that the experimental treatment is superior to the control treatment. If the score statistic is too small, the trial is stopped and, depending on the way in which the test is constructed, it may either be concluded that the experimental treatment is inferior to the control or that there is insufficient evidence to distinguish between the two treatments. If neither criterion is met, that is for intermediate values of the score statistics, the trial continues to the next interim analysis. Graphically, the observed values of the score statistic may be plotted against the values of the information. As the information available increases throughout the trial the plotted points form what is called a *sample path*. At each interim analysis, the sample path is compared with upper and lower critical values, with the trial stopped as soon as the score statistic lies either above the upper critical value or below the lower critical value. The critical values, which, in general take different values at the different interim analyses, thus define a continuation region. As already explained, the problem of sequential analysis is the calculation of the critical values so as to give a specified Type I error rate, for example of 5%.

As the choice of critical values to achieve this aim is not unique, problems of appropriate choices for use in a sequential clinical trial setting are also of interest. In particular, in contrast to fixed sample size hypothesis tests, asymmetric sequential methods are possible. A fixed sample size test that is designed to have specified power, say 90%, to detect a treatment effect of given size, say $\theta = \theta_1$, has equal power to detect the opposite treatment effect of the same magnitude, that is $\theta = -\theta_1$. A sequential test may be constructed to have power 0.9 to detect $\theta = \theta_1$, but lower power to detect $\theta = -\theta_1$. Such a sequential test may have smaller expected sample size when $\theta = -\theta_1$ than when $\theta = \theta_1$. This is sometimes desirable in clinical trials, when it is advantageous to stop a trial as soon as possible if the experimental treatment appears to be inferior to the control and there is no desire to continue recruiting patients to test whether or not this inferiority is statistically significant.

The method based on the score statistic is a very flexible one, since, as shown by Scharfstein, Tsiatis and Robins (1997), for a wide range of problems, conditional on the observed information values, the score statistics at the interim analyses are approximately normally distributed. This means that critical values can be obtained based on this normality to provide sequential tests that can be used for many different types of data and choices of measure for the treatment difference. Two distinct approaches to the calculation of the critical values with which the efficient score statistics are compared have been developed. The first, which is sometimes called the *boundaries approach*, is based on modelling a continuous sample path. The second uses the assumed normality of the score statistics directly, evaluating the critical values via a recursive numerical integration technique, with the form of the sequential test often specified by what is called a *spending function*. The two approaches are described in detail later. A more general approach, the adaptive design method, which is not based on the asymptotic normality of the score statistics, is also briefly described. After a brief example, the problem of analysis at the end of a sequential trial is then discussed. We then continue with a description of the related area of response-driven designs and end with some comments on the role of a DATA AND SAFETY MONITORING COMMITTEE in a sequential clinical trial.

In the boundaries approach, the approximate normal distribution of the score statistics evaluated at the interim analyses means that the observed values can be considered as points on a Brownian motion with drift equal to the treatment difference, observed at times given by the observed information. This has led to the consideration of the abstract concept of continuous monitoring, in which the value of the test statistic is taken to be observed at all times rather than at the discrete times given by the interim analyses. The plotted sample path thus forms a continuous line, which is compared with continuous boundaries, that may be expressed as functions of the information level. Many of the theoretical developments in sequential analysis have been based on consideration of this problem. A consequence of this formulation is that, since the sample path is considered to be continuous, the trial stops exactly on a boundary, whereas for a discretely monitored trial, there is some overshoot of the critical value when the trial stops.

The boundaries approach stems from the work of Wald (1947) who developed the sequential probability ratio test (SPRT) for the testing of armaments during the Second World War. In Wald's SPRT after each observation, the likelihood ratio for the simple alternative hypothesis relative to the null hypothesis is calculated and the test continues so long as this likelihood ratio falls within some fixed range, equivalent to the plotted values of the score statistic lying between two parallel straight boundaries. Wald derived stopping limits so as to give a test with specified Type I error rate and power under the assumption of continuous monitoring. Among all tests with the same properties, the SPRT minimises the expected sample size when either the null or alternative hypothesis holds. However, the parallel boundaries give a test that, although it terminates with probability 1, has no finite maximum sample size. This feature makes it unsuitable for many clinical trials.

Following the work of Wald, a number of alternative forms for boundaries that maintain the overall Type I error rate have been proposed. Whitehead (1997) describes a wide range of such tests. One form that is particularly commonly used in sequential clinical trials is the *triangular test*. This test has straight boundaries that form a triangular-shaped continuation region. The test approximately minimises the maximum expected sample size among all tests with the same error rates and has a high probability of stopping with a sample size below that of the equivalent fixed sample size test.

The critical values obtained using the boundaries approach maintain the overall Type I error rate for a continuously monitored test. In practice, monitoring is necessarily discrete, since even if an interim analysis is conducted after observation of each patient, the information will increase in small steps. This means that if the critical values from the boundaries approach are used, the Type I error rate will be less than the planned level of, for example, 5%. Whitehead (1997) has proposed a correction to modify the continuous boundaries to allow for the discretely monitored sample path. This correction brings in the critical values by an amount equal to the expected overshoot of the discrete sample path. The correction is particularly accurate for the triangular test.

In general, specialist software is needed for the construction of critical values using the boundaries approach. A commercially available software package, Planning and Evaluation of Sequential Trials (PEST), has been developed by the Medical and Pharmaceutical Statistics Research Unit at the University of Reading for the calculation of the boundaries.

An alternative approach was a recursive numerical integration method for calculation of the overall Type I error rate for a sequential trial with specified critical values under the assumption that the score statistics observed at the interim analyses are normally distributed (Armitage, McPherson and Rowe, 1969). As well as demonstrating the effect of conducting interim analyses without adjusting for the multiple testing, this method allows the construction of critical values to maintain an overall Type I error rate of, say, 5%. Using this approach, Pocock (1977) and O'Brien and Fleming (1979) calculated critical values for sequential tests that preserve the overall Type I error rate to be 5% when, for O'Brien and Fleming's design, the critical values with which the score statistics are compared are the same at each interim analysis, and, for Pocock's design, the critical values correspond to the same *P-VALUE* for a conventional analysis performed at each interim analysis. The critical values obtained were tabulated to allow easy implementation without the need for additional computation. Although these methods, particularly that proposed by O'Brien and Fleming, remain in use, they are not always the most appropriate designs in the clinical trial setting. Pocock's design has been criticised because it has a relatively high chance of leading to rejection of the null hypothesis very early in the trial. O'Brien and Fleming's design, in contrast, is unlikely to stop early in the trial unless there is very strong evidence of a treatment difference. If the two treatments are very similar, both designs are likely to lead to a trial requiring more patients than the equivalent fixed sample size trial.

A more flexible design approach is provided by the spending function method proposed by Lan and DeMets (1983). In this approach, the total overall Type I error rate of, say, 5%, is considered to be spent through the course of the trial, with the rate at which it is spent controlled by the specified spending function. Not only does this introduce flexibility in the choice of the shape of the stopping boundaries, it also, in contrast to the tests of Pocock and O'Brien and Fleming, allows construction of a test that maintains the Type I error rate if interim analyses are not taken at the planned times. Many forms can be used for the spending function, but families of functions to give tests with certain properties have been proposed. A thorough review of the approach is given by Jennison and Turnbull (2000). As with the boundaries approach, specialist software is required to calculate the critical values. The software package EaSt produced by Cytel Software Corporation, and the S-PLUS module SeqTrial produced by MathSoft perform the necessary calculations.

An alternative to the sequential design approaches based on the assumption of normality for score statistics just described is the adaptive design approach described by Bauer and Köhne (1994). Although the ideas can be extended to trials with greater numbers of stages, Bauer and Köhne focus on a two-stage design and assume that the data from each stage are independent of those from the other stage. Suppose that a standard hypothesis test of the null hypothesis that there is no treatment difference is conducted based on the data obtained from each stage, leading to two P-values, p_1 and p_2. A result of Fisher cited by Bauer and Köhne, shows that, if there is no treatment difference, $-2 \log(p_1 p_2)$ follows a CHI-SQUARE DISTRIBUTION on 4 DEGREES OF FREEDOM, allowing the data from the two stages to be combined in a single test.

The fact that the only assumption made is the independence of data from the two stages means that this approach has great flexibility, enabling changes to many features of the trial design without invalidating the final test. The most common change discussed is modification of the sample size of the second stage based on the predicted power of the trial at the end of the first stage, but possible changes go far beyond this to include changes of the endpoint being measured and the null hypothesis being tested. The adaptive design approach has been criticised, however, for the fact that the test statistic, $-2 \log(p_1 p_2)$, is not a sufficient statistic for the treatment difference. This leads to a lack of power for the test, so that, if the flexibility of the adaptive design is not utilised, a sequential test based on the boundaries approach or the spending function method can be found that is as powerful and has smaller expected sample size.

As an example of a sequential analysis, the Figure shows results from the analysis of a small trial to assess the efficacy of Viagra in men suffering erectile dysfunction as a result of spinal cord injury. Eligible men with a regular female partner, who were attending clinics in Southport, Belfast and Stoke Mandeville, were randomised between Viagra and a matching placebo pill. After four weeks they were asked whether the treatment received had improved their erections. The trial was designed using the boundaries approach with the triangular test being chosen as an appropriate design. The solid lines on the Figure illustrate the continuation region for this test when the efficient score statistic, Z, is plotted against the observed Fisher's information, V. The trial continues until the values of Z and V lead to a point outside this triangular region.

At the first interim analysis, 12 men had completed four weeks' treatment with 5/6 on Viagra and 1/6 on placebo reporting improvement. The first plotted point on the Figure represents these data. To allow for the fact that the trial is not monitored continuously, the boundaries are adjusted using the so-called Christmas tree correction, so that the plotted point is compared with the inner dotted boundaries shown. As the point is between these bound-

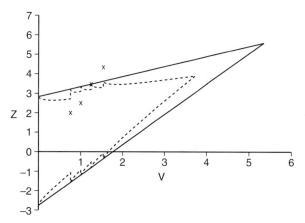

sequential analysis *Continuation region and sample path for a clinical trial of Viagra in men with spinal cord injury*

aries, recruitment to the trial continued. At the third interim analysis, the observed improvement rates were 8/10 on Viagra and 1/10 on placebo. On the basis of these data, the upper boundary was reached and recruitment closed. When the results on the 6 men under treatment were added, the improvement rates became 9/12 and 1/14 respectively, leading to the fourth plotted point. The design allowed a strong positive conclusion to be drawn after only 26 men had been treated. This is in comparison with a conventional fixed sample size trial, for which 57 subjects, more than twice as many, would have been required for a design of the same power.

The methods described earlier mainly lead to tests conducted at a number of interim analyses of the data obtained in a clinical trial with the possibility of stopping the trial as soon as sufficient evidence of a treatment effect, or the lack or such an effect, is obtained. Much more general methods can be envisaged in which many aspects of a clinical trial design may be reconsidered following an interim analysis. Such methods are sometimes referred to as DATA-DEPENDENT DESIGNS, or response-driven designs or, rather confusingly given that the same terms are used for the different approaches described here, as either sequential designs or ADAPTIVE DESIGNS. A review of response-driven design methods is given by Rosenberger (1996).

A simple response-driven design is the play-the-winner design for a clinical trial comparing two treatments on the basis of a success/failure endpoint. The purpose of this design is to replace the random allocation of treatment to patients with a method that leads to more patients receiving the superior treatment. Since, of course, it is not known at the beginning of the trial which treatment is superior, the first patient may be assigned to a treatment at random. If a success is observed from the treatment of this patient, the next patient receives the same treatment. If a failure is observed, the next patient receives the other treatment. Each subsequent patient receives the same treatment as the previous one if a success was observed and the other treatment if a failure was observed. In practice, the simple play-the-winner rule is generally modified to include some random element. Several other rules with different properties, but with the common aim of assigning more patients to the most successful treatment arm, have also been suggested.

Response-driven designs have found most use in early-phase clinical trials for dose finding. Here, the dose of the experimental treatment that is to be given to each patient in the trial is determined depending on the responses from patients treated earlier. Often the aim is to determine a dose that leads to a certain proportion of patients experiencing some event; in trials in oncology, for example, toxicity rates of 20% are often considered optimal. The use of response-driven designs in such trials means that the optimal dose can be efficiently estimated without exposing patients to large doses that may be highly toxic.

The use of a sequential stopping rule in a clinical trial means that many of the standard analysis methods are no longer appropriate. Suppose that a sequential trial has stopped at some interim analysis with the test statistic exceeding the upper critical value, that is, with the conclusion that the experimental treatment is superior to the control treatment. The trial has stopped precisely because of the large observed value of the random score statistic. This means that a standard unbiased estimate of the treatment difference based on the observed value of test statistic, for example the common maximum likelihood estimate will, on average, overestimate the true value of the treatment difference. The P-value from a standard analysis will, in a similar way, on average be too small, that is, it will overstate the evidence against the null hypothesis. Special methods of analysis allowing for the sequential monitoring have been developed. These are described in detail by Whitehead (1997) and Jennison and Turnbull (2000) and are implemented in the software packages PEST, EaSt and SeqTrial.

In large-scale clinical trials, monitoring of accumulating data is commonly undertaken by an independent DATA AND SAFETY MONITORING COMMITTEE (DMC). The primary role of such a committee is to ensure the safety of patients recruited to the trial. It is therefore natural, in a sequential clinical trial, that the DMC should be involved in the interim analyses conducted to assess the treatment difference and in decisions of whether or not the study should be stopped. The involvement of a DMC, the use of a carefully chosen sequential stopping rule, approved by the DMC before start of the study, and a final analysis that allows for the sequential monitoring provide a clinical trial that can be stopped when appropriate without compromising the statistical integrity of the results obtained. *NS*

Armitage, P., McPherson, C.K. and Rowe, B.C. 1969: Repeated significance tests on accumulating data. *Journal of the Royal Statistical Society Series A* 132, 235–44. **Bauer, P. and Köhne, K.** 1994: Evaluation of experiments with adaptive interim analyses. *Biometrics* 50, 1029–41. **Jennison, C. and Turnbull, B.W.** 2000: *Group sequential methods with applications to clinical trials.* Boca Raton: Chapman & Hall/CRC. **Lan, K.K.G. and DeMets, D.L.** 1983: Discrete sequential boundaries for clinical trials. *Biometrika* 70, 659–63. **O'Brien, P.C. and Fleming, T.R.** 1979: A multiple testing procedure for clinical trials. *Biometrics* 35, 549–56. **Pocock, S.J.** 1977: Group sequential methods in the design and analysis of clinical trials. *Biometrika* 64, 191–9. **Rosenberger, W.F.** 1996: New directions in adaptive designs. *Statistical Science* 11, 137–49. **Scharfstein, D.O., Tsiatis, A.A. and Robins, J.M.** 1997: Semiparametric efficiency and its implications on the design and analysis of group-sequential studies. *Journal of the American Statistical Association* 92, 1342–50. **Wald, A.** 1947: *Sequential analysis.* New York: John Wiley & Sons. **Whitehead, J.** 1997: *The design and analysis of sequential clinical trials.* Chichester: John Wiley & Sons.

SeqTrial   See SEQUENTIAL ANALYSIS

shrinkage   See MULTILEVEL MODELS

sign test   One of the oldest non-parametric methods and one of the most simple. It is so named because it uses the sign of the differences rather than their magnitude and is therefore less sensitive than the WILCOXON SIGNED RANK TEST. It can be used for two samples that are matched or paired with a null hypothesis that the MEDIANS are not different between the two groups. Alternatively, it can be used in the one sample case to compare to a particular value, for example the median, where the null hypothesis is that the group median is not different to the proposed median. It is a non-parametric version of both the paired and the one sample t-test.

For the two-sample case, find the sign of the difference between the two values in the pair. Calculate N, the number of differences showing a sign. For the one-sample case, find the sign of the difference between each subject's value and the value of interest. Calculate N, the number of observations that are different to the value of interest. Then for both cases let x be the number of fewer signs, $x = min(+s, -s)$, compare x to the critical region of the binomial distribution, N, ½. Reject the null hypothesis if x is less than or equal to the critical value.

As part of a study, the general health section of the SF-36 was collected. The subject's values (shown in the first Table) are to be compared to the expected value of 72 within the population.

There are 5 plus signs, 9 minus signs and 1 tie, therefore $x = 5$ and $N = 14$. From the tables of the binomial distribution ($N = 14$, $p = ½$) the critical value is 3. As 5 is greater than 3 there is insufficient evidence to reject the null hypothesis, so it is concluded that this group's general health scores are not different from those expected in the population.

General health scores were collected on this group of subjects at a second time point; the scores at this time point are shown in the second Table (see page 323).

This time, there are 7 plus signs, 8 minuses and *no* ties. Therefore $x = 7$ and $N = 15$. Compare $x = 7$ to the critical value of the binomial distribution 15, ½. This value is 3, as 7 is greater than 3 there is insufficient evidence to reject the null hypothesis. Therefore the general health scores are not different at the two time points.   *SLV*

sign test *Subject's values for general health section of the SF-36, using signs from the sign test*

GH value	60	55	75	100	55	60	50	60	72	40	90	75	70	75	55
Sign	−	−	+	+	−	−	−	−	=	−	+	+	−	+	−

sign test *Second recording of subject values in general health section of the SF-36*

Time 1	60	55	75	100	55	60	50	60	72	40	90	75	70	75	55
Time 2	40	45	100	50	70	95	95	65	85	55	70	45	75	65	50
Sign	+	+	−	+	−	−	−	−	−	−	+	+	−	+	+

Pett, M.A. 1997: *Nonparametric statistics for health care research.* Thousand Oaks: Sage. **Siegel, S. and Castellan, N.J.** 1998: *Nonparametric statistics for the behavioral sciences*, 2nd edn. New York: McGraw-Hill.

significance tests and significance levels

Significance tests were introduced by R.A. Fisher (1925) as a means of assessing the evidence against a *null hypothesis*. Often, such a null hypothesis states that there is no association between two variables: for example, between hypertension and subsequent heart disease. Significance tests are conducted by calculating the P-VALUE, defined as the probability, if the null hypothesis were true, that we would have observed an association as large as we did by chance. The term significance level is sometimes used as a synonym for the P-value. If the P-value is small we have evidence *against* the null hypothesis: the entry on P-values describes their calculation and interpretation in more detail. Fisher suggested that if the P-value is sufficiently small then the result of the test should be regarded as providing evidence against the null hypothesis. He advocated that a conventional line be drawn at 5% significance (although he rejected fixed rules) and described results of experiments in which the P-value was sufficiently small as *statistically significant*. Sterne and Davey Smith (2001) have argued that in situations typical of modern medical research, P-values of around 0.05 provide only modest evidence against the null hypothesis.

A different use of the phrase significance level arises from the hypothesis testing approach to the interpretation of experiments advocated by Neyman and Pearson (1933), who showed how to find optimal rules that would minimise the TYPE I and TYPE II ERROR rates over a series of many experiments. We make a Type I error if we reject the null hypothesis when it is in fact true, while we make a Type II error if we accept the null hypothesis when it is, in fact, false (see HYPOTHESIS TESTS).

The Type I error rate, usually denoted as α, is closely related to the P-value since if, for example, the Type I error rate is fixed at 5%, then we will reject the null hypothesis when $P < 0.05$. Therefore, researchers using the Neyman-Pearson approach often report simply that the P-value for their test was less than their chosen *significance level*. There is, however, an important distinction between the use of the term significance level to refer to the evidence against the null hypothesis provided by a particular experiment (Fisher's approach) and the choice of a fixed significance level that, together with the Type II error rate, will be used to determine our behaviour with regard to the results. Goodman (1999) discusses the confusion caused by the failure to appreciate this distinction in more detail. *JS*

Fisher, R.A. 1925: *Statistical methods for research workers.* Edinburgh: Oliver and Boyd. **Goodman, S.N.** 1999: Toward evidence-based medical statistics. 1: The P-value fallacy. *Annals of Internal Medicine* 130, 995–1004. **Neyman, J. and Pearson,**

E. 1933: On the problem of the most efficient tests of statistical hypotheses. *Philosophical Transactions of the Royal Society Series A* 231, 289–337. **Sterne, J.A. and Davey Smith, G.** 2001: Sifting the evidence – what's wrong with significance tests? *British Medical Journal* 322, 226–31.

simple random sample

This is the most basic sampling technique. It is where a smaller group, a sample, is chosen by chance from a population. Each member of the population has an equal and known probability of being chosen to be in the sample. Each sample of a given size also has an equal probability of being chosen from the population. Sampling is usually done without replacement, so that each member of the population can only be selected for inclusion in the sample once.

To choose a random sample, first a list is needed of every member of the population to be sampled: this is the sampling *frame*. Each member of this list is then assigned a number from 1 to N (where N is the total size of the population) in any order. Each member of the sample then has a probability of $1/N$ of being in the sample. A random number generator, or table, is then used to select a random number. The member of the population assigned that number is then selected to be included in the sample. This process is repeated until a sample of the required size is obtained.

For example, suppose that a survey of doctors' opinions is to be carried out. There are 500 doctors in a hospital and a 10% sample is to be collected. First, the sampling frame needs to be obtained, a list of all doctors in the hospital. Next, each doctor is assigned a number from 1 to 500, e.g. in alphabetical order or the order on the list. Now look at a random number table, which gives the following numbers, say:

28049	11632	68254	14217	44612	05049
16831	13213	76103	07222	31852	43501

Therefore, the sample would include doctors numbered 280, 491, 163, 268, 254, 142, 174, 461, 205, 49, 168, 311, 321, 376, 103, 72, 223, 185, 243, 501. As 501 is outside the range of the numbers assigned it is ignored. Care is needed so as not to ignore leading zeros or else some numbers might be inadvertently overlooked.

The main advantage of this method of sampling is the lack of classification error, as no information needs to be known about items except that they are in the population. It is useful when little is known about the population, only that it is likely to be homogenous. The main disadvantage is it might not be possible to find the sampling frame. In the example given earlier, there might not be a list of all the doctors in the hospital meaning a different method would need to be used. *SLV*

Crawshaw, J. and Chambers, J. 1994: *A concise course in A level statistics*, 3rd edn. Cheltenham: Stanley Thornes Publishers Ltd.

simple randomisation   See RANDOMISATION

Simpson's paradox   The observation that a measure of association between two categorical variables may be identical within the levels of a third categorical variable, but can take on an entirely different value when the variable is disregarded and the association measure calculated from the pooled data.

As an example consider the three-way CONTINGENCY TABLE shown in the table. Infants born in two clinics during a certain time period were categorised according to survival and amount of pre-natal care received.

Simpson's paradox *Three-way classification of infant survival and amount of pre-natal care in two clinics, taken from Everitt (1992)*

Clinic	Amount of pre-natal care	Infant survival Died	Infant survival Survived
A	Less	3	176
	More	4	293
B	Less	17	197
	More	2	23

Calculated within clinics the odds of survival vary little between the two pre-natal care groups (odds ratio for survival, OR, comparing higher with lower amount of care, clinic A: OR=1.25, clinic B: OR=0.99) and the corresponding CHI-SQUARED TESTS of independence of survival and amount of care do not reach significance. If, however, the data are collapsed over clinics the odds ratio becomes OR=2.82 and is statistically significant according to a chi-squared test and the conclusion would be that amount of care and survival are related.

Such a situation occurs when the third variable is associated with both the other variables and, therefore, confounds the association between the variables of interest. Here, relatively more pre-natal care is given in clinic A and the survival percentage is also higher in clinic A than B. Therefore, to some extent the pooled measure of association between survival and pre-natal care measures both the association with prenatal care as well as that with clinics.

To take account of the levels of a confounding variable, such as clinic, a pooled within-level measure of association can be constructed (see MANTEL-HAENSZEL METHODS) or a statistical model can be used to adjust the association of interest for the confounder (see LOGISTIC REGRESSION, LOG-LINEAR MODELS).   *SL*

Everitt, B.S. 1992: *The analysis of contingency tables*, 2nd edn. Boca Raton: Chapman & Hall/CRC.

skewness   Data are described as skewed if they have an asymmetric distribution. When the tail of the distribution is on the right-hand side (see (a) in first Figure) the data have positive or right-hand skew. When the tail of the distribution is on the left-hand side (see (b) in the first Figure) the data have negative or left-hand skew.

Many distributions encountered in analyses of medical data are positively skewed. For example, leptin, a fat-related growth hormone, was measured in umbilical cord blood samples taken from 407 babies born at 37 weeks' gestation or later. The distribution of the results is given in

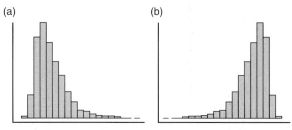

skewness   *Example of right-hand and left-hand skew*

the second Figure; the data are positively skewed since relatively few babies have cord leptin levels above 20 ng/ml.

Analysis of skewed data can proceed either using the ranks of the data or using transformed values. Analyses using ranks are known as nonparametric or distribution-free methods, because they make no assumptions about the distribution of the data. When describing skewed data using non-parametric methods the MEDIAN is a suitable MEASURE OF LOCATION.

Alternative analysis techniques are based on transformed values. These use parametric methods, which rest on the assumption that the data have a particular distribution, usually a NORMAL DISTRIBUTION. Although skewed data do not conform to this assumption, it may be possible to apply a mathematical transformation to the data so that they do. When the data are positively skewed it is often found that the logarithmic (log) TRANSFORMATION is appropriate. If the leptin data are logged they have an approximately normal distribution, as shown in the third Figure, on page 325. When describing skewed data in this situation then the GEOMETRIC MEAN is an appropriate parametric measure of location.

Mathematical measures of skewness can be used to describe distributions. Data with a symmetric distribution, such as the normal distribution have a skewness of zero. Positive values for skewness indicate a positively skewed distribution whereas negative values for skewness indicate a negative skew. The skewness of the raw cord leptin measurements is 2.7, whereas that of the log-transformed measurements is 0.2, which is considerably closer to zero.   *SRC*

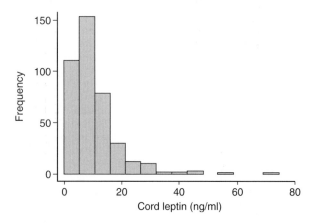

skewness *Recordings of leptin in umbilical cord blood samples*

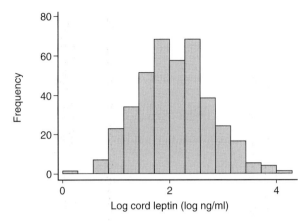

skewness *Logarithmic transformation of leptin readings*

software See STATISTICAL PACKAGES

spatial epidemiology The analysis of epidemiological or public health data that are geographically referenced. Typically the data arises in two forms: either the residential address of cases of disease are known or arbitrary small areas such as census tracts, zip codes or postcodes have counts of disease observed within them. The locational information is used in the analysis usually to make inferences about spatial health effects.

Often hypotheses of interest in spatial epidemiology focus on whether the residential address of cases of disease yields insight into aetiology of the disease or, in a public health application, whether adverse environmental health hazards exist locally within a region (as exemplified by local increases in disease risk). For example, in a study of the relationship between malaria endemicity and diabetes in Sardinia a strong negative relationship has been found. This relation had a spatial expression and the geographical distribution of malaria was important in generating explanatory models for the relation (Bernadelli *et al.*, 1999).

In public health practice, it is of considerable importance to be able to assess whether localised areas that have larger than expected numbers of cases of disease are related to any underlying environmental cause. Here spatial evidence of a link between cases and a source is fundamental in the analysis. Evidence such as a decline in risk with distance from the putative source of hazard or elevation of risk in a preferred direction is important in this regard (see, for example, Lawson and Williams, 2001: ch. 7; Lawson, Biggeri *et al.*, 1999).

There are four main areas where statistical methods have seen development in spatial epidemiology: disease mapping, DISEASE CLUSTERING, ecological analysis and disease map surveillance. Before looking in detail at each of these areas, it is appropriate to consider some common themes or issues that arise in all areas of the subject.

A fundamental feature of data available for analysis in spatial epidemiology is that it is usually discrete (either in the form of a point process or counting process) and the cases of concern arise from within a local human population that varies in spatial density and in susceptibility to the disease of interest. Hence any model or test procedure must make allowance for this background (nuisance) population effect. The background population effect can be allowed for in a variety of ways.

For count data, it is commonplace to obtain expected rates for the disease of interest based on the age–sex structure of the local population and some crude estimates of local relative risk are often computed from the ratio of observed to expected counts (e.g. standardised mortality/incidence ratios: SMRs). For case event data, expected rates are not available at the resolution of the case locations and the use of the spatial distribution of a control disease has been advocated. In that case, the spatial variation in the case disease is compared to the spatial variation in the control disease. One major issue in this approach is the correct choice of control disease. It is important to choose a control that is matched to the age–sex structure of the case disease but is unaffected by the feature of interest. For example, in the analysis of cases around a putative health hazard, a control disease should not be affected by the health hazard. Counts of control disease cases could also be used instead of expected rates when analysing count data. The first and second Figures display case event and control data maps for a region of the UK for a fixed time period. The third Figure displays a typical count data example.

Case event locations often represent residential addresses of cases and the cases arise from a heterogeneous population that varies both in spatial density and in susceptibility to disease. A heterogeneous Poisson process (see Kingman, 1998) model is often assumed as a starting point for further analysis. The focus of interest for making inference regarding parameters describing excess risk lies in a relative risk function that is included in the first order intensity of the Poisson process.

It is possible that population or environmental heterogeneity may be unobserved in the dataset. This could be because either the population background hazard is not directly available or the disease displays a tendency to cluster (perhaps due to unmeasured covariates). The heterogeneity could be spatially correlated, or it could lack CORRELATION in which case it could be regarded as a type

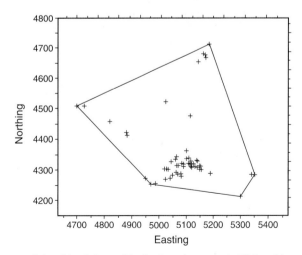

spatial epidemiology *Distribution of cases of childhood lymphoma and leukaemia in Humberside, UK, 1974–1986*

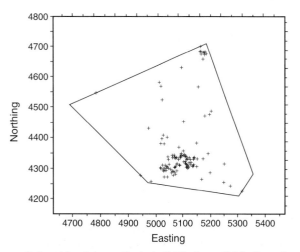

spatial epidemiology *Control distribution: distribution of a sample of live births from the birth register in Humberside, UK, 1974–1986*

of overdispersion. One can include such unobserved heterogeneity within the framework of conventional models as a RANDOM EFFECT.

A considerable literature has developed concerning the analysis of count data in spatial epidemiology (e.g. see reviews in Elliot, Wakefield *et al.*, 2000; Lawson, 2001; Lawson and Williams, 2001; Lawson, Browne *et al.*, 2003).

The usual model adopted for the analysis of region counts assumes that the counts are independent Poisson random variables with parameter λ_i in the ith region. This model may be extended to include unobserved heterogeneity between regions by introducing a prior distribution for the log relative risks ($\log \lambda_i$). Incorporation of such heterogeneity has become a common approach and the Besag, York and Mollié (BYM) (see Lawson, 2001) model is now a standard model. A full Bayesian analysis

using this model is available on WinBUGS (see BAYESIAN METHODS). *AL*

Bernardinelli, L., Pascutto, C. et al. 1999: Ecological regression with errors in covariates: an application. In Lawson, A.B., Biggeri, A., Boehning, D., Lesaffre, E. *et al. Disease mapping and risk assessment for public health.* New York: John Wiley & Sons. **Elliott, P., Wakefield, J. et al.** (eds) 2000: *Spatial epidemiology: methods and applications.* London: Oxford University Press. **Kingman, J.F.C.** 1998: Poisson process. In Armitage, P. and Colton, T. (eds), *Encyclopedia of biostatistics.* Chichester: John Wiley & Sons. **Lawson, A.B.** 2001: *Statistical methods in spatial epidemiology.* New York: John Wiley & Sons. **Lawson, A.B. and Williams, F.L.R.** 2001: *An introductory guide to disease mapping.* New York: John Wiley & Sons. **Lawson, A.B., Biggeri, A. et al.** 1999: A review of modelling approaches in health risk assessment around putative sources. **Lawson, A.B., Biggeri, A., Boehning, D., Lesaffre E. et al.** *Disease mapping and risk assessment for public health.* New York: Wiley. **Lawson, A.B., Browne, W. et al.** 2003: *Disease mapping in WinBUGS and MLwiN.* New York: John Wiley & Sons.

Spearman's rank correlation coefficient See CORRELATION

Spearman's rho (ρ) Also known as *Spearman's rank correlation coefficient*, this is a measure of the relationship between two variables that uses only the rankings of the observations. If the ranked values of the two variables for a set of n individuals are a_i and b_i, with $d_i = a_i - b_i$, then the coefficient is defined explicitly as:

$$\rho = 1 - \frac{6 \sum_{i=1}^{n} d_i^2}{n^3 - n}$$

In essence, ρ is simply Pearson's product moment correlation coefficient between the rankings a and b. We can illustrate the coefficient on the data shown in the Table on page 327, which were collected to investigate the relationship between mean annual temperature and the mortality rate for a type of breast cancer in women. The data relate to certain regions of Great Britain, Norway and Sweden

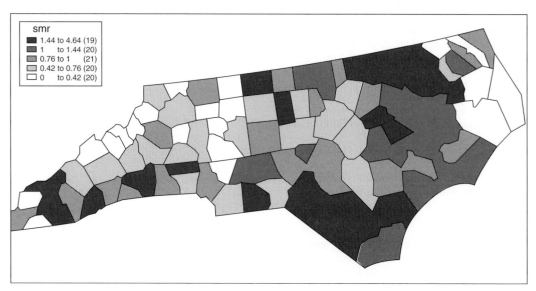

spatial epidemiology *Distribution of counts of sudden infant death (SID) within the counties of North Carolina, USA, 1974–1978*

Spearman's rho (ρ) *Breast cancer mortality and temperature*

Mean annual temperature (°F)	Mortality index
51.3	102.5
49.9	104.5
50.0	100.4
49.2	95.9
48.5	87.0
47.8	95.0
47.3	88.6
45.1	89.2
46.3	78.9
42.1	84.6
44.2	81.7
43.5	72.2
42.3	65.1
40.2	68.1
31.8	67.3
34.0	52.5

(see Lea, 1965). Here, the Spearman correlation is 0.90 and Pearson's product moment correlation 0.87. In general, the Spearman coefficient is more robust against the presence of OUTLIERS. *BSE*

[See also CORRELATION, NONPARAMETRIC METHODS – AN OVERVIEW]

Lea, A.J. 1965: New observations on distribution of neoplasms of female breast cancer in certain European countries. *British Medical Journal* 1, 488–90.

specificity A measure of how well an alternative test performs when it is compared with the reference of 'gold' standard test for diagnosis of a condition. Specificity is the proportion of patients correctly identified as free from the condition by the diagnostic test out of all patients who do not have the condition. Specificity may also be expressed as a percentage and is the counterpart to SENSITIVITY.

The reference standard may be the best available diagnostic test or may be a combination of diagnostic methods, including following up patients until all patients with the disease have presented with clinical symptoms. It follows that the best design when a diagnostic test is evaluated against a reference standard is a COHORT STUDY. Investigators should consider whether verification bias is present: this occurs when obtaining a negative result on one diagnostic test influences the chances of a patient going on to have further tests, so that some patients with the condition never receive the correct diagnosis.

When the data are set out as in the Table,

$$specificity = \frac{d}{b + d}.$$

specificity *General table of test results among a + b + c + d individuals sampled*

	Disease		
	Present	Absent	Total
Positive	a	b	a + b
Negative	c	d	c + d
Total	a + c	b + d	a + b + c + d

Specificity should be presented with confidence intervals, typically set at 95%, calculated using an appropriate method such as that of Wilson (described in Altman *et al.*, 2000) that will not produce impossible values, i.e. that will not give values for the upper confidence interval > 1 when specificity approaches 1 and the sample size is small.

Where a test result is a continuous measurement, for example, HDL cholesterol, a cut-off point for abnormal values is chosen. If a higher value is chosen, then specificity will be relatively high, but sensitivity relatively low. The impact of all possible cut-off points can be displayed graphically in a RECEIVER OPERATING CHARACTERISTIC (ROC) CURVE. The choice of cut-off point is not, however, solely a statistical decision, as the balance between the FALSE POSITIVE RATE and the FALSE NEGATIVE RATE should be related to the clinical context and consequences of wrong diagnosis both for the patient and the healthcare system.

A sample size calculation for specificity can be made by stipulating a CONFIDENCE INTERVAL (for example, 95%) and an acceptable width for the lower bound of the confidence interval. Where the anticipated specificity is high and the sample size is small, a 'small sample' method should be used: a sample size table is included in Machin *et al.* (1997). *CLC*

[See also NEGATIVE PREDICTIVE VALUE, POSITIVE PREDICTIVE VALUE, TRUE POSITIVE RATE]

Altman, D.G., Machin, D., Bryant, T.N. and Gardner, M.J. 2000: *Statistics with confidence*, 2nd edn. London: BMJ Books. **Machin, D., Campbell, M., Fayers, P. and Pinol, A.** 1997: *Sample size tables for clinical studies*, 2nd edn. Oxford: Blackwell Sciences Ltd.

spending function See SEQUENTIAL ANALYSIS

spline function See SCATTERPLOT SMOOTHERS

S-PLUS See STATISTICAL PACKAGES

SPSS See STATISTICAL PACKAGES

stable population See DEMOGRAPHY

stacked bar chart See BAR CHART

standard deviation A MEASURE OF SPREAD intended to give an indication of the spread of a series of values $(x_1, x_2, ..., x_n)$ about their MEAN $(\bar{x})$.

Taking the average of the differences from the mean may initially seem a good measure of their spread, but in fact this is always zero. Therefore, the standard deviation is based on the average of the squared differences from the mean, since these are all positive. Taking the square root of this result gives a measure that is in the same units as the original values. Thus, the standard deviation is calculated using the following formula. Here n is the number of observations, i takes values from 1 to n, and the $\sum$ notation denotes the sum i.e. $(x_1 - \bar{x})^2 + (x_2 - \bar{x})^2 + ... + (x_n - \bar{x})^2$:

$$s = \sqrt{\frac{\sum (x_i - \bar{x})^2}{n - 1}}$$

Note that the formula indicates division by $n - 1$, rather than n, when taking the average of the squared differences. This gives a result that is a better estimate of the standard deviation in the whole population, which is being estimated from the sample available.

The standard deviation can be denoted SD, *sd*, *s* or σ,

although the last technically refers to the standard deviation of a population, rather than a sample. To calculate the standard deviation by hand there is a more convenient and mathematically equivalent formula:

$$s = \sqrt{\frac{\sum x_i^2 - \left[\left(\sum x_i\right)^2 / n\right]}{n-1}}$$

As an example, the bone mineral content (BMC) of 10 babies was measured using dual energy X-ray absorptiometry (DXA). The measurements in grams were: 46.6, 46.9, 49.2, 49.8, 53.2, 61.1, 68.1, 73.1, 77.1 and 78.6.

It is simple to calculate that the sum of the observations $\sum x_i = 603.7$ and the sum of the squares of the observations $\sum x_i^2 = 37938.89$. Thus:

$$s = \sqrt{\frac{37938.89 - [(603.7)^2 / 10]}{9}} = 12.88 \text{ g}$$

The VARIANCE of a set of measurements is the square of their standard deviation. Although the variance has many uses, the standard deviation is a more meaningful descriptive statistic because it is in the same units as the raw data. Whereas square millimetres, mm^2, may have an obvious interpretation, square millimetres of mercury, $mmHg^2$, does not. Altman (1991) suggests that standard deviations may be quoted with one or two more decimal places than the original values.

The standard deviation is typically used as a measure of spread alongside the mean and is most appropriate when the data are approximately symmetrically distributed. It has the useful property that when the data follow a NORMAL DISTRIBUTION then approximately 95% of the observations will be within two standard deviations of the mean. The Figure shows the case of a standard normal distribution, which has a mean of 0 and a standard deviation of 1.   *SRC*

Altman, D.G. 1991: *Practical statistics for medical research.* London: Chapman & Hall.

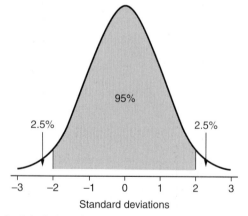

standard deviation *Standard normal distribution, with mean of 0 and SD of 1*

standard error The standard deviation of the sampling distribution of a statistic. For example, the standard error of the sample mean of n observations is $\sigma/\sqrt{n}$, where σ^2 is the variance of the original observations.

A useful aide-memoire to distinguish when to use STANDARD DEVIATION (SD) and when to use standard error (SE) is to recall: 'SD for description, SE for estimation.' In particular, when describing patient characteristics in a sample, as in a research paper's typical Table 1, means and SDs should be reported, whereas when seeking to learn from the sample and apply results to the relevant population, that is performing statistical inference either by HYPOTHESIS TESTS or estimation by CONFIDENCE INTERVALS, then the standard error is used. The SE is necessarily smaller than the SD and it is wrong to use SE as a MEASURE OF SPREAD when describing samples.

More generally, standard errors can be attached to any sample-based quantity, not just the mean of a single sample of continuously distributed data, as just discussed.

The general form of a large-sample 95% confidence interval for a population parameter (numerical characteristic) is the sample-based point estimate ± 1.96 (standard errors), where 1.96 arises from the standard NORMAL DISTRIBUTION and the standard error is that of the point estimate, itself the best sample-based guess for the value of the parameter. For two-sample inference, this is usually a quantity such as the difference in population means, for continuous data, or the difference in population proportions, for categorical data.   *BSE*

standard population See DEMOGRAPHY

statistical consulting See CONSULTING A STATISTICIAN

standardised mortality ratio (SMR) See DEMOGRAPHY

STATA See STATISTICAL PACKAGES

statistical methods in molecular biology Molecular biology is the branch of biology that studies the structure and function of biological macromolecules of a cell and especially with their genetic role. Three types of macromolecules are the main subjects of interest: deoxyribonucleic acids (DNA), ribonucleic acids (RNA) and proteins. Genetic information is encoded in the DNA and inherited from parents to children and when expressed, a gene, the basic unit of inheritance, is first transcribed to messenger RNA, which then carries the information to a cellular machinery (ribosome) for protein production. This basic principle of the information flow in biology is often referred to as the 'central dogma', put forward by Francis Crick in 1958. A central goal of molecular biology is to decipher the genetic information and understand the regulation of protein synthesis and interaction in cellular processes.

The rapid advance of biotechnology in the past few decades has facilitated manipulation of these important biopolymers and allowed scientists to clone, sequence and amplify DNA. As a result, a large amount of biological sequence and structural information has been generated and deposited into public accessible databases. The phenomenal growth of biological data is underpinned by the developments of high-throughput DNA sequencing and microarray technologies and the recent progresses in giant research projects such as the human genome project that produced the sequence of the human genome.

The word 'genome' refers to the entire collection of genetic material of an organism. These advances result in many complex and massive datasets, sometimes decoupled from specific biological questions under investigation. The need to extract scientific insights from these rich data by computational and analytic means has spawned the new field of bioinformatics and computational molecular biology, which deals with storage, retrieval and analysis of biological data. These can consist of information stored in the genetic code, but also experimental results from various sources, patient statistics and scientific literature. Bioinformatics is highly interdisciplinary, using techniques and concepts from informatics, statistics, mathematics, physics, chemistry, biochemistry and linguistics. Nowadays, various biological databases and practical applications of bioinformatics are readily available through the internet and are widely used in biological and medical research.

A wide spectrum of statistical methods has been successfully applied in bioinformatics, ranging from the basic summary statistics and exploratory data analysis tools, to sophisticated hidden Markov models and Bayesian resampling methods (see BAYESIAN METHODS, MARKOV CHAIN MONTE CARLO). Analyses in bioinformatics focus on three types of datasets: genome sequences, macromolecule structures and large-scale functional genomics experiments. Various other data types are also involved, such as taxonomy trees, sequence polymorphisms, relationship data from metabolic pathways, patient statistics, text from scientific literature and so on.

DNA sequences are the primary data from the sequencing projects and they only become really valuable through multiple layers of annotation and organisation. Several areas of bioinformatics analysis are relevant when dealing with DNA and protein sequences: sequence assembly: to establish the correct order of sequence contigs for a contiguous sequence; prediction of functional units: to identify subsets of sequences that code for various functional signals such as protein coding genes, promoters, splice sites, regulatory elements; and sequence comparison and database search: to retrieve data efficiently from organised databases.

Most of these analyses involved *sequence alignment*, one of the classic problems in the early development of bioinformatics. Sequence alignment is the basic tool that allows us to determine the similarity of two or more sequences

and infer components that might be conserved through evolution and natural selection. To align two protein sequences, similarity scores are assigned to all possible pairs of residues and the sequences are aligned to each other so as to maximise the sum total of scores in the sequence pairings induced by the alignment. *Dynamic programming*-based algorithms were developed to overcome the large search space for the solution of optimal global and local alignment problem (Needleman and Wunsch, 1970; Smith and Waterman, 1981).

Dynamic programming is a general algorithmic technique that solves an optimisation problem by recursively 'divide and conquer' its sub-problems. Faster heuristic word-based alignment algorithms were later introduced for large database similarity searches (BLAST by Altschul *et al.*, 1990; FASTA by Pearson and Lipman, 1988). These algorithms build alignments by extending or joining common short patterns ('words') that are computationally efficient, but often yield suboptimal solutions. The interpretation of alignment scores and database search results was aided by statistical significance derived from simulations and probability theory of extreme value distributions under the framework of standard statistical hypothesis testing (Karlin and Altschul, 1990). These classic results have become indispensable tools for biomedical researchers and computational biologists to analyse molecular sequence data.

Statistical models are also routinely used to construct probabilistic profiles to characterise the regularity of biological signals based on collections of pre-aligned sequences and to increase sensitivity of searches. For example, a block-based product multinomial model can be used to describe the position-specific base distributions of the 5′ splice site (exon-intron junction) signal in humans (see Figure), which gives a richer representation of the sequence motif than the consensus CAG|GTGAG ('|' indicates the exon-intron junction). A *position-specific scoring matrix* can be derived subsequently using logarithms of the odds ratio of the signal to background base to evaluate matches of new query sequences to the sequence motif and to quantify the *information content* of the signal sequence pattern. The information content of a signal is defined as the average score of random sequence

```
AAGGTGCTGTG
CAGGTGAGTGG
AATGTACGTGT
CAGGTGAGCGG
CAGGTATGCGG
AAGGTAAAGTT
CAGGTGAGCCC
GCGGTAAGAGG
GGGGTGAGTCA
GAGGTGTGTGC
CAGGTAATCAA
ACGGTAAGCCC
GTGGTGAGCGG
AAGGTGGGTGC
GAGGTGAGAGG
AAGGTGAGGGC
CAGGTAAGGCA
CAGGTGAGCCT
    . . .
```

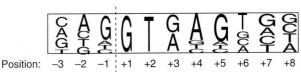

Position:	−3	−2	−1	+1	+2	+3	+4	+5	+6	+7	+8
A	0.34	0.65	0.10	0.00	0.00	0.61	0.70	0.09	0.18	0.29	0.22
C	0.36	0.10	0.03	0.00	0.01	0.03	0.07	0.05	0.15	0.19	0.25
G	0.18	0.11	0.81	1.00	0.00	0.34	0.11	0.78	0.19	0.30	0.24
T	0.11	0.14	0.07	0.00	0.99	0.03	0.12	0.08	0.49	0.22	0.29

statistical methods in molecular biology *The human 5′ splice site (exon-intron junction signal)*

matches, measured in 'bits' using the log (base two) odds-ratio scores that represent the number of 0–1s necessary to code for this signal in a binary coding system. For instances, the human 5′ splice site depicted in the figure contains 8 bits of information, meaning that 'decoy' splice sites will be observed roughly every $2^8 = 256$ bases in random sequence. Note that the information content can also be formulated as the *relative entropy* (or *Kullback-Leibler distance*) of the signal to background nucleotide frequency distributions in the context of information theory. More sophisticated models and scoring matrices are also available to capture dependencies among neighbouring positions using *Markov models* and others.

Another area of biological sequence analysis that relies heavily on statistical reasoning is gene finding or, more generally, predicting complex features from a sequence. The goal of protein-coding gene finding is to locate gene features such as exons and introns in a DNA genomic sequence, which is the essential first-pass annotation of the genome project products. In addition to inferring *homologous* (evolutionarily related) gene structures from database similarity searches, statistical *ab initio* gene-finding programs have been developed to integrate all known features and 'grammars' of protein-coding genes in a probabilistic model.

Hidden Markov models (HMMs) are at the heart of the most popular gene finders (Genscan by Burge and Karlin, 1997 (reviewed in Durbin *et al.*, 1998)). HMMs were originally developed in early 1970s by electrical engineers for the problem of speech recognition – to identify what sequence of phonemes (or words) was spoken from a long sequence of category labels representing the speech signal. The resemblance of the gene-finding problem to speech recognition and the way HMMs are formulated make them especially suited in this context. In addition, HMMs are theoretically well-founded models, combining probabilistic modelling and formal language theory that guarantees 'sensible' predictions that obey specified grammatical rules even though they might not be the correct genes.

There are also well-documented and computational efficient methods for parameter estimation (e.g. expectation-maximisation) and optimisation (Viterbi algorithm). A Markov chain is a series of random events occurring with probabilities conditionally dependent on the state of the preceding event(s). A hidden Markov model is a Markov chain in which each state generates an observation according to some rule (usually stochastic). The objective is to infer the hidden state sequence that maximises the posterior probability of the observed event sequence given the model. For example, the hidden states may represent words or phonemes and the observations are the acoustic signal.

Motif discovery is an area under active research and has benefited from sophisticated modern statistical techniques. In a typical setting, a collection of sequences derived from MICROARRAY EXPERIMENTS or various sources are believed to share common sequence motifs that often represent functional domains or regulatory elements and the challenge is to find the unknown signals and locate them in individual sequences. One approach is to formulate the multiple alignment information as missing data and infer them together with other parameters of the statistical model, given only the sequences as observables. Advanced statistical modelling and iterative computation

techniques such as the EM algorithm and Markov chain Monte Carlo are typically used for simultaneous model estimation (Liu, Neuwald and Lawrence, 1999).

The function of a protein is determined by its three-dimensional (3-D) structure and the problem of predicting the 3-D structure of a protein from its amino-acid sequence (or the protein-folding problem, because proteins are capable of quickly folding into their stable, unique 3-D structure starting from a random coil conformation without additional genetic mechanisms) is one of biggest challenges in bioinformatics. There are three major lines of approaches for protein structure prediction: comparative modelling, fold recognition and *ab initio* prediction.

Comparative modelling makes use of sequence alignment and database searches and builds on the fact that evolutionarily related proteins with similar sequences have similar structure. For proteins without homologous sequence of known structure, the approach of 'threading' has been developed. It is assumed that a small collection of 'folds', perhaps several hundreds in number, can be used to model the majority of protein domains in all organisms. The protein-folding problem is thus reduced to the tasks of classifying the query protein based on its primary sequence into one of the folding classes in a database of known 3-D structures. This classification is often accomplished using complicated statistical models such as Gibbs sampling and HMMs to parameterise the fit of a sequence to a given fold and solve the optimisation problem accordingly.

Analogous to the gene-finding problem, one may attempt to directly compute a protein's structure from its sequence based on biophysical understanding of how the 3-D structure of proteins is attained. The challenge can be broken down into two components: devising a scoring function that can distinguish between correct and incorrect structures and a search method to efficiently explore the conformational space. If successful, direct folding certainly would give deeper insight than the 'top-down' threading or homology modelling approaches. However, currently no reliable method has yet emerged in this category.

During the past few years, the development of DNA array technology has scaled up the traditionally one-gene-at-a-time functional studies to allow the monitoring of hundreds of thousands of genes simultaneously. A large number of statistical issues arise in connection with these studies and these have fostered unprecedented conversation and collaborations between biologists and statisticians to establish means to plan, process and analyse these massive datasets. Many branches of statistics have been revived and/or extended by their recent applications in the analysis of functional genomics and molecular data, including *data-mining* methods to discover and classify patterns, *multiple testing procedures* to adjust P-VALUES to control false discovery rates and *meta-analysis* (see SYSTEMATIC REVIEWS AND META-ANALYSIS) to combine experimental results from various sources. New statistical methods will soon be needed when combining information from multiple distinct data types (sequence, gene expression, protein structures, sequence variation and phenotypes) for the same subjects. *RFY*

Altschul, S.F., Gish, W., Miller, W., Myers, E.W. and Lipman, D. 1990: Basic local alignment search tool. *Journal of*

Molecular Biology 215, 403–10. **Burge, C.B. and Karlin, S.** 1997: Prediction of complete gene structures in human genomic DNA. *Journal of Molecular Biology* 268, 78–94. **Durbin, R., Eddy, S., Krogh, A. and Mitchison, G.** 1998: *Biological sequence analysis: probabilistic models of proteins and nucleic acids.* Cambridge: Cambridge University Press. **Karlin, S. and Altschul, S.F.** 1990: Methods for assessing the statistical significance of molecular sequence features by using general scoring schemes. *Proceedings of the National Academy of Sciences of the United States of America* 87, 2264–8. **Liu, J.S., Neuwald, A. and Lawrence, C.** 1999: Markovian structures in biological sequence alignments. *Journal of the American Statistical Association* 94, 1–15. **Needleman, S.B. and Wunsch, C.D.** 1970: A general method applicable to the search for similarities in the amino acid sequence of two proteins. *Journal of Molecular Biology* 48, 443–53. **Pearson, W.R. and Lipman, D.J.** 1988: Improved tools for biological sequence comparison. *Proceedings of the National Academy of Sciences of the United States of America* 85, 2444–8. **Smith, T.H. and Waterman, M.S.** 1981: Identification of common subsequences. *Journal of Molecular Biology* 147, 195–7.

statistical packages In 2004 the Association for Survey Computing (ASC) website (www.asc.org.uk) listed some 187 statistical packages. Many of these have been under development for nearly 40 years and therefore it is both a very mature and diverse software market.

While many of these 187 packages are developed for niche markets, there are still several generic software suites. It seems almost invidious to try to select and discuss individual packages. However, there are clearly some well-known and long established packages, and to many the term 'statistical package' is almost synonymous with SPSS™ or possibly SAS™. Given the variety of analyses that these packages offer they can meet most user needs. It would seem likely that a virtual monopoly should exist, but in fact there have been new entrants gaining popularity. Comparing these is instructive about trends in the development of statistical software. The packages in the first table are the ones on which we will concentrate here.

statistical packages *Major statistical packages*

Major statistical packages	
SPSS	www.spss.com
SAS	www.sas.com
STATA	www.stata.com
S-Plus	www.insightful.com

The prevalence of these major packages notwithstanding, there are other packages, as listed in the second table, although these will not be further discussed. Competition has been good for the development of programs and potential purchasers should always be aware of options outside the norm that may well fit their requirements. Together with the ASC website (given earlier), it will always be profitable to make comparisons when purchasing.

statistical packages *Other major statistical packages*

Other major statistical packages	
Genstat	www.vsn-intl.com
STATISTICA	www.statsoft.com
NCSS	www.ncss.com
SYSTAT	www.systat.com

Naturally enough, one wants a statistical package to do statistics and the leading packages cover a wide range. These include basic descriptive statistics, including EDA-style charting, comprehensive cross-tabulation analysis, means testing, the general linear model, multivariate methods, data reduction and clustering, non-parametrics, log-linear modelling, time series – and more.

The conversion in the late 1980s–early 1990s of the packages SPSS and SAS to run on desktop PCs seemed to cause a hiatus in the development of statistical methodology within these suites. Quite possibly, one of the main reasons for this was the need to develop new user interfaces, as an alternative the command-line format previously used on mainframe and minicomputers. With the DOS interface model being rapidly succeeded by that of Windows™, major consecutive design changes were needed. This did seem to leave a window of opportunity for new entrants to the market, which could write directly using modern programming architectures.

S-PLUS is perhaps the earliest example of this, initially written for the UNIX system and then subsequently ported to PCs. The design was conceptually novel, based on the notion of an extensible statistical calculator. It provides advanced graphics facilities and has become popular with professional statisticians for its ability to develop analysis methodologies, rather than being tied to a rigid framework. Over time S-PLUS has developed to add extensive user interface enhancements as well as larger statistical libraries. The public domain 'R' (www.r-project.org) is based on a similar philosophy to S-PLUS (see R).

STATA has become a very popular alternative for similar reasons. Starting out as a command-line-driven program, it has matured over the years to offer a windowing interface in addition. Its attractiveness to researchers has been a modern approach to statistical testing, as well as its ability to incorporate new methodologies quickly. Not only do the developers have an architecture that permits easy incremental expansion, users themselves can program their own procedures. This has gained the support of the professional statistical community, who through their educative role have promoted the package's popularity.

Partly as a result of competition, packages have also begun to differentiate themselves in terms of extending extra support to the whole data analysis process. While the actual test result remains the core of any analysis, data management is far more demanding in terms of time. The resources needed to support data management in a MULTI-CENTRE clinical TRIAL are significantly larger than those for a classical experiment. In these scenarios, managing and manipulating data prior to analysis becomes very important.

SAS has long specialised in data management support, with flexible procedures for merging and manipulating datasets, as well as links to database packages. In the pharmaceutical industry SAS is almost a de facto standard for major analyses, reflecting its ability to support the strong audit requirements in the industry. To a certain extent other packages have been restricted to the rectangular data model (or spreadsheet) view of data, although all are now improving these features.

One direct effect of the development of statistical packages has been to introduce the possibility of statistical data analysis to a wider audience than just statisticians. Since these users are often in finance and commerce, they represent a significant revenue stream to package producers and making the program user friendly for non-specialist audiences has become a priority for some. SPSS's menu-driven 'point-and-click' interface for example, epitomises this model. In contrast, the command-line models of SAS, STATA or SPLUS require more dedicated training, although as noted earlier all have developed similar facilities. (STATA 8 introduced a menu-driven interface in 2003 to complement its traditional command-line orientation.)

Integrating advanced data-entry features with a statistical analysis package is common. The predominant spreadsheet data entry model can be enhanced to include data-entry forms, data checking and audit. The large packages such as SPSS and SAS provide 'add-on' programs for this. Other programs provide direct database links so that data entry can be provided in a normal programming package such as Microsoft Access and then directly imported for analysis.

While traditionally the results of an analysis are interpreted and then incorporated into a final report, packages have begun to differentiate themselves on their ability to produce tables and results that can be directly pasted into a presentation quality report. Packages vary widely on their ability to do this and support can be patchy. SPSS provides a very good ability to move results tables, but the exported graphics are not of such a good quality. STATA, by contrast, does not offer sophisticated export of results, but has in its latest versions excellent graphical output. SAS offers full programmable reporting features which are very flexible, but challenging for the naive user.

While the main focus of any statistical user is on the large packages, dedicated packages still have a role. As an example, programs such as NQUERY (www.statsol.ie), dedicated to sample size estimation, do one particular job very well and are popular as a result. The lone, innovative researcher (an example perhaps being MX found at www.vcu.edu/mx/) is also a likely producer of innovative software.

An important dimension for the individual consumer can be price. Some of the major packages have prices that match their capabilities: the single researcher, particularly in the commercial sector, may find this an important factor in choice. All the relevant websites can give guidance on obtaining price quotations.

Rather than ossifying, the marketplace for statistical software is healthy and researchers can find themselves well supported with a choice of diverse packages.   *CS*

statistical parametric map See STATISTICS IN IMAGING

statistical refereeing There are hundreds of review articles published in the biomedical literature that point out statistical errors in the design, conduct, analysis, summary and presentation of research studies. The contents of every general medical journal (most notably *Annals of Internal Medicine, British Medical Journal, Journal of the American Medical Association, Lancet* and *New England Journal of Medicine*), as well as of many specialist ones, have been subjected to this intense scrutiny sometimes frequently. These review articles have focused on particu-

lar statistical tests, frequency of usage and correct application of techniques of statistical analysis, design of clinical trials and epidemiological studies, use of power calculations and CONFIDENCE INTERVALS and many other aspects.

Their almost universal conclusion is that a substantial percentage of research studies, perhaps as many as 50%, published in the biomedical literature, contain errors of sufficient magnitude to cast some doubt on the validity of the conclusions that have been drawn. This does not mean that the conclusions are wrong, but it does imply that they may not be right and this inevitably leads to serious concern about the consequences both for understanding of disease and for the treatment of patients.

One solution to this problem has been the introduction of medical statisticians into the peer review process. Some have advocated that all submitted papers should be scrutinised in this way, arguing that statistical review of those that are not published, no matter how poor, will at least lead to higher standards in research and improvement in future papers. In view of the very large number of biomedical journals and the huge numbers of papers submitted for publication every year, such a remedy is impracticable. An alternative, now used by several journals, is to divide the peer review process into two stages whereby papers considered by the editors as candidates for publication, are sent first to subject matter referees (physicians, surgeons, epidemiologists etc.) and those recommended for publication by them, are then sent to statisticians for further specialist review.

The process of statistical review is complex, requires sophisticated judgement and varies considerably in its application to every section of a paper (abstract, introduction, methods, results and discussion). Altman (1998) reviews some of the difficulties and provides practical examples of both definite errors and matters of judgement, within study design, analysis, presentation and interpretation. There are 12 broad aims of statistical review that can be summarised as follows: to prevent publication of studies that have a fundamental flaw in design; to prevent publication of papers that have a fundamental flaw in *interpretation*; to ensure that key aspects of background, design and methods of analysis are reported clearly; to ensure that key features of the design are reflected in the analysis; to ensure that the best methods of analysis, appropriate to the data, are used; to ensure that the presentation of results is adequate and employs summary statistics, that are justified by the design, the data and the analysis; to ensure that tables are accurate, are consistent both with the text and with each other; to ensure that the style of figures is appropriate, that they are consistent with text and tables and not unduly repetitious of other content; to guard against excessive analysis and spurious accuracy; to ensure that conclusions are justified by the results; to ensure that content of the discussion is justified by the results and, in particular, that it avoids generalisation far beyond the confines of the paper; and, finally, to ensure that the abstract accords with the paper.

The statistical reviewer may also comment on subject matter when expert within the medical specialty of the paper, but will not indicate typos, except when these are critical for accuracy within formulae or text. Indeed, pointing out inconsequential typos is not part of any aspect of any review process; they should be disregarded by expert reviewers and left entirely to the journal's copy editor!

Since statistical review is complicated and, for the reviewer, sometimes excessively tedious with the necessity of making very similar, sometimes the same, comments about manuscript after manuscript, detailed statistical guidelines and checklists have been written with the specific intention of helping authors (and reviewers). These have been supported by the editors of many biomedical journals and referred to in the journal's guidelines to authors. Examples can be found in Altman *et al.* (2000) and Gardner *et al.* (2000). Those most widely used for clinical trials are the CONSORT guidelines (Moher, Schulz and Altman, 2001), for which there is accompanying explanation (Altman *et al.*, 2001) and recent extension to cluster trials (Campbell, Elbourne and Altman, 2004). The checklist that forms part of the CONSORT statement is intended to accompany a submitted paper and to indicate where in the manuscript each item in the checklist has been addressed, thus serving as a useful reminder to authors and an aide to referees.

Statistical review is intended to be helpful and constructive; it should also reassure authors and readers that published papers are sound. However, it is not always seen from this perspective and editors of journals need to be vigilant in ensuring that it does not become a focus for controversy and dispute, as can happen, for example, when authors parade the views of 'their own statistician' to counter comments from a referee. There is at present little incentive for statisticians to engage in such review – it does not enhance their careers, there is no specific training for it, small (if any) remuneration, it is time consuming and 'the only likely concrete consequence of good reviewing is future requests for more reviews' (Bacchetti, 2002). Bacchetti also points out that statistics is a rich area for finding mistakes and, when coupled with 'the notion that finding flaws is the key to high quality peer review', can lead to 'finding flaws that are not really there'. This reinforces the need for sound statistical judgement. Statisticians may also have to counter mistaken criticisms from subject matter reviewers with limited statistical knowledge (Bacchetti, 2002).

The final part of statistical review is usually a recommendation to the journal's editor either to accept, accept with revision, revise and resubmit or reject the paper. The distinction between the second and third is sometimes difficult and can only be made by balancing the extent and nature of the revisions against the capabilities of the authors as evinced from the submitted paper. Rejection by the statistician can also lead to provocation especially as authors will be aware that their 'subject matter' peers have already judged it sound. In 1937 the *Lancet*'s leading article that heralded the series of classic papers by Bradford Hill on *The Principles of Medical Statistics* forewarned: 'It is exasperating, when we studied a problem by methods that we have spent laborious years in mastering, to find our conclusions questioned, and perhaps refuted, by someone who could not have made the observations himself. It requires more equanimity than most of us possess to acknowledge that the fault is in ourselves.'

Authors of papers are advised to read statistical reviews carefully, put them aside for 48 hours and only then start to think about how to respond.   *TJ*

Altman, D.G. 1998: Statistical reviewing for medical journals. *Statistics in Medicine* 17, 2661–74. **Altman, D.G., Gore, S.M., Gardner, M.J. and Pocock, S.J.** 2000: *Statistical guidelines for contributors to medical journals.* In Altman, D.G., Machin, D., Bryant, T.N. and Gardner, M.J. (eds), *Statistics with confidence*, 2nd edn. London: BMJ Books, 171–90. **Altman, D.G., Schulz, K.F., Moher, D., Egger, M., Davidoff, F., Elbourne, D., Gotzsche, P.C. and Lang, T. for the CONSORT Group** 2001: The revised CONSORT statement for reporting randomised trials: explanation and elaboration. *Annals of Internal Medicine* 134, 663–94. **Bacchetti, P.** 2002: Peer review of statistics in medical research: the other problem. *British Medical Journal* 324: 1271–3. **Campbell, M.K., Elbourne, D.R. and Altman, D.G. for the CONSORT Group** 2004: CONSORT statement: extension to cluster randomised trials. *British Medical Journal* 328, 702–8. **Gardner, M.J., Machin, D., Campbell, M.J. and Altman, D.G.** 2000: *Statistical checklists.* In Altman, D.G., Machin, D., Bryant, T.N. and Gardner, M.J. (eds), *Statistics with confidence*, 2nd edn. London: BMJ Books, 191–201. **Moher, D., Schulz, K.F. and Altman, D.G. for the CONSORT Group** 2001: The CONSORT statement: revised recommendations for improving the quality of reports of parallel-group randomised trials. *Annals of Internal Medicine* 134, 657–62.

statistics in imaging The use of statistical techniques to analyse and quantify information contained in digital image format. Imaging is widely used in medicine to visualise objects, structures and even physical processes *in vivo* and *in vitro*. A significant advantage in medical imaging is the ability to visualise structures or processes without relying on surgical operations. Thus, animals may be recycled in drug discovery and development or patients may not suffer from intrusive procedures. The ability to acquire information without intrusive procedures is also a disadvantage to medical imaging. This raises the issue of surrogate imaging endpoints (or *surrogacy*); that is, how well do the conclusions from an imaging experiment correspond to physical properties obtained from an intrusive procedure?

Although the human visual system is very good at extracting information from images, the sheer amount of data being produced creates the common problem of 'not enough time to look at everything'. Statistical techniques using computers enable researchers and clinicians to summarise large numbers of images rapidly so that patterns, trends, regions of activation etc. may be identified and quantified. Besides the amount of information, medical imaging systems also see beyond the visible light spectrum and are able to process information from a wide range of the electromagnetic spectrum.

Examples of medical imaging systems include conventional radiology (X-rays), angiography (imaging of a system of blood vessels using X-rays), positron emission tomography (PET), X-ray transmission-computed tomography (CT), magnetic resonance imaging (MRI), microscopy, single photon emission (computed) tomography (SPET or SPECT), spectroscopy and ultrasound imaging. Even electroencephalograms (EEGs) or magnetoencephalograms (MEGs) are examples of imaging systems, albeit with very poor spatial resolution when compared to MRI or PET.

An image is a two-dimensional function that depends on spatial coordinates, where the amplitude of the function represents the brightness or grey level of the image at a particular point. Individual elements of the image are known as picture elements, pixels for short. Images may be collected to form a three-dimensional data structure, or volume, where the individual elements are called voxels. This is common in, for example, MRI and PET, where an experiment on a single subject will involve acquiring information in three spatial dimensions and in time.

Traditional statistical techniques in image analysis include areas such as signal and morphological processing. Signal processing applications include image enhancement, image restoration, colour image processing, wavelets and compression. Morphological processing assumes that set theory may be applied to manipulate structures present in an image.

A relatively new area of research in imaging is the use of MRI in functional or pharmacological studies of the brain. Functional MRI (fMRI) is now well developed and seeks to associate brain functions (human or animal) with specific regions of the brain. Pharmacological MRI (phMRI) is relatively new and seeks to associate pharmacokinetics with specific regions of the (animal) brain. Although group studies are widespread, consider a single-subject analysis from a typical fMRI experiment. After data acquisition, a set of images associated with distinct slices of the brain is available for analysis. Each slice will have a time sequence associated with it; that is, the imaging experiment contains both spatial and temporal information. Given knowledge of the study design, the goal is to identify regions of the brain where significant activation was observed where activation is measured by the intensity of the signal observed in the fMRI experiment. Signal intensity is related to the ratio of oxygenated and deoxygenated blood locally in the brain.

The time course in the Figure shows a typical slice from an MRI experiment and the study design of on/off sequences for visual (dashed line) and auditory (dotted line) stimuli. Each voxel in the image has an associated time course, a mask that eliminates non-brain voxels is typically used to focus the data analysis. Linear regression, or more fully, fitting the GENERALISED LINEAR MODEL (GLM), is performed on each voxel using the experimental design, convolved with a function to model the haemo-dynamic response of the patient, as the independent variable. Trend removal is an important step and may be applied as a pre-processing step or by incorporating low-frequency terms explicitly in the GLM. The typical assumption of independence between observations is not true in fMRI data, methods such as pre-whitening, autoregressive modelling and least squares with adjustment for correlated errors are attempts to overcome the limitations of ordinary least squares.

Fitting the GLM to fMRI data may be performed on an individual voxel, on a cluster of voxels known as a region of interest (ROI) where the data are averaged in space to produce a single time course or on every brain voxel in the image. For the first two cases, standard theory for statistical inference on regression models may be applied. For the third case, techniques such as Gaussian random field theory, resampling (see BOOTSTRAP) and adjustments by multiple comparison procedures have been used. Regardless of which method is applied, a set of voxels is obtained where significant activation during the experiment was detected. Researchers then relate the images to the anatomical regions identified in the activation image, also known as a statistical parametric map, SPM.

Information from a group of patients may be combined or compared by first registering all images with a standard brain. The most common brain atlas used is the Talairach atlas. Then, a random effects or fixed effects model (see LINEAR MIXED EFFECTS MODELS) may be used to apply a statistical hypothesis test between groups of subjects in the experiment. *BW*

Glasbey, C.A. and Horgan, G.W. 1995: *Image analysis for the biological sciences*. Chichester: John Wiley & Sons. **Gonzalez, R.C. and Woods, R.E.** 2002: *Digital image processing*, 2nd edn. Englewood Cliffs, NJ: Prentice Hall. **Moonen, C.T.W. and Bandettini, P.A. (eds)** 1999: *Functional MRI*. Berlin: Springer-Verlag. **Serra, J.** 1982: *Image analysis and mathematical morphology*. London: Academic Press. **Worsley, K.J., Liao, C.H., Aston, J., Petre, V., Duncan, G.H., Morales, F. and Evans, A.C.** 2002: A general statistical approach for fMRI data. *NeuroImage* 15, 1, 1–15.

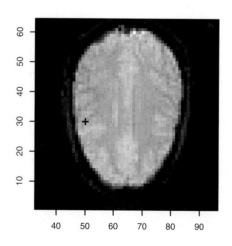

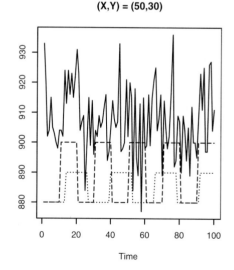

(X,Y) = (50,30)

Time

statistics in imaging *Example of an MRI slice (left) and voxel time course (right). The experimental design has been superimposed on the time course plot where the visual stimulation is shown by a dashed line and the audio stimulation is shown by a dotted line (data provided by the Brain Mapping Unit, Department of Psychiatry, University of Cambridge)*

StatXact A specialised software package for the exact analysis of small-sample categorical and nonparametric data with special emphasis on data in the form of contingency tables. The term 'small-sample' applies equally to datasets with only a few observations, to large but unbalanced datasets or to CONTINGENCY TABLES with zeros and small cell counts in some of the cells but large cell counts in other cells.

In these settings, StatXact produces exact P-VALUES and exact confidence intervals instead of relying on possibly unreliable large-sample theory for its inferences. The inference is based on generating permutation distributions of the appropriate test statistics in a conditional reference set.

Different reviews of StatXact are given by Lynch, Landis and Localio (1991), Wass (2000) and Oster (2002). The current version, StatXact 6, offers exact P-values for one, two and K-sample problems, 2×2, $2 \times c$ and $r \times c$ contingency tables and measures of association. The data may be either unstratified or stratified. Both independent and blocked samples are accommodated. This version computes the exact confidence interval for odds ratios that arise from 2×2 and $2 \times c$ contingency tables, as well as an exact confidence interval for the median shift parameter in an ordered $2 \times c$ contingency table. StatXact offers procedures that cater explicitly to binomial data, Poisson data, nominal categorical data, ordered categorical data, ordered correlated categorical data, continuous complete data and continuous right-censored data. For comparing two proportions (either from dependent or independent samples), StatXact provides the exact unconditional confidence interval for a difference in proportions or the ratio of two proportions and computes exact P-values for tests of equivalence and non-inferiority.

In addition to tools for exact inference, StatXact also provides exact power and sample-size calculations for study designs involving one, two or several binomial populations. In the two-binomial case, these features include exact power and sample-size calculations for designing non-inferiority and equivalence studies.

In case the computation of an exact P-value becomes infeasible due to the lack of either time or computing memory, StatXact produces an unbiased estimate of the exact P-value to at least two decimal digits of accuracy using efficient Monte Carlo simulation strategies (see MARKOV CHAIN MONTE CARLO). The user can arbitrarily increase the number of Monte Carlo simulations in order to increase the accuracy.

StatXact 6 runs on Microsoft Windows NT/2000/XP as a stand-alone product. In addition, a special version, StatXact PROCs for SAS Users, is available as external SAS procedures for both the Microsoft Windows and Unix operating systems. *CCo/PSe/CM/NP*

Lynch, J.C., Landis, J.R. and Localio, A.R. 1991: StatXact. *The American Statistician* 45, 2, 151–4. **Oster, R.A.** 2002: An examination of statistical software packages for categorical data analysis using exact methods. *The American Statistician* 56, 3, 235–46. **Wass, J.A.** 2000: StatXact 4 for Windows. *Biotech Software & Internet Report* 1, 1, 17–23.

stem-and-leaf plot Essentially, an enhanced HISTOGRAM in which the actual data values are retained for inspection. Observed values are each divided into a suit-

```
14 : 2
14 : 555
14 : 67777
14 : 889
15 : 000000111111
15 : 22222222222233333333333333333
15 : 4444444444445555555555555555555555
15 : 6666666666666666666666777777777777777777777
15 : 888888888888888888888888888888889999999999999999999
16 : 0000000000000000000011111111111111111111
16 : 22222222222222222222333333333333333333333333333333
16 : 44444444444444444455555555555555555555
16 : 666666666667777777
16 : 888888999999
17 : 00000000000111
17 : 333
17 : 4
17 : 67
17 : 88
```

stem-and-leaf plot *A stem-and-leaf plot for the heights in centimetres of 351 elderly women*

able 'stem' and 'leaf', for example, the tens figure and the units figure in many examples, and then all the leaves corresponding to a particular stem are listed (usually horizontally) next to the value of the stem. An example is shown in the Figure.

The plot combines the visual picture of the data provided by the histogram with a display of the ordered data values. The design of stem-and-leaf plots is discussed in Velleman and Hoaglin (1981). It is important to use a typeface for which each digit occupies equivalent space, otherwise a key feature of being 'a histogram on its side' is lost. *BSE*

Velleman, P.F. and Hoaglin, D.C. 1981: *Applications, basics, and computing of exploratory data analysis.* Boston: Duxbury.

stepwise regression See LOGISTIC REGRESSION, MULTIPLE LINEAR REGRESSION

stochastic process Any system that develops in accordance with probabilistic laws, usually in time but sometimes in space and possibly even in both time and space. For example, the spread of an epidemic is a stochastic process and its development can be tracked in time, across some terrain or at the conjunction of both time and position.

The constituents of a stochastic process are its *state*, X say, and its *indexing variable(s)*, s or t. The state is the primary measure of interest, such as number of individuals ill, while the indexing variable denotes either the time (t) or the position (s) at which the state is measured. A discrete indexing variable is usually shown as a subscript, but a continuous index appears within traditional function notation. For example, suppose that the state of the epidemic is the number of individuals who are ill. Then X_t would denote the number of individuals ill at time t if observations were taken at the start of each day, while $X(s)$ would denote the number of individuals ill at position s measured continuously in space. Of course, the state of the process can also be either discrete (e.g. number of individuals ill) or continuous (e.g. ECG reading of a cardiac patient).

An essential ingredient in a stochastic process is the *dependence* of either successive or neighbouring observations. Different assumptions about the dependence structure lead to different types of stochastic process that can be used as models for many observations collected in practice. The objective is usually to derive theoretical probabilities for the various states of the system and thus to use these probabilities either for predicting the future behaviour of the system or for gaining some understanding of its mechanism. Many practical systems can be modelled adequately by assuming a Markovian dependence structure, in which the probability distribution of X depends only on the most recent or neighbourly value. Standard stochastic processes that accord with such an assumption include random walks, Markov chains, branching processes, birth-and-death processes, queues and Poisson processes. Jones and Smith (2001) provide an accessible introduction to the mathematics of such processes. Some classical applications of stochastic models to medicine are described in Gurland (1964).

Successful uses of Markov models in medical contexts range in time and application from the planning of patient care (Davies, Johnson and Farrow, 1975) to resource provision (Davies and Davies, 1994) and the cost-effectiveness of vaccines (Byrnes, 2002). Many more examples can be found in journals such as *Health Care Management Science*. *WK*

Byrnes, G.B. 2002: A Markov model for sample size calculation and inference in vaccine cost-effectiveness studies. *Statistics in Medicine* 21, 3249–60. **Davies, R. and Davies, H.T.O.** 1994: Modelling patient flows and resource provision in health systems. *Omega, International Journal of Management Science* 22, 123–31. **Davies, R., Johnson, D. and Farrow, S.** 1975: Planning patient care with a Markov model. *Operational Research Quarterly* 26, 599–607. **Gurland, J. (ed.)** 1964: *Stochastic models in medicine and biology*. Madison, WI: University of Wisconsin Press. **Jones, P.W. and Smith, P.** 2001: *Stochastic processes, an introduction*. London: Arnold.

stratified randomisation   See RANDOMISATION

stratified sampling

Sampling within defined strata of some population. This should be carried out when the population contains easily identifiable subpopulations. If the sizes of the strata are different then proportional allocation should be used. If the standard deviations are known in advance then optimal or Neyman allocation can be used to minimise the variance of the estimate of the population mean. If they are unknown it is possible to use a pilot study to estimate the standard deviations.

The method is as follows. Define the strata that the population falls into. Decide if the strata are similar sizes and if the standard deviations are known. For similar sized strata use simple random sampling to select members of each stratum. If the sizes are different then the number in each stratum is proportional to stratum size. Then simple random sampling is used to obtain the correct number in each stratum. If the standard deviation is known in advance then for a fixed population size, n is obtained by choosing n_j so that:

$$\frac{n_j}{n} \approx \frac{N_j S_j}{\sum_{m=1}^{s} N_m S_m}$$

where N_j is the number in the stratum; S_j is the standard deviation of values of items within the strata; n is the fixed population size; n_j is the number to be chosen by simple random sampling from the stratum; and s is the number of strata.

Thornhill *et al.* (2000) used stratified sampling in a study of disability following head injury. The patients were stratified according to the Glasgow coma score. The mild and unclassified patients were further stratified by presenting hospital and a simple random sample was taken.

In general, if the population can be separated into distinguishable strata then the estimates from stratified sampling will be more precise than from a simple random sample, therefore it can be efficient. The disadvantages are that it can be difficult to choose the strata, it is not useful without homogeneous subgroups, it can require accurate information about the population and it can be expensive. *SLV*

Crawshaw, J. and Chambers, J. 1994: *A concise course in A level statistics*, 3rd edn. Cheltenham: Stanley Thornes Publishers Ltd. **Thornhill, S., Teasdale, G.M., Murray, G.D., McEwen, J., Roy, C.W. and Penny, K.I.** 2000: Disability in young people and adults one year after head injury: prospective cohort study. *British Medical Journal* 320, 1631–5. **Upton, G. and Cook, I.** 2002: *Dictionary of statistics*. Oxford: Oxford University Press.

structural equation modelling software

The three most commonly used packages for fitting structural equation models are EQS (www.mvsoft.com/ eqsorderforms.htm), LISREL (www.ssicentral.com/ prices/price.htm) and MPLUS (www.statmodel.com/ order.html).

All three allow the fitting of complex models relatively easily, although MPLUS is possibly the most flexible. Each package's website provides specific information on their capabilities, as well as availability and cost. *BSE*

structural equation models

The operational definition provided by Pearl (2000: 160) states: 'An equation $y = \beta x + \varepsilon$ is said to be *structural* if it is to be interpreted as follows: In an ideal experiment where we control X to x and any other set Z of variables (not containing X or Y) to z, the value of Y is given by $\beta x + \varepsilon$, where ε is not a function of the settings x and z.'

The key word here is 'control'. We are observing values of Y after manipulating or fixing the values of X. The model implies that the values of Y, in fact, are determined by the values of X. A structural equation model is a description of the causal effect of X on Y. It is a CAUSAL MODEL and the parameter β is a measure of the causal effect of X on Y. It should be clearly distinguished from a linear regression equation that simply describes the association between two random variables, X and Y. If we are able, in practice, to intervene and control the values of X (by random allocation, for example) then it is straightforward to use the resulting data to obtain a valid estimate of β. If, however, we do not have control of X, but can only observe the values of X and Y (and Z), as in an epidemiological or other type of observational study, for example, this does not invalidate the above operational definition, but the challenge for the data analyst is to find a valid (i.e. unbiased) estimate of the causal parameter β under these circumstances.

The equation $y = \beta x + \varepsilon$ is, of course, a description of a very simple structural model. It is common to collect data on several response variables (Ys) and several explanatory variables (Xs) and to construct a series of structural equations of the following form:

$$y_j = \Sigma_i \beta_i x_i + \Sigma_{k \neq j} \beta_k y_k + \varepsilon_j \quad (i = 1 \text{ to } I; j,k = 1 \text{ to } J) \quad (1)$$

in which several of the βs will be fixed to be zero, *a priori*. The others are to be estimated from the data. The form of the equations defined in (1) – i.e. the structural theory that determines the pattern of βs to be estimated and those fixed at zero – is determined by the investigator's prior knowledge or hypotheses concerning the causal processes generating the data. Quoting Byrne (1994: 3): 'Structural modeling (SEM) is a statistical methodology that takes a hypothesis-testing (i.e. confirmatory) approach to the multivariate analysis of a structural theory bearing on some phenomenon.'

Typically, SEM involves (a) the specification of a set of structural equations, (b) representation of these structural equations using a graphical model (a path diagram – see later) and (c) simultaneously fitting the set of structural equations to a given set of data in order to estimate the βs and to test the adequacy of the model. If the model fails to fit then the investigator may revise the model and try again. The success of the exercise is likely to be highly dependent on the quality of the investigator's prior knowledge of the likely causal mechanisms under test and how much thought he or she has given to the design of the study in the first place. Good design and subsequent statistical analyses require technical knowledge, skill and experience. For technical knowledge, readers are referred to introductory texts by Byrne (1994), Dunn, Everitt and Pickles (1993) and Shipley (2000) and to the advanced monograph by Bollen (1989). Discussion of SEM in the context of recent work on causal inference can be found in Pearl (2000) and, again, in Shipley (2000). Traditionally, SEM has concentrated on structural models for quantitative data, which are usually assumed to be multivariate normal. Extensions from the traditional linear structural equations (i.e. linear regression) to generalised linear structural equations are discussed by Skrondal and Rabe-Hesketh (2004).

It is frequently the case that we cannot measure constructs directly or at least not without considerable measurement error. This gives rise to the idea of LATENT VARIABLES. These are characteristics that are not directly observable. They may be straightforward concepts such as height, weight, amount of exposure to a known toxin or concentration of a given metabolite in blood or urine, but we explicitly acknowledge that they cannot be measured without error. The observed measurement is a manifest or indicator variable, while the corresponding unknown, but true, value is a latent variable. However, latent variables may be more abstract theoretical constructs that are introduced to explain covariance between manifest or indicator variables.

An example of this last type is the set of scores on a battery of cognitive tests that are assumed in some way to reflect a subject's cognitive ability or general intelligence. Another example could be a set of symptom severity scores (the manifest variables) that are assumed to be indicators of a patient's overall degree of depression (the latent variable). Typically, a data analyst will propose a formal measurement model (usually equivalent to some form of factor analysis representation) to relate the observed measurements with the underlying latent variables. We can then proceed to propose structural or causal hypotheses involving the latent variables instead of the fal-

lible (error-prone) indicators. We start, for example, with a covariance matrix for the observed variables and we fit a general structural equations model to this covariance or moments matrix and this procedure will involve the simultaneous fitting of the measurement equations for the relevant latent variables and their corresponding indicators and of the structural equations thought to reflect the assumed causal relationships between the latent variables. Specialist software packages are now widely available for such analyses (see SOFTWARE FOR STRUCTURAL EQUATIONS MODELLING).

Structural equation models are very often represented by a graphical structure known as a path diagram (see PATH ANALYSIS). In a path diagram, the proposed relationships between variables (whether manifest or observed) are represented either by a single-headed arrow (indicating the direction of a causal effect) or a double-headed one (indicating CORRELATION). The observed or manifest variables are usually placed within a rectangular square box, while latent variables are placed within an oval or a circle. Random measurement errors and residuals from structural equations, although they are strictly speaking latent variables, are not traditionally placed within a circle or oval. Path diagrams are very closely related to the graphical representations (directed acyclic graphs, or DAGS, for example (see GRAPHICAL MODELS)) that have relatively recently been developed elsewhere (see Pearl, 2000). Simple examples of path diagrams are shown in the Figures.

For an example, Permutt and Hebel (1989) describe a trial in which pregnant women were randomly allocated to receive encouragement to reduce or stop their cigarette smoking during pregnancy (the treatment group) or not (the control group) – indicated by the binary variable, Z. An intermediate outcome variable (X) was the amount of cigarette smoking recorded during pregnancy. The ultimate outcome (Y) was the birth weight of the newborn child. Smoking is likely to have been reduced in the group subject to encouragement, but also in the control group (but, presumably, to a lesser extent). There are also likely to be hidden confounders (e.g. other health promoting behaviours) that are associated both with mothers smoking during pregnancy and the children's birth weight. Smoking (X) is an endogenous treatment variable – the confounding will result in the residual from a structural equation model to explain the level of smoking by randomisation to receive encouragement being correlated with the residual from the structural equation linking observed levels of smoking to the birth weight of the child. We assume that the only effect of randomisation (Z) on outcome (Y) is through its effect on smoking (X) – that is, Z is an INSTRUMENTAL VARIABLE. Ignoring the intercept terms, the two structural equations are the following:

$$X = \gamma Z + D_X \quad \text{and} \quad Y = \beta X + D_Y$$

In fitting these two models to the appropriate data we acknowledge the correlation (ρ) between the residuals, D_X and D_Y. The overall model is illustrated by the first Figure (see page 338). Now, what if we acknowledge that smoking levels cannot be measured accurately and we decide to obtain two different measurements on each person in the trial ($X1$ and $X2$, say, being self-reported numbers of packs per day, obtained at 6 months and 8 months into the pregnancy)? The true level of smoking is now represented by the variable T_X. Our measurement model is represented by the two equations:

$$X1 = T_X + E1 \quad \text{and} \quad X2 = T_X + E2$$

We assume that the $E1$ and $E2$ measurement errors are uncorrelated and that there is no change in the true level of smoking between the two times. The revised structural equations now use T_X rather than X, as follows:

$$T_X = \gamma Z + D_X \quad \text{and} \quad Y = \beta T_X + D_Y$$

The corresponding path diagram is shown in the second Figure.

Note that not all of the model parameters implied by the model in the second figure can be estimated. The model is too complex for the data at hand. The model as a whole is said to be under-identified, but the good news is that we can still estimate β, the parameter most likely to be of interest to the investigator. Problems of under-identification are beyond the scope of this section, but are covered by any standard textbook on structural equation modelling.   *GD*

Bollen, K.A. 1989: *Structural equations with latent variables*. New York: John Wiley & Sons. **Byrne, B.M.** 1994: *Structural equation modeling with EQS and EQS/Windows*. Thousand Oaks, CA: Sage. **Dunn, G., Everitt, B.S. and Pickles, A.** 1993: *Modelling covariances and latent variables using EQS*. London: Chapman &

Hall. **Pearl, J.** 2000: *Causality*. Cambridge: Cambridge University Press. **Permutt, T. and Hebel, J.R.** 1989: Simultaneous-equation estimation in a clinical trial of the effect of smoking and birth weight. *Biometrics* 45, 619–22. **Shipley, B.** 2000: *Causes and correlation in biology*. Cambridge: Cambridge University Press. **Skrondal, A. and Rabe-Hesketh, S.** 2004: *Generalized latent variable modeling: multilevel, longitudinal and structural equations models*. Boca Raton: Chapman & Hall/CRC.

Student's t-distribution   See t-DISTRIBUTION

Student's t-test

William Sealy Gosset, who worked under the pseudonym of 'Student', developed the Student's t-test. The Student's t-test is commonly referred to merely as the t-test. The simplest use of the t-test is in comparing the mean of a sample to some specified population mean this is usually called the one-sample t-test. The t-test can be modified to compare the means of two independent samples (the two-sample t-test) and for paired data to compare the differences between the pairs (the paired t-test).

Student's t-test is a parametric test and certain assumptions are made about the data. These are that the observations within each group (with independent samples) or the differences (with paired samples) are approximately normally distributed and for the two-sample case we also require the two groups to have similar variances. If the sample data does not meet these assumptions then the analysis is seriously flawed. However, the t-test is 'robust' and is not greatly affected by a moderate failure to meet the assumptions.

The one-sample t-test can be used to compare the mean of a sample to a certain specified value. This value is usually the population MEAN. The null hypothesis states that there is no significant difference between the sample mean and the population mean and the alternative hypothesis states that there is a significant difference between the sample mean and the population mean. The assumption we make is that the data are a random sample of independent observations from an underlying normal distribution. The test statistic t is given by:

$$t = \frac{\text{sample mean} - \text{hypothesised mean}}{\text{standard error of sample mean}}$$

This is compared against the t-distribution with $n-1$ DEGREES OF FREEDOM, where n is the sample size. So t is the deviation of a normal variable from its hypothesised mean measured in standard error units. The standard error of the sample mean is given by $\sqrt{\left(s^2/n\right)}$ where s is the sample standard deviation.

For example, suppose BMI values for a sample of 25 people were measured and a mean value of 24.5 was found with a sample standard deviation of 2.5. To test if this sample mean BMI is significantly different from a population mean BMI of 26 we can use the one-sample t-test, where our null hypothesis is that there is no difference between the sample mean of 24.5 and the population mean of 26. This allows us to calculate the test statistic as follows:

$$t = \frac{24.5 - 26}{\sqrt{\dfrac{6.25}{25}}} = -3.0$$

Using tables for t-distribution with $(n-1) = 24$ degrees of freedom. We find a *P*-VALUE of 0.0062. The result is

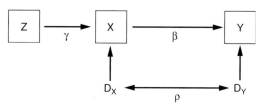

structural equation models *Path diagram to represent the structural equations model linking encouragement to stop smoking during pregnancy (Z), the amount smoked during pregnancy (X) and the birth weight of the child (Y). D_X and D_Y are randomly distributed residuals*

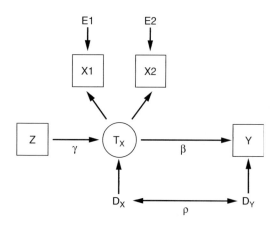

structural equation models *Path diagram to represent the structural equations model linking encouragement to stop smoking during pregnancy (Z), the true amount smoked during pregnancy (T_X) and the birth weight of the child (Y). D_X and D_Y are randomly distributed residuals. X1 and X2 are error-prone indicators of smoking, with uncorrelated measurement errors E1 and E2, respectively*

statistically significant and we therefore accept the alternative hypothesis that the mean BMI of the sample is significantly different from 26.

We can use the two-sample t-test to determine the statistical significance of an observed difference between the mean values of some variable between two subgroups or between separate populations. For example, we could look at the differences in heights between males and females. The test statistic for the two-sample t-test is given by:

$$t = \frac{\text{(difference in sample means)} - \text{(difference in hypothesised means)}}{\text{standard error of the difference in the two sample means}}$$

Frequently the null hypothesis of interest is whether the two groups have equal means and the corresponding two-sided alternative hypothesis is that the means are in fact different. For example, when comparing the mean outcome for two different treatments is the difference in means observed a statistically significant one. In this case the test statistic reduces to:

$$t = \frac{\text{difference in the two sample means}}{\text{standard error of the difference in the two sample means}}$$

This is then compared to the t-distribution with $n_1 + n_2 - 2$ degrees of freedom, where n_1 is the sample size for the first group and n_2 is the sample size for the second group. The standard error of the difference in the two-sample means is given by

$$SE(\overline{x}_1 - \overline{x}_2) = \sqrt{\frac{s_p^2}{n_1} + \frac{s_p^2}{n_2}}$$

$$\text{where } s_p = \frac{(n_1 - 1)\, s_1^2 + (n_2 - 1)s_2^2}{n_1 + n_2 - 2}$$

s_1 and s_2 are the standard deviations for groups one and two respectively.

For the paired t-test, the data are dependent, i.e. there is a one-to-one correspondence between the values in the two samples. Paired data can occur from two measurements on the same person, for example, before and after treatment or the same subject measured at different times. It is incorrect to analyse paired data ignoring the pairing in such circumstances, as important information is lost. Some factors you do not control in the experiment will affect the before and the after measurements equally, so they will not affect the difference between before and after. By looking only at the differences, a paired t-test corrects for these factors.

The two-sample paired t-test usually tests the null hypothesis that the population mean of the paired differences of the two samples is zero. We assume that the paired differences are independent. To perform the paired t-test we calculate the difference between each set of pairs and then perform a one-sample t-test on the differences with the null hypothesis that the population mean of the differences is equal to zero.   *MMB*

Altman, D.G. 1991: *Practical statistics for medical research.* London: Chapman & Hall.

subgroup analysis

A form of analysis often employed in CLINICAL TRIALS in an attempt to identify particular subgroups of patients for whom a treatment works better (or worse) than for the overall patient population. For example, does a treatment work better for men than for women? Such a question is a natural one for clinicians

to ask since they do not treat 'average' patients and, when confronted with a female patient with a certain condition, would like to know whether the accepted treatment for the condition works, say, less well for women.

Assessing whether the effect of treatment varies according to the value of one or more patient characteristics is relatively straightforward from a statistical viewpoint involving nothing more than testing a treatment by covariate interaction. But many statisticians would caution against such analyses and, if undertaken at all, suggest that they are interpreted extremely cautiously in the spirit of 'exploration' rather than anything more formal. The reasons for such caution are not difficult to identify.

First, trials can rarely provide sufficient power to detect such subgroup/interaction effects; clinical trials accrue sufficient participants to provide adequate precision for estimating quantities of primary interest, usually overall treatment effects. Confining attention to subgroups almost always results in estimates of inadequate precision. A trial just large enough to evaluate an overall treatment effect reliably will almost inevitably lack precision for evaluating differential treatment effects between different population subgroups.

Second, RANDOMISATION ensures that the overall treatment groups in a clinical trial are likely to be comparable. Subgroups may not enjoy the same degree of balance in patient characteristics.

And, finally, there are often many possible prognostic factors in the baseline data, for example, age, gender, race, type or stage of disease, from which to form subgroups, so that analyses may quickly degenerate into 'data dredging', from which arises the potential for post-hoc emphasis on the subgroup analysis giving results of most interest to the investigator, with undue emphasis given to results deemed 'statistically significant' contributing, in turn, to a preponderance of '$p < 0.05$' results published in the medical literature (an excess of false positive findings, therefore).

Other potential dangers of subgroup analysis can be found in detail in Pocock *et al.* (2002).   *BSE*

Pocock, S.J., Assmann, S.E., Enos, L.E. and Kasten, L.E. 2002: Subgroup analysis, covariate adjustment and baseline comparisons in clinical trial reporting: current practice and problems. *Statistics in Medicine* 21, 2917–30.

sufficient-component cause model

See CAUSAL MODELS

summary measure analysis

A relatively straightforward approach to the analysis of LONGITUDINAL DATA, in which the repeated measurements of a response variable made on each individual in the study are reduced in some way to a single number that is considered to capture an essential feature of the response over time. In this way, the multivariate nature of the repeated observations is transformed to a univariate measure. The approach has been in use for many years – see, for example, Oldham (1962) and Matthews *et al.* (1989). The most important consideration when applying a summary measure analysis is the choice of a suitable summary measure, a choice that needs to be made before any data are collected. The measure chosen needs to be relevant to the particular questions of interest in the study and in the broader scientific context in which the study takes place. A wide range of

summary measure analysis *Possible summary measures (from Matthews et al., 1989)*

Type of data	Question of interest	Summary measure
Peaked	Is overall value of outcome variable the same in different groups?	Overall mean (equal time intervals) or area under curve (unequal intervals)
Peaked	Is maximum (minimum) response different between groups?	Maximum (minimum) value
Peaked	Is time to maximum (minimum) response different between groups?	Time to maximum (minimum) response
Growth	Is rate of change of outcome different between groups?	Regression coefficient
Growth	Is eventual value of outcome different between groups?	Final value of outcome or difference between last and first values or percentage change between first and last values
Growth	Is response in one group delayed relative to the other?	Time to reach a particular value (e.g. a fixed percentage of baseline)

summary measures has been proposed as shown in the first Table. According to Frisson and Pocock (1992), the average response over time is often likely to be the most relevant, particularly in CLINICAL TRIALS.

Having chosen a suitable summary measure, analysis will involve nothing more complicated than the application of STUDENT'S t-TEST or calculation of a CONFIDENCE INTERVAL for the group difference when two groups are being compared or a one-way analysis of variance when there are more than two groups. If considered more appropriate because of the distributional properties of the selected summary measure, then analogous NONPARAMETRIC METHODS might be used.

The summary measure approach can be illustrated using the data shown in the second Table that come from a study of alcohol dependence. Two groups of subjects, one with severe dependence and one with moderate dependence on alcohol, had their salsolinol excretion levels (in millimoles) recorded on four consecutive days.

Using the mean of the four measurements available for each subject as the summary measure leads to the results

summary measure analysis *Salsolinol excretion data*

Subject	Day 1	2	3	4
Group 1 (moderate dependence)				
1	0.33	0.70	2.33	3.20
2	5.30	0.90	1.80	0.70
3	2.50	2.10	1.12	1.01
4	0.98	0.32	3.91	0.66
5	0.39	0.69	0.73	3.86
6	0.31	6.34	0.63	3.86
Group 2 (severe dependence)				
7	0.64	0.70	1.00	1.40
8	0.73	1.85	3.60	2.60
9	0.70	4.20	7.30	5.40
10	0.40	1.60	1.40	7.10
11	2.50	1.30	0.70	0.70
12	7.80	1.20	2.60	1.80
13	1.90	1.30	4.40	2.80
14	0.50	0.40	1.10	8.10

summary measure analysis *Results from using the mean as a summary measure for the data in the second table*

	Moderate	Severe
Mean	1.80	2.49
sd	0.60	1.09
n	6	8

$t = -1.40$, df = 12, $P = 0.19$
95% CI: $[-1.77, 0.39]$

shown in the third Table. There is no evidence of a group difference in salsolinol excretion levels.

A possible alternative to the use of the mean as summary measure is to use the maximum excretion rate recorded over the four days. Applying the WILCOXON RANK SUM TEST to this summary measure results in a test statistic of 36 and associated P-VALUE of 0.28.

The summary measure approach to the analysis of longitudinal data can accommodate MISSING DATA but the implicit assumption is that these are missing completely at random (see DROPOUTS). *BSE*

[See also AREA UNDER CURVE]

Frison, L. and Pocock, S.J. 1992: Repeated measures in clinical trials: analysis using mean summary statistics and its implications for design. *Statistics in Medicine* 11, 1685–704. **Matthews, J.N.S., Altman, D.G., Campbell, M.J. and Royston, P.** 1989: Analysis of serial measurements in medical research. *British Medical Journal* 300, 23–35. **Oldham, P.D.** 1962: A note on the analysis of repeated measurements of the same subjects. *Journal of Chronic Disorders* 15, 969–77.

support vector machines Algorithms for learning complex classification and regression functions, belonging to the general family of 'kernel methods' discussed later. Their computational and statistical efficiency recently made them one of the tools of choice in certain biological data-mining applications.

SVMs work by embedding the data into a feature space by means of kernel functions (the so-called 'kernel trick'). In the binary classification case, a separating hyperplane that separates the two classes is sought in this feature space. New data points will be classified into one of both classes according to their position with respect to this

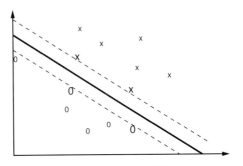

support vector machines *A typical SVM*

hyperplane. SVMs owe their name to their property of isolating a (often small) subset of data points called 'support vectors', which have interesting theoretical properties.

The SVM approach has several important virtues, when compared with earlier approaches: the choice of the hyperplane is founded on statistical arguments; the hyperplane can be found by solving a convex (quadratic) optimisation problem, which means that training an SVM is not subject to local minima; when a non-linear kernel function is used, the hyperplane in the feature space can correspond to a complex (non-linear) decision boundary in the original data domain. Even more interestingly, kernel functions can be defined not only on vectorial data but on virtually any kind of data, making it possible to classify strings, images, trees or nodes in a graph; the classification of unseen data points is generally computationally cheap and depends on the number of support vectors.

First introduced in 1992, support vector machines are now one of the standard tools in pattern recognition applications, mostly due to their computational efficiency and statistical stability. In recent years, extensions of this algorithm to deal with a number of important data analysis tasks have been proposed, resulting in the general family of 'kernel methods' (Shawe-Taylor and Cristianini, 2004) (see DENSITY ESTIMATIONS).

The kinds of relation detected by kernel methods include classifications, regressions, clustering (see CLUSTER ANALYSIS IN MEDICINE), principal components (see PRINCIPAL COMPONENT ANALYSIS), canonical correlations and many others. In the same way as with SVMs, the kernel trick allows to apply these methods in a feature space that is induced by this kernel, making kernel methods applicable to virtually any kind of data.

Elegantly, development of kernel methods can always be decomposed into two modular steps: the kernel design on the one hand, and the choice of the algorithm on the other hand. The kernel design part implicitly defines the feature space, which should contain all available information that is relevant for the problem at hand. The choice of the algorithm (that needs to be written in terms of kernels) can be done independently from the kernel design.

As with SVMs, most kernel methods reduce their training phase to optimising a convex cost function or to solving a simple eigenvalue problem, hence avoiding one of the main computational pitfalls of NEURAL NETWORKS. However, since they often implicitly make use of very high dimensional spaces, kernel methods run the risk of overfitting. For this reason, their design needs to incorporate principles of statistical learning theory, that help

identify the crucial parameters that need to be controlled in order to avoid this risk (see Vapnik, 1995). For further reference on SVMs, see Cristianini and Shawe-Taylor (2000). *NC/TDB*

Cristianini, N. and Shawe-Taylor, J. 2000: *An introduction to support vector machines.* Cambridge: Cambridge University Press (www.support-vector.net). **Shawe-Taylor, J. and Cristianini, N.** 2004: *Kernel methods for pattern analysis.* Cambridge: Cambridge University Press (www.kernel-methods.net). **Vapnik, V.** 1995: *The nature of statistical learning theory.* New York: Springer.

surrogate endpoints   See ENDPOINTS

survival analysis – an overview   Methods for the analysis of time-to-event data, for example, survival times. Survival data occur when the outcome of interest is the time from a well-defined time origin to the occurrence of a particular event or endpoint. If the endpoint is the death of a patient the resulting data are, literally, survival times. However, other endpoints are possible, for example, the time to relief or recurrence of symptoms. Such observations are often referred to as time-to-event data although survival data is commonly used as a generic term. Standard statistical methodology is not usually appropriate for such data, for two main reasons.

First, the distribution of survival time in general is likely to display positive SKEWNESS and so assuming normality for an analysis (as done for example by a t-test or a regression) is probably not reasonable.

Second, more critical than doubts about normality, however, is the presence of censored observations, where the survival time of an individual is referred to as censored when the endpoint of interest has not yet been reached (more precisely right censored). For true survival times this might be because the data from a study are analysed at a time point when some participants are still alive. Another reason for censored event times is that an individual might have been lost to follow-up for reasons unrelated to the event of interest, for example due to moving to a location which cannot be traced or due to accidental death (see DROPOUTS). When censoring occurs all that is known is that the actual, but unknown, survival time is larger than the censored survival time.

Specialised statistical techniques developed to analyse such censored and possibly skewed outcomes are known as survival analysis. An important assumption made in standard survival analysis is that the censoring is non-informative, that is that the actual survival time of an individual is independent of any mechanism that causes that individual's survival time to be censored. For simplicity, this description also concentrates on techniques for continuous survival times – the analysis of discrete survival times is described in Collett (2003).

As an example, consider data that arise from a double-blind, randomised controlled CLINICAL TRIAL (RCT) to compare treatments for prostate cancer (placebo vs 1.0 mg of diethylstilbestrol (DES) administered daily by mouth). The full dataset is given in Andrews and Herzberg (1985) and the first Table (see page 342) shows the first seven of a subset of 38 patients used here and discussed in Collett (2003).

In this study, the time of origin was the date on which a cancer sufferer was randomised to a treatment and the

survival analyisis *Survival times of prostate cancer patients*

Patient number	Treatment (1= placebo, 2 = DES)	Survival time (months)	Status (1 = died, 0 = censored)	Age (years)	Serum haem. (gm/100 ml)	Size of tumour (cm²)	Gleason index
1	1	65	0	67	13.4	34	8
2	2	61	0	60	14.6	4	10
3	2	60	0	77	15.6	3	8
4	1	58	0	64	16.2	6	9
5	2	51	0	65	14.1	21	9
6	1	51	0	61	13.5	8	8
7	1	14	1	73	12.4	18	11
...	...	...	...	...	...	...	...

endpoint is the death of a patient from prostate cancer. The survival times of patients who died from other causes or were lost during the follow-up process are regarded as right censored. The 'status' variable in the first table takes the value unity if the patient has died from prostate cancer and zero if the survival time is censored. In addition to survival times, a number of prognostic factors were recorded, namely the age of the patient at trial entry, their serum haemoglobin level in gm/100 ml, the size of their primary tumour in cm² and the value of a combined index of tumour stage and grade (the Gleason index with larger values indicating more advanced tumours). The main aim of this study was to compare the survival experience between the two treatment groups.

In general, to describe survival two functions of time are of central interest – the *survival function* and the *hazard function*. These are described in some detail next. The survival function $S(t)$ is defined as the probability that an individual's survival time, T, is greater than or equal to time t, i.e.:

$$S(t) = \text{Prob}(T \geq t)$$

The graph of $S(t)$ against t is known as the survival curve. The survival curve can be thought of as a particular way of displaying the frequency distribution of the event times, rather than by, say, a HISTOGRAM. When there are no censored observations in the sample of survival times, the sur-

vival function can be estimated by the empirical survivor function:

$$\hat{S}(t) = \frac{\text{Number of individuals with survival times} \geq t}{\text{Number of individuals in the data set}}$$

Since every subject is 'alive' at the beginning of the study and no one is observed to survive longer than the largest of the observed survival times then:

$$\hat{S}(0) = 1 \quad \text{and} \quad \hat{S}(t_{\max}) = 0.$$

Furthermore the estimated survivor function is assumed constant between two adjacent death times, so that a plot of $\hat{S}(t)$ against t is a step function that decreases immediately after each 'death'.

This simple method cannot be used when there are censored observations since the method does not allow for information provided by an individual whose survival time is censored before time t to be used in the computing of the estimate at t. The most commonly used method for estimating the survival function for survival data containing censored observations is the product-limit or KAPLAN-MEIER ESTIMATOR. The essence of this approach is the use of a product of a series of conditional probabilities. One alternative estimator for censored survival times, derived differently but in practice often similar, is the Nelson-Aalen estimator. Approximate standard errors and pointwise symmetric or asymmetric confidence intervals for the

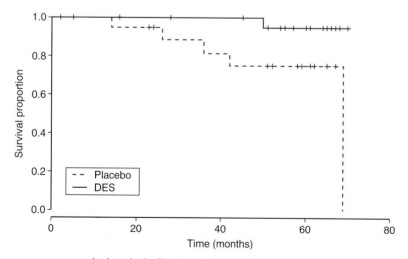

survival analysis *Display of Kaplan-Meier survivor curves*

survival function at a given time can be derived to determine the precision of the estimator – details are given in Collett (2003).

The Kaplan-Meier estimators of the survivor curves for the two prostate cancer treatments are shown graphically in the Figure on page 342. The survivor curves are step functions that decrease at the time points when participants died of the cancer. The censored observations in the data are indicated by the 'cross' marks on the curves. In our patient sample there is approximately a difference of 20% in the proportion surviving for at least 50 to 60 months between the treatment groups.

Since the distribution of survival times tends to be positively skewed the median is the preferred summary measure of location. The median survival time is the time beyond which 50% of the individuals in the population under study are expected to survive and, once the survivor function has been estimated by $\hat{S}(t)$, can be estimated by the smallest observed survival time, t_{50}, for which the value of the estimated survivor function is less than 0.5. The estimated median survival time can be read from the survival curve by finding the smallest value on the x axis for which the survival proportion reaches less than 0.5. The figure shows that the median survival in the placebo group can be estimated as 69 years while an estimate for the DES group is not available since survival exceeds 50% throughout the study period. A similar procedure can be used to estimate other percentiles of the distribution of the survival times and approximate confidence intervals can be found once the variance of the estimated percentile has been derived from the variance of the estimator of the survivor function.

In the analysis of survival data, it is often of some interest to assess which periods have the highest and which the lowest chance of death (or whatever the event of interest happens to be) among those people alive at the time. The appropriate quantity for such risks is the hazard function, $h(t)$, defined as the (scaled) probability that an individual experiences an event in a small time interval δt, given that the individual has survived up to the beginning of the interval. The hazard function therefore represents the instantaneous death rate for an individual surviving to time t. It is a measure of how likely an individual is to experience an event as a function of the age of the individual. The hazard function may remain constant, increase or decrease with time or take some more complex form. The hazard function of death in human beings, for example, has a 'bathtub' shape. It is relatively high immediately after birth, declines rapidly in the early years and then remains relatively constant until beginning to rise during late middle age.

A Kaplan-Meier type estimator of the hazard function is given by the proportion of individuals experiencing an event in an interval per unit time, given that they have survived to the beginning of the interval. However, the estimated hazard function is generally considered 'too noisy' for practical use. Instead, the cumulative or integrated hazard function, which is derived from the hazard function by summation, is usually displayed to describe the change in hazard over time.

In addition to comparing survivor functions graphically, a more formal statistical test for a group difference is often required in order to compare survival times analytically. In the absence of censoring a nonparametric test, such as

the Mann-Whitney test could be used (see MANN-WHITNEY RANK SUM TEST). In the presence of censoring the log-rank or Mantel-Haenszel test is the most commonly used non-parametric test (see MANTEL-HAENSZEL METHODS). It tests the null hypothesis that the population survival functions $S_1(t)$, $S_2(t)$, ..., $S_k(t)$ are the same in k groups.

Briefly, the test is based on computing the expected number of deaths for each observed 'death' time in the dataset, assuming that the chances of dying, given that subjects are at risk, are the same in the groups. The total number of expected deaths is then computed for each group by adding the expected number of deaths for each failure time. The test finally compares the observed number of deaths in each group with the expected number of deaths using a CHI-SQUARE TEST with $k - 1$ degrees of freedom (see Hosmer and Lemeshow, 1999).

The log-rank test statistic, X^2, weights contributions from all failure times equally. Several alternative test statistics have been proposed that give differential weights to the failure times. For example, the generalised Wilcoxon test (or Breslow test) uses weights equal to the number at risk. For the prostate cancer data in the first table the log-rank test ($X^2 = 4.4$ on 1 degree of freedom, $P = 0.036$) detects a significant group difference in favour of longer survival on DES treatment while the Wilcoxon test, that puts relatively more weight on differences between the survival curves at earlier times, fails to reach significance at the 5% test level ($X^2 = 3.4$ on 1 degree of freedom, $P = 0.065$).

Modelling survival times is useful especially when there are several explanatory variables to consider. For example, in the prostate cancer trial patients were randomised to treatment groups so that the theoretical distributions of the diagnostic factors were the same in the two groups. However, empirical distributions in the patient sample might still vary and if the prognostic variables are related to survival they might confound the group difference. A survival analysis that 'adjusts' the group difference for the prognostic factor(s) is needed. The main approaches used for modelling the effects of covariates on survival can be divided roughly into two classes – models based on assuming proportional hazards and models for direct effects on the survival times.

The main technique used for modelling survival times is due to Cox (1972) and known as the *proportional hazards model* or, more simply, Cox's regression (see COX'S REGRESSION MODEL). In essence, the technique acts as the analogue of multiple regression for survival times containing censored observations, for which multiple regression itself is clearly not suitable. Briefly, the procedure models the hazard function and central to it is the assumption that the hazard functions for two individuals at any point in time are proportional, the so-called proportional hazards assumption. In other words, if an individual has a risk of 'death' at some initial time point that is twice as high as another individual, then at all later times the risk of death remains twice as high. Cox's model is made up of an unspecified baseline hazard function, $h_0(t)$, which is then multiplied by a suitable function of an individual's explanatory variable values, to give the individual's hazard function. The interpretation of the regression parameter of the ith covariate, β_i, is that $\exp(\beta_i)$ gives the hazard or incidence rate change associated with an increase of one unit in the ith covariate, all other explanatory variables remaining constant.

Cox's regression is considered a semi-parametric procedure because the baseline hazard function, $h_0(t)$, and by implication the probability distribution of the survival times does not have to be specified. The baseline hazard is left unspecified; a different parameter is essentially included for each unique survival time. These parameters can be thought of as NUISANCE PARAMETERS whose purpose is merely to control the parameters of interest for any changes in the hazard over time.

Cox's regression can be used to model the prostate cancer survival data. To start with a model containing only the single treatment factor is fitted. The estimated regression coefficient of a DES indicator variable is -1.98 with a standard error of 1.1. This translates into an (unadjusted) hazard ratio of $\exp(-1.98) = 0.138$. In other words, DES treatment is estimated to reduce the hazard of immediate death by 86.2% relative to placebo treatment. According to a likelihood ratio (LR) test, the unadjusted effect of DES is statistically significant at the 5% level ($X^2 = 4.55$ on 1 degree of freedom, $P = 0.033$).

For the prostate cancer data, it is of interest to determine the effect of DES after controlling for the other prognostic variables. Likelihood ratio tests showed that dropping age and serum haemoglobin from a model that contains the treatment indicator variable and all four prognostic variables did not significantly worsen the model fit (at the 10% level) and the fit of the final model is shown in the second table. After adjusting for the effects of tumour size and stage the hazard reduction for DES relative to placebo treatment is reduced to 67.1% and no longer statistically significant (LR test: $X^2 = 0.48$ on 1 degree of freedom, $P = 0.49$). Both tumour size and Gleason index have a hazard ratio above unity indicating that increases in tumour size and advanced stages are estimated to increase the chance of death.

Cox's model does not require specification of the probability distribution of the survival times. The hazard function is not restricted to a specific form and as a result the semi-parametric model has considerable flexibility and is widely used. However, if the assumption of a particular probability distribution for the data is valid, inferences based on such an assumption are more precise. For example, estimates of hazard ratios or median survival times will have smaller standard errors.

A fully parametric proportional hazards model makes the same assumptions as Cox's regression but in addition also assumes that the baseline hazard function, $h_0(t)$, can be parameterised according to a specific model for the distribution of the survival times. Survival time distributions that can be used for this purpose, i.e. that have the pro-

portional hazards property, are principally the exponential, Weibull and Gompertz distributions. Different distributions imply different shapes of the hazard function, and in practice the distribution that best describes the functional form of the observed hazard function is chosen – for details see Collett (2003).

A family of fully parametric models that accommodate direct multiplicative effects of covariates on survival times and hence do not have to rely on proportional hazards are *accelerated failure time models*. A wider range of survival time distributions possesses the accelerated failure time property, principally the exponential, Weibull, log-logistic, generalised gamma or LOGNORMAL DISTRIBUTIONS. In addition, this family of parametric models includes distributions (e.g. the log-logistic distribution) that model unimodal hazard functions while all distributions suitable for the proportional hazards model imply hazard functions that increase or decrease monotonically. The latter property might be limiting, for example for modelling the hazard of dying after a complicated operation that peaks in the post-operative period.

The general accelerated failure time model for the effects of p explanatory variables, $x_1, x_2, \ldots, x_p$, can be represented as a log-linear model for survival time, T, namely:

$$\ln(T) = \alpha_0 + \sum_{i=1}^{p} \alpha_i x_i + \text{error}$$

where $\alpha_1, \ldots, \alpha_p$ are the unknown coefficients of the explanatory variables and α_0 an intercept parameter. The parameter α_i reflects the effect that the ith covariate has on log-survival time with positive values indicating that the survival time increases with increasing values of the covariate and vice versa. In terms of the original timescale, the model implies that the explanatory variables measured on an individual act multiplicatively and so affect the speed of progression to the event of interest.

The interpretation of the parameter α_i then is that $\exp(\alpha_i)$ gives the factor by which any survival time percentile (e.g. the median survival time) changes per unit increase in x_i, all other explanatory variables remaining constant. Expressed differently, the probability, that an individual with covariate value $x_i + 1$ survives beyond t, is equal to the probability, that an individual with value x_i survives beyond $\exp(-\alpha_i)t$. Hence $\exp(-\alpha_i)$ determines the change in the speed with which individuals proceed along the timescale and the coefficient is known as the acceleration factor of the ith covariate.

Software packages typically use the log-linear formulation. The regression coefficients from fitting a log-logistic accelerated failure time model to the prostate cancer survival times using treatment, size of tumour and Gleason index as predictor variables are shown in the third table.

survival analysis *Parameter estimates from Cox regression of survival on treatment group, tumour size and Gleason index*

Predictor variable	Effect estimate			95% CI for $\exp(\beta)$	
	Regression coefficient ($\hat{\beta}$)	Standard error ($\sqrt{\text{var}(\hat{\beta})}$)	Hazard ratio ($\exp(\hat{\beta})$)	Lower limit	Upper limit
DES	−1.113	1.203	0.329	0.031	3.47
Tumour size	0.0826	0.048	1.086	0.990	1.19
Gleason index	0.7102	0.338	2.034	1.049	3.95

survival analysis *Parameter estimates from log-logistic accelerated failure time model of survival on treatment group, tumour size and Gleason index*

Predictor variable	Effect estimate			95% CI for $\exp(-\alpha)$	
	Regression coefficient ($\hat{\alpha}$)	Standard error ($\sqrt{\mathrm{var}(\hat{\alpha})}$)	Acceleration factor ($\exp(-\hat{\alpha})$)	Lower limit	Upper limit
DES	0.628	0.550	0.534	0.182	1.568
Tumour size	−0.031	0.022	1.031	0.988	1.077
Gleason index	−0.335	0.203	1.393	0.939	2.080

The negative regression coefficients suggest that the survival times tend to be shorter for larger value of tumour size and Gleason index. The positive regression coefficient for the DES treatment indicator suggests that survival times tend to be longer for individuals assigned to the active treatment after adjusting for the effects of tumour size and stage. The estimated acceleration factor for an individual in the DES group compared with the placebo group is $\exp(-0.628) = 0.534$, i.e. DES is estimated to slow down the progression of the cancer by a factor of about 2. While possibly clinically relevant, this effect is, however, not statistically significant (LR test: $X^2 = 1.57$ on 1 degree of freedom, $P = 0.211$).

In summary, survival analysis is a powerful tool for analysing time-to-event data. The classical techniques Kaplan-Meier estimation, Cox's regression and accelerated failure time modelling are implemented in most general purpose statistical packages, with the S-PLUS package having particularly extensive facilities for fitting and assessing non-standard Cox models.

The area is complex and one of active current research. For more recent advances such as frailty models to include random effects, multistate models to model different transition rates and models for competing risks the reader is referred to Andersen (2002), Crowder (2001) and Hougaard (2000).   *SL*

Andersen, P.K. (ed.) 2002: *Multistate models, statistical methods in medical research 11.* London: Arnold. **Andrews, D.F. and Herzberg, A.M.** 1985: *Data.* New York: Springer. **Collett, D.** 2003: *Modelling survival data in medical research*, 2nd edn. London: Chapman & Hall/CRC. **Cox, D.R.** 1972: Regression models and life tables (with discussion). *Journal of the Royal Statistical Society Series B* 74, 187–220. **Crowder, K.J.** 2001: *Classical competing risks.* Boca Raton: Chapman & Hall/CRC. **Hosmer, D.W. and Lemeshow, S.** 1999: *Applied survival analysis.* New York: John Wiley & Sons. **Hougaard, P.** 2000: *Analysis of multivariate survival data.* New York: Springer.

survival curve See KAPLAN-MEIER ESTIMATION, SURVIVAL ANALYSIS

survival function See SURVIVAL ANALYSIS

systematic reviews and meta-analysis An approach to the combining of results from the many individual CLINICAL TRIALS of a particular treatment or therapy that may have been carried out over the course of time. Such a procedure is needed because individual trials are rarely large enough to answer the questions we want to answer as reliably as we would like. In practice, most trials are too small for adequate conclusions to be drawn about potentially small advantages of particular therapies. Advocacy of large trials is a natural response to this situa-

tion, but it is not always possible to launch very large trials before therapies become widely accepted or rejected prematurely. An alternative possibility is to examine the results from all relevant trials, a process that involves two components, one *qualitative*, i.e. the extraction of the relevant literature and description of the available trials, in terms of their relevance and methodological strengths and weaknesses (the *systematic review*), and the other *quantitative*, i.e. mathematically combining results from different studies, even on occasions when these studies have used different measures to assess outcome. This component is known as a *meta-analysis* (Normand, 1999).

Informal synthesis of evidence from different studies is, of course, nothing new, but it is now generally accepted that meta-analysis gives the systematic review an objectivity that is inevitably lacking in the classical review article and can also help the process to achieve greater precision and generalisability of findings than any single study. There remain sceptics who feel that the conclusions from a meta-analysis often go far beyond what the technique and the data justify, but despite such concerns, the demand for systematic reviews of healthcare interventions has developed rapidly during the last decade, initiated by the widespread adoption of the principles of EVIDENCE-BASED MEDICINE both among healthcare practitioners and policymakers. Such reviews are now increasingly used as a basis for both individual treatment decisions and the funding of healthcare and healthcare research worldwide. This growth in systematic reviews is reflected in the current state of the COCHRANE COLLABORATION database containing as it does more than 1200 complete systematic reviews, with a further 1000 due to be added soon.

Systematic reviews and the subsequent meta-analysis have a number of aims: to review systematically the available evidence from a particular research area; to provide quantitative summaries of the results from each study; to combine the results across studies if appropriate – such combination of results leads to greater statistical power in estimating treatment effects; to assess the amount of variability between studies; to estimate the degree of benefit associated with a particular study treatment; to identify study characteristics associated with particularly effective treatments.

Ideally, the trials included in a systematic review should be clinically homogeneous. For example, they might all study a similar type of patient for a similar duration with the same treatment in the two arms of each trial. In practice, of course, the trials included are far more likely to differ in some aspects, such as eligibility criteria, duration of treatment, length of follow-up and how ancillary care is used. On occasions, even treatment itself may not be identical in all the trials. This implies that, in most circumstances, the objective of a systematic review *cannot* be equated with that of a single large trial, even if that trial has wide eligibility. While a single trial focuses on the effect of a specific treatment in specific situations, a meta-analysis aims for a more generalisable conclusion about the effect of a generic treatment policy in a wider range of areas.

When the trials included in a systematic review do differ in some of their components, therapeutic effects may very well be different, but these differences are likely to be in the *size* of the effects rather than their direction. It would, after all, be extraordinary if treatment effects were exactly the same when estimated from trials in different countries, in different populations, in different age groups or under different treatment regimens. If the studies were big enough it would be possible to measure these differences reliably, but in most cases this will not be possible. But meta-analysis allows the investigation of sources of possible heterogeneity in the results from different trials as we shall see later and discourages the common, simplistic and often misleading interpretation that the results of individual clinical trials are in conflict because some are labelled 'positive' (i.e. statistically significant) and others 'negative' (i.e. statistically non-significant). A systematic approach to synthesising information can often both estimate the degree of benefit from a particular therapy and whether the benefit depends on specific characteristics of the studies.

The selection of studies is the greatest single concern in applying meta-analysis and there are at least three important components of the selection process, namely, breadth, quality and representativeness (Pocock, 1996). Breadth relates to the decision as to whether to study a very specific narrow question (e.g. the same drug, disease and setting for studies following a common protocol) or a more generic problem (e.g. a broad class of treatments for a range of conditions in a variety of settings). The broader the meta-analysis, the more difficulty there is in interpreting the combined evidence as regards future policy. Consequently, the broader the meta-analysis, the more it needs to be interpreted qualitatively rather than quantitatively.

Quality and reliability of a systematic review is dependent on the quality of the data in the included studies, although criticisms of meta-analyses for including original studies of questionable quality are typical examples of shooting the messenger who bears bad news. Aspects of quality of the original articles that are pertinent to the reliability of the meta-analysis include, valid randomisation process (we are assuming that in meta-analysis of clinical trials, only randomised trials will be selected), minimisation of potential biases introduced by DROPOUTS, acceptable methods of analysis, level of blinding and recording of adequate clinical details. Several attempts have been made to make this aspect of meta-analysis more rigorous by using the results given by applying specially constructed quality assessments scales to assess the candidate trials for inclusion in the analysis. Determining quality would be helped if the results from so many trials were not so poorly reported. In the future, this may be improved by the CONSORT statement (consolidation of standards for reporting trials).

The representativeness of the studies in a systematic review depends largely on having an acceptable search strategy. Once the researcher has established the goals of the systematic review, an ambitious literature search needs to be undertaken, the literature obtained and then summarised. Possible sources of material include the published literature, unpublished literature, uncompleted research reports, work in progress, conference/symposia proceedings, dissertations, expert informants, granting agencies, trial registries, industry and journal hand searching. The search will probably begin by using computerised bibliographic databases of published and unpublished research review articles, for example, MEDLINE. This is clearly a sensible strategy, although there is some evidence of deficiencies in MEDLINE when searching for randomised controlled trials.

Ensuring that a meta-analysis is truly representative can be problematic. It has long been known that journal articles are not a representative sample of work addressed to any particular area of research. Research with statistically significant results is potentially more likely to be submitted and published than work with null, or non-significant results, particularly if the studies are small. The problem is made worse by the fact that many medical studies look at multiple outcomes and there is a tendency for only those outcomes suggesting a significant effect to be mentioned when the study is written up. Outcomes that show no clear treatment effect are often ignored and so will not be included in any later review of studies looking at those particular outcomes. Publication bias is likely to lead to an over representation of positive results.

Clearly it becomes of some importance to assess the likelihood of publication bias in any meta-analysis reported in the literature. A well-known informal method of investigating this potential problem is the so-called FUNNEL PLOT, usually a plot of a measure of a study's precision (for example, one over the standard error), against effect size. The most precise estimates (e.g. those from the largest studies) will be at the top of the plot, and those from less precise or smaller studies at the bottom. The expectation of a 'funnel' shape in the plot relies on two empirical observations. First, the variances of studies in a meta-analysis are not identical, but are distributed in such a way that there are fewer precise studies and rather more imprecise ones and, second, at any fixed level of variances, studies are symmetrically distributed about the mean.

Evidence of publication bias is provided by an absence of studies on the left-hand side of the base of the funnel. The assumption is that, whether because of editorial policy or author inaction or other reason, these studies (which are not statistically significant) are the ones that might not be published. An example of a funnel plot suggesting the possible presence of publication bias is given in the Figure (taken from Duval and Tweedie, 2000).

Various proposals have been made as to how to test for publication bias in a systematic review although none of these is wholly satisfactory. The danger of the testing approach is the temptation to assume that, if the test is not significant, there is no problem and the possibility of publication bias can be conveniently ignored. In practice, however, publication bias is very likely endemic to all empirical research and so should be assumed present, whatever the result of some testing procedures with possibly low power.

Once the studies for systematic review have been selected and the possible problems of publication bias

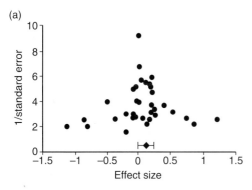
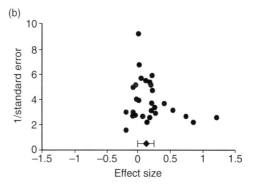

systematic reviews *(a) Funnel plot of 35 simulated studies and meta-analysis with true effect size of zero: estimated effect size is 0.080 with a 95% confidence interval of [–0.018,0.178]; (b) funnel plot as in (a) with five 'leftmost' studies suppressed; overall effect size is now estimated as 0.124 with a 95 % confidence interval of [0.037,0.210].* Reprinted with permission from The Journal of the American Statistical Association. *Copyright 2000 by the American Statistical Association. All rights reserved*

addressed, effect sizes and variance estimates are extracted from the selected papers, reports etc. and subjected to a meta-analysis, in which the aim is to provide a global test of significance for the overall null hypothesis of no effect in all studies and to calculate an estimate and a confidence interval of the overall effect size.

Two models are usually considered, one involving FIXED EFFECTS and the other RANDOM EFFECTS (Fleiss, 1993; Sutton *et al.*, 2000). The former assumes that the true effect is the same for all studies whereas the latter assumes that individual studies have different effect sizes that vary randomly around the overall mean effect size. Thus the random effects model specifically allows for the existence of both between study heterogeneity and within-study variability. When the research question concerns whether treatment has produced an effect, on the average, in the set of studies being analysed, then the fixed effects model for the studies may be the more appropriate; here there is no interest in generalising the results to other studies. Many statisticians believe, however, that the random effects model is more appropriate than a fixed effects model for meta-analysis, because between-study variation is an important source of uncertainty that should not be ignored, in assigning uncertainty into pooled results. Tests of homogeneity are available, i.e. a test that the between-study variance component is zero – if it is, a fixed effects model is considered justified. Such a test is, however, likely to be of low power for detecting departures from homogeneity and so its practical consequences are probably quite limited.

The essential feature of both the fixed and random effects models for meta-analysis is the use of a weighted mean of treatment effect sizes from the individual studies, with the weights usually being the reciprocals of the associated variances. Effect sizes might be standardised mean differences for continuous response variables or relative risks or odds ratios for binary outcomes. Both fixed effects and random effects models result in a test of zero effect size and a confidence interval for effect size. But it should be remembered that, in general, a more important aspect of meta-analysis is often the exploration of the likely heterogeneity of effect sizes from the different studies. Random effect models, for example, allow for such heterogeneity but they do not offer any way of exploring and

potentially explaining the reasons study results vary. In other words, random effects models do not 'control for', 'adjust for' or 'explain away' heterogeneity. Understanding heterogeneity should perhaps be the primary focus of the majority of meta-analyses carried out in medicine.

The examination of heterogeneity may begin with formal statistical tests for its presence, but even in the absence of statistical evidence of heterogeneity, exploration of the relationship of effect size to study characteristics may still be valuable. The question of importance is, what causes heterogeneity in systematic reviews of clinical trials? Study of the causes of heterogeneity of treatment effects in a meta-analysis often involves the technique generally known as META-REGRESSION. Essentially, this is nothing more than a weighted regression analysis with effect size as the dependent variable, a number of study characteristics as explanatory variables and weights usually being the reciprocal of the sum of the estimated variance of a study and the estimated between study variance, although other more complex approaches have been described. Meta-regression can, like SUBGROUP ANALYSIS within a single clinical trial, quickly become little more than data dredging. This danger can be partially dealt with at least, by pre-specification of the covariates that will be investigated as potential sources of heterogeneity.

As an example of the systematic review and associated meta-analysis we shall consider transcranial magnetic stimulation (TMS) for the treatment of depression. Such treatment involves placing a high-intensity magnetic field of brief duration at the scalp surface to induce an electrical field at the cortical surface that can alter neuronal function. Repetitive TMS (rTMS) involves applying trains of these magnetic pulses. In humans rTMS has been shown to produce changes in frontal lobe blood flow and to normalise the response to dexmethasone in depression. Since trials in the late 1990s, rTMS has been proposed as a treatment for drug-resistant depression, schizophrenia and mania. McNamara *et al.* (2001) report a systematic review of the published data, in which randomised controlled trials were searched for using a variety of databases, including Medline and Embase. Sixteen published clinical trials of rTMS for depression were identified, but eight were excluded because there was no

systematic reviews and meta-analysis *Data for five RCTs of rTMS*

		rTMS	Placebo
Trial 1	Improved	11	6
	Not improved	6	11
Trial 2	Improved	7	1
	Not improved	1	4
Trial 3	Improved	8	2
	Not improved	4	4
Trial 4	Improved	4	1
	Not improved	6	10
Trial 5	Improved	17	8
	Not improved	18	24

randomised control group and a further three excluded for reasons given in the original paper. The results from the five trials accepted for the meta-analysis are shown in the Table.

The results from both the fixed effects and random effects model are, for these data, exactly the same. The overall effect size (log odds ratio) is estimated to be 1.33 with a standard error of 0.37, leading to an estimated odds ratio of 3.78 with 95% confidence interval (1.83, 7.81). *BSE*

[See also FOREST PLOT]

Duval, S. and Tweedie, R.L. 2000: Nonparametric 'trim and fill' method of accounting for publication bias in meta-analysis. *Journal of the American Statistical Association* 95, 89–98. **Fleiss, J.L.** 1993: The statistical basis of meta-analysis. *Statistical Methods in Medical Research*, 2, 121–45. **MacNamara, B., Ray, J.L., Arthurs, O.J., and Boniface, S.** 2001: Transcrannial magnetic stimulation for depression and other psychiatric disorders. *Psychological Medicine* 31, 1141–6. **Normand, S.T.** 1999: Meta-analysis: formulating, evaluating, combining and reporting. *Statistics in Medicine* 18, 321–59. **Pocock, S.J.** 1996: Clinical trials: a statistician's perspective. In Armitage, P. and David, H.A. (eds), *Advances in biometry*. Chichester: John Wiley & Sons. **Sutton, A.J., Abrams, K.R., Jones, D.R. and Sheldon, T.A.** 2000: *Methods for meta-analysis in medical research*. Chichester: John Wiley & Sons.

systematic sample Every *k*th element in a list is included in the sample. To obtain such a sample, begin with the sampling frame and arrange in an order, which may be alphabetical or some other order. Then select the number of samples to be taken. Select a random starting point in the list. Divide the size of the population by the number of samples to be taken. This is the length of interval, *k*. Then every *k*th unit, depending on the starting point, is included in the sample until the number of samples to be taken is reached. This may mean starting again from the beginning of the list.

For example, Little, Keefe and White (1995) used a systematic sample when studying melanoma patients in a general practice. Every 125th patient on the general practice register was selected to be included; this was to yield a minimum of 60 individuals.

The main advantage of systematic sampling is that it is a quick and easy-to-use sampling method, particularly when dealing with large samples, where it is often used in preference to simple random samples. However, if there is a periodic cycle within the sampling frame then estimates obtained from systematic sampling may be incorrect. If the periodic cycle is recognised then the starting point and the length of interval between chosen items can be varied. Systematic sampling can often only be used when there is a sampling frame available that can be ordered in some way. *SLV*

Crawshaw, J. and Chambers, J. 1994: *A concise course in A level statistics*, 3rd edn. Cheltenham: Stanley Thornes Publishers Ltd. **Little, P., Keefe, M. and White, J.** 1995: Self-screening for risk of melanoma: validity of self-mole counting by patients in a single general practice. *British Medical Journal* 310, 912–16. **Upton, G. and Cook, I.** 2002: *Dictionary of statistics*. Oxford: Oxford University Press.

T

t-distribution Also known as Student's t-distribution, this is the distribution of the estimate of the mean of a normal distribution when the standard error has also been estimated. The distribution is used when performing STUDENT'S t-TEST. If we have a NORMAL DISTRIBUTION of known VARIANCE σ^2, then we can test to see if the mean of a set of observations $x_1, x_2, \ldots x_n$, denoted m, is consistent with a hypothesised mean μ by calculating a confidence interval for μ. This is done by considering that:

$$N = \frac{m - \mu}{\sqrt{(\sigma^2/n)}}$$

will have an approximately standard normal distribution mean (mean 0, standard deviation 1), denoted N(0,1) and calculating a 95% CONFIDENCE INTERVAL for μ as:

$$\left(m - 1.96\sqrt{\sigma^2/n}\right) < \mu < \left(m + 1.96\sqrt{\sigma^2/n}\right)$$

where 1.96 is the critical value from the standard normal distribution.

If the variance is also being estimated, instead of knowing the population variance σ^2, we must use the sample estimate s^2. Now if we construct the statistic:

$$T = \frac{m - \mu}{\sqrt{(s^2/n)}}$$

will have a t-distribution with $n - 1$ DEGREES OF FREEDOM, written $t(n - 1)$. A 95% confidence interval for μ can then be expressed as:

$$\left(m + t_{0.025}\sqrt{s^2/n}\right) < \mu < \left(m + t_{0.975}\sqrt{s^2/n}\right)$$

where $t_{0.025}$ and $t_{0.975}$ are the critical values from the t(n − 1) distribution. These values, which are chosen to ensure 2.5% of the probability density lies in each tail, can be found from tables or computer packages. As long as n is at least three, like the standard normal distribution, the t-distribution has a zero mean and is symmetric, but the variance is $(n - 1)/(n - 3)$. As the sample size, n, increases, the variance approaches 1, but for small sample sizes, the variance will be greater, which reflects the large uncertainty in the estimate of σ^2.

The t-distribution is related to other common distributions. If we compare the statistics N and T, we will see that T is merely N divided through by $\sqrt{s^2/\sigma^2}$. Now, $(n - 1)\, s^2/\sigma^2$ is known to have a CHI-SQUARE DISTRIBUTION with $n - 1$ degrees of freedom and we see that more generally, the t-distribution with $n - 1$ degrees of freedom arises when a standard normal variable is multiplied by the square root of $(n - 1)$ and divided by the square root of a $\chi^2(n - 1)$ variable.

Having observed this, if we now square T, we can see that it is $(n - 1)$ times the square of a standard normal variable divided by a $\chi^2(n - 1)$ variable. Now the square of a standard normal variable is a $\chi^2(1)$ variable, so the square of T is $(n - 1)$ times a $\chi^2(1)$ variable divided by 1 times a $\chi^2(n - 1)$ variable. The division of one chi-square variable by another with the correct multipliers is known to generate an F-distribution, and so we can see that the square of a t-distributed variable (with $n - 1$ degrees of freedom) will have an F-DISTRIBUTION (with 1 and $n - 1$ degrees of freedom). *AGL*

Altman, D.G. 1991: *Practical statistics for medical research.* London: Chapman & Hall. **Grimmet, G.R. and Stirzaker, D.R.** 1992: *Probability and random processes*, 2nd edn. Oxford: Clarendon Press. **Leemis, L.M.** 1986: Relationships among common univariate distributions. *The American Statistician* 40, 2, 143–6. **Lindley, D.V. and Scott, W.F.** 1984: *New Cambridge elementary statistical tables.* Cambridge: Cambridge University Press.

teaching medical statistics

Four main groups of people are expected to learn medical statistics: undergraduate students of medicine and other healthcare professional subjects, healthcare practitioners, researchers in healthcare and would-be medical statisticians. For all these groups we must select the most appropriate material from the huge amount available (even to master the contents of the journal *Statistics in Medicine* would take me several lifetimes). This material will, in turn, partly determine the teaching method.

Students rarely have much time in their crowded curriculum for statistics and rarely have much natural sympathy for the subject. They see their futures as practical people busy saving lives and caring for the sick, not analysing data or reading journals. They are also usually at the age of maximum confidence in their own infallibility and hence difficult to persuade that they might be mistaken in their image of their future role. It is easier to persuade them of the relevance of reading evidence than number crunching, and such courses do better if they concentrate on the understanding of research publications. I have found that my conventional lectures are of little value to this group and seminars where they discuss papers, backed up by printed notes or web pages on the statistical principles, are more effective.

Lectures work better when students who have been challenged with this material are then able to ask a statistician to explain things that puzzle them. The concepts acquired in this way are more likely to be backed up by other parts of their course than the calculation of CHI-SQUARED TESTS. If students can be equipped with the basic ideas of variability, measurement, RANDOMISATION, estimation and significance, we have done well. The machines can do the sums.

Increasing numbers of healthcare students are taught by problem-based learning (PBL), a system intended to prepare students for a life of evidence-based practice. Statistics is rarely taught as part of the core PBL programme, but is instead taught as a separate addition to PBL cases, or in a separate, parallel lecture- or seminar-based course or not at all. This is bad news not only for medical statistics (and those who teach it) but also for medicine. Surely the skills needed for the interpretation of evidence should be central in a course preparing students for evidence-based practice. It happens because tutors, mainly laboratory scientists or clinicians, feel insecure about teaching statistics and because the 'problems' of PBL are usually descriptions of a patient. Tutors need to be convinced that they do not need to know the subject to facilitate students' mutual education and course organisers need to be convinced that problems can be a publication or a community problem, that the patient case is not the only way.

Healthcare practitioners are usually taught statistics as part of study for a higher professional qualification. The key application is still the interpretation of numerical evidence, mainly in the context of published research. However, they often have the more immediate goal of passing a demanding examination with a high failure rate. Some of these examinations include some quite advanced statistics, such as those in radiotherapy or public health. The teacher can make use of this by collaborating with the students to defeat the examiner and concentrating on past questions. I find that starting with a few multiple-choice questions to identify areas of difficulty and then explaining the answers the students get wrong works very well. Once the basics have been covered in this way, past examination questions form the ideal motivator. It is for the examiners to design their tests so that in order to pass them the students must learn what the examiners think they need to know.

For those who do not have to satisfy an examiner but simply wish to understand their own subject's literature better, indirect teaching is frequently used. Many journals have carried long series of articles on statistics intended to help their readers understand what is published, a practice which began with the early ground-breaking *Lancet* articles by Bradford Hill in the 1930s and continues still.

Researchers have very different needs from practitioners. They must acquire the skills to design studies and analyse data. Understanding of concepts, while still central, is not enough. Practical skills are usually developed in hands-on computing practical classes, preferably using software of the type that they will use in their own research. Lectures have more natural place in this teaching, as methods and their applications and limitations can be described. We can even risk a few mathematical formulae without too much discouragement of well-motivated students. The opportunity to discuss their own projects is very attractive to these students.

Textbooks are particularly important to this group. At one time the market was flooded with poor books on medical statistics (Bland and Altman, 1987), but there are now many good ones. Another source of statistical education for researchers comes from individual discussions of their projects with a statistician. This is a two-way street, as they educate the statistician about the research topic and medicine in general. I have learned so much from the people who have come to me for help.

For new statisticians, statistics is usually a master's course taken by graduates in mathematics or other quantitative subjects. It is possible to study statistics as a branch of mathematics without real data making much of an appearance, but if students have chosen to study med-

ical statistics specifically we would expect them to want a practical course with the focus on application to real problems. Clearly, they must become familiar with the common techniques of design and analysis and should be able to analyse data within both the frequentist and the Bayesian frameworks (see BAYESIAN METHODS). As nearly all statistical analysis is now done using general-purpose statistical software, they should learn the basics of the software they are likely to meet. At the time of writing, SAS, Stata and BUGS would be contenders for the programs of choice, but familiarity with other widely used or specialist software could be included. Statisticians need not only technical skills, but also the ability to collaborate with and give advice to members of other disciplines. Experience is the best teacher, but experience is what you get just after you needed it. We would like to give our students a bit of experience before they are plunged into real-life problems. Medicine and other healthcare professions have much to teach us here. I used to run a session for MSc students in medical statistics where I invited clinical researchers who sought my advice to come and get it in front of a live audience. I pointed out to them that if I went to consult them, they would do it with an audience of medical students. Perhaps we could incorporate this type of advisory clinic into our teaching.

We want to enable our students not only to use the current set of statistical methods, but also to develop new ones where these are needed. To this end they need some theory as well as the practice of statistics. I think that statisticians should also have a secure basis for thinking that the statistical methods that we routinely use are in some way the best methods we could use and for this reason a theoretical course will provide valuable grounding, even though they may never use it again.

We should not think that students will learn and retain all we teach them or that if we do not teach them something they will never know it. Being taught is only a part of learning and good students will continue to learn throughout their careers. What we must try to do is to give them the desire to retain what they have learned already and the ability to add to their knowledge whenever they need to.

JMB

Bland, J.M. and Altman, D.G. 1987: Caveat doctor: a grim tale of medical statistics textbooks. *British Medical Journal* 295, 979.

tetrachoric correlation coefficient See CORRELATION

thrive lines See GROWTH CHARTS

time-dependent variables Time-dependent covariates also known as time varying covariates or updating covariates. These are variables that can change their value over time. They are particular important for prognostic models, such as COX'S REGRESSION MODEL. They should be distinguished from fixed covariates, which are measurable at baseline and do not change with time. Examples of fixed covariates are race and sex. Age varies with time, but is completely predictable from baseline data and so is not included among time-dependent covariates. Time-dependent covariates may be classed as being internal and external (Altman and de Stavola, 1994). External factors impact on outcome but do not explicitly reference time,

for example half-life of a drug treatment; whereas internal factors are measurements taken at set times relating to the individual or their condition, for example, blood pressure or blood markers.

The reason for considering the inclusion of time-dependent covariates is that including only baseline variables may ignore a great deal of potential prognostic information. Therefore, the inclusion of time-dependent covariates may substantially increase the potential detail and accuracy in a model. For example, increases (or decreases) over time in patients' blood pressure may be a better predictor of future prognosis than a single baseline value of blood pressure.

The Cox model can be extended to include time-dependent covariates instead of, or in addition to, fixed covariates. In simplest terms, the hazard for a time-dependent covariate takes the form: $h(t) = \exp[\gamma z(t)]$ where $h(t)$ is the hazard at time t and z is a time-dependent covariate and γ is its coefficient value. As for fixed covariates, all data types can be entered as time-dependent covariates into a Cox regression model. It is important to assess the assumption of PROPORTIONAL HAZARDS, once any time-dependent covariate has been taken into account.

These variables do add additional complications to any model. First, they require the dataset being analysed to contain additional variables or additional observations (depending on the dataset's structure). Second, it can be difficult to obtain complete data on these variables, especially with increasing time. MISSING DATA can be problematic. Third, these variables effectively increase the choice of Cox models available for consideration. One must ensure that issues of multiplicity of testing are addressed. Finally, there are issues of interpretation. Including time-dependent covariates in a model may be practically simple, but the greater difficulty lies in interpreting the data: one must be sure how any variable would be interpreted before including it in a model. Simply, the hazard ratio for a time-dependent covariate represents an additional change in risk associated with a change in this variable over time. For example, when considering bone pain as an outcome after treatment for prostate cancer, one may wish to record the development of osteoarthritis over time as the second condition may increase the risk of bone pain. When interpreting output it can be complicated trying to tease cause from effect with such variables.

MS/MP

Altman, D.G. and de Stavola, B.L. 1994: Practical problems in fitting a proportional hazards model to data with updated measurements of the covariates. *Statistics in Medicine* 13, 4, 301–41. **Cleves, M.A., Gould, W.W. and Gutierrez, R.G.** 2003: *An introduction to survival analysis using Stata®*, rev. edn. Texas: Stata Press. **Machin, D. and Parmar, M.K.B.** 1995: *Survival analysis: a practical approach.* London: John Wiley & Sons. **Piantodosi, S.** 1997: *Clinical trials.* New York: Wiley Interscience.

time series in medicine Chatfield (1989) has defined a time series as 'a sequence of observations ordered in time'. In medicine and medical research, observations are often ordered in time and special techniques have evolved to deal with them. It is helpful to think of three types of time series: (1) single series, often long; (2) more than one series, each of moderate length; and (3) many shorter series.

There are at least three reasons for collecting a single time series:

(i)   to predict some future event. An example might be measuring creatinine clearance from kidney failure patients where the main aim is to predict complete kidney failure;

(ii) to test whether some event in time has an effect on subsequent outcomes. These are sometimes called before-and-after studies or interrupted times series (Glass, Wilson *et al.*, 1975). Examples include the effect of seat belt legislation on deaths due to car accidents, effect of NHS Direct on consultation to a general practitioner and behavioural experiments in psychology;

(iii) to look for trends and rhythms in the series. An example would be a spectral analysis of the EEG signal to measure the strength of alpha waves.

For series of more moderate length a common theme is to examine whether there is an *association* between two series. Examples include studies to examine relationships between cot deaths and environmental temperature and daily deaths from heart disease and air pollution.

Shorter series are often dealt with under the term 'repeated measures'. The reason for measuring observations over time is that a series would more accurately reflect the action of treatment than a single measure at one point in time. A typical example would be repeated measures in clinical trial, such as blood pressure measured monthly for a year. Summary measures (Matthews *et al.*, 1990) such as the AREA UNDER CURVE or the slope of the response over time are often the outcomes of interest. Repeating observations can improve the accuracy of the estimates of treatment effects.

The most basic time series model is the autoregressive (AR(1)) model. Given a time series x_t, from which mean value has been subtracted an AR(1) is given by:

$$x_t = ax_{t-1} + \varepsilon_t \quad \text{where } -1 < \alpha < 1.$$

This model is often called a *Markov* model because the value at one point in time only depends on the value at the point immediately preceding it. The model is easily extended to AR(p) where $p > 1$. For $p = 2$, certain values of the coefficients can give models in which cycles appear. Some forecasting models use autoregressive models, but in medicine these are rarely used because usually one is more interested in estimating trends, which are more easily fitted using convention models.

The complementary model to the AR(1) is the moving average model MA(1)

$$x_t = \varepsilon_t + \beta\varepsilon_{t-1} \quad \text{where } -1 < \beta < 1.$$

This model is less commonly used than an AR(1) but again can be easily extended to an MA(q), $q > 1$.

These models can be combined to produce an autoregressive, moving average ARMA model. This has been found to model many time series and requiring only low values of p and q. The procedure of fitting these models is often known as *Box-Jenkins* modelling (Box and Jenkins, 1976). In general, this type of modelling is more common in the forecasting and control of industrial processes, although on occasion it has been applied in medicine.

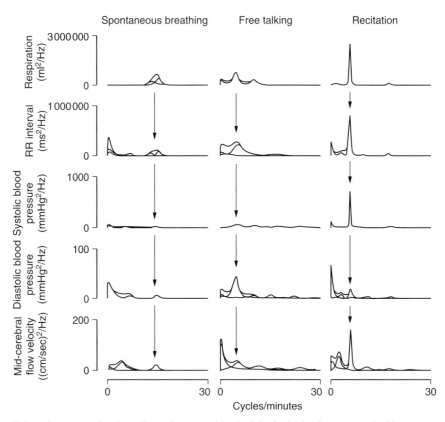

time series in medicine *Spectrum showing effects (in one subject) of rhythmic rituals compared with spontaneous breathing, on respiratory and cardiovascular rhythms. Note slow rhythmic oscillations (approximately 6/min) in all signals during recitation (Bernardi et al., 2001, British Medical Journal 323, 1446–9, with permission from the BMJ Publishing Group)*

Perhaps the most common feature of the analysis of clinical signals is to look for regularly occurring features or rhythms (Campbell, 1996). For humans to maintain stable bodily functions, clinical signals must be constrained to lie within certain limits and this is done using nonlinear feedback loops and this tends to make patterns within signals recur regularly. A simple example will illustrate the point. To remain healthy, humans must maintain blood pressure to within certain narrow limits. Blood pressure is mediated through the baroreceptors, located in the wall of the aortic arch and in the wall of the carotid sinus. If blood pressure is too high, then signals from the baroreceptors result in vasodilation, which drops the blood pressure. If pressure is too low, then vasoconstriction occurs to increase the blood pressure. The feedback mechanism is thought to be nonlinear and incorporates a delay and, for these reasons, at rest rhythms can occur spontaneously.

Periodogram analysis involves decomposing a signal into individual frequency components where the amplitude of these components is proportional to the 'energy' of the signal at that frequency. It is a convenient method for summarising a long time series and is a natural procedure if we believe there are rhythms in the data. Periodogram analysis is the method of choice for the analysis of clinical signals.

The problem with the periodogram is that it is an inconsistent estimator, in that its variance does not reduce as the sample size increases. To achieve a consistent estimator various smoothing techniques (known as 'windows') are applied to the periodogram, so that it estimates what is known as the *spectrum*.

There are three major components to be found in a typical heart rate spectrum and these are also present in the blood pressure spectrum. A region of activity occurs at around 0.25 Hz, which is attributable to respiration (respiratory sinus arrhythmia) and this is thought to be a marker of vagal (parasympathetic) activity. A second component at around 0.1 Hz arises from spontaneous vasomotor activity within the blood pressure control system and is mediated by vagal and sympathetic activity. A third, low-frequency component at around 0.04 Hz is thought to arise from thermoregulatory activity. An example is given in the first Figure (Bernardi *et al.*, 2001) that shows the effect of recitation of mantras or prayers on the spectrum of respiration, heart rate (RR interval) blood pressure and mid-cerebral blood flow. It can be seen that recitation concentrates the power of the signal at a cycle with a frequency of about 6 cycles per minute (0.1 Hz).

Some signals are essentially continuous, whereas others are discrete. For example, the heart rate is measured from surface electrodes on the chest from the ECG. Although the ECG is continuous, the heart rate is usually derived from the 'R' wave in the ECG, which is a sudden spike just preceding the ventricular contraction. Thus, the heart beat signal is essentially a point process. Some authors have analysed the interbeat intervals, thus arriving at a spectrum, which estimates frequencies per beat, rather than per unit time. Others sample the heart rate (or RR interval) signal at regular intervals or filter the point process to produce a continuous signal that can be sampled.

The electroencephlogram (EEG) is electrical activity of the brain measured by electrodes at the surface of the skull. There is an immense amount of literature devoted to the spectral analysis of EEGs. In particular, six spectral peaks can be identified. These peaks, with a typical range of frequencies are: delta 1 (0.5–2.0 Hz), delta 2 (2.0–4.0 Hz), theta (4.0–8.0 Hz), alpha (8.0–12.0 Hz), sigma (12.0–14.0 Hz) and beta (14.0–20.0 Hz). The peaks can be used, for example, to classify different levels of sleep. Recently there has been interest in describing neural processes in the context of nonlinear dynamics and, in particular, in the rapidly evolving field of *deterministic chaos*.

An assumption before applying spectral analysis is that the signal is stationary (i.e. the mean and variance do not change). However, medical signals are not stationary in the usual sense. They contain rhythms that may come and go in the time interval, the frequencies may vary or amplitudes of cycles at certain frequencies increase or decrease. Spectral analysis considers the entire time interval and so cycles that only occur in part of the interval will have their spectral peaks attenuated by the low power in other parts of the interval. One solution is to divide the series up into sections and compute the spectrum for each section. The difficulty here is that it is not realistic to think of a signal being stationary in sections. A better intuitive model is one in which the signal 'evolves' slowly so that the non-stationary component is slow in comparison with the signal in which we are interested. The newly developed field of WAVELET ANALYSIS is used to analyse signals of this kind.

The main problem with time series is that serial correlation invalidates one of the main assumptions of conventional regression, namely that the errors in the model are independent of each other. The second problem is that if we are interested in the relationship between two time dependent variables y_t and x_t, any other variable associated with time will be a confounder between them. For example, if both series increase with time, then they will appear correlated. This has been the source of much amusement, with positive correlations such as those between the annual population of Holland and the number of storks' nests and sales of ice cream and deaths by drowning being quoted as evidence of causation!

To make progress one has to try and fit a model that removes the confounder variables.

For a continuous outcome suppose the model is $y_t = \beta'x_t + \upsilon_t$, $t = 1,..., n$ where y_t is the dependent value measured at time t, x_t a vector of confounder and predictor variables, and β a vector of regression coefficients.

If the residuals are serially correlated, then ordinary least squares does not provide valid estimates of the standard errors of the parameters. If we assume that x_t and υ_t are generated by AR(1) processes with parameters α and γ then using ordinary least squares to estimate β, the ratio of the estimated variance to the true variance is approximately $(1 - \alpha\gamma)/(1 + \alpha\gamma)$. In general, x_t and υ_t are likely to be positively correlated. Thus the effect of ignoring serial correlation is to give artificially low estimates of the standard error of the regression coefficients. This means declaring significance more often than the significance level would suggest, under the null hypothesis of no association.

Assuming α is known, a method of generalised least squares known as the Cochrane-Orcutt procedure (Cochrane and Orcutt, 1949) can be employed.

Write $y_t^* = y_t - \alpha y_{t-1}$ and $x_t^* = x_t - \alpha x_{t-1}$.

Obtain an estimate of β using ordinary least squares on y_t^* and x_t^*. However, since α will not usually be known it

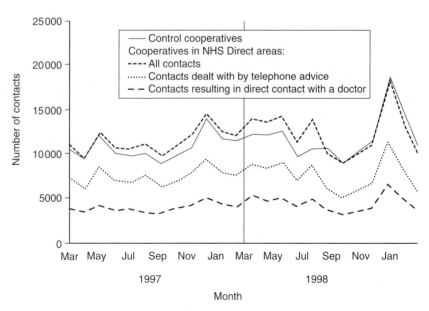

time series in medicine *Monthly number of contacts with GPs before and after introduction of NHS Direct (Munro et al., 2000, British Medical Journal 321, 150–3, with permission from the BMJ Publishing Group)*

can be estimated from the ordinary least squares residuals e_t by:

$$a = \sum_{t=2}^{n} e_t e_{t-1} \Big/ \sum_{t=2}^{n} e_{t-1}^2$$

This leads to an iterative procedure in which we can construct a new set of transformed variables and thus a new set of regression estimates and so on until convergence.

The iterative Cochrane-Orcutt procedure can be interpreted as a stepwise algorithm for computing maximum likelihood estimators of α and β where the initial observation y_1 is regarded as fixed. If the residuals can be assumed to be normally distributed then full maximum likelihood methods are available, which estimate α and β simultaneously and this can be generalised to higher order autoregressive models. These models can be fitted using (say) PROC AUTOREG or AUTOREGRESSION in the computer packages SAS and SPSS, respectively (see STATISTICAL PACKAGES). However, autocorrelation of residuals can appear because the wrong model is being fitted. For example, if the true response was quadratic and a linear model was fitted, the errors would appear as a group of negative errors, a group of positive errors and then a group of negative errors. It is a better strategy to obtain a good model than using an autoregressive error model as a panacea for models that simply do not fit.

Interrupted time series are often either before-and-after treatment for single subjects or before-and-after intervention for populations. An important question for the analysis is whether the data are correlated. The main reason for correlation might be because the same subject is measured before and after. However if we removed the subject effect, the data may be independent and so, for example, a two-sample STUDENT'S t-TEST would be valid.

One could look for three different sorts of effect on an outcome of an intervention at one point in time: (i) a change in slope, (ii) a change in level or (iii) a combination of a change in slope and a change in level.

NHS Direct is a telephone system designed to relieve pressure on general practitioners (GPs). It was introduced into the UK in 2001 (Munro et al., 2000). We are interested whether it has an effect on the number of telephone calls to GPs.

The most likely model is change in slope (see second Figure). One simple method is the following. We make the origin for time the point at which the intervention occurred.

The model is $y_t = \alpha + \beta_1 t + \beta_2 t' + \varepsilon_t$, where y_t is the monthly number of calls to selected practices in month t and $t' = 0$ if $t < 0$, $t' = t$ if $t > 0$. Thus a test of the effect is to test whether $\beta_2 = 0$. As stated earlier, conventional regression will give invalid results if the errors are serially correlated and so we need to check the serial correlation of ε_t. Again, we can use certain statistical packages to fit the model assuming the errors are generated by an autoregressive process.

Many epidemiological series consist of counts and require Poisson regression rather than ordinary linear regression. We can also employ a method similar to the Cochrane-Orcutt method to allow for serial correlation and use GENERALISED ESTIMATING EQUATIONS to estimate the parameters.

Campbell (1994) analysed the dependence of daily deaths from sudden infant death syndrome (SIDS) in England and Wales from 1979 to 1983 on mean daily environmental temperature measured in London. The input was mean daily temperature and the output daily deaths due to SIDS. There is clear seasonality in the mortality series but this does not mean that there is a causal relationship between temperature and cot deaths since many factors behave seasonally, such as length of day and rainfall. It is only when these effects are removed can we deduce a possible relationship. A model was fitted which removed seasonality and then included a linear temperature effect. The coefficient associated with mean temperature 3–5 days before the death was –0.041 (SE 0.005). We interpret this as saying that a 1°C drop in temperature is associated with a rise in SIDS by about 4%. Further investigations demonstrated that the relationship was approximately linear.

We can test the residuals for autocorrelation, using tests such as the Durbin-Watson test (1st order AR) and the Ljung-Box (general order). However, one should ask if it is sensible to test for serial correlation and only include serial correlation in the model if the test is significant. One should also ask why the data are serially correlated.

Serial correlation could be split into *intrinsic* correlation (endogenous) and *extrinsic* correlation (exogenous). Intrinsic correlation means the value at a particular time depends directly on value at an earlier time. Examples include: serum cholesterol at different times, population in age groups in successive years, epidemics of measles. Extrinsic correlation occurs because both variables depend on some third (time-dependent) variable. Examples include daily SIDS, where the deaths are not caused by epidemics and are really unrelated to each other except through (say) the weather.

We will not cover repeated measures in detail here. Commonly they arise when individuals have measurements taken repeatedly over time (see REPEATED MEASURES ANALYSIS OF VARIANCE). Often the serial correlation aspect of the data can be removed by the simple expedient of using summary measures (Matthews et al., 1990). If not, usually either a simple AR(1) model is assumed, or what is known as an exchangeable correlation model or compound symmetry. This is generated by a model of the form

$$y_{it} = \mu + \alpha_i + \varepsilon_{it}$$

where y_{it} is an outcome at time t on subject i, α_i is the effect of subject i and this is assumed normally distributed with variance σ_α^2, $E(\alpha_i \alpha_j) = 0$ when $i \neq j$ and ε_{ij} has variance σ^2.

The effect of this is to generate a covariance matrix with σ_α^2 on the off diagonal and $\sigma^2 + \sigma_\alpha^2$ on the diagonal terms. Although one would expect measurements made further away to be less correlated (i.e. perhaps an AR(1)), in practice compound symmetry has been found to be a reasonable assumption in many cases.

We need to distinguish between methods where serial correlation is an important part of the model, such as for prediction, and where it is simply a nuisance. If it is a nuisance, then we need to examine intrinsic and extrinsic correlation. We should allow for serial correlation in regression modelling. Often serial correlation can be 'made to go away' and so the time series aspect is not a major concern. Compound symmetry is a useful assumption for repeated measures in randomised controlled trials.   *MJC*

Bernardi, L., Sleight, P., Bandinelli, G., Cencetti, S., Fattorini, L., Wdowczyc-Szulc, J. and Lagi, A. 2001: Effect of rosary prayer and yoga mantras on autonomic cardiovascular rhythms: comparative study. *British Medical Journal* 323, 1446–9. **Box, G.E.P. and Jenkins, G.** 1976: *Time series analysis: forecasting and control.* San Francisco: Holden Day. **Campbell, M.J.** 1994: Time series regression for counts: an investigation into the relationship between sudden infant death syndrome and environmental temperature. *Journal of the Royal Statistical Society Series A* 157, 191–208. **Campbell, M.J.** 1996: Spectral analysis of clinical signals: an interface between medical statisticians and medical engineers. *Statistical Methods in Medical Research* 5, 51–66. **Chatfield, C.** 1989: *The analysis of time series: An introduction,* 4th edn. London: Chapman & Hall. **Cochrane, D. and Orcutt, G.H.** 1949: Application of least squares regression to relationships containing autocorrelated error terms. *Journal of the American Statistical Association* 44, 32–61. **Diggle, P.J.** 1990: *Time series. A biostatistical introduction.* Oxford: Oxford Science Publications. **Glass, G.V., Wilson, V.L. and Gottman, J.M. et al.** 1975: *Design and analysis of time series experiments.* Colorado: Colorado Associated Press. **Matthews, J.N.S., Altman, D.G., Campbell, M.J. and Royston, J.P.** 1990: Analysis of serial measurements in medical research. *British Medical Journal* 300, 230–5. **Munro, J., Nicholl, J., O'Cathain, A. and Knowles, E.** 2000: Impact of NHS Direct on demand for immediate care: observational study. *British Medical Journal* 321, 150–3.

time trade-off technique See VON-NEUMAN-MORGENSTERN STANDARD GAMBLE

total fertility rate (TRF) See DEMOGRAPHY

transformations The use of transformations in statistics has a long history. For example, the Wilson-Hilferty cube root transformation for chi-square distributions, the Fisher z transformation for correlations, the use of logarithms for biological data and the arc-sine root transformations for proportions are well known procedures. In most cases the use of transformations is not an end in itself, but rather a means to an end. The ultimate benefit is usually not what the transformation directly achieves, but rather that it allows subsequent analysis to be simpler, more revealing or more accurate. What is most important is how the transformation aids in the interpretation and description of the data.

The transformations may be applied to observations, either response or explanatory variables, or to parameters or statistics, or they might be an explicit part of a statistical model. The purposes of using transformations include (i) to reduce non-additivity or non-normality in ANOVA, or more generally to improve the agreement between the observations and the assumptions in a model, (ii) to reduce skewness or achieve approximate symmetry, (iii) to describe the structure of observations and (iv) to simplify the relationship between variables.

The power transformation x^λ or Box-Cox transformation $x^{(\lambda)} = (x^\lambda - 1)/\lambda$ are simple monotonic transformations that are frequently used; however, they can be applied only to non-negative x. The Box-Cox transformation has the advantage that the limiting transformation as $\lambda \to 0$ is log (x). To ease interpretation, it is sometimes preferable to limit λ to a finite set, such as $(-2, -1, -1/2, 0, 1/4, 1/3, 1/2, 2/3, 1, 2)$. A general discussion of a variety of aspects in the use of power transformations can be found in Box and Cox (1964), the review article by Sakia (1992) and the book by Carroll and Ruppert (1988).

A common use of transformations is in a regression or ANOVA setting. It is common for the variance of the response to increase as the expected value increases. In such cases a power transformation of the response variable can sometimes achieve approximate homogeneity of variance. Also when the variance does increase with the mean it is fairly common for the observations, or residuals from the mean, to be positively skewed, for which the same transformation may have the added benefit of substantially reducing the skewness.

Overall in regression settings, transformations of the response variable are used in the hope that they will give a correct structure in the systematic part of the model and also achieve homogeneous and Gaussian error distributions. It is unlikely that a single transformation will achieve all of these exactly. It is the correct systematic that is the most important of the three aspects to achieve.

For a set of observations $\mathbf{Y}^T = (Y_1, \ldots, Y_n)$ Box and Cox proposed the model

$$Y_i^{(\lambda)} = \mathbf{X}_i\beta + e_i \qquad (1)$$

where $\mathbf{X}_i$ is the ith row of the design matrix $\mathbf{X}$, e_i are independent, $e_i \sim N(0, \sigma^2)$. In this model a single λ is assumed to achieve the three objectives of a simple systematic structure, homogeneity of variance and normal errors.

A problematic aspect of (1) is that the interpretation of the parameter β depends on λ. However, various aspects of β, in particular, the direction of β (represented by $\beta/(length(\beta))$, say) or the ratio of two regression coefficients, β_1/β_2, which measures the relative importance of one explanatory variable to another, both have interpretations that are not dependent on λ.

For models involving transformations some aspects of inference for the regression coefficient, β, have been controversial. In an unconditional approach λ is treated as a parameter on equal footing with all the other parameters; however, the interpretation of β depends on the estimated λ, and the variance of β is very large. In the conditional approach inference about β is made on the estimated transformed scale, ignoring the fact that λ has been estimated from the observations, which is not entirely satisfactory because it ignores the uncertainty associated with the estimation of λ. Aspects of inference which are less controversial are tests of $\beta = 0$, hypotheses which have an interpretation irrespective of λ.

In some applications transformations back to the original Y scale are desirable and can be particularly useful for graphical display. Caution is necessary in transforming interpretations from one scale to the other; for example, a lack of interaction on the transformed scale should not be interpreted as a lack of interaction on the original scale. Power transformations allow predictions back to the original scale because they are monotonic. For model (1), the quantity $1 + \lambda(\mathbf{X}_0\beta)^{1/\lambda}$, when $\lambda \neq 0$ or $\exp(\mathbf{X}_0\beta)$ when $\lambda = 0$, is the predicted median of the distribution of Y given $\mathbf{X}_0$.

In multiple regression modelling it is common to consider transformations of explanatory variables. In the model

$$Y_i = \alpha + \beta X_i^{(\lambda)} + e_i \qquad (2)$$

for scalar X, where $e_i \sim N(0, \sigma^2)$, the purpose of adding the extra parameter λ is to better fit the systematic structure of the model, with the requirement of homogeneity of variance and normality of e_i playing a lesser role. Whether the transformation achieves symmetry or normality of the marginal distribution of $X^{(\lambda)}$ is usually of less importance, other than to reduce the sensitivity of outliers in X or unless one needs to model the X distribution.

Carroll and Ruppert (1988) have developed an approach for non-linear regression models in which the systematic part of the model, $f(\mathbf{X}, \beta)$, is known through subject matter considerations. For example, the Michaelis-Menten equation for enzyme reactions is $Y = \beta_0 X/(\beta_1 + X)$. The same transformation is applied to both sides of this equation, by assuming the model $Y_i^{(\lambda)} = (f(\mathbf{X}_i, \beta))^{(\lambda)} + e_i$ where $e_i \sim N(0, \sigma^2)$. The model assumes that the untransformed relationship already fits the median of the data adequately, but that the residuals exhibit heteroscedasticity and/or non-normality. The main aim of the transform-both-sides approach is to make the residuals normal with constant variance, hence improving properties and inference associated with estimates of β. An important aspect of the approach is that the interpretation of β does not depend on λ.

The accelerated failure time model for censored survival data, $\log(T_i) = \mathbf{X}_i\beta + e_i$, where $e_i \sim N(0, \sigma^2)$, can be viewed as a special case of the power transformation model. In the extension of the Box-Cox procedure to multivariate data a separate power transformation parameter is assumed for each component of the multivariate vector. Solomon and Taylor (1999) considered Box-Cox transformations for components of variance models.

Power transformations have been used to assist in estimating regression centiles, which have application in establishing reference ranges. In the LMS method at each fixed value of a scalar variable x the distribution of Y is assumed to be normal following a power transformation, from this the percentiles can be easily calculated. The model assumes that the median of Y, the power transformation parameter and the scale parameter of the normal distribution all vary smoothly as a function of x.

In AIDS studies, viral load and CD4 count, a measure of the immune system, are frequently measured and are important indicators of disease progression. Both these variables are highly skewed. Relatively complicated longitudinal and joint longitudinal-survival models have been applied to serial measurements of these markers. Nearly everyone uses the logarithm of viral load, either $\log_e$, $\log_{10}$ or $\log_2$. For CD4 counts some authors use the log for ease of interpretation, whereas others use $CD4^{1/4}$ or $CD4^{1/2}$ to ensure that the assumptions in their models, such as homogeneity of variance and symmetry for the measurement error, were satisfied for their data.

PSA is a common blood test used in prostate cancer studies both for screening and to monitor disease progression. PSA is quite skew and it is natural to consider a logarithm transformation because the PSA value is thought to be roughly proportional to the volume of the tumour, which grows approximately exponentially. In practice log(PSA+1) has been used, because PSA can be close to or even equal to zero, causing a standard log transformation to produce too many large negative values or not be calculable. *JMGT*

Box, G.E.P. and Cox, D.R. 1964: An analysis of transformations, (with discussion). *Journal of the Royal Statistical Society B*, 26, 211–52. **Carroll, R.J. and Ruppert, D.** 1988: *Transformation and weighting in regression.* London: Chapman and Hall. **Cole, T.J. and Green, P.J.** 1992: Smoothing reference centile curves: the LMS method and penalized likelihood. *Statistics in Medicine* 11, 1305–19. **Sakia, R.M.** 1992: The Box-Cox transformation technique: a review. *The Statistician*, 41, 169–78. **Slate, E.H. and Cronin, K.A.** 1997: Changepoint modeling of longitudinal PSA as a biomarker for prostate cancer. *Case Studies in Bayesian Statistics* III, Springer-Verlag, 435–56. **Solomon, P.J. and Taylor, J.M.G.** 1999: Orthogonality and transformations in variance components model. *Biometrika* 86, 289–300. **Tsiatis, A.A., DeGruttola, V. and Wulfsohn, M.S.** 1995: Modeling the relationship of survival to longitudinal data measured with error. Applications to survival and CD4 counts in patients with AIDS. *Journal of the American Statistical Association* 90, 27–37. **Wang, Y. and Taylor, J.M.G.** 2001: Jointly modeling longitudinal and event time data: application in AIDS studies. *Journal of the American Statistical Association* 96, 895–905.

tree-structured methods (TSM)

Methods designed to produce interpretable prediction rules by subdividing data into subgroups that are homogenous with respect to both covariates and outcome. Predictions flow from this outcome constancy, with simple subgroup summaries sufficing. The interpretability of the attendant prediction rules derives from the simple, recursive fashion by which the covariates are employed in eliciting the subgroups. As a consequence of this simplicity tree-structured methods have enjoyed widespread popularity, particularly in biomedical settings. But, of course, all this simplicity belies a number of issues, especially pertaining to prediction performance, that have spawned considerable recent research activity.

TSM prediction rules can be developed for both categorical and continuous outcomes, reflecting classification and regression problems respectively. It was the correspondingly named monograph 'Classification and regression trees' by Breiman *et al.* (1984) that, by way of establishing a methodological framework and providing several compelling applications, fuelled the subsequent popularity of TSM. Indeed, tree-structured methods are frequently referred to by the monograph's title-based acronym, CART. The terminology 'recursive partitioning' is also commonplace, with another relevant monograph being that by Zhang and Singer (1999). The 'tree' terminology itself derives from the companion graphical depictions of the fitted models (see first Figure on page 357). As an historical note, the forerunners of TSM date to the 1960s.

The basic TSM paradigm, as developed by Breiman *et al.* (1984) and outlined later, has been extended in many directions. Of particular importance from a biomedical standpoint are extensions to survival outcomes and longitudinal data. The resultant methods are described in an overview article (Segal, 1995). Here, illustration of TSM will make recourse to the SURVIVAL ANALYSIS applications since this allows exposition of TSM fundamentals, as well

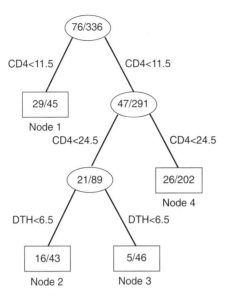

tree-structured methods *Log-rank survival tree*

as showcasing a setting for which tree concepts seem particularly well suited.

The central thrust of tree techniques is the elicitation of subgroups. Within these subgroups covariates are homogenous and between subgroups outcomes are distinct. So, in clinical settings with survival outcomes, interpretation in terms of prognostic group identification is frequently possible. Creation of the subgroups according to a tree structure (binary recursion) mimics, at least simplistically, medical decision making: if the patient is female, has a family history of breast cancer and is over 40, then annual mammograms are recommended. Similarly, given a survival tree, it is straightforward to classify a new patient to a prognostic group by simply answering the sequence of yes/no (binary) questions or splits that give rise to each subgroup or node.

It is reasonable to assess whether this goal of subgroup extraction requires new methodology. Could not, for

example, the COX REGRESSION MODEL (1972) be employed for this purpose? Suppose, without loss of generality, that in fitting a PROPORTIONAL HAZARDS model with 3 continuous covariates we obtain positive coefficients for each. That is, each variable is adverse: increased values of each are associated with elevated risk. Thus, we might try to create a high-risk group by combining individuals who have high values for all 3 covariates. However, this approach may fail due to no patients possessing such a covariate profile.

Alternatively, we could compute a risk score for each member of the sample based on substitution of the actual covariate profiles into the log-linear model using the fitted coefficients. Then a high-risk stratum could be obtained by selecting the desired percentile of the sample risk scores. The difficulty here is that individuals with potentially disparate covariate values are combined and hence the resultant risk group is hard to label or interpret.

In addition to identifying important prognostic groups, which can be thought of as local interactions, survival tree techniques can also be informative about individual covariates. This derives from single splitting (subdivision) being revealing about threshold effects for time-independent covariates or change points in the case of time-dependent covariates. Also, repeated splitting on a given covariate can be revealing about more complex nonlinearities. However, use of (smoothed) martingale residual plots (Therneau, Grambsch and Fleming, 1990) is arguably a more direct way for determining appropriate functional form. Further, tree methods in general are not geared toward making global assessments of a covariate's importance. This is for a variety of reasons.

First, if a covariate is used (to define a split) in just one branch of the tree, then it is problematic trying to gauge its overall importance. Second, masking whereby a covariate selected as (the best) split variable precludes another, almost as good, covariate from emerging complicates covariate evaluation. (Splitting criteria are discussed later; these allow determination as to which covariate constitutes the best split variable. Most software implementations of TSM provide output detailing several of the top competing splits (not just the best), as well as measures of overall

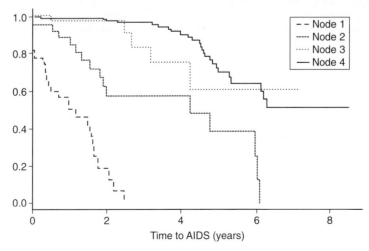

tree-structured methods *Kaplan-Meier curves: log-rank tree*

covariate importance. The related issue of instability is further discussed in the context of improving TSM predictive performance.) Finally, covariate splits are selected by optimising a split criterion and are therefore highly adaptive. While some corresponding distributional results have been obtained, difficulties remain in assigning significances to a sequence of splits, and hence to formally appraising covariate importance.

The prescription for tree construction advanced by Breiman *et al.* (1984) has served as the foundation for many extensions and refinements and is so worth detailing. Their approach features four constituent components: a set of questions, or splits, phrased in terms of the covariates that serve to partition the covariate space. A tree structure derives from the recursive application of these questions and a binary tree results if the questions are binary (yes/no). The subgroups created by assigning cases according to these splits are termed *nodes*; a split function (or split criterion) $\phi(s, t)$ that can be evaluated for any split s of any node t. The split function is used to assess the worth of the competing splits; a means for determining appropriate tree size; statistical summaries for the nodes of the tree.

The first item defines what sort of subdivisions are permitted – these are the allowable splits. Binary splits are generally used, mostly for computational reasons. These have the flavour: '*Is age less than 45?*' or '*Is ethnicity Asian, black or Hispanic?*'. The answers to such questions induce a partition, or split, of the covariate space: cases for which the answer is 'yes' belong to the corresponding region while those for which the answer is 'no' belong to the complementary region. The allowable splits satisfy the following constraints: each split depends on the value of only a single covariate; for ordered (continuous or categorical) covariates, X_j, only splits resulting from questions of the form '*Is $X_j \leq c$?*' for $c \in$ domain (X_j) are considered. Thus ordering is preserved (see first question); for unordered categorical predictors all possible splits into disjoint subsets of the categories are allowed (see second question).

The allowable splits are formulated in this fashion in order to balance flexibility and interpretability of the fitted models with computational feasibility. While variants and extensions have been subsequently promoted, this formulation underlies most implementations.

Given a set of allowable splits a tree is grown as follows: for each subgroup or node (i) examine every allowable split on each predictor variable, (ii) select and execute (create left and right daughter nodes) the best of these splits.

The initial or root node comprises the entire sample. Steps (i) and (ii) are then reapplied to each of the daughter nodes and so on. It is this reapplication that gives rise to the *recursive partitioning* terminology. The determination of tree size (how many splits), the third component of the paradigm, is important yet complicated – details are deferred to Breiman *et al.* (1984) and Segal (1995). Thus, it remains to define what constitutes a best split; this is the province of the second component.

Best splits are decided by optimising a split function $\phi(s, g)$ that can be evaluated for any splits of any node g. For regression (i.e. continuous outcomes) Breiman *et al.* (1984) describe two possibilities: least squares (LS), detailed later and least absolute deviations. Let g designate

a node of the tree. That is, g contains a sub-sample of cases $\{(x'_i, y_i)g$ where $x'_i = (x_{i1}, x_{i2}, ..., x_{ip})$ is the vector of observed covariate values and y_i is the observed outcome for the ith case. Let N_g be the total number of cases in g and let $\bar{y}(g) = (1/N_g)\sum_{i \in g} y_i$ be the outcome average for node g. Then the within node sum of squares is given by $SS(g) = \sum_{i \in g}(y_i - \bar{y}(g))^2$. Now suppose a split s partitions g into left and right daughter nodes g_L and g_R. The LS split function is $\phi(s, g) = SS(g) - SS(g_L) - SS(g_R)$ and the best split $s^\star$ of g is the split such that $\phi(s^\star, g) = \max_{s \in \Omega}(s, g)$ where Ω is the set of all allowable splits s of g. An LS regression tree is constructed by recursively splitting nodes so as to maximise the above ϕ function. The function is such that we create smaller and smaller nodes of progressively increased homogeneity on account of the non-negativity of ϕ: $\phi \geq 0$ since $SS(g) \geq SS(g_L) + SS(g_R) \ \forall \ s$.

It is worth noting that a tree grown in accordance with this LS split function will coincide with a tree grown using a two-sample t-statistic as split function if the latter uses a pooled estimate of variance. Selecting the split that makes the resultant t-statistic maximal can be viewed as optimising node separation as measured by the difference in the respective node averages.

Modifications to the split function are a primary means for expanding the scope of TSM. Several such modifications have been proposed to enable handling of (censored) survival outcomes. One suite of such split functions is based on notions of between-node separation, analogous to use of the t-statistic. The log-rank statistic provides a familiar and readily implemented example. The resultant rewarding of subgroups that are internally homogenous with regard covariates (as imparted by allowable splits), yet externally different, dovetails with the objective of identifying distinct prognostic groups. Further, use of the log-rank statistic as split function allows additional accommodation of left-truncated survival times as well as time-dependent covariates (see TIME-DEPENDENT VARIABLES).

We present an illustrative example of TSM with survival endpoints that pertains to HIV disease progression. The latency or incubation period for AIDS (i.e. the time from HIV infection to an AIDS diagnosis) is both long and variable. In order to try to explain this variability in terms of immune function decay, markers of immune function are regularly measured on longitudinally followed cohorts of HIV seropositive and seroconverting individuals. In particular, counts of CD4+T lymphocytes have been widely used both to follow the course of immune function loss and to predict time to AIDS or death. Here we consider an additional marker, delayed-type hypersensitivity (DTH) skin tests, as a putative supplement to CD4.

Use of DTH is motivated in part by deficiencies of CD4: quantification of peripheral blood CD4 depletion underestimates the severity of the HIV-induced loss of antigen-specific cellular immunity and provides no guide as to which antigen-specific responses have been lost. More sensitive measures of antigen-specific cellular immunity are therefore required as an adjunct to the monitoring of CD4 counts. Testing of cutaneous DTH responses to recall antigens provides a direct measure of cell mediated antigen-specific responses *in vivo*.

Assessment of these markers made recourse to the Western Australian HIV database. Patients in Western

Australia with HIV infection have been managed at a single specialist referral centre since the first AIDS case was confirmed in August 1983. Both HIV-infected and at-risk individuals were followed regularly. The closely scheduled (bimonthly) visits and early inception of the cohort provides a good opportunity for marker evaluation. Further details on the cohort, markers, handling sero-prevalent (HIV positive at enrolment) subjects in the context of survival analysis, treating markers as time-dependent covariates and complementary Cox proportional hazards results are given in Segal *et al.* (1995).

Results from a TSM analysis of the survival endpoint time-to-AIDS are presented in the Figures on page 357. The log-rank statistic was used as a split function, although results were insensitive to this choice. The covariates used were age, CD4 and DTH, all measured at enrolment. CD4 is expressed as the percentage of T-lymphocytes that are CD4 positive, is in accord with studies that while noting strong correlations between this and other measures (CD4 count, CD4/CD8 ratio), found CD4% to be most prognostic for time-to-AIDS and exhibiting smallest variability on repeated determinations.

The initial sample features 336 individuals, 76 of whom progressed to AIDS, as depicted in the uppermost (root) node. This sample is subdivided on the basis of CD4%, the optimal cut-off point being 11.5%, as shown on the emanating branches. In determining this split all possible cut-off points on all three (continuous) covariates were evaluated; i.e. corresponding log-rank statistics computed. The selected split was maximal among all these statistics. The 291 individuals with CD4% exceeding 11.5% are also subdivided on the basis of CD4% – covariates can be used repeatedly. Examination of these CD4-based splits affirms the anticipated: the subgroups with higher CD4% have superior survival.

Indeed, the Kaplan-Meier curves (seen in the second Figure on page 357) for the respective terminal nodes (rectangles in the first Figure) showcase dramatic differences between the CD4 extremes, with survival prospects for the low CD4 group (Node 1) being dismal in comparison with the high group (Node 4). The 89 individuals with intermediary CD4% (11.5 < CD4 < 24.5) are further partitioned, this time on the basis of DTH. The optimal cut-off point is at a DTH value of 6.5mm. The second Figure again reveals survival differences for those in the two DTH-defined subgroups (Node 2 vs Node 3). Thus, it is possible that DTH can serve to augment CD4% as a marker for HIV progression: for individuals whose CD4% values are intermediary, rather than extreme, additional prognostic information may be obtained from their DTH values. It is interesting to contrast the splits with smoothed martingale residual plots obtained from a null Cox proportional hazards model. Such graphics are useful for informing appropriate covariate functional form (Therneau, Grambsch and Fleming, 1990). Each split conforms to a step function approximation of the smoothed martingale residuals, which in turn are suggestive of threshold effects.

Of course, TSM are not without shortcomings. The primary deficiencies pertain to the interrelated concerns of instability, modest prediction performance and inefficiency in capturing underlying smooth response surfaces. Instability refers to the frequently large impact (on tree topology – selected covariates and cut-off points) that can

result from small changes in data and/or inputs. This instability in part leads to relatively modest prediction performance by way of the associated large prediction variances that are exhibited when applying a TSM to independent test data.

A number of so-called committee or ensemble prediction methods have recently emerged that improve performance by reducing this variability by way of strategic creation and combination of (many) individual TSMs. Bagging, boosting and random forests are examples; see Breiman (2001). Nonetheless, by virtue of their ready interpretability, TSMs remain a valuable tool for a wide range of biomedical problems.   *MRS*

Breiman, L. 2001: Statistical modelling: the two cultures. *Statistical Science* 16, 199–215. **Breiman, L., Friedman, J.H., Olshen, R.A. and Stone, C.J.** 1984: *Classification and regression trees.* Belmont: Wadsworth. **Cox, D.R.** 1972: Regression models and life-tables (with discussion). *Journal of the Royal Statistical Society Series B* 34, 187–220. **Segal, M.R.** 1995: Extending the elements of tree-structured regression. *Statistical Methods in Medical Research* 4, 219–36. **Segal, M.R., James, I.R., French, M.A.H. and Mallal, S.** 1995: Statistical issues in the evaluation of markers of HIV progression. *International Statistical Review* 63, 179–97. **Therneau, T.M., Grambsch, P.M. and Fleming, T.R.** 1990: Martingale-based residuals for survival models. *Biometrika* 77, 147–60. **Zhang, H. and Singer, B.** 1999: *Recursive partitioning in the health sciences.* New York: Springer.

trellis graphics An approach to examining high-dimensional structure in data by means of one-, two- and three-dimensional graphs. The problem addressed is how observations on one or more variables depend on the values of other variables. The essential feature of the approach is the multiple conditioning that allows some type of graphic involving one or more variables to be displayed several times, each time as it appears when one or more other variables take particular values. The simplest example of a trellis graphic is the coplot, which is a SCATTERPLOT of two variables conditioned on the values taken by a third variable.

For example, the first Figure on page 360 shows a coplot of mortality versus latitude conditioned on population size. In this diagram, the panel at the top of the Figure is known as the 'given' panel; those below are 'dependence' panels. Each rectangle in the given panel specifies a range of values of population size. On a corresponding dependence panel, mortality is plotted against latitude for those countries whose population sizes lie in the particular interval. To match population size intervals to dependence panel, the latter are examined in order from left to right in the bottom row and then again from left to right in subsequent rows. The association between higher values of mortality and lower values of latitude (and vice versa) is seen to hold for all levels of population size.

A more complex example of a trellis graphic is shown in the second Figure on page 360; here a three-dimensional plot of mortality, latitude and longitude is given for four ranges of population size.

Several other examples of the use of trellis graphics are given in Verbyla *et al.* (1999).   *BSE*

[See also SCATTERPLOT MATRICES]

Verbyla, A.P., Cullis, B.R., Kenward, M.G. and Welham, S.J. 1999: The analysis of designed experiments and longitudinal data using smoothing splines (with discussion). *Applied Statistics* 48, 269–312.

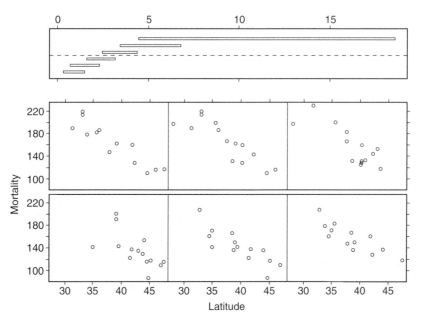

trellis graphics *Coplot of mortality versus latitude conditioned on population size*

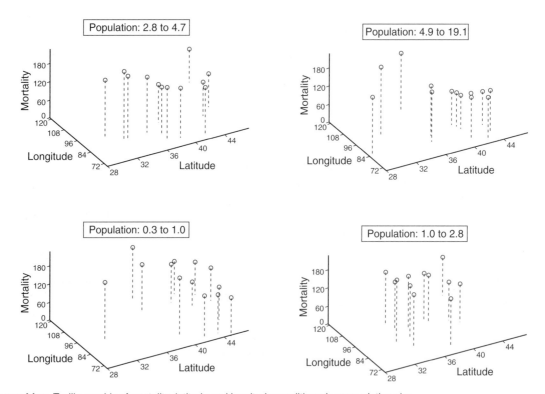

trellis graphics *Trellis graphic of mortality, latitude and longitude conditioned on population size*

triangular test See SEQUENTIAL ANALYSIS

t-test See STUDENT'S t-TEST

twin analysis The analysis of diseases or other pheno-types in twins is an important tool in genetic epidemiology. Twins may be either monozygotic (MZ; that is, arising from the same fertilised egg) or dizygotic (DZ). MZ twins are genetically identical to one another. DZ twins, contrariwise, are genetically equivalent to siblings and share, on average, half their genetic material. Since both MZ and DZ twin pairs share the same environment (at least *in utero* and early life) they provide a well-controlled study design to evaluate genetic influences; for any phenotype that has a genetic component, MZ twins will tend to be more similar than DZ twins. MZ and DZ may be distinguished in studies by questionnaire (e.g. '*Are you like two peas in a pod?*') or more objectively by DNA analysis.

For quantitative traits, the extent of concordance between MZ and DZ twins can be expressed in terms of *intraclass correlations*. Simple comparisons can then be made using F-tests. Since these tests assume normality, some transformation of the trait may be required.

More general analysis of twin data is usually conducted in the framework of a variance components analysis. Thus, we think of the trait X as being decomposed into a sum of components:

$$X = G + E + R$$

where G is the genetic component, E is a component due to shared environmental factors and R is a residual component. The proportion of the trait variance due to genetic component G is called the *heritability* of the trait (often written H). The genetic component can be further decomposed into an *additive* genetic component, A, and a non-additive (or *dominance*) component D. An additive component in this sense is such that the value for any individual is the mean of the values in their two parents. If the proportions of the trait variance due to additive and non-additive genetic factors and shared environment are ρ_A, ρ_D and ρ_E, then the correlations between MZ and DZ twin pairs will be given by:

$$\rho_{MZ} = \rho_A + \rho_D + \rho_E$$

$$\rho_{MZ} = 1/2\rho_A + 1/4\rho_D + \rho_E$$

Since twin studies only allow two correlations to be estimated, it is not possible to estimate the additive, dominance and shared environmental components simultaneously. A common assumption is that the dominance component is zero, so that genetic component is purely additive. Data on other relatives may allow all three components to be estimated. Where necessary, other covariates may be included in this framework. Age may be a particularly important covariate to include since twin pairs are identical in age.

An important assumption in these analyses is that the shared environment component E is identical in MZ and DZ twins. This assumption may sometimes be violated if certain *in utero* effects are important.

Twin data for binary traits are often expressed in terms of concordance rate, defined as the proportion of twins of affected individuals who are themselves affected. A higher concordance rate in MZ twins is expected for traits with a genetic component. Concordance rates may be calculated in two ways. If the starting point is a series of affected individuals (for example from hospital records), the concordance rate can be estimated straightforwardly by identifying those individuals with twins and calculating the rates in the co-twins. If, however, the starting point is a register of twins, the concordance rate can be calculated from the number of pairs where both twins are affected (concordant) and where only one twin is affected (discordant), thus:

$$\frac{2 \times \text{\# concordant pairs}}{2 \times \text{\# concordant pairs} + \text{\# discordant pairs}}$$

The factor of two is necessary to allow for the fact that concordant twins may be ascertained through either twin. Studies based on twin registers can be seriously biased if concordant twin pairs are more likely to be identified. For this reason, the best twin data on disease come from population-based registers with record linkage to medical records, as are available, for example, in Scandinavia.

More general methods of analysing binary twin data have been developed. A common approach is to extend the ideas of LOGISTIC REGRESSION or, for a chronic disease, Poisson or Cox regression. The genetic and shared environmental effects are modelled by including RANDOM EFFECTS terms in the model in addition to any fixed covariates.   *DE*

[See also GENETIC EPIDEMIOLOGY, GENOTYPE, PHENOTYPE]

Balding, D.J., Bishop, M. and Cannings, C. (eds) 2001: *Handbook of statistical genetics*. Chichester: John Wiley & Sons. **Sham, P.** 1998: *Statistics in human genetics*. London: Arnold.

two-dimensional contingency table   See CONTINGENCY TABLES

two-sample t-test   See STUDENT'S t-TEST

two-sided tests   In hypothesis tests we try to distinguish between chance variation in a dataset and a genuine effect. We do this by comparing the null hypothesis, which states that there is no difference between the populations in which the data arose, and the alternative hypothesis, which states that there is, in fact, a difference. If no direction for the difference is specified by either the null hypothesis or the alternative hypothesis, we have a two-sided test, sometimes referred to as a two-tailed test. So we are looking for a difference but are equally interested in differences in either direction.

For instance, when comparing a new treatment to an existing one we would be interested in detecting differences both in favour of or against the new treatment. In the majority of cases, the two-sided alternative is the appropriate one as it allows for the uncertainty about the direction of an effect that is often present. Whether or not to use a two-sided test should be decided based on the design of the study. Unless the study specifically seeks to detect an upward or downward change determined in advance two sided tests should be used. It is usually assumed that the *P*-VALUE reported from a specific statistical test is two-sided unless stated otherwise.   *MMB*

Bland, J.M. and Altman, D.G. 1994: Statistics notes: one- and two-sided tests of significance. *British Medical Journal* 309, 248.

[See also ONE-SIDED TESTS]

two-way analysis of variance   A test to see if the mean varies with either (or both) of two categorical factors. The one-way ANALYSIS OF VARIANCE seeks to partition the variation in a sample into that due to the group factor (the between-groups sum of squares) and the residual variation that cannot be explained by a factor (the within-groups sum of squares).

In a two-way analysis of variance, there are two factors that define the groups and each factor explains some of

two-way analysis of variance *Two-way ANOVA table for main factor effects only. Entries in bold must be calculated directly from the data; other entries follow in the manner indicated*

Source of variance	Degrees of freedom	Sums of squares	Mean squares	F	P-value
Factor A	k–1	A SS	A MS = A SS/(k–1)	$\dfrac{\text{A MS}}{\text{Res MS}}$	p
Factor B	j–1	B SS	B MS = B SS/(j–1)	$\dfrac{\text{B MS}}{\text{Res MS}}$	p
Residual	N–k–j+1	Res SS = Total SS – (A SS + B SS)	Res MS = Res SS/(N–k–j+1)		
Total	N–1	Total SS			

two-way analysis of variance *Two-way ANOVA table when an interaction effect is included. Entries in bold must be calculated directly from the data; the other entries follow in the manner indicated*

Source of variance	Degrees of freedom	Sums of squares	Mean squares	F	P-value
Factor A	k–1	A SS	A MS = A SS/(k–1)	$\dfrac{\text{A MS}}{\text{Res Ms}}$	p
Factor B	j–1	B SS	B MS = B SS/(j–1)	$\dfrac{\text{B MS}}{\text{Res MS}}$	p
Interaction	(k–1)(j–1)	Int SS	Int MS = Int SS/((k–1)(j–1))	$\dfrac{\text{Int MS}}{\text{Res MS}}$	p
Residual	N–kj	Res SS = Total SS – (Int SS + A SS + B SS)	Res MS = Res SS/(N–kj)		
Total	N–1	Total SS			

the variation. It is therefore necessary to partition the variation in the sample into that due to Factor A, that due to Factor B and the residual variation.

The total variation/sum of squares (total SS) can be calculated in the same way as for one-way analysis of variance. The sum of squares due to Factor A is the sum over all individuals of the squared differences between the overall mean and the mean value associated with the level of the factor appropriate to the individual. The sum of squares due to Factor B can be calculated in a similar manner. The residual sum of squares is then calculated as the total sum of squares minus the sums of squares due to Factors A and B.

If we wish to calculate the sum of squares due to the interaction between the factors, then this is calculated as the sum over all individuals of the squared difference between the mean for the appropriate combination of the factors and the sum of the means associated with the relevant levels of the individual factors less the overall mean.

Like the one-way flavour, the two-way ANOVA can be presented as a table. If Factor A has k levels and Factor B has j levels, then the statistics to test for factor effects are presented in the first table. The F-statistic associated with Factor A will be compared to an F distribution with $k – 1$ and $N – k – j + 1$ DEGREES OF FREEDOM. That associated with Factor B will be compared to an F distribution with

$j – 1$ and $N – k – j + 1$ degrees of freedom.

If the interaction term is required, then the analysis is as shown in the second table.

Reneman *et al.* (2001) use two-way ANOVA to compare alcohol use in eight groups defined by gender ($k = 2$) and four levels of ecstasy use ($j = 4$). With 69 people in the study and no interaction being considered, the test for a gender effect is conducted by comparing the F-statistic to an F distribution with 1 and 64 degrees of freedom.

AGL

[See also GENERALISED LINEAR MODEL]

Armitage, P. and Berry, G. 1987: *Statistical methods in medical research*. Oxford: Blackwell. **Reneman, L.** *et al.* 2001: Effects of dose, sex, and long-term abstention from use on toxic effects of MDMA (ecstasy) on brain serotonin neurons. *Lancet* 358, 1864–9.

Type I error After every hypothesis test, the decision to accept or reject the null hypothesis is made. This decision can, however, lead to two possible errors. First, we can obtain a significant result and thus reject the null hypothesis, when the null hypothesis is, in reality, true. This is termed a Type I error and can be considered as a false positive result. Second, we may obtain a non-significant result and thus accept the null hypothesis when the null hypothesis is not true. In this case the error is called a Type II error, which may be considered a false negative result. The Type I error rate is no more than the so-called significance level, frequently denoted by alpha, α. Thus the significance level represents the chance that the null hypothesis is rejected when it is actually true. For every hypothesis test the significance level should be decided beforehand, the typical value chosen for this is 0.05. Consequently, over many trials, 5% or one in 20 are expected to yield false positive results.

Sometimes, however, smaller values for alpha are used in particular to help deal with the problem of multiple testing.   *MMB*

Altman, D.G. 1991: *Practical statistics for medical research.* London: Chapman & Hall.

Type II error   After every hypothesis test, the decision to accept or reject the null hypothesis is made. This decision can however lead to two possible errors. First, we can obtain a significant result and thus reject the null hypothesis, when the null hypothesis is in reality true. This is termed a Type I error and can be considered as a false

positive result. Type II error, in contrast, refers to a mistaken failure to reject the null hypothesis when the alternative hypothesis is true and there is a real difference between the study groups, which may be considered a false negative result. The probability of making a Type II error is represented by beta, β.

The Type II error is closely related to the power of a test. The statistical power of a test can be thought of as the chance or probability that a study of a given size would detect as statistically significant a real difference of a given magnitude defined as $1 - \beta$ or, more usually, power = $100(1 - \beta)\%$. For example when $\beta = 0.2$, there is only an 80% chance of the test detecting the particular alternative hypothesis when actually true. In designing a study, both types of error should ideally be minimised.

It is common to fix beta in advance by choosing an appropriate sample size. We do this by calculating the necessary sample size for a study to have a high probability of finding a true effect of a given magnitude.   *MMB*

Altman, D.G. 1991: *Practical statistics for medical research.* London: Chapman & Hall.

U

uncle test for randomisation   See ETHICS AND CLINICAL TRIALS

uniform distribution   The PROBABILITY DISTRIBUTION whereby all outcomes (within a range) are equally likely. There is a discrete uniform distribution and a continuous uniform distribution (also known as the rectangular distribution), and we consider the discrete version first. If a random variable has a discrete uniform distribution on the integers from a to a+b, then we can write the probability mass function as:

$$P(X = x) = \frac{1}{b+1} \quad a \leq x \leq b$$

Expressed in this way, the distribution has a MEAN of a + b/2 and variance of $(b^2+2b)/12$. As all probabilities are the same, it is of course symmetric about the mean.

The discrete uniform distribution is used in assessing DIGIT PREFERENCE. If durations of operations are being recorded to the nearest minute, and the operations typically take between two and four hours, then it might be presumed that the distribution of the terminal digit of the minutes would be approximately uniform from 0 to 9. The observed digits can be compared to the uniform distribution to detect any bias. The most common use of the uniform distribution in the medical sciences is perhaps in generating random sequences for clinical trials.

The probability density function of the continuous uniform distribution appears as a rectangle on a graph (hence its alternative name), since the area of the rectangle must be equal to 1, the value of the density function is defined by the range of plausible observations (to keep the area of the rectangle constant, the height is defined by the width). The probability density function for the continuous uniform distribution is:

$$f(x) = \frac{1}{b-a} \quad a \leq x \leq b$$

In this formulation, the mean is (a+b)/2, and the VARIANCE is $(b-a)^2/12$. As with the discrete uniform, the distribution is symmetric about the mean. Note that when a=0 and b=1, this is a special case of the BETA DISTRIBUTION.

The cumulative distribution function maps observations from a distribution to probabilities that should be uniformly distributed between 0 and 1. Conversely the inverse of the cumulative distribution function maps uniform observations between 0 and 1 to observations from the distribution in question. The first property provides a useful check of model fit. The second allows us to generate random observations from many distributions, if we can generate random uniformly distributed data and write out the inverse of the cumulative distribution function.

AGL

Altman, D.G. 1991: *Practical Statistics for Medical Research.* London: Chapman and Hall.

V

variance The variance is the square of the STANDARD DEVIATION. It is calculated using the following formula, in which n is the number of observations, i takes values from 1 to n and the Σ notation denotes the sum i.e. $(x_1 - \overline{x})^2 + (x_2 - \overline{x})^2 + \ldots + (x_n - \overline{x})$:

$$s^2 = \frac{\sum(x_i - \overline{x})^2}{n-1}$$

Both s^2 and σ^2 are used to indicate the variance. Technically, the former refers to the variance of the sample and the latter to the variance of the population, which is being estimated by the sample and is marginally smaller, since the divisor is n instead of $n-1$ in the formula. When quoting a mean to summarise data, it is also customary to quote a sample standard deviation. This is the square root of the sample variance, and is in the same units as the raw data. *SRC*

variance components See COMPONENTS OF VARIANCE

variogram A procedure that provides a description of the autocorrelation in line series or spatial clusters. It is the latter that forms the focus for the following account. It is important to describe and model this autocorrelation so as to incorporate it into estimation and prediction procedures. For example, consider disease incidences measured at spatial locations. To construct a map, one would need to interpolate the incidence value for the locations at which it was not observed and in the absence of large-scale spatial trend such predictions should give larger weights to nearby locations if the autocorrelation were increasing with decreasing distances.

The variogram is based on the semi-variance $\gamma(x, y; h_x, h_y)$, which measures half the variance of the difference between two values of an outcome, Z, observed at two spatial locations referenced by the spatial coordinates (x, y) and $(x + h_x, y + h_y)$. Strictly speaking, the theoretical variogram is defined as twice the semi-variance, i.e.:

$$2\gamma(x, y; h_x, h_y) = E\big[[Z(x, y) - Z(x + h_x, y + h_y)]^2\big]$$

but the semi-variance itself is usually referred to as the variogram. It represents an (inverse) measure of the statistical dependency of the variables at locations (x, y) and $(x + h_x, y + h_y)$.

In all generality, the variogram is a function of both the location (x, y) and the distance and direction (h_x, h_y). Hence, to estimate it replicate observations at each location would be needed. In practice, only one such realisation is available. To overcome this, the intrinsic hypothesis is introduced that makes assumptions about the difference $Z(x, y) - Z(x + h_x, y + h_y)$. It states that for the spatial area under investigation (1) the expectation of the difference is zero – i.e. that there is no spatial trend and that (2) the variance of the difference depends only on the distance vector (h_x, h_y) and not the location. For variograms that reach an asymptote (so-called *bounded* variograms) this hypothesis is equivalent to assuming second-order stationarity of the measures themselves.

Under this assumption it is possible to estimate the variogram from the data. For simplicity further assuming that the variogram is isotropic, that is that it only depends on the distance, h, between two locations and not the direction of (h_x, h_y), the variogram can be estimated by the empirical variogram $\hat{\gamma}(h) = \frac{1}{2|N(h)|} \sum_{N(h)} (z_i - z_j)^2$, where $N(h)$ is the set of distinct location pairs (i, j) that are distance h apart, $|N(h)|$ the number of such pairs and z_i and z_j the observed values at these locations. To achieve reasonable numbers estimation is carried out at discrete lags and distance bins are allowed for. Care has to be taken when choosing the number of lags, lag increments and bin widths (see Cressie, 1993).

Since the main goal of variogram analysis is to find a parsimonious description of the spatial autocorrelation structure of a variable a variogram of a particular functional form is usually fitted to the empirical variogram. Suitable monotonically increasing functions for bounded variograms are defined through three parameters: the *nugget effect* represents micro-scale variation or measurement error; the *sill* represents the variance of the outcome measure; and the *effective range* is the distance at which autocorrelation becomes negligible.

For an example, the open symbols in the Figure show an empirical variogram to which a spherical variogram function (a particular choice of functional form) was fitted. The curve is fully described by the parameter estimates (effective range = 0.8, sill = 1.75, nugget = 0.7) and indicates small-scale spatial autocorrelation up to a distance of 0.8.

Once a variogram function has been identified and

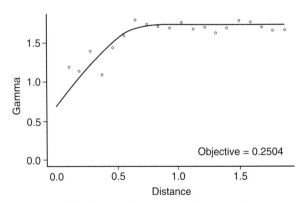

variogram *Spherical variogram model (curve) fitted to an empirical variogram (open symbols) by optimising an objective function*

fitted this function is usually considered as known and fed into a prediction routine to specify the interpolation weights (see Lawson, 1998), although simultaneous MAXIMUM LIKELIHOOD ESTIMATION of the variogram parameters and possible trend parameters is considered preferable (see Cressie, 1993).   *SL*

Cressie, N.A.C. 1993: *Statistics for spatial data.* New York: John Wiley & Sons. Lawson, A.B. 1998: Statistical map. In Armitage, P. and Colton, T. (eds), *Encyclopedia of biostatistics.* Chichester: John Wiley & Sons.

velocity charts   See GROWTH CHARTS

visual analogue scale   Scales used to measure a subjective assessment, such as 'amount of pain' or 'level of anxiety', particularly when the assessment is believed to lie along a continuum rather than only taking a discrete set of values. The item consists of a line, typically 10cm in length, with lowest and highest values indicated by labels at each end. The subject is expected to place a mark on the line to represent his or her assessment. An example follows (with a cross indicating where a subject has placed a mark):

How much pain do you feel?

No pain |————×————| Unbearable pain

The data from a visual analogue scale are recorded by measuring how far along the line from the left end the subject has placed a mark.

It is important to remember that, although it is possible to record the data from a visual analogue scale with great accuracy, the value is very subjective. In the example, the subject's response may be recorded as 1.1 (because it is 1.1cm from the left-hand end of the line), but there is no objective unit on this value. If another subject records a value of 2.1, it is not necessarily the case that this subject experiences more pain than the first subject. However, if the first subject is measured again (say, after a month) and gives a score of 2.1, it is possible to interpret this to mean that the first subject is now experiencing more pain than previously.

It is also important to remember that a visual analogue scale is unlikely to be linear. For example, a distance of 1cm at one end of the scale does not necessarily represent the same difference as a distance of 1cm at the other end of the scale. This cautions against the use of standard methods for continuous data; a common recommendation is to analyse ranks of the scores rather than the raw scores.   *PM*

Altman, D.G. 1991: *Practical statistics for medical research.* London: Chapman & Hall. Streiner, D.L. and Norman, G.R. 1995: *Health measurement scales: a practical guide to their development and use,* 2nd edn. Oxford: Oxford University Press.

Von Neumann-Morgenstern standard gamble

The classic method of measuring preferences in health economics first presented in von Neumann and Morgenstern (1953). The methods uses hypothetical lotteries as a means of measuring people's preferences when faced with a choice between treatment that offers potential benefit in quality of life (see QUALITY OF LIFE MEASUREMENT), but with the trade-off that there is a finite possibility that the patient will not survive treatment. An individual might be asked to choose between the certainty of surviving for a fixed period in a particular state of ill health and a gamble between surviving for the same period without disability, on the one hand, and immediate death, on the other. The probability of surviving without disability, as opposed to dying, is then varied until the person shows no preference between the certain option and the gamble. This probability then defines the utility of an individual for the disabled state between 0 and 1, whose endpoints are death and perfect health.

Because few patients are accustomed to dealing in probabilities, an alternative procedure called the time trade-off technique is often suggested. This begins by estimating the likely remaining years of life for a healthy subject, using actuarial tables and then the following question is asked: 'Imagine living the remainder of your natural span (an estimated number of years would be given) in your present state. Contrast this with the alternative that you remain in perfect health for fewer years. How many years would you sacrifice if you could have perfect health?'

An example of the use of the standard gamble approach is given in Petrou and Campbell (1997) who use it to estimate utilities for a range of health states in colorectal carcinoma. They were able to demonstrate that the quality of life benefits of stabilisation in the treatment of advanced metastatic colorectal cancer were rated almost as highly as those of partial response. They also showed that the benefits of irinotecan, a drug licensed for the treatment of metastatic colorectal cancer in patients who had failed an established 5-FU-containing regimen, outweighed the short-term impact of toxicity in those patients who achieved at least stabilisation of their disease.   *BSE*

Petrou, S. and Campbell, N. 1997: Stabilisation in colorectal cancer. *International Journal of Palliative Nursing* 3, 275–80. Von Neumann, J. and Morgenstern, O. 1953: *Theory of games and economic behavior.* New York: Wiley.

W

washout period   See CROSS-OVER TRIALS

wavelet analysis   A method of representing a function by projecting it onto a collection of basis functions derived from a single wavelet (often referred to as the mother wavelet $\psi(t)$). All basis functions (wavelets) required in the analysis are translated (shifted) and dilated (stretched) versions of the mother wavelet. Unlike the Fourier transform (see Subba Rao, 1998), whose basis functions are derived from sine and cosine waves with persistent oscillations, the basis functions for the wavelet transform are non-zero and oscillate for a short interval. As a result, the wavelet transform simultaneously localises information from a function in both time and frequency. For functions with time-varying characteristics or sudden changes, the wavelet transform has proved quite useful.

Two main flavours of the wavelet transform are the continuous wavelet transform (CWT) and the discrete wavelet transform (DWT). They differ by the fact that the transform works with continuous or discrete translations and dilations, respectively, of the wavelet function. The CWT is a highly redundant transform with the family of wavelets being computed via $\psi(at + b)$ where a and b are real numbers. In general, the number of wavelet coefficients is much greater than the number of observations. Popular continuous wavelet functions include the Morlet, Mexican hat and first derivative of a Gaussian density function (top row of Figure). Notice that all the wavelet functions oscillate – that is, they have both positive and negative values – and the Morlet wavelet is complex valued (the real and imaginary portions are plotted using different line types).

The DWT uses a wavelet that is translated and dilated by discrete values, that is, of the form $\psi(2^j t + k2^j)$ where j and k are integers. The parameter j is commonly referred to as the *scale*. The DWT may be an orthogonal or biorthogonal transform depending on the wavelet function. Popular orthogonal discrete wavelet functions include the Haar and Daubechies families of wavelets (bottom row of Figure). Although the discrete wavelet functions displayed look continuous they are derived from two, four and eight unique values – from left to right. Notice, the discrete wavelet functions are not symmetric, except for the Haar wavelet, and much less smooth when compared to continuous wavelet functions.

A compromise between the CWT and DWT is partially achieved by using the translation invariant DWT where a discrete wavelet function is applied to all possible integer shifts of the data in time via $\psi(2^j t + k)$. This results in a redundant (*not* orthogonal) transform in time with the same number of scales as the DWT; each scale is a distinct range of frequencies.

The DWT is most commonly used in nonparametric regression (see Hazelton, 1998) (using a technique known as *wavelet denoising*). The key contribution of the wavelet transform is that both smooth and abrupt changes in the signal will result in a few large wavelet coefficients while the noise will be dispersed throughout the entire vector of wavelet coefficients. Thus, thresholding all wavelet coefficients will eliminate the noise and preserve the features of interest. Wavelet denoising has been adapted to cases where the noise exhibits autocorrelation and may be non-Gaussian (e.g. Poisson distributed). It is very important when performing a wavelet analysis to select the wavelet

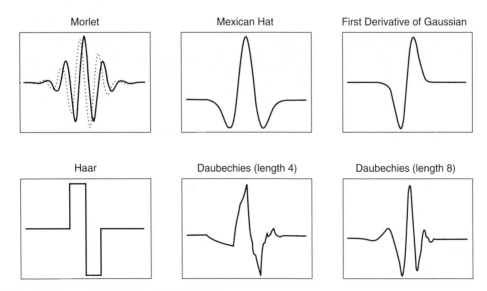

wavelet analysis *Continuous and discrete wavelet functions*

function (discrete or continuous) that best matches the features inherent in the function of interest. This will concentrate the function into a small number of wavelet coefficients, simplifying the analysis.

The wavelet transform may be applied to data of several dimensions, for example, in time series analysis (one dimension), image analysis (two dimensions) or spatio-temporal analysis (three or more dimensions). For further details behind the theory and applications to medicine and time series, see Aldroubi and Unser (1996), Chui (1997) and Percival and Walden (2000).   *BW*

Alroubi, A. and Unser, M. (eds) 1996: *Wavelets in medicine and biology*. Boca Raton: Chapman & Hall/CRC. Chui, C.K. 1997: *Wavelets: a mathematical tool for signal analysis*. SIAM monographs on mathematical modeling and computation. Philadelphia: Society for Industrial and Applied Mathematics. Hazelton, M.L. 1998: Nonparametric regression. In Armitage, P. and Colton, T. (eds), *Encyclopedia of biostatistics*. Chichester: John Wiley & Sons. Percival, D.B. and Walden, A.T. 2000: *Wavelet methods for time series analysis*. Cambridge: Cambridge University Press. Subba Rao, T. 1998: Fast Fourier transform. In Armitage, P. and Colton, T. (eds) *Encyclopedia of biostatistics*. Chichester: John Wiley & Sons.

web resources in medical statistics
The growth of the internet has revolutionised access to information for everyone from academics to the general public. The potential uses of the internet in the area of medical statistics are vast and here we can only provide an overview of these uses as they currently stand. As the internet continues to develop, its potential for use in this area can only increase.

Internet resources in medical statistics can be grouped loosely under the following headings: sources of routinely collected data; reference (online encyclopaedias, dictionaries, lecture notes); email discussion lists; statistical software, reviews and downloads; e-journals; and datasets for use in teaching

For routinely collected data, the World Health Organization (WHO) website (www.who.int/en) is a good place to start. As well as providing a wide range of links to related sites, the WHO Statistical Information System (WHOSIS) can be accessed directly. This is the guide to health and health-related epidemiological and statistical information available from the WHO.

Many countries have their own websites for routinely collected data, for example: National Statistics Online for the UK as a whole, which incorporates health statistics (www.statistics.gov.uk), Scottish Health Statistics (www.isdscotland.org), and the CDC National Centre for Health Statistics in the United States (www.cdc.gov/nchs). Data are routinely available from all of these sites in summary tables and charts and some sites allow access to some of the data in the form of Excel spreadsheets that can be customised by the user. Most national sites provide information from censuses, mortality data, morbidity data and information on usage and performance of health services. If any of these links become redundant in the future, many university libraries will continue to maintain up-to-date, accessible links to the latest information on their web pages. For example, the Glasgow University Library website (www.lib.gla.ac.uk/Depts/MOPS/Stats/medstats.shtml), which can be accessed by anyone, has an excellent page of links to local, national and international data sources and is regularly updated.

The internet is increasingly a source of good reference material in medical statistics. There are many online dictionaries, glossaries, encyclopaedias, sets of lecture notes, lists of statisticians, interactive training websites (Computer-Assisted Statistics Teaching: http://cast.massey.ac.nz), Java applets for use in teaching (www.stat.sc.edu/~west/javahtml; Rice Virtual Lab in Statistics: www.ruf.rice.edu/~lane/rvls.html), free statistical software (e.g. StatCrunch, formerly Webstat Software: www.statcrunch.com) and e-journals. It is likely that links to materials of this sort, especially lecture notes and teaching materials, will be volatile but there are a few sites that are likely to maintain up-to-date lists of available materials. The website of the Learning and Teaching Support Network (LTSN) for Maths, Statistics and OR (www.mathstore.gla.ac.uk) maintains useful links to medical statistics topics. Another useful site with up-to-date links is the US-based MedBioWorld (www.medbioworld.com). The Royal Statistical Society (www.rss.org.uk) maintains a page of links to statistics journals, publishers, mailing lists, glossaries of statistical terms and software providers that are kept up to date.

Most leading journals have their own websites with useful links. They also generally allow free access to abstracts of papers and sometimes also to the full text of papers. The *British Medical Journal* website (www.bmj.com) allows free access to the full text of most articles published since 1994 (with restrictions on certain articles published in the previous 12 months). Perhaps the most useful feature of this site for medical statisticians is the 'collected resources' feature. These are collections of BMJ articles by speciality and under the heading of 'statistics and research methods' there are collections of articles on randomised controlled trials, systematic reviews, Bayesian statistics and other statistics and research methods. These collections are an invaluable resource of material for teaching and research.

Finally the role of generally available search engines such as Google (www.google.com) in finding resources for medical statistics should not be underestimated. The majority, if not all, of the links mentioned earlier could be located by a careful search in Google using appropriate keywords and phrases. There are many other widely available search engines including some that are dedicated to resources in the area of health and medicine, such as Omni (www.omni.ac.uk).

The development and use of the internet has taken place at such a phenomenal rate that it is difficult to predict what further changes will take place in the future. The one thing that is certain is that its importance as a resource for all those with an interest in medical statistics will increase.   *WHG*

weighted kappa   See KAPPA AND WEIGHTED KAPPA

weighted least squares estimator (WLSE)   See LEAST SQUARES ESTIMATION

Wennberg's design   See RANDOMISATION

when to use which test?
This is a question raised by many clinical researchers wanting to grasp basic statistics and hence feel equipped to analyse their own data. However, there are several reasons why it may not be the

when to use which test? *When to use which test, according to number and type of samples and outcome (or response) variable measured. Some entries contain alternative tests. Last two rows indicate circumstances to use various approaches for assessing association or agreement. The table is not a complete categorisation of all possible tests and data types but includes those referred to elsewhere under individually named entries*

		Nominal (categorical)	*Ordered categorical or continuous and non-normal*	*Continuous and normally distributed*
One sample		χ^2-test	Kolmogorov-Smirnov test, Sign test	Student's test
Two samples	Independent	χ^2-test $(2 \times k)$, Fisher's exact test	Mann-Whitney rank sum test	Unpaired t-test
	Paired	McNemar's test	Wilcoxon signed rank test, Sign test	Paired t-test
Multiple samples (k>2)	Independent	χ^2-test $(r \times k)$	Kruskal-Wallis test, Jonckheere-Terpstra test	Analysis of variance (ANOVA)
	Related	Cochran Q-test	Friedman test	Repeated measures ANOVA
Association between two variables		Contingency coefficient	Spearman's rank correlation, Kendall's tau correlation	Pearson product-moment correlation
Agreement between two variables		Kappa coefficient	Weighted kappa coefficient	Limits of agreement

most appropriate question to ask and it is instructive to begin by considering why not.

First, many medical statisticians, and informed medical journal editors, nowadays prefer analyses by CONFIDENCE INTERVALS instead of hypothesis tests. There are numerous reasons for this, some of which are intrinsic problems with the inferential procedure of hypothesis testing, while others are due to this procedure's historical misuse, overuse or abuse. Thus, first advice is to counter the question with: 'Are you sure you want to do a hypothesis test?'

Second, the question betrays a false view of statistics as if there were a formulaic approach with one size fitting all. Unfortunately for those seeking quick answers to apparently simple questions, this is not the case, as doctors may know from their own experiences calling differential diagnoses from outwardly similar signs and symptoms. Equally, medical statistics is a diverse discipline with no two research studies being quite the same and hence different analytical strategies may apply in similar looking circumstances.

Third, it may be inappropriate to perform a hypothesis test if the topic of investigation is only raised by the data themselves and not by a pre-existing research question (see PITFALLS IN MEDICAL STATISTICS).

Fourth, research must never be seen as a chase to get a *P*-VALUE and preferably one less than 0.05, for among other things such confuses CLINICAL VS STATISTICAL SIGNIFICANCE.

Consequently, we may here not fully answer the question as posed, but with suitable precautions and having decided a test is appropriate, will go as far as identifying the proper test to use in commonly encountered univariate situations. Fuller details concerning methods and applications of each test procedure mentioned can be found under their specific entry. Note too one can easily find guides about choice of statistical procedures on the internet (see WEB RESOURCES IN MEDICAL STATISTICS), for example www.whichtest.info/index.htm may prove helpful.

Three factors influence choice of statistical test: the nature of the response (type of data being analysed); the number of groups sampled (one, two or many); and, if more than one, the nature of the sampling (matched or independent).

The response or outcome variable can be continuous and approximately normally distributed or dichotomous (a binary 'yes/no' outcome) or intermediate to these in a variety of ways. For example, the response variable could be in ordered categories (see ANALYSIS OF ORDINAL DATA). Otherwise, the response variable could be continuous and non-normally distributed, being skewed or containing OUTLIERS, perhaps. In either of these latter cases it is appropriate to apply one of the many NON-PARAMETRIC METHODS.

In the special case of the response variable being the time until an event, which may or may not have occurred by the time of analysis (strictly, database closure) then survival methods would be used to handle the CENSORED OBSERVATIONS. Notably, this entails a version of the log-rank test or one of its alternatives and can be stratified or not depending on the structure of the data (see SURVIVAL ANALYSIS).

The number of groups being sampled is generally obvious, although sometimes care must be taken about analysing the correct statistical unit. In a cluster randomised study, for instance, it is the clusters that need to be analysed, not the individuals forming the clusters. When repeated measurements are taken, while more sophisticated approaches can be adopted, the simplest is to convert each individual's data into a suitable summary statistic prior to analysis. For example, this statistic might be area under the curve, slope of regression line or mean observation etc. depending on whatever was previously decided to be the most clinically meaningful. In practice, note that statistical convenience should not be the criteria for choosing among possible summary statistics (see SUMMARY MEASURE ANALYSIS).

Lastly, the relationship among groups is crucial for deciding on the correct testing procedure. In the simplest case involving two groups, one needs to know whether sample data were *paired* (also known as *matched, related* or *dependent*) or unpaired (unmatched, unrelated or independent). This is usually straightforward, for example, whenever data are collected on the same patients before and after an intervention or when a pair of organs (ear, eye, hand, kidney etc.) is measured within the same person or when twins are studied within a controlled experiment. It can be less clear how best to analyse data in certain CASE-CONTROL STUDIES, matched by sex and age to within a fixed number of years, however. This is because, here, the purpose of matching is to create broadly comparable groups according to basic demographic status, rather than attempting to achieve precisely well-matched pairs (see MATCHING).

The Table on page 369 shows, according to the three basic criteria, when to use which test method in the simplest cases. For completion, it also indicates which procedure applies when assessing association or agreement. Again, further details can be found under individually named entries.

However, as emphasised throughout, confidence intervals are preferred to tests and for more informative analyses still, modelling or regression techniques can be better still. These provide mutually adjusted results for important confounders, an altogether more satisfactory approach to handling data and superior to expecting it to be adequately described by a P-value, as if relationships within the data could possibly be encapsulated by a single number, a hopelessly false ambition. Nevertheless, viewed positively and correctly, the right hypothesis test can serve to rule out chance as an explanation for discrepant data apparent in one or more random samples and lead the investigator on towards a fuller analysis of the data collected and, in turn, a deeper clinical understanding. *CRP*

[See also EXACT METHODS FOR CATEGORICAL DATA, HYPOTHESIS TESTS]

Wilcoxon rank sum test See MANN-WHITNEY RANK SUM TEST

Wilcoxon signed rank test A non-parametric version of the paired t-test (see STUDENT'S t-TEST) used for two groups that are either matched or paired. It is more sensitive than the SIGN TEST as it uses the magnitude of the differences between the pairs not simply the sign of the difference. It gives more weight to pairs that show large differences than those that show small differences. The Wilcoxon signed rank test tests the assumption that the sum of the positive ranks equals the sum of the negative ranks. The test statistic is the smaller of the sum of the

Wilcoxon signed rank test *Mcm2 and Ki67 values, data from a study of patients with cancer*

Patient	Mcm2	Ki67	Difference	Rank of difference	Signed rank of difference
1	14.78	14.78	0	–	–
2	7.96	8.68	−0.72	1	−1
3	10.89	1.57	9.32	2	+2
4	12.10	1.85	10.25	3	+3
5	18.23	5.84	12.39	4	+4
6	16.40	3.04	13.36	5	+5
7	18.02	3.96	14.06	6	+6
8	23.35	8.16	15.19	7	+7
9	26.70	8.40	18.30	8	+8

positive and the sum of the negative ranks. The data should be continuous or ordinal in nature. The paired differences should be independent and symmetrical about the true median difference.

First, find the difference in values for each pair (variable 1 – variable 2). Then rank the magnitude of the differences, smallest to largest, assigning the average rank to ties in the differences and no rank to zero differences. Find the sum of the ranks for the positive differences, W^+ and the sum of the ranks for the negative differences, W^-. Find N, the total number of differences not including ties. Find the critical value from standard tables and compare $W = \min(W^+, W^-)$ reject the null hypothesis if W is less than or equal to the critical value. If $W^+ > W^-$, then variable one tends to be greater than variable two and vice versa.

As part of a study Mcm2 and Ki67 values were compared to see if there was a difference between the values in patients with cancer. Data are shown in the Table. A plot of the differences shows that they are plausibly symmetric so the assumption of symmetry holds.

$W^+ = 35$, $W^- = 1$. $W = \min(W^+, W^-) = 1$, $N = 8$. From standard tables ($N = 8$, $\alpha = 0.05$) and the critical value is 3. As 1 is less than 3, there is sufficient evidence to reject the null hypothesis. Therefore there is a difference between Mcm2 and Ki67 values. Mcm2 values tend to be higher than Ki67 values. *SLV*

Pett, M.A. 1997: *Non-parametrics for health care research.* Thousand Oaks: Sage. **Siegel, S. and Castellan, N.J.** 1998: *Nonparametric statistics for the behavioral sciences*, 2nd edn. New York: McGraw-Hill. **Swinscow, T.D.V. and Campbell, M.J.** 2002: *Statistics at square one*, 10th edn. London: BMJ Books.

WinBUGS See BUGS AND WinBUGS

WLSE Abbreviation for weighted least squares estimator. See LEAST SQUARES ESTIMATION

Y

Yates' correction An adjustment made to a CHI-SQUARE TEST when the number of observations is small. Yates' correction is an example of a continuity correction and is designed specifically for 2×2 frequency tables.

The chi-square test uses the CHI-SQUARE DISTRIBUTION to determine whether a set of observed counts from a study (the number of observations in each cell of a frequency table) differ significantly from the expected counts predicted by a hypothesis. This use of the chi-square distribution is an approximation based on the use of the NORMAL DISTRIBUTION to approximate the distribution of the number of observations in each cell of the frequency table.

The use of the normal distribution is only an approximation because the number of observations in a cell of a frequency table is a discrete value (it can only take non-negative integer values: 0, 1, 2, ...) whereas the normal distribution is continuous (it can take any value). When the number of observations is large, this difference becomes irrelevant (the approximation becomes very good), but when the number of observations is small the approximation can mean that the standard chi-square test result is invalid (the P-VALUE reported by the test may be too low).

Yates' correction is an attempt to take account of the approximation in the calculation of the chi-square test statistic, χ^2. The effect of the correction is to decrease the size of χ^2, which increases the P-value from the test. This means that Yates' correction will always give a more conservative test; it will be less likely to report a significant result.

There is no universal agreement on when Yates' correction should be applied. With modern computer processing speeds and memory capacity it is now usually feasible to use EXACT METHODS instead, which avoid approximations altogether (e.g. FISHER'S EXACT TEST). *PM*

Altman, D.G. 1991: *Practical statistics for medical research.* London: Chapman & Hall.

Z

z-score The standardised value of an observation, X, obtained by subtracting the sample MEAN and dividing by sample STANDARD DEVIATION. The z-score of a sample value gives, therefore, the number of standard deviations, s, above or below the sample mean, $\bar{x}$:

$$z = \frac{X - \bar{x}}{s}$$

so that the PROBABILITY DISTRIBUTION of the z-score has mean 0 and variance 1.

CRP

z-transformation A TRANSFORMATION of the sample CORRELATION coefficient, r, proposed by R.A. Fisher and hence also known as Fisher's transformation. Mathematically, it is expressible in two equivalent ways, either $z = 0.5\ln[(1 + r)/(1 - r)]$ or $z = \tanh^{-1} r$, the latter being more convenient to evaluate using a scientific calculator with hyperbolic functions.

Even with moderate-sized samples the transformed correlation, z, has superior theoretical properties compared with the untransformed correlation coefficient, r, notably that z is a better approximation to the NORMAL DISTRIBUTION. The variance of z is $1/(n - 3)$, where n is the sample size, and hence for reasonably sized samples the 95% confidence interval for the transformed correlation is given by:

$$z \pm 1.96/\sqrt{(n - 3)}.$$

Back-transforming these limits to the usual $[-1,1]$ scale is achieved by use of the equation $r = [(e^{2z} - 1)/(e^{2z} + 1)]$ or, more simply, $r = \tanh (z)$.

CRP